Textbook of Neuromodulation

Helena Knotkova • Dirk Rasche
Editors

Textbook of Neuromodulation

Principles, Methods and Clinical Applications

Springer

Editors
Helena Knotkova
MJHS Institute for Innovation in Palliative Care
New York, NY, USA

Dirk Rasche
Department of Neurosurgery
University Hospital Schleswig-Holstein
University of Lübeck
Lübeck, Germany

ISBN 978-1-4939-1407-4 ISBN 978-1-4939-1408-1 (eBook)
DOI 10.1007/978-1-4939-1408-1
Springer New York Heidelberg Dordrecht London

Library of Congress Control Number: 2014950891

Printed on acid-free paper

Springer is part of Springer Science+Business Media (www.springer.com)

Foreword

This book has brought together scientists, clinicians, and bioengineers in order to present a constitutive overview of invasive and noninvasive neuromodulatory approaches and their potential for the treatment of various pathological states and conditions.

Over the past two decades, the field of neuromodulation has enormously expanded in the means of understanding neural changes in the central nervous system that represent functional targets for neuromodulation, mechanisms that underlie the neuromodulatory effects, as well as available evidence supporting clinical applications of various neuromodulatory methods. In parallel, the field has witnessed escalating interest of medical professionals, scientists, biomedical industry, and patients—the final "consumers" of neuromodulatory procedures. Hand-in-hand with growing knowledge, new open questions and challenges have emerged, facilitating further technological progress, translational research, clinical applications, and education in this exciting expertise of neuromodulation.

As reflected in the title, this book encompasses the basic principles, methods, and current clinical applications of neuromodulation, presenting both invasive and noninvasive approaches. We thank all contributors to this book and to Springer-Verlag for generously sharing their expertise, experience, and support, reaching out to readers interested in this field.

New York, NY, USA — Helena Knotkova
Lübeck, Germany — Dirk Rasche

Preface

There is something both mundane and exotic about the use of stimulation to treat human disease and distress. Common human behaviors that are inborn or learned from early childhood suggest potential benefits from stimulation after injury. After painful trauma to bones, joints, or soft tissues, the painful part often is grasped or rubbed. Abdominal cramps lead to rubbing or pressure on the abdominal wall. With lumbar strain, a closed fist against the sacrum or spine is often observed. These behaviors offer clues about the existence of neural systems by which stimulation can produce salutary effects.

The medical application of electrical stimulation for the treatment of pain and other disorders has a very long history. Ancient Egyptian practitioners used electrical shocks produced by specific species of fish to treat pain. With the advent of machines to produce electrostatic charges in the 1700s, the medical use of technology to deliver electric shocks to the skin began. With the development of the battery by Volta, which used chemical means to produce electricity, "electrotherapy" evolved as a treatment for both medical and psychiatric disorders. Direct current (galvanism) was used by the early 1800s, and the heat and tissue damage that it produced was harnessed to treat tumors, uterine fibroids, and other maladies. Within a short time, however, Faraday developed a safer alternating current and the medical use of electrical stimulation advanced greatly with the development of "faradic" devices.

Guillaume Duchenne (1806–1875), a prominent French neurologist, has been credited as the "father of electrotherapy," popularizing the use of interrupted and alternating currents to treat a wide variety of medical and psychiatric ills during the mid-1800s. By the end of this century, the medical use of electrical stimulation via electrodes and needles was commonplace in many countries. The nonpsychiatric focus of this effort was in the treatment of musculoskeletal disorders, including paralysis and pain.

Not surprisingly, growing demand for the treatment created a marketplace for devices and practitioners. Many physicians acquired or constructed their own machines and offered electrotherapy routinely. Nonphysicians, some who were technically adept and some who sold nostrums, created lucrative businesses. Fraud and quackery increased and became recognized as a serious threat to the development of medicine, which by the early twentieth century was formally adopting a more scientific approach to patient care. The famous Flexner report in 1910 identified the teaching of treatments with no known biological basis as a major impediment to the standardization of high-quality medicine, and in the years that followed its publication, medical schools dropped electrotherapy from curriculums.

The pendulum swung away from the view of stimulation as a mainstream allopathic therapy for more than 50 years, even as neuroscience made stunning advances in discerning the anatomy of the nervous system and the role of electricity in its physiology. In pain management, the 1966 publication of the gate control theory by Melzack and Wall initiated a renewed interest in the potential therapeutic effects of peripherally applied stimulation. Although the specific predictions of this theory have required numerous alterations, the underlying concept—that activation of endogenous non-nociceptive neural systems can potentially suppress nociceptive afferent input—was broadly and profoundly heuristic. It generated hypotheses about the potential for multiple segmental and suprasegmental pain-modulating systems, and touched on a biomedical understanding of analgesic therapies as diverse as ancient acupuncture techniques and a variety of approaches subsumed by the electrotherapy rage of the prior century.

The use of electrical stimulation to relieve pain regained scientific and clinical credibility, and is itself now subsumed under the broader strategy of neuromodulation. The latter term was coined to remind clinicians of the biological or practical linkages among a rapidly growing number of interventions undergoing investigation and development for pain and other disorders. From the clinical perspective, neuromodulation has had a flexible definition that has broadened in tandem with extraordinary advances in technology and the adoption by pain specialists of interventions that involve placement of both electrical leads and catheters to specific sites in the body. The International Neuromodulation Society now endorses the view that neuromodulation encompasses any therapy that targets specific sites in the nervous system and delivers either electricity or drugs in an effort to reduce symptoms or restore function.

From the clinical perspective, neuromodulation techniques are currently important in the treatment of an array of disorders. In addition to diverse types of chronic pain, neuromodulation techniques are used for refractory epilepsy and movement disorders; hearing loss; and dysmotility disorders involving gastrointestinal tract, bladder, or diaphragm. The future in restorative medicine may be the realization of the science fiction of decades ago.

Like so much of medicine, the clinical advances in the use of neuromodulation for pain have represented the combination of clinical practices developed from observations, clinical trials of new tools created to accomplish specific technical goals, and translational work drawn from an increasingly robust understanding of neurophysiology. Some techniques, such as "old-fashioned" transcutaneous electrical nerve stimulation and new-fashioned transcranial electrical or magnetic stimulation, are seemingly so safe that clinical use has (in the first instance) and will (in the second) advance before either the biological basis or trials-based efficacy is ascertained. Other interventional approaches that involve more risky and expensive implants likely will be used in a small segment of the population with pain unless evidence grows to justify broader uptake. For all these treatments, the future will depend in part on the emerging scientific evidence pertaining to the neural basis of chronic pain, most notably the nature and impact of neuroplasticity and genetics.

Two things are clear. First, stimulation of sites in the body for therapeutic purposes related to pain management has returned from the historical dust heap to a place of importance in the science and practice of pain medicine. A clinical interest in pain requires knowledge of neuromodulation.

Second, the world of neuromodulation is changing very rapidly and there is a compelling need for accessible compendia that can update scientists and clinicians alike about the current status. This volume, nicely edited by Drs. Knotkova and Rasche, provides a broad background, explaining the science and offering a snapshot of clinical neuromodulation circa 2014. It explores the role of neuroplastic changes in the effects produced by stimulation and describes the large variation that characterizes all human responses to these treatments. It is both a brief history of a period with extraordinary scientific motion and a jumping off point for the next set of advances and issues. It will not be the last word on neuromodulation, but is an excellent work to prepare for a future of change.

New York, NY, USA Russell Portenoy, M.D.

Contents

List of Contributors

Margaret Altemus, M.D. Department of Psychiatry, Weill Medical College, Cornell University, New York, NY, USA

Andrea Antal, Ph.D. Department of Neurophysiology, University Medical Center, Goettingen, Goettingen, Germany

Marom Bikson, Ph.D. Neural Engineering Laboratory, Department of Biomedical Engineering, The City College of New York of CUNY, New York, NY, USA

André R. Brunoni, M.D., Ph.D. Department and Institute of Psychiatry, University of São Paulo, São Paulo, Brazil

Christian P. Bührle, M.D., Ph.D. Laboratory for Electrophysiology and Computational Neuroscience (Stereotactic and Functional Neurosurgery), Department of Stereotactic and Functional Neurosurgery, University Hospital of Cologne, Cologne, Germany

Alexios G. Carayannopoulos, D.O., M.P.H. Spine Center, Department of Neurosurgery, Rhode Island Hospital, Providence, RI, USA

Anne P. Caruso, P.A-.S. Seton Hill University's Physician Assistant Program, Seton Hill University, Greensburg, PA, USA

Quirino Cordeiro, M.D., Ph.D. Department of Psychiatry, Santa Casa Medical School, São Paulo, Brazil

Ricardo A. Cruciani, M.D., Ph.D. Center for Comprehensive Pain Management and Palliative Care, Capital Health Medical Center, Pennington, NJ

Martin Diers, Ph.D., M.Sc. Department of Cognitive and Clinical Neuroscience, Central Institute of Mental Health, Medical Faculty Mannheim\Heidelberg University, Mannheim, Germany

Marc J. Dubin, M.D., Ph.D. Department of Psychiatry, Weill Medical College, Cornell University, New York, NY, USA

Felipe Fregni, M.D., Ph.D., M.P.H. Department of Physical Medicine and Rehabilitation, Berenson-Allen Center for Noninvasive Brain Stimulation, Harvard Medical School, Boston, MA, USA

Kliment Gatzinsky, M.D., Ph.D. Department of Neurosurgery, Sahlgrenska University Hospital, Gothenburg, Sweden

Aaron Greenberg, B.A. Department of Pain Medicine and Palliative Care, Institute for Non-Invasive Brain Stimulation, Beth Israel Medical Center, New York, NY, USA

Berkan Guleyupoglu, B.E. Department of Biomedical Engineering, The City College of New York, New York, NY, USA

Louise Jones, M.C.S.P. Faculty of Health and Applied Sciences, University of the West of England, Bristol, UK

Helena Knotkova, Ph.D. MJHS Institute for Innovation in Palliative Care, New York, NY, USA

Imre P. Krabbenbos, M.D. Department of Anaesthesiology, Intensive Care and Pain Medicine, St. Antonius Hospital Nieuwegein, Nieuwegein, The Netherlands

Jeffery Kramer, Ph.D. Spinal Modulation Inc., Menlo Park, CA, USA

College of Medicine, University of Illinois, Peoria, IL, USA

Jens Kuhn, M.D. Department for Psychiatry and Psychotherapy, University of Cologne, Cologne, Germany

Min-Fang Kuo, M.D., Ph.D. Department of Clinical Neurophysiology, Georg-August-University Goettingen, Goettingen, Germany

Michal Lavidor, Ph.D. Department of Psychology, Bar-Ilan University, Ramat Gan, Israel

Doris Lenartz, Dr. med. Department of Stereotactic and Functional Neurosurgery, University of Cologne, Cologne, Germany

A. Liong Liem, M.D. Department of Anaesthesiology, Intensive Care and Pain Medicine, St. Antonius Hospital Nieuwegein, Nieuwegein, The Netherlands

Candida S. McCabe, Ph.D., R.G.N. Faculty of Health and Applied Sciences, University of the West of England, Bristol, UK

The Royal National Hospital for Rheumatic Diseases, Bath, UK

Janet Mindes, Ph.D. Department of Psychiatry, Center for Bioethics, College of Physicians and Surgeons, Columbia University, New York, NY, USA

Preet Minhas, B.E. Department of Biomedical Engineering, The City College of New York, New York, NY, USA

Albert Mokrejs Stuyvesant High School, Class of 2016, New York, NY, USA

Michaela Möller, Dip. Psych. Department for Psychiatry and Psycotherapy, University of Cologne, Cologne, Germany

Michael A. Nitsche, M.D. Clinical Neurophysiology, University Medical Center, Georg-August-University, Goettingen, Germany

Nam-Jong Paik, M.D., Ph.D. Department of Rehabilitation Medicine, Seoul National University College of Medicine, Bundang Hospital, Seoul National University, Seongnam, Republic of Korea

Walter Paulus, M.D. Department of Clinical Neurophysiology, Georg-August-University, Goettingen, Germany

Monica A. Perez, P.T., Ph.D. Department of Physical Medicine and Rehabilitation, Systems Neuroscience Institute, Center for the Neural Basis of Cognition, University of Pittsburgh, Pittsburgh, PA, USA

Mark Plazier, M.D. Department of Neurosurgery, University Hospital Antwerp, Edegem, Antwerp, Belgium

Russell Portenoy, M.D. MJHS Institute for Innovation in Palliative Care, New York, NY, USA

Dirk Rasche, M.D. Department of Neurosurgery, University Hospital of Schleswig-Holstein, University of Lübeck, Lübeck, Germany

Rosamaria Raza, M.D. Department of Psychiatry, Santa Casa Medical School, São Paulo, Brazil

Dirk De Ridder, M.D., Ph.D. Section of Neurosurgery, Department of Surgical Sciences, Dunedin Public Hospital, Dunedin, Otego, New Zealand

Pedro Schestatsky, M.D., Ph.D. Department of Internal Medicine, Universidade Federal do Rio Grande do Sul, Capes, Brazil

Tal Sela, Ph.D. Department of Psychology, Bar-Ilan University, Ramat Gan, Israel

Pedro Shiozawa, M.D. Laboratory of Clinical Neuromodulation, Santa Casa Medical School, Sao Paulo, Brazil

Konstantin V. Slavin, M.D. Department of Neurosurgery, University of Illinois at Chicago, Chicago, IL, USA

Eliezer Soto, M.D. Anesthesia Pain Care Consultants, Tamarac, FL

Veronika Stock, M.D. Dissociative Disorders and Trauma Program, McLean Hospital, Belmont, MA, USA

Volker M. Tronnier, M.D., Ph.D. Department of Neurosurgery, University Hospital Lübeck, University of Lübeck, Lübeck, Germany

Dennis Truong, M.S. Department of Biomedical Engineering, The City College of New York, New York, NY, USA

Sven Vanneste, Ph.D. School for Behavioral and Brain Sciences, University of Texas at Dallas, Dallas, TX, USA

Veerle Visser-Vandewalle, M.D., Ph.D. Department of Stereotactic and Functional Neurosurgery, University Hospital of Cologne, Cologne, Germany

Nicola E. Walsh, Ph.D. Faculty of Health and Life Sciences, University of the West of England, Bristol, United Kingdom

Part I

Basic Aspects

Principles of Neuromodulation

1

Veronika M. Stock, Helena Knotkova, and Michael A. Nitsche

Neuroplasticity and Neuromodulation

Until several decades ago, it was thought that the human brain is modifiable only during early stages of ontogenesis. However, neurophysiological and neuroimaging studies indicated that the mature human brain is, under certain conditions, capable of substantial long-lasting changes in neural pathways and synapses which are due to changes in behavior, previous experience, physiological demand, or environmental pressures, as well as changes resulting from bodily injury [1, 2]. The encompassing term for these changes is neuroplasticity or brain plasticity, which includes synaptic plasticity (strengthening or weakening of synaptic connections or formation or abolition of spines over time in response to increases or decreases in their activity) and nonsynaptic plasticity that involves functional modification of ion channels in the neuronal axon, dendrites, and cell body that results in a modification of the intrinsic excitability of the neuron. Nonsynaptic plasticity affects fundamental mechanisms of neuronal functioning at the cellular level. In interaction with synaptic plasticity, these individual neuronal alterations can then result in changes in higher brain functions [3–7].

In the past few decades, advanced imaging methods have made it possible to examine how the human nervous system changes in response to various stimuli and physiological demands. It has been shown that neuroplastic changes can be adaptive, for example, helping the organism to compensate for lost function due to injury or facilitating recovery after injury, or maladaptive, contributing to the development and/or maintenance of various pathological conditions and diseases [6, 8–10].

Neuromodulation encompasses a broad range of invasive and noninvasive interventions that aim for an alteration of neuronal activity, or excitability. The rationale for explorations and use of neuromodulation for research and therapeutic purposes builds on growing evidence indicating that besides acute alteration of cortical activity, neuromodulation results also in enduring alterations of neural activity and connectivity [11–14], i.e., induces neuroplastic changes, and therefore can be used to attempt a reversal of maladaptive neuroplastic changes already occurring in the brain, or to prevent the development of maladaptive neuroplastic changes, or to enhance adaptive neuroplastic changes occurring in the brain, for example, during functional recovery after damage to the central nervous system [11, 15].

Below we discuss an example of neuroplastic changes in the brain, a phenomenon called cortical reorganization [16–18], in the context of illustrating the rationale for a potential use of neuromodulation.

Cortical Reorganization

In general, cortical reorganization reflects adaptive or maladaptive changes involving neuroplastic changes of the connectivity, excitability, and activity of functionally defined brain regions.

For the somatosensory and motor cortices, the cortical and subcortical systems contain two distinct neural maps—one for the recognition and processing of somatosensory input and the other for the delivery of motor commands [19]. Somatosensory and motor maps (sensory homunculus and motor homunculus, Fig. 1.1) have an orderly,

V.M. Stock (✉)
Dissociative Disorders and Trauma Program, McLean Hospital, 115 Mill Street, Belmont, MA 02478, USA
e-mail: vmstock@partners.org

H. Knotkova
MJHS Institute for Innovation in Palliative Care, 39 Broadway, New York, NY, USA
e-mail: hknotkov@mjhs.org

M.A. Nitsche
Clinical Neurophysiology, University Medical Center, Georg-August-University, Goettingen, Germany

H. Knotkova and D. Rasche (eds.), *Textbook of Neuromodulation*,
DOI 10.1007/978-1-4939-1408-1_1, © Springer Science+Business Media, LLC 2015

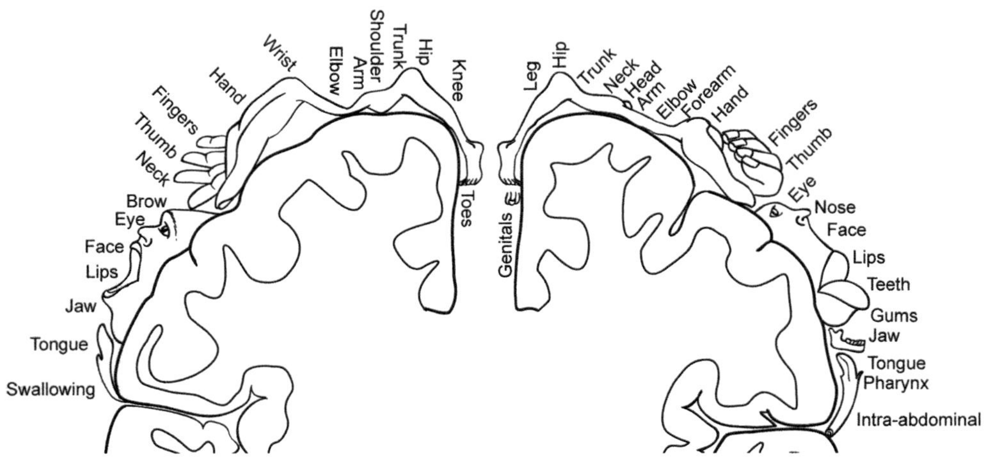

Fig. 1.1 Somatotopic organization within the somatosensory motor cortices. Somatosensory and motor maps (the somatosensory and primary motor homunculi) have an orderly arrangement of neural connections to represent each area of the body. The maps reflect an allocation of the cortical space representing specific parts of the body (Adapted from ref. 29)

somatotopic arrangement of neural connections to represent each area of the body.

These functional maps are able to respond to changes in afferent input, experience, practice, or injury. Neural plasticity in the somatotopic organization is manifested as the preferential allocation of cortical space to those peripheral areas proportionately most in use [19]. By these means, somatotopic reorganization reflects changes in allocation of the cortical space representing specific parts of the body and occurs most commonly in response to a change in sensory input whether it is an increase, a reduction, or a cessation of afferent information [3]. Jones [5] reviewed available data on neuroplastic responses to an increased sensory input as well as responses to a loss of sensory input. The findings suggest that enhanced stimulation of a body part may result in an enlargement of the cortical representational map of that body part. In contrast, sensory loss may result in a maladaptive invasion of the deafferented cortical representational map by adjacent areas of the homunculus, accompanied by increased neural activity of these representations. Under certain conditions, cortical reorganization may reflect an adaptive change, for example, in brain injury when the function of a damaged area is supplemented by other nondamaged areas of the brain. However, cortical reorganization is complex, and adaptive and maladaptive changes may occur in parallel. Further, even years after injury, the human brain may still retain the ability to reorganize in response to interventions that may influence recovery of lost or damaged function [7, 20–22]. Therefore, neuromodulation in such conditions may facilitate reversal of the maladaptive changes back to normal as well as facilitate the adaptive reorganization toward recovery. For example, extensive reorganization has been observed in patients after stroke as compared to healthy subjects [15, 21]. In healthy subjects, unilateral hand movements were associated predominantly with activation contralateral motor areas, involving the primary motor cortex, and performance of complex tasks when acquiring novel motors skills involved a larger extent of bihemispheric activation. In poststroke patients, simple hand movements using the stroke-affected (weak) hand led to activation of widespread bilateral motor network including both primary motor cortices. Therefore, it was hypothesized that promoting cortical reorganization that leads to activation and inhibitory interhemispheric interactions that resemble those observed in healthy subjects may contribute to recovery of motor function [21]. Accordingly, Ward and Cohen [21] proposed a model of poststroke interactions between motor cortices and suggested that either facilitating activity of the ipsilesional primary motor cortex or downregulating activity of the contralesional primary motor cortex in association with motor training could facilitate functional recovery after stroke [21, 23]. Indeed, results of several studies employing neuromodulation confirmed this model and proved that both suggested approaches lead to an improvement of motor function after stroke (for review see Fregni and Pascual-Leone [24]).

Further, there is ample evidence showing that changes associated with cortical reorganization may be associated with specific symptoms, such as pain. For example, in amputees, maladaptive cortical reorganization of an amputated limb representation in the somatosensory and motor cortices is prominent in patients suffering from phantom limb pain, but not in pain-free amputees [25, 26]. In amputees with phantom limb pain, Lotze and colleagues [26] found a shift of the lip representation into the deafferented primary motor and somatosensory areas of the hand displacement of the lip representation in the primary motor and somatosensory cortices was positively correlated with the intensity of phantom limb pain and was not present in pain-free amputees or healthy controls. Notably, the application of neuromodulatory methods, such as spinal cord stimulation [27], transcranial magnetic stimulation [28], or visual feedback (mirror-box therapy) and motor imagery [29], resulted in the relief of phantom limb pain. In the study by MacIver [29], following training in mental

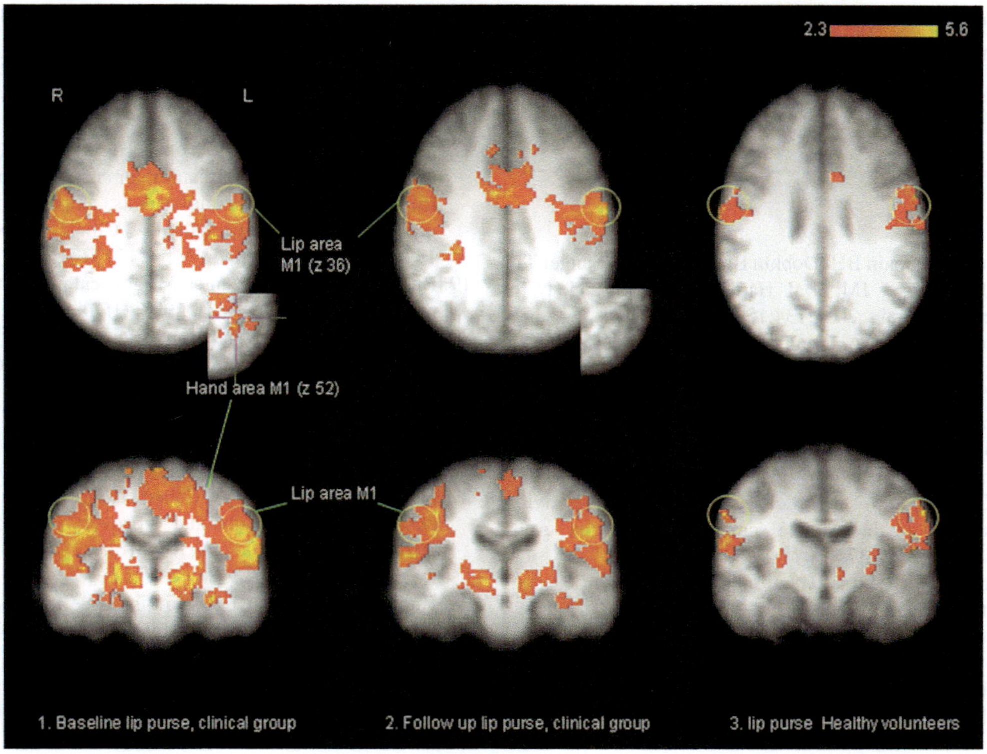

Fig. 1.2 Functional brain imaging of lip pursing movement in upper-limb amputees with phantom limb pain and healthy subjects. A cortical reorganization presented as a shift of activation from somatotopic representation of the lip toward deafferented areas of the hand has been observed in the phantom limb pain patients. Mental imagery training resulted in a significant pain relief and a corresponding reversal of cortical reorganization (From ref. 29; with permission)

imagery, the phantom limb pain patients reported a significant reduction of the intensity of constant pain, as well as relief of pain in exacerbations, with a corresponding reversal of cortical reorganization (Fig. 1.2).

Similarly, neuroimaging studies in patients with chronic pain due to carpal tunnel syndrome [30, 31] (Fig. 1.3) have shown signs of cortical reorganization, including cortical hyperexcitability and changes in the somatotopic organization of digits, as compared with healthy subjects. These maladaptive changes reversed toward normal after acupuncture treatment and were paralleled by functional improvement and pain relief.

The concept of neuromodulation builds on growing evidence indicating that (1) the human neural system can undergo neuroplastic changes that may be associated with altered functional outcomes and/or symptoms and pathological conditions; (2) various neuromodulatory approaches can induce neuroplasticity in the means of enduring alterations of neural activity and connectivity and therefore can be used to attempt a reversal (or prevention) of maladaptive neuroplastic changes occurring in the brain or to facilitate adaptive neuroplasticity; and (3) facilitation of adaptive neuroplastic changes and reversal of maladaptive ones have been shown to be associated with functional improvement.

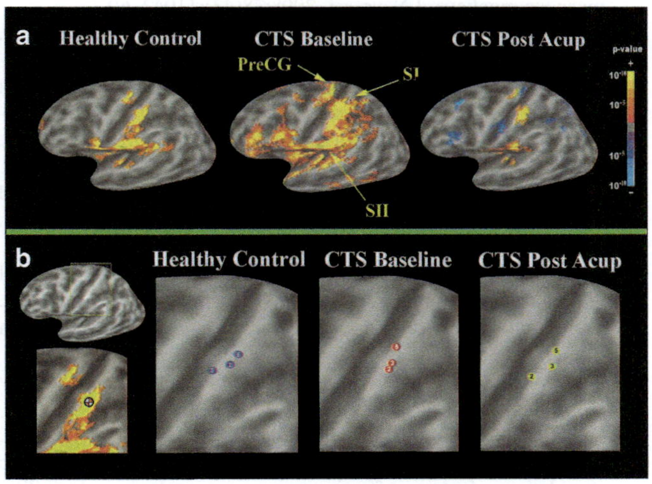

Fig. 1.3 Cortical reorganization in carpal tunnel syndrome. (**a**) Functional MRI has shown that carpal tunnel syndrome leads to electrical stimulation for digit 3 (D3), a median nerve innervated digit. Following treatment with acupuncture, hyperactivation was found to decrease. (**b**) Multi-digit stimulation found that carpal tunnel syndrome is also characterized by somatotopic changes in the primary somatosensory cortex, where median nerve innervated digits 2 and 3 have cortical receptive fields with center of mass closer to one another, compared to healthy adults. Treatment with acupuncture increased this D3/D2 separation distance, now resembling the one in healthy subjects (From ref. 31; with permission)

Overall, these principles constitute the rationale for therapeutic applications of neuromodulation in medical disciplines.

References

1. Cramer SC, Sur M, Dobkin BH, Dobkin BH, O'Brien C, Sanger TD, Trojanowski JQ, Rumsey JM, et al. Harnessing neuroplasticity for clinical applications. Brain. 2011;134:1591–609.
2. Pascual-Leone A, Amedi A, Fregni F, Merabet LB. The plastic human cortex. Annu Rev Neurosci. 2005;28:377–401.
3. Hickmott PW, Merzenich MM. Local circuit properties underlying cortical reorganization. J Neurophysiol. 2002;88:1288–301.
4. Engelman HS, MacDermott A. Presynaptic ionotropic receptors and control of transmitter release. Nat Rev Neurosci. 2004;5:135–45.
5. Jones EG. Cortical and subcortical contributions to activity-dependent plasticity in the primate somatosensory cortex. Annu Rev Neurosci. 2000;23:1–37.
6. Kelly C, Garavan H. Human neuroimaging of brain changes associated with practice. Cereb Cortex. 2005;15:1089–102.
7. Kantak SS, Stinear JW, Buch ER, Cohen LG. Rewiring the brain: potential role of the premotor cortex in motor control, learning, and recovery of function following brain injury. Neurorehabil Neural Repair. 2012;26(3):282–92. doi:10.1177/1545968311420845. PMID: 21926382.
8. Frost SB, Barbay S, Friel KM, Plautz EJ, Nudo RJ. Reorganization of remote cortical regions after ischemic brain injury: a potential substrate for stroke recovery. J Neurophysiol. 2003;89(6):3205–14.
9. Flor H. Cortical reorganization and chronic pain: implications for rehabilitation. J Rehabil Med. 2003;Suppl 41:66–72.
10. Jain N, Qi HX, Collins CE, Kaas JH. Large-scale reorganization in the somatosensory cortex and thalamus after sensory loss in macaque monkeys. J Neurosci. 2008;28(43):11042–60.
11. Lefaucher JP. Methods of therapeutic cortical stimulation. Neurophysiol Clin. 2009;39:1–14.
12. Liebetanz D, Nitsche MA, Tergau F, Paulus W. Pharmacological approach to the mechanisms of transcranial DC-stimulation-induced after-effects of human motor cortex excitability. Brain. 2002;125:2238–47.
13. Nitsche MA, Paulus W. Sustained excitability elevations induced by transcranial DC motor cortex stimulation in humans. Neurology. 2001;57:1899–901.
14. Nitsche MA, Cohen LG, Wassermann EM, Priori A, Lang N, Antal A, Paulus W, Hummel F, Boggio PS, Fregni F, Pascual-Leone A. Transcranial direct current stimulation: state of the art 2008. Brain Stimul. 2008;1:206–23.
15. Sharma N, Cohen LG. Recovery of motor function after stroke. Dev Psychobiol. 2012;54:254–62.
16. Brasil-Neto JP, McShane LM, Fuhr P, Hallett M, Cohen LG. Topographic mapping of the human motor cortex with magnetic stimulation: factors affecting accuracy and reproducibility. Electroencephalogr Clin Neurophysiol. 1992;85(1):9–16. PMID: 1371748.
17. Chen R, Cohen LG, Hallett M. Nervous system reorganization following injury. Neuroscience. 2002;111(4):761–73. PMID: 12031403.
18. Cohen LG, Bandinelli S, Topka HR, Fuhr P, Roth BJ, Hallett M. Topographic maps of human motor cortex in normal and pathological conditions: mirror movements, amputations and spinal cord injuries. Electroencephalogr Clin Neurophysiol Suppl. 1991;43:36–50. PubMed PMID: 1773774.
19. Buonomano DV, Merzenich M. Cortical plasticity: from synapse to maps. Annu Rev Neurosci. 1998;21:149–86.
20. Cramer SC, Riley JD. Neuroplasticity and brain repair after stroke. Curr Opin Neurol. 2008;21(1):76–82. doi:10.1097/WCO.0b013e3282f36cb6. Review, PMID: 18180655.
21. Ward NS, Cohen LG. Mechanisms underlying recovery of motor function after stroke. Arch Neurol. 2004;61(12):1844–8. Review. PMID: 15596603.
22. Sharma N, Classen J, Cohen LG. Neural plasticity and its contribution to functional recovery. Handb Clin Neurol. 2013;110:3–12. doi:10.1016/B978-0-444-52901-5.00001-0. Review, PMID: 23312626.
23. Hummel FC, Cohen LG. Non-invasive brain stimulation: a new strategy to improve neurorehabilitation after stroke? Lancet Neurol. 2006;5(8):708–12.
24. Fregni F, Pascual-Leone A. Hand motor recovery after stroke: tuning the orchestra to improve hand motor function. Cogn Behav Neurol. 2006;19(1):21–33.
25. Flor H, Nikolajsen L, Staehelin JT. Phantom limb pain: a case of maladaptive CNS plasticity? Nat Rev Neurosci. 2006;7(11):873–81. Review. PubMed PMID: 17053811.
26. Lotze M, Flor H, Grodd W, Larbig W, Birbaumer N. Phantom movements and pain. An fMRI study in upper limb amputees. Brain. 2001;124(Pt 11):2268–77. PMID: 11673327.
27. Viswanathan A. Use of spinal cord stimulation in the treatment of phantom limb pain: case series and review of literature. Pain Pract. 2010;10(5):479–84.
28. Ahmed MA, Mohamed SA, Sayed D. Long-term antalgic effects of repetitive transcranial magnetic stimulation of motor cortex and serum beta-endorphin in patients with phantom pain. Neurol Res. 2011;33(9):953–8. PMID: 22080997.
29. MacIver K, Lloyd DM, Kelly Roberts SN, Nurmikko T. Phantom limb pain, cortical reorganization and the therapeutic effect of mental imagery. Brain. 2008;131(8):2181–91. PMCID: PMC2494616.
30. Napadow V, Dhond RP, Kim J, LaCount L, Vangel M, Harris RE, Kettner N, Park K. Brain encoding of acupuncture sensation-coupling on-line rating with fMRI. Neuroimage. 2009;47(3):1055–65. doi:10.1016/j.neuroimage.2009.05.079. PubMed PMID: 19500677.
31. Napadow V, Maeda Y, Audette J, Kettner N. Chapter IX. Neuroplasticity in carpal tunnel syndrome. In: Knotkova, Cruciani, Merrick, editors. Neural plasticity in chronic pain. New York, USA: Nova Science Publishers, Inc.; 2012, p. 153-184.

Methods and Technologies for Low-Intensity Transcranial Electrical Stimulation: Waveforms, Terminology, and Historical Notes

2

Berkan Guleyupoglu, Pedro Schestatsky, Felipe Fregni, and Marom Bikson

Scope and Approach

Transcranial electrical stimulation (tES) encompasses all forms of research and clinical applications of electrical currents to the brain noninvasively using (at least one) electrodes on the head. The dose of tES is defined by the electrode montage and the stimulation waveform applied to the electrode [1]. There has been a resurgence of interest since 2000, but "modern" tES developed incrementally over a century. This review provides the first comprehensive organization of approaches and doses used in modern tES since 1900.

This process involves defining the litany of terminology that has developed and evolved around tES. We make no attempt to re-define or qualify any approaches used, but explain the terminology as used contemporarily by researchers. Particular attention is paid to historically linked categories of tES, "streams," of which we identify four that span decades plus "contemporary" approaches (Fig. 2.1).

1. Cranial electrical stimulation (CES) descended from electrosleep (ES) through cranial electro-stimulation therapy (CET), transcerebral electrotherapy (TCET), and neuroelectric therapy (NET).
2. Electroanesthesia (EA) went through several periods of waning interest and resurgence when new waveform variations were proposed, including transcutaneous cranial electrical stimulation (TCES), Limoge, and interferential stimulation (IS).
3. Polarizing or direct current stimulation includes recent transcranial direct current stimulation, transcranial micropolarization, high-definition transcranial direct current stimulation (HD-tDCS), and galvanic vestibular stimulation (GVS).
4. Electroconvulsive therapy (ECT), initially called *electroshock therapy*, evolved in technique and dose, such as focal electrically administered seizure therapy (FEAST).
5. Finally, we categorize "contemporary" approaches that have been explored intensely over the last decade, such as transcranial alternating current stimulation (tACS), transcranial sinusoidal direct current stimulation (tSDCS), and transcranial random noise stimulation (tRNS). Though analogues to these contemporary approaches can be identified in earlier literature, contemporary approaches contain dose features that motivate us to consider them novel. Contemporary approaches to some extent reflect a "re-boot" of the tES approach, typically employing basic, well-documented, and well-defined waveforms (e.g., one sinusoid [1] in contrast to the increasingly complex waveforms developed [though not always justified] over decades in some streams.

As our technical focus is on dose clarification and classification, we minimize comments on the clinical efficacy or safety of any approaches except in special cases where findings resulted in historically notable and sudden changes in dose or terminology. We note specific conferences and regulatory agencies that helped identify and shape the field of tES including establishing terminology. Commercial (brand) names of devices are noted ad hoc for context and linked to dose terms where appropriate. We do not comment directly on mechanisms but emphasize that dose determines electric field in the brain [2] which, in turn, gives rise to neurophysiological responses [3]; thus

B. Guleyupoglu (✉)
Department of Biomedical Engineering, The City College of New York, 160 Convent Avenue, 463 Steinman Hall, New York, NY 10031, USA
e-mail: bguleyup@gmail.com

P. Schestatsky
Department of Internal Medicine, Universidade Federal do Rio Grande do Sul, Capes, Brazil

F. Fregni
Department of Physical Medicine and Rehabilitation, Harvard Medical School, Berenson-Allen Center for Noninvasive Brain Stimulation, Boston, MA, USA

M. Bikson
Neural Engineering Laboratory, Department of Biomedical Engineering, The City College of New York of CUNY, New York, NY, USA

H. Knotkova and D. Rasche (eds.), *Textbook of Neuromodulation*,
DOI 10.1007/978-1-4939-1408-1_2,

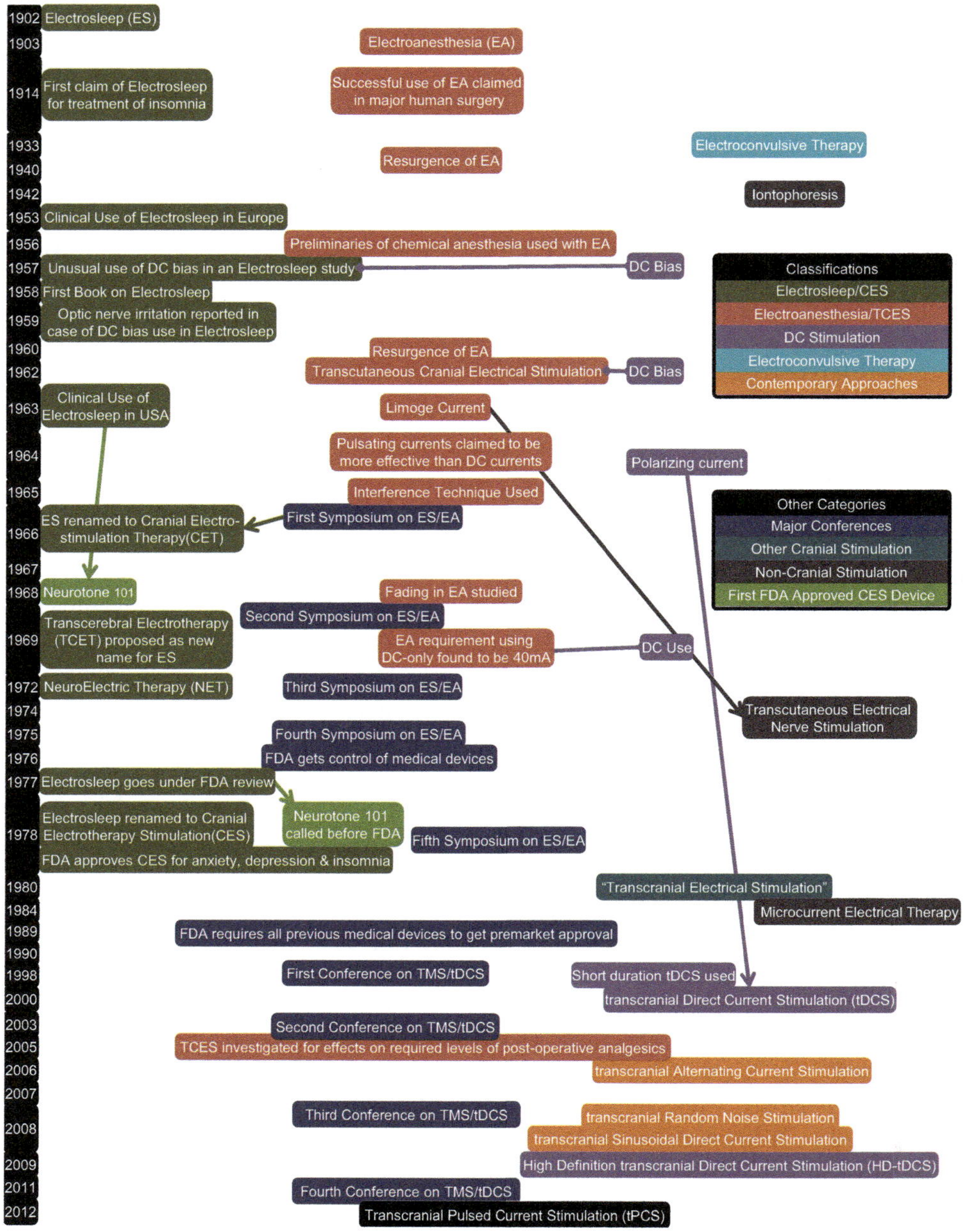

Fig. 2.1 A general timeline of ES/EA noting key points in the history from 1902 until 2011 as well as their relation to DC stimulation. A brief history of DC stimulation is also presented in this table. Other cranial therapies are mentioned for a complete cranial stimulation history and noncranial therapies are mentioned for their connection to ES/EA. *Arrows* are used to connect historically related points while the *horizontal purple lines* are used to point out DC use in historically pulsed applications

understanding the dose is a prerequisite to understanding mechanisms.

We do not address magnetic stimulation approaches or electrical stimulation approaches not targeting the brain, or nonelectrical therapies, except in specific cases to indicate the terminology used in these other approaches for the purpose of overall clarity of nomenclature. We did not attempt to perform an exhaustive cataloging of tES publications.

Though we do not comment on efficacy, the nominal indications for tES use (intended clinical outcomes) are noted when contextually relevant, especially for many historical streams (defined above). There are instances in which researchers used terminology to describe a dose in a manner potentially inconsistent with typical historical norms of dose associated with that terminology; when these papers provide sufficient dose details, these deviations are noted. Our summary aims to reflect the most typical doses used across the majority of studies (Figs. 2.2, 2.3, and 2.4). In addition, to promote a more comprehensive and systematic dose classification, we propose new categories for those waveforms using pulsed stimulation in Fig. 2.5 (transcranial pulsed current stimulation [tPCS]).

It is important to emphasize that the specifics of tES dose (electrode montage and waveform) determine brain modulation—evidently the given therapy name is incidental and often reflects a historical bias and varying intended use. In this sense, a strict approach would involve ignoring all historical nomenclature and consideration of specific dose.

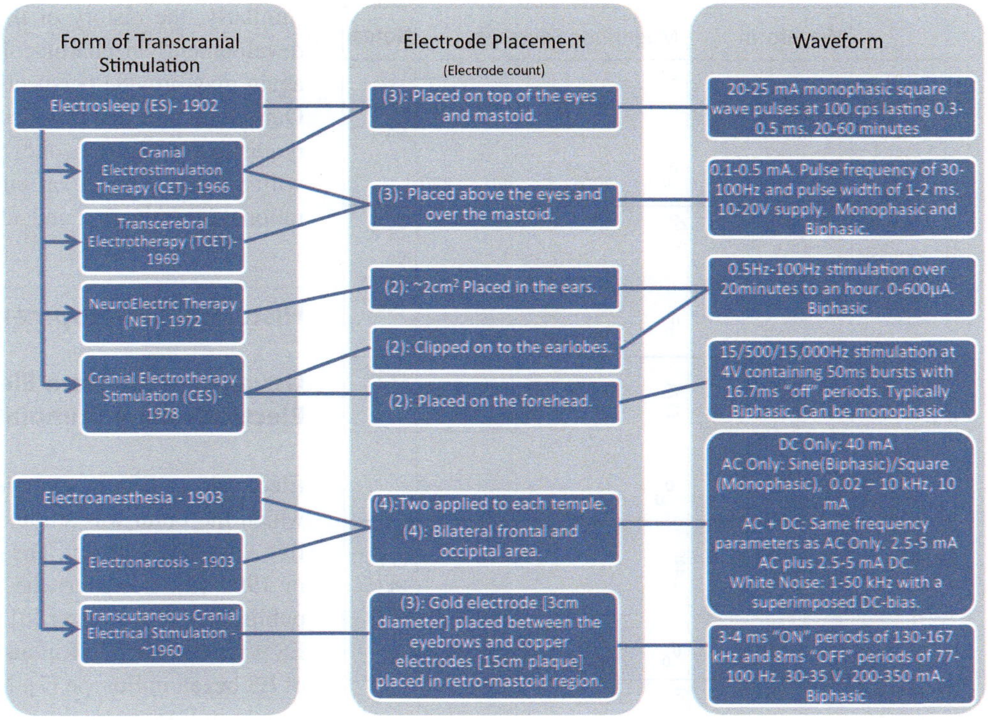

Fig. 2.2 Electrosleep and Electroanesthesia Dosage. These are a mixture of low- and high-intensity stimulation waveforms. The year at which the form of stimulation came about is written with the stimulation method. Each method is connected to an electrode placement as well as a waveform used

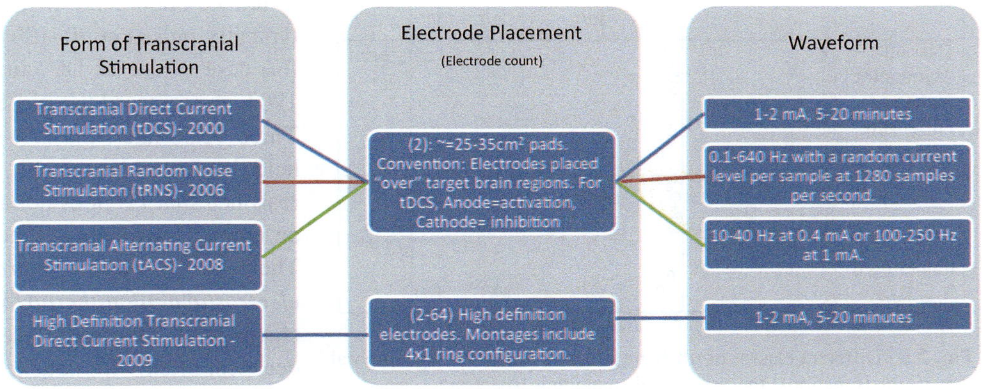

Fig. 2.3 Contemporary Approaches Dosages. These are primarily low-intensity stimulation waveforms. The year at which the form of stimulation came about is written with the stimulation method. Each method is connected to an electrode placement as well as a waveform used

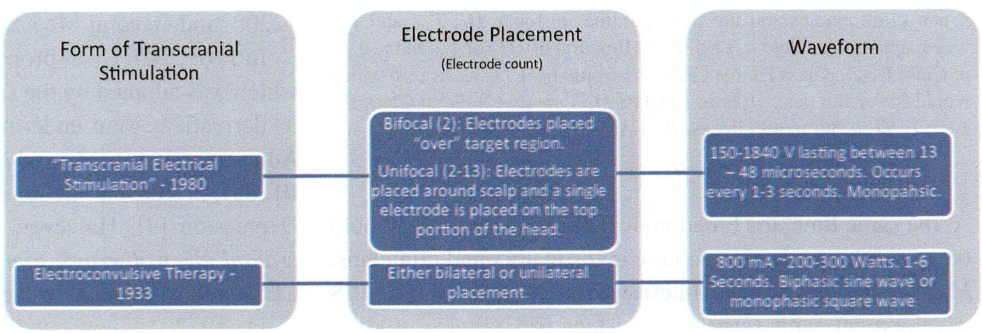

Fig. 2.4 "TES" and ECT Dosages. These are primarily high-intensity stimulation waveforms. The year at which the form of stimulation came about is written with the stimulation method. Each method is connected to an electrode placement as well as a waveform used

However, this ideal approach is problematic due to the following reasons: (1) In most cases, the complete dose details are not provided (e.g., electrode size, waveform details, etc.); (2) investigators often adjusted dose, resulting in hundreds of potential categories.

Ultimately, this review should serve as a road map for further investigation of classical techniques and appreciation of the origin of recent techniques. Even experienced researchers may remain unclear about basic features in classical literature; for instance, did ES use direct current (DC)?

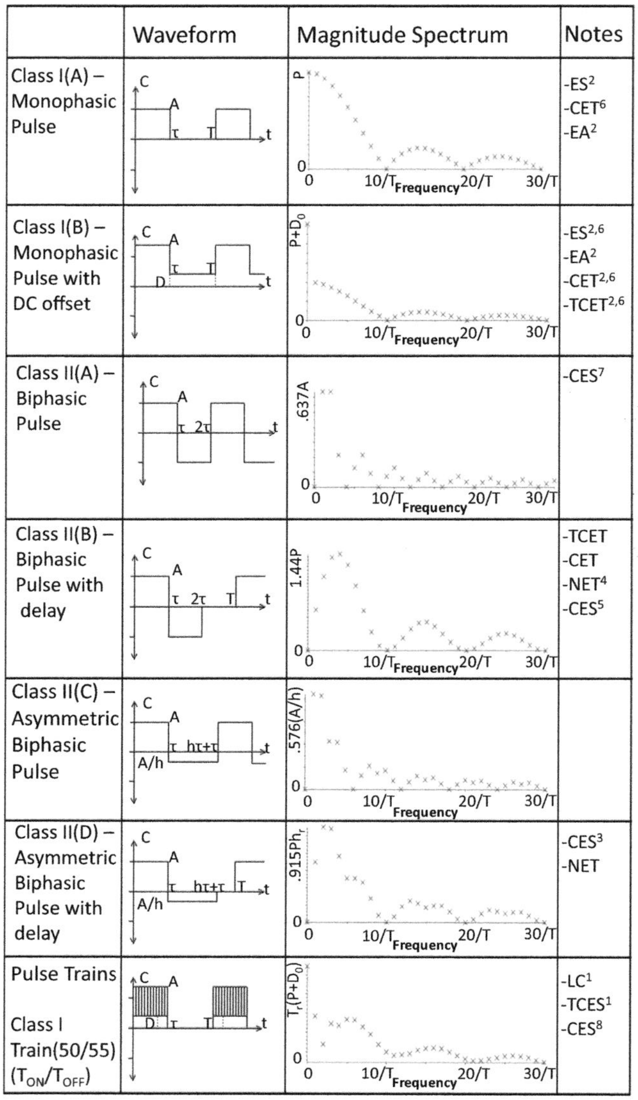

Fig. 2.5 Different classes of tPCS are summarized including temporal waveform (function), the associated magnitude spectrum (frequency content), and clinical references including dose using "CES." The Fourier series were generated using the same parameters for T, τ, and A across all classes and the same parameters for h, D_0, T_{on}, and T_{off} where applicable. Note n is a discrete function of $1/T$ (or T_{off} in the case of Class III). In Class III, the CES case would have D_0 set to zero which would lower the peak at zero. In Class II, $h_r = (h + 1)/h$, in Class III, $T_r = T_{on}/T_{off}$ and in all classes, $P = A(\tau/T)$. Data from [6, 13, 63]

At the same time, the broad view taken in this review should be a useful introduction to new investigators and clinicians. More generally, we are interested in the narrative of tES development with respect to current tES clinical studies. Research into tES mechanisms in clinical outcomes has been active for over a century. Some specific dose approaches (with indications) generated increased interest only later to be largely abandoned—the context for such waxing and waning of enthusiasm for specific historical approaches may be relevant for current clinical efforts. Similarly, the history of tES development reflects parallel developments in pharmacology including narcotics, which again may provide perspective on current clinical trials [4]. Our intention is that this historical dose analysis of tES, with requisite clarification and definition of dose terminology, will provide context on current approaches and facilitate rational investigation and adoption.

Historical Development

Developments from Electrosleep to Cranial Electrotherapy Stimulation

Electrosleep (ES), in short, is the name for tPCS methods by which the brain was stimulated in order to induce a sleep-like state in the subject. The first studies on ES were initiated in 1902 [5]; however, the first clinical report of ES was published 12 years later [6]. Most of the research regarding ES was conducted in Russia up until 1953, when clinical use of ES began in Europe [7]. New approaches were developed mostly in Europe, such as changing electrode position from covering the eyes to locations around the eyes, presumably to reduce optic nerve irritation [6]. ES dose waveform was typically pulsed at 30–100 Hz, but at least one (unsuccessful) case of use of DC current was documented [6]. After 1963, an increased use of ES in the United States was noted. Three years later, the first symposium on ES and EA was held in Graz, Austria [7, 8]. At this symposium it was reasoned that ES does not actually induce sleep, rather it is an indirect side effect of the relaxing effects of stimulation. Therefore, the term *electrosleep* was changed to *cranial electrostimulation therapy* [8]. This was the first of several changes of the term "electrosleep" over the next few decades, often with notable changes in dose. Some devices that were used during this time were Jungbluth CET-1, Tritronics 100, Somatron 500, Lafayette 72000, Lafayette 72200, and General Medical Industry 1-1007-1 [6].

In 1969, TCET was proposed as another alternative name, which was adopted by the same authors [6]. In 1977, ES and its derivatives went under review by the US Food and Drug Administration (FDA) and in 1978 were classified as a Class III device for the treatment of Anxiety, Insomnia, and Depression [9]. However, such devices were renamed as *cranial electrotherapy stimulation* [10]. The FDA status of CES remains debated to the present day [9].

In 1972, a new method and device of ES called NeuroElectric Therapy (NET) [11, 12] was developed in England. Though NET preceded many modern CES devices (see below) it may have influenced the doses they used decades later. Another notable device, produced after the name change to CET, was the Neurotone 101, which was based on a Russian ES device brought to the United States.

Although the Neurotone 101 is no longer in production, it was the first device to be approved by the FDA as a CES device [10] and all subsequent CES devices approved by the FDA were through a 510 k process claiming equivalency, either direct or descendent, to the Neurotone 101. This equivalency is not reflected in identical dose of current CES devices, which in fact are often claimed to be a novel dose.

Modern CES is thus a historical descendant of ES even as dose and indications have continuously evolved.

Developments from Electroanesthesia to Limoge Currents and Other Related Methods

Electroanesthesia, in short, was intended to induce anesthesia in the subject so that chemicals did not have to be used presurgery. EA studies started in 1903 but were first known as electronarcosis (EN) [6, 13]. Russian scientists used the term "electroanesthesia" to describe local anesthesia while "electronarcosis" described general anesthesia [6]. However, EA stopped being referred to as local, applied to the periphery, and began to be known as general anesthesia, now applied to the brain. Therefore, in this review, EA will refer to general anesthesia. One of the earliest published claims of success in regards to EA during surgery was made in 1914 by Leduc [6, 14]. Safety and tolerability concerns, and the development of early chemical anesthetics, may have contributed to quelling interest in EA. In the 1940s, research on EA focused on chemical primers being used in conjunction with EA [6]. Soon after, research appeared to largely halt again presumably due to severe side effects. For example, severe side effects such as cardiac arrest, respiratory arrest, and apoplexy were observed [15, 16]. A third wave of research in EA initiated after a study was published in 1960, proposing a new EA approach to reduce side effects: "...a combination of pulsed and direct currents ... the very slow increase of current levels ... and ... the use of a generator that minimized changes in electrode impedance resulting from polarization [6]" [16].

Research into EA dosage continued and the term *transcutaneous cranial electrical stimulation* was adopted around 1960–1963, with the intended use to "potentiate some drug effects, especially opiates and neuroleptics, during anesthetic clinical procedures...[with the goal of] drastic reduction in pharmacologic anesthetic agent and reducing post-operative complications" [13]. Even though the term TCES was not adopted until the early 1960s, similar protocols were used as early as 1902 by Leduc [13]. In 1951, Denier proposed that high-frequency trains of 90 kHz could be used to avoid muscular contraction [13]. Three years later, Knutson (1954) claimed that alternating currents at 700 Hz should be applied, but this was abandoned in 1958 due to cardiovascular complications [13]. In 1957, investigators in the Soviet Union attempted to add a DC component to Leduc's currents but, as claimed by an American scientist Robert Smith, it resulted in a collection of undesirable side effects [16]. In 1963, Aimé Limoge modified the TCES dose and called it *Limoge current* [13]. In 1964, a study claimed pulsating currents are more effective than direct currents for the induction of EA [6]. Another study suggested that the use of pure DC for EA required high intensity of approximately 40 mA [6].

In 1965, IS was proposed by Russian scientists and consisted of having two pairs of electrodes energized with sine waves of slightly shifted frequencies [6]. Through pulsation the higher frequencies would create a lower frequency, where the two frequencies intersect. This was done because low frequencies were more desirable in inducing EA, whereas higher frequencies were more desirable when it came to patient comfort (e.g., reduced pain, sensation, etc.) [6, 14]. In this way lower frequencies were indirectly combined with high frequencies—an approach also hinted at in some CES technologies. Even though power is modulation, under the assumption that the time-constant in neuronal membranes effectively filters out high-frequency signals (>100 Hz [3]) then regardless of how they are combined and modulated, these signals would be neurophysiologically inactive.

In the development of EA, *Fading* has two different meanings: decrease in anesthetic state [17] or increase in tolerability. In the first case, fading indicated a decrease in the subjects' anesthetic state while the dosage was kept steady [17]. Maintenance of anesthetic state was accomplished by either reduction of frequency or increase of current [17]. Fading, more recently, has been used to increase tolerability by incremental increase to the maximum dosage under the premise that sensation at the skin adapts to current flow. Indeed, fading is a common method used in many contemporary tES approaches such as tDCS. TCES has been studied to reduce postoperative analgesic requirements [18], as are other contemporary tES approaches [19].

Contemporary tES is also concerned with the treatment of a broad range of neuropsychiatric disorders, including pain [4, 20, 21]. Historically, EA/TCES used current intensities typically well above those used in contemporary tES. Nonetheless, these relatively high-intensity EA/TCES approaches provide insight into (upper) safety limits and approaches to enhance tolerability, and broad indications of responsive conditions when applied alone or with pharmacotherapy.

Direct Current Stimulation

Direct current stimulation has been used intermittently as a component in both ES and EA. In 1957, a DC bias was added to ES which is traditionally applied using only alternating current (AC). The advent of TCES, around 1960–1963, in the third resurgence of EA research, also incorporated a DC bias. In 1969, pure direct current stimulation was investigated for inducing anesthesia [6]. However, it was not until 1964 that preliminary studies heralding modern tDCS were published.

In 1964, Redfearn and Lippold investigated polarizing current for treatment of neuropsychiatric diseases [22], their use of prolonged (minutes) or stimulation was motivated by animal studies showing that prolonged direct current stimulation could produce lasting changes in excitability. Short-duration tDCS was investigated by Priori and colleagues in 1998 [23]. Nitsche and Paulus established that prolonged tDCS could produce lasting and polarity-specific changes in cortical excitability [24] followed by pilot clinical studies [25]. Transcranial micropolarization is a technique investigated in Russia which is a modified version of tDCS using small electrodes instead of pads [26]. In 2007, HD-tDCS was proposed as a focalized form of tDCS [27]. HD-tDCS uses specially optimized electrodes [28], arranged in arrays that can be optimized per indication [29], including the 4 × 1 configuration [30].

Galvanic vestibular stimulation is being investigated for effects on ocular and postural movement [31]. Alongside GVS, caloric vestibular stimulation (CVS) is under investigation due to similar areas being targeted by stimulation. However, CVS does not utilize electricity, rather irrigation of the ear canal using cold or warm water [32].

Electroconvulsive Therapy

Initially developed circa 1933, ECT [5, 33] used repetitive high-intensity pulses to trigger seizures. A common term used for ECT is electroshock therapy (EST). ECT was cleared by the FDA for Depression in 1976 as a "pre-amendment device" ("grandfathered" similar to the process for CES). In 2011 the FDA summarized:

The ECT procedure was first conducted in 1938 [34]. Two Italian physicians, UgoCerletti and LucioBini, guided by a theory holding an antagonistic relationship between seizures and psychosis, became the first to use electricity to induce a therapeutic seizure in humans [35]. They reported on the first treatment of a patient using this method in 1939 [36]. Joining a number of other somatic-based therapies of the era (prior to the advent of modern pharmacotherapy), ECT became a popular intervention for psychiatric conditions. Since that time, the use of ECT has waxed and waned. In the 1950s and 1960s, with the development of drug therapies for psychiatric conditions, and due to concern for serious device-related adverse events, the use of ECT in the United States declined [37]. However, in recent years, interest in, and use of, ECT has experienced resurgence; ECT use in the United States has been estimated at 100,000 individuals receiving this treatment annually [38]. Reflecting the greater proportion of women who suffer from major depression, two thirds of patients who receive ECT are women [39]. In clinical practice, ECT is generally considered after failure of one or more antidepressant medication trials, or when there is a need for a rapid and definitive response (APA 2001; p. 23–24). ECT has been used to treat a variety of psychiatric disorders. These disorders include: Depression (unipolar and bipolar), Schizophrenia, Bipolar manic (and mixed) states, Catatonia, and Schizoaffective disorder. The evidence supporting the effectiveness of ECT for each of these indications is variable.

Contemporary Approaches

Two contemporary forms of tES are transcranial alternating current stimulation (tACS) and transcranial random noise stimulation (tRNS) [2]. Both tACS and tRNS use relatively low-intensity current and are being investigated for therapeutic effects [2]. A modified protocol for tACS is transcranial sinusoidal direct current stimulation (tSDCS) [40] where the stimulation is monophasic due to a DC bias added to the sinusoid.

Another form of tES that was used by Marshall and colleagues [41] consisted of monophasic trapezoidal pulses with a DC bias, frequency of .75 Hz. The pulses used by Lisa Marshall were investigated for their effects on learning. The subject would learn the task before sleeping, and be tested on the task the next morning. The stimulation would occur 4 min after stage 2 sleep occurred for the first time, without reversion to stage 1, and stimulation continued at 5 min intervals with a 1 min break throughout the night [41].

Transcranial Alternating Current Stimulation

The first mention of "TES" was 1980 in a study by Morton and Merton [42]. "TES" uses single (isolated) high-intensity pulses to typically activate motor cortex and stimulate motor response. This early use of "TES" resulted in many contemporary investigators associating "TES" with only supra-threshold low-frequency pulses. In this review, we use tES in the broader sense and "TES" (quotes and capitals) to specify the use of supra-threshold low-frequency pulses. "TES" technique can be painful and was not investigated for therapeutic applications, but remains used for diagnostic purposes under anesthesia [43–45]. For the purposes of experimental with low-frequency supra-threshold stimulation in awake subjects, contemporary investigators often use transcranial magnetic stimulation (TMS) instead, as it is more tolerated for these purposes. "TES" continues to be used for intraoperative evaluation in anesthetized subjects and "TES" was first "cleared" by the FDA in 2002 for monitoring.

Noncranial Therapies

Noncranial electrical therapies are mentioned here only in context of historical relevance to cranial therapies. The advent of Limoge currents became the basis for the release of transcutaneous electrical nerve stimulation (TENS) in 1974. Microcurrent electrical therapy (MET) was developed approximately in 1984 and was incorporated into CES devices such as the Alpha-stim 100 [10, 13]. Another noncranial therapy, electroacupuncture, is indicated for local anesthesia in combination with anesthetic primers and combines EA (in this case local EA) and acupuncture [46].

Dosage

This section aims to further clarify the stimulation dose associated with select approaches. It is noteworthy that even early in TES development it was recognized that: (1) stimulation waveform along with electrode positions (stimulation dose [1]) can be varied to change efficacy and safety; (2) the value of current controlled stimulation in contrast to voltage controlled stimulation; and (3) electrode design including the use of a fluid/gel (electrolyte) buffer between the metal electrode and skin increases skin tolerability [47]. Nonetheless, ad hoc and often poorly documented variations in dose are coming in the literature, a matter that remains of concern to this date [1]. Unless otherwise stated, we presume that stimulation was current controlled.

Though we divide dose by category below, certain overarching developments can be noted for both electrode design and waveforms. "Active" and "return" terminology for electrodes reflect only the brain target of interest with "active" being places nearer the target; evidently both electrodes will affect brain function and indeed the position of the return determines "active" current flow [48]. Early approach to stimulation the brain involved two "active" electrodes placed directly over the eyes with two "return" return electrodes, presumably to facilitate active current deliver through the optic foramina. Active electrode positions around the eye (e.g., supraorbital) were explored, as well as reducing the number of active electrodes (e.g., single electrode on the forehead) or using just one return electrode. After 1970, approaches using electrodes on or around the ears were explored (though much earlier examples of ear electrodes are noted), with presumed current flow to deeper brain structures [49]. In the 1980s, approaches using tES showed that current could be delivered focally using small closely spaced electrodes on the scalp (e.g., as indicated by motor responses). After 2000, contemporary approaches (e.g., tDCS, tACS, etc.) used reduced currents and large-sponge electrodes [24] with an "active" electrode placed "over" the nominal target, though the use of larger electrodes and distant electrodes precludes focal stimulation [27] of cortex or avoidance of deep brain structures [50] though functional effects may be shaped [51]. Current approaches using arrays of small high-definition electrodes are intended to allow focal cranial stimulation.

In the context of waveform, a notable overarching progression was: (1) from basic waveforms (often limited to existing stimulation hardware) to increasingly complex and customized waveforms motivated by the perception that increased efficacy, safety, or tolerability was needed; (2) with complexity and (proprietary) uniqueness especially developed in commercial devices (e.g., CES); (3) leading to a reversion to the most basic waveform after 2000, associated with a resurgence of clinical interest using standardized and defined approaches. Early intended uses focused on short-term effects motivated investigators to explore increased intensities (e.g., sleep, anesthesia, etc.), while interest in chronic diseases (e.g., depression) is consistent with efforts using reduced (well tolerated) current intensities and increasingly prolonged (repeated session) use (Fig. 2.1).

Electrosleep and Derivative Techniques

The dosage for ES has evolved since it first was investigated in 1902 [5]. Dosage used for ES consisted of electrode placement over each eye and a return electrode over the mastoid, with a waveform consisting of 100 Hz pulses between 20 and 25 mA [8]. The pulse width was between 0.3 and 0.6 ms and stimulation duration lasted from 20 to 60 min [8]. In 1966, the name changed to CET and shortly afterward a new dosage was developed. Due to patient discomfort and the changing perception that penetration of current into the brain (including deep brain structures) did not require placement of electrodes directly on top of the eyes [6, 52]. Under this CET electrode montage, the stimulation waveform was pulsed at 30–100 Hz, pulse width of 1–2 ms, at 0.1–0.5 mA [52]. TCET was proposed as a new name for ES/CET but under this new nomenclature the dose for TCET was unchanged in regards to electrode placement or waveform [6].

A notable change in dosage occurred with the advent of NET and CES after 1970. In NET and CES, the number of electrodes was reduced from 3 to 2 [10, 53, 54]. The electrode placement for NET was in the subjects' ears [53]—an approach later adopted by some CES devices with electrodes clipped onto the ears [10]. The waveform used in NET, and also in some later CES devices, was 0.5–100 Hz stimulation at up to 600 μA over a period of 20 min [10, 53]. The other variant for CES devices uses two electrodes placed on top of the forehead. The waveform for this variant of CES uses 15, 500 or 15,000 Hz at 4 V with 50 ms pulses and "off" periods of 16.7 ms [49, 54, 55].

Electroanesthesia and Derivative Techniques

The dose for EA evolved since the early 1900s. An early electrode placement for EA/EN consists of four electrodes with either two electrodes applied to each temple or to the bilateral frontal and occipital areas [6]. There are a wide range of frequencies and current intensities that were evaluated. As noted, EA has been tested with pure DC requiring current approximately 40 mA to induce EA [6]. Under AC-only conditions, the frequency ranged from 10 to 20 kHz with intensities approximately 10 mA; higher current intensities were claimed to be needed with higher frequencies and currents of 500 mA and frequencies around 200 kHz have been used. When biased by DC, AC frequencies typically remained in the same range with the AC component ranges from 2.5 to 5 mA with the DC component also ranging from 2.5 to 5 mA. In some instances, waveforms with a high-frequency "ON" periods were incorporated into TCES. TCES uses three electrodes rather than the four in EA; the electrodes are positioned with a single electrode between the eyebrows and two return electrodes on the retromastoid region [6]. TCES waveform consists of frequency trains. The high-frequency portion of the train is "ON" for 3–4 ms at 130–167 kHz and "OFF" for 8-ms periods. The low-frequency portion ("ON"/"OFF") was ~77–100 Hz and the overall waveform uses 200–350 mA with 30–35 V [13] (Fig. 2.3).

Transcranial Direct Current Stimulation/ Transcranial Random Noise Stimulation/ Transcranial Alternating Current Stimulation

Developed over the last decade, tDCS, tRNS, and tACS are three different distinct forms of "contemporary" tES as far as waveform, but all share the same approach to electrode number and shape. Though each applies a distinct waveform, in all cases the duration of stimulation is typically 20 min with a peak current of a few mA. Conventionally, two electrodes are used with one positioned "over" the target region and the other elsewhere on the scalp (often the contralateral [40, 56]). Electrodes are typically saline-soaked sponge material wrapped around a conductive rubber electrode, though gel may also be used. In tDCS, the (positive) anode and (negative) cathode are distinguished for their actions on cortical excitability: 1–2 mA is applied over 5–20 min [2]. For tACS, a single sinusoid at 10–40 Hz with a peak intensity of 0.4–1 mA has been tested [2, 40, 56]. The waveform parameter for tRNS includes: "a frequency spectrum between 0.1 and 640 Hz… [and]… a normally distributed random level of current generated for every sample at a sampling rate of 1,280 samples per second with no overall DC offset." [2, 57].

High-Definition Transcranial Direct Current Stimulation

High-definition transcranial direct current stimulation shares the same waveform with tDCS, 1–2 mA at 5–20 min; however, the large sponge electrodes used for tDCS (as for tACS/tRNS) are replaced with an array of smaller electrodes. The electrode montage is then optimized for brain targeting; for example, the 4 × 1-Ring montage uses a center electrode which determines the polarity of stimulation (anode or cathode) and four return electrodes at ~4–7 cm radius. More broadly, HD-tES spans all efforts to focalize prior diffuse tES protocols by using arrays of HD electrodes to rationally guide current flow [29] (Fig. 2.4).

Transcranial Electrical Stimulation

"Transcranial electrical stimulation" uses high-intensity pulses (150–1,840 V, presumed to be voltage controlled) lasting between 13 and 48 μs at an intermittent frequency of 1–3 s or less [43, 45, 58, 59]. Typically, stimulation is applied using a bifocal (and bipolar) montage, but a "unifocal" montage has also been explored with an active electrode over the target a "ring" of return electrodes, either as a single band or 12 separate electrodes, around the width of the scalp [45, 58, 59].

Electroconvulsive Therapy

The waveforms for ECT are high-intensity, ~800 mA, with trains lasting 1–6 s per cycle. The electrodes are placed either unilaterally or bilaterally on the cranium and current intensity is typically increased by varying the number of pulses per train, pulse duration, or intensity until a seizure is triggered [5, 60]. Modern efforts to refine dose have focused on minimizing memory loss, for example through focused stimulations [61, 62] (Fig. 2.5).

Conclusion

The field of electromedicine has evidently evolved through the past 100 years. Early technology evaluated very basic waveforms, continued on to increasingly complicated waveforms (i.e., pulse trains; *see* Fig. 2.5), returning to more defined and simple waveforms at the turn of the century (i.e., tDCS and tACS). Although techniques and protocols have constantly been adjusted (with many waxing and waning in popularity), it is not prudent to globally conclude that early approaches were ineffective or that they should be automatically ignored; rather, both experience with efficacy (even when anecdotal or not fully documented by modern standard) as well as findings on safety (which were significant enough to warrant dose changes) should be considered to inform ongoing efforts. In this sense, the history on electrical stimulation may guide ongoing rational advancement.

Reporting the stimulation dosage used as well as the specific device used is and continues to be important for reproducibility. Descriptions of waveforms can at times be convoluted and we proposed ongoing efforts to carefully define the dosages and devices as well as using a form of standardized terminology (such as the one stated in Fig. 2.5) can be extremely useful in furthering research at a faster pace. The focus on terminology and dose in this review is intended to disambiguate the historical narrative, which is necessary if past experience with specific dose is to inform ongoing efforts.

References

1. Peterchev AV, Wagner TA, Miranda PC, Nitsche MA, Paulus W, Lisanby SH, Pascual-Leone A, Bikson M. Fundamentals of transcranial electric and magnetic stimulation dose: definition, selection and reporting practices. Brain Stimul. 2012;5:435–53.
2. Paulus W. Transcranial electrical stimulation (tES – tDCS; tRNS, tACS) methods. Neuropsychol Rehabil. 2011;21:602–17.
3. Bikson M, Inoue M, Akiyama H, Deans JK, Fox JE, Miyakawa H, Jefferys JG. Effects of uniform extracellular DC electric fields on excitability in rat hippocampal slices in vitro. J Physiol. 2004;558:175–90.
4. Brunoni AR, Ferruci R, Bortolomasi M, Scelzo E, Boggio PS, Fregni F, et al. Interactions between transcranial direct current stimulation (tDCS) and pharmacological interventions in the Major Depressive Episode: findings from a naturalistic study. Eur Psychiatry. 2013;28:114–9.
5. Gilula FM, Kirsch DL. Cranial electrotherapy stimulation review: a safer alternative to psychopharmaceuticals in the treament of depression. J Neurother. 2005;9:7–26.
6. Brown CC. Electroanesthesia and electrosleep. Am Psychol. 1975;30:402–10.
7. Smith RB. Cranial electrotherapy stimulation: its first fifty years, plus three: a monograph. Mustang, OK: Tate Publishing and Enterprises; 2006.
8. Knutson RC. First international symposium on electrosleep therapy and electroanesthesia. Anesth Analg. 1967;46:333–9.
9. FDA Executive Summary. Prepared for the February 10th, 2012 meeting of the neurological devices panel meeting to discuss petitions to request change in classification for cranial electrotherapy stimulators.
10. Kirsch DL. Low level brain stimulation for anxiety: a review of 50 years of research and supporting data. 2010. http://www.cesultra.cn/pdf/6%E3%80%81Low%20Level%20Brain%20Stimulation%20for%20Anxiety%20A%20Review.pdf.
11. Patterson MA. Effects of neuro-electric therapy (N.E.T.) in drug addiction: interim report. Bull Narc. 1976;28:55–62.
12. Patterson MA. Electrotherapy: addictions and neuroelectric therapy. Nurs Times. 1979;75:2080–3.
13. Limoge A, Robert C, Stanley TH. Transcutaneous cranial electrical stimulation (TCES): a review 1998. Neurosci Biobehav Rev. 1999;23:529–38.
14. Smith RH. Electroanesthesia (EA). Anesthesiology. 1971;34: 60–72.
15. Knutson RC, Tichy FY, Reitman JR. Use of electrical current as an anesthetic agent. Anesthesiology. 1956;17:815–25.
16. Smith RH, Tatsuno J, Zouhar RL. Electroanesthesia : a review – 1966. Anesth Analg. 1967;46:109–25.
17. Smith RH, Andrew JH, Suzuki H, Tatsuno J. Electroanesthesia studies: a new current pattern and control of fading. Anesth Analg. 1968;47:627–32.
18. Nekhendzy V, Lemmens HJ, Tingle M, Nekhendzy M, Angst MS. The analgesic and antihyperalgesic effects of transcranial electrostimulation with combined direct and alternating current in healthy volunteers. Anesth Analg. 2010;111:1301–7.
19. Borckardt JJ, Romagnuolo J, Reeves ST, Madan A, Frohman Y, Beam W, George MS. Feasibility, safety, and effectiveness of transcranial direct current stimulation for decreasing post-ERCP pain: a randomized, sham-controlled, pilot study. Gastrointest Edosc. 2011;73:1158–64.
20. Zaghi S, Thiele B, Pimentel D, Pimentel T, Fregni F. Assessment and treatment of pain with non-invasive cortical stimulation. Restor Neurol Neurosci. 2011;29:439–51.
21. Brunoni AR, Valiengo L, Baccaro A, Zanão TA, de Oliveira FJ, Goulart A et al. The sertraline vs electrical current therapy for treating depression clinical study: results from a factorial, randomized, controlled trial. JAMA Psychiatry. 2013;30:646–653. doi: 10.1001/2013.jamapsychiatry.32. [Epub ahead of print].
22. Redfearn JW, Lippold OC, Costain R. Preliminary account of the clinical effects of polarizing the brain in certain psychiatric disorders. Br J Psychiatry. 1964;110:773–85.
23. Priori A, Berardelli A, Rona S, Accornero N, Manfredi M. Polarization of the human motor cortex through the scalp. Neuroreport. 1998;9:2257–60.
24. Nitsche MA, Paulus W. Excitability changes induced in the human motor cortexes by weak transcranial direct current stimulation. J Physiol. 2000;527:633–9.
25. Bolognini N, Pascual-Leone A, Fregni F. Using non-invasive brain stimulation to augment motor training-induced plasticity. J Neuroeng Rehabil. 2009;6:1–13.
26. Shelyakin A, Preobrazhenskaya I. Principles of the weak direct current therapy. https://sites.google.com/site/micropolarization/principles.
27. Datta A, Bansal V, Diaz J, Patel J, Reato D, Bikson M. Gyri-precise head model of transcranial direct current stimulation: improved spatial focality using a ring electrode versus conventional rectangular pad. Brain Stimul. 2009;2:201–7.
28. Minhas P, Bansal V, Patel J, Ho JS, Diaz J, Datta A, Bikson M. Electrodes for high-definition transcutaneous DC stimulation for applications in drug delivery and electrotherapy, including tDCS. J Neurosci Methods. 2010;190:188–97.
29. Dmochowski JP, Datta A, Bikson M, Su Y, Parra LC. Optimized multi-electrode stimulation increases focality and intensity at target. J Neural Eng. 2011;8:1–16.
30. Edwards D, Cortes M, Datta A, Minhas P, Wassermann EM, Bikson M. Physiological and modeling evidence for focal transcranial electrical brain stimulation in humans: A basis for high-definition tDCS. Neuroimage. 2013; doi: pii: S1053-8119(13)00089-X. 10.1016/j.neuroimage.2013.01.042. [Epub ahead of print].
31. Watson SRD, Colebatch JG. EMG responses in the soleus muscles evoked by unipolar galvanic vestibular stimulation. Electroencephalogr Clin Neurophysiol. 1997;105:476–83.

32. Miller SM, Ngo TT. Studies of caloric vestibular stimulation: implications for the cognitive neurosciences, the clinical neurosciences and neurophysiology. Acta Neuropsychiatr. 2007; 19:183–203.
33. Abrams R. Electroconvulsive therapy. New York: Oxford University Press; 2002.
34. Rudorfer MV, Henry ME, Sackeim HA. Electroconvulsive therapy. In: Tasman A, Kay J, Lieberman JA, editors. Psychiatry, vol. 2. Philadelphia: W.B. Saunders; 1997.
35. Faedda GL, Becker I, Baroni A, Tondo L, Aspland E, Koukopoulos A. The origins of electroconvulsive therapy: Prof Bini's first report on ECT. J Affect Disord. 2010;120:12–5.
36. Bini L. Professor Bini's notes on the first electro-shock experiment. Convuls Ther. 1995;11:260–1.
37. Lisanby SH. Electroconvulsive therapy for depression. N Engl J Med. 2007;357:1939–45.
38. Hermann RC, Dorwart RA, Hoover CW, Brody J. Variation in ECT use in the United States. Am J Psychiatry. 1995;152:869–75.
39. Olfson M, Marcus S, Sackeim HA, Thompson J, Pincus HA. Use of ECT for the inpatient treatment of recurrent major depression. Am J Psychiatry. 1998;155:22–9.
40. Antal A, Boros K, Poreisz C, Chaieb L, Terney D, Paulus W. Comparatively weak after-effects of transcranial alternating current stimulation (tACS) on cortical excitability in humans. Brain Stimul. 2008;1:97–105.
41. Marshall L, Helgadottir H, Molle M, Born J. Boosting slow oscillations during sleep potentiates memory. Nature. 2006;444: 610–3.
42. Merton PA, Morton HB. Stimulation of the cerebral cortex in the intact human subject. Nature. 1980;285:227.
43. Zentner J, Kiss I, Ebner A. Influence of anesthetics—nitrous oxide in particular—onelectromyographic response evoked by transcranial electrical stimulation of the cortex. Neurosurgery. 1989;24:253–6.
44. Macdonald DB. Safety of intraoperative transcranial electrical stimulation motor evoked potential monitoring. J Clin Neurophysiol. 2002;19:416–29.
45. Kalkman CJ, Drummond JC, Kennelly NA, Patel PM, Partridge BL. Intraoperative monitoring of tibialis anteriro muscle motor evoked responses to transcranial electrical stimulation during partial neuromuscular blockade. Anesth Analg. 1992;75:584–9.
46. Christensen PA, Rotne M, Vedelsdal R, Jensen R, Jacobsen K, Husted C. Electroacupuncture in anesthesia for hysterectomy. Br J Anesth. 1993;71:835–8.
47. Merrill D, Bikson M, Jefferys JGR. Electrical stimulation of excitable tissue: design of efficacious and safe protocols. J Neurosci Methods. 2005;141:171–98.
48. Bikson M, Datta A, Rahman A, Scaturro J. Electrode montages for tDCS and weak transcranial electrical stimulation: role of "return" electrode's position and size. Clin Neurophysiol. 2010;121:1976–8.
49. Datta A, Dmochowski JP, Guleyupoglu B, Bikson M, Fregni F. Cranial electrotherapy stimulation and transcranial pulsed current stimulation: a computer based high-resolution modeling study. Neuroimage. 2013;65:280–7.
50. Dasilva AF, Mendonca ME, Zaghi S, Lopes M, Dossantos MF, Spierings EL, et al. tDCS-induced analgesia and electrical fields in pain-related neural networks in chronic migraine. Headache. 2012;52:1283–95.
51. Nitsche MA, Doemkes S, Karakose T, Antal A, Liebetanz D, Lang N, et al. Shaping the effects of transcranial direct current stimulation of the human motor cortex. J Neurophysiol. 2007;97:3109–17.
52. von Richthofen CL, Mellor CS. Cerebral electrotherapy: methodological problems in assessing its therapeutic effectiveness. Psychol Bull. 1979;86:1264–71.
53. NET Device Corp Information. About NET. http://www.netdevice.net/aboutnet.php.
54. Liss Body StimulatorManual (M), Monopolar Model No. SBL-501-M Manual. http://charlesmccusker.com/pdf/Liss-Waveforms.pdf.
55. Liss Body StimulatorManual (B), Bipolar Model No. SBL-502-B Manual. http://charlesmccusker.com/pdf/Liss-Waveforms.pdf.
56. Zaehle T, Rach S, Herrmann CS. Transcranial alternating current stimulation enhances individual alpha activity in human EEG. PLoS One. 2010;5:1–7.
57. Chaieb L, Kovacs G, Cziraki C, Greenlee M, Paulus W, Antal A. Short-duration transcranial random noise stimulation induces blood oxygenation level dependent response attenuation in the human motor cortex. Exp Brain Res. 2009;198:439–44.
58. Rossini PM, Marciani MG, Caramia M, Roma V, Zarola F. Nervous propagation along "central" motor pathways in intact man: characteristics of motor responses to "bifocal" and "unifocal" spine and scalp non-invasive stimulation. Electroencephalogr Clin Neurophysiol. 1985;61:272–86.
59. Rothwell J, Burke D, Hicks R, Stephen J, Woodforth I, Crawford M. Transcranial electrical stimulation of the motor cortex in man: further evidence for the site of activation. J Physiol. 1994;481: 243–50.
60. Sackeim HA, Prudic J, Devanand DP, Nobler MS, Lisanby SH, Peyser S, Fitzsimons L, Moody BJ, Clark J. A prospective, randomized, double-blind comparison of bilateral and right unilateral electroconvulsive therapy at different stimulus intensities. Arch Gen Psychiatry. 2000;57:425–34.
61. Spellman T, Peterchev AV, Lisanby SH. Focal electrically administered seizure therapy: a novel form of ECT illustrates the roles of current directionality, polarity, and electrode configuration in seizure induction. Neuropsychopharmacology. 2009;34: 2002–10.
62. Datta A, Elwassif M, Battaglia F, Bikson M. Transcranial current stimulation focality using disc and ring electrode configurations: FEM analysis. J Neural Eng. 2008;5:163–74.
63. Bystritsky A, Kerwin L, Feusner J. A pilot study of cranial electrotherapy stimulation for generalized anxiety disorder. J Clin Psychiatry. 2008;69:412–7.

Part II

Methods

Peripheral Nerve Stimulation

3

Konstantin V. Slavin, Alexios G. Carayannopoulos, Mark Plazier, Sven Vanneste, and Dirk De Ridder

Introduction

Within the family of neuromodulation procedures, peripheral nerve stimulation (PNS) has a unique place. Despite several decades of clinical use, PNS struggles to become a widely used and, to some extent, legitimate counterpart to its more established siblings, which include deep brain (DBS) and spinal cord stimulation (SCS). PNS is defined as electric stimulation performed on the peripheral nervous system and applied to a specific nerve [1]. Electrical current can be delivered to nerves transcutaneously (transcutaneous electrical nerve stimulation: TENS), percutaneously with a temporary electrode (the so-called percutaneous electrical nerve stimulation: PENS), and with help of surgically or percutaneously implanted electrodes (PNS).

Historically, the first published report of PNS for treatment of neuropathic pain described procedure performed on October 9, 1965 when Drs. Wall and Sweet implanted electrodes around the median and ulnar nerves of a 26-year-old woman with a clinical presentation consistent with complex regional pain syndrome (CRPS). Electrical stimulation of the median nerve provoked pleasant paresthesias and modulated pain in the medial three fingers [2]. During that same year, Drs. Melzack and Wall published the seminal "gate-control" theory of pain in their article in *Science*, postulating that innocuous sensory information may suppress the transmission of pain [3]. This was the scientific foundation for the development of a new treatment modality, coined neuromodulation, which subsequently grew in its number of indications and types of procedural applications. Soon thereafter, the famous 1969 book "Pain and the neurosurgeon" by White and Sweet was published and detailed a description and an X-ray image of a PNS device implanted on the ulnar nerve of a patient with post-traumatic neuropathy [2]. Shortly after, dozens of clinical reports detailed various aspects of PNS in the 1970s thru 1990s, and PNS has remained relatively unchanged since: the target nerve was exposed, and a paddle-type electrode lead was placed in direct contact with the nerve trunk [4]. To facilitate this procedure, a specially designed paddle lead was created; it had an integrated mesh attached to the paddle, allowing the surgeon to wrap the electrode around the nerve, rather than to struggle with suturing it in situ.

Introduction of a percutaneous PNS insertion technique in the late 1990s [5] has since revolutionized the PNS field. Although the approach initially appeared to be most applicable to craniofacial stimulation, it gradually spread to use in the lower parts of the body, including the extremities, abdomen, chest wall, upper and lower back, groin area, and neck. The next development was introduction of the peripheral nerve field stimulation (PNFS) concept (sometimes called subcutaneous nerve stimulation, subcutaneous target stimulation, or peripheral field stimulation). Considered a variation of PNS, PNFS targets more distal neural structures, including unnamed nerve branches and subcutaneous nerve endings [1]. More recently, the PNS approach was augmented by addition of ultrasound

K.V. Slavin
Department of Neurosurgery, University of Illinois at Chicago, 912 South Wood Street, M/C 799, Chicago, IL 60612
e-mail: kslavin@uic.edu

A.G. Carayannopoulos
Spine Center, Department of Neurosurgery, Lahey Clinic, 41 Mall Road, 7 Central, Burlington, MA 01805
e-mail: Alexios.G.Carayannopoulos@Lahey.org

M. Plazier
Department of Neurosurgery, University Hospital Antwerp, Wilrijkstraat 10, Edegem, Antwerp 2650, Belgium
e-mail: Mark.plazier@uza.be

S. Vanneste
School for Behavioral and Brain Sciences, University of Texas at Dallas, 1966 Inwood Rd, Dallas, TX 75235, USA
e-mail: sven.vanneste@utdallas.edu

D. De Ridder (✉)
Department of Surgical Sciences, Section of Neurosurgery, Dunedin Public Hospital, 201 Great King Street, Dunedin, Otago 9016, New Zealand
e-mail: dirk.deridder@otago.ac.nz

H. Knotkova and D. Rasche (eds.), *Textbook of Neuromodulation*,
DOI 10.1007/978-1-4939-1408-1_3, © Springer Science+Business Media, LLC 2015

guidance, which helps in visualization of peripheral nerves during percutaneous lead insertion [6]. Finally, progress in PNS was facilitated by technical innovations of several new companies, each of which came up with surgical techniques specifically developed for PNS applications.

The Spectrum of Peripheral Nerve Stimulation

Transcutaneous Electrical Nerve Stimulation

TENS is an external neuromodulation modality that involves delivery of electrical current through intact skin, over the course of a nerve. Generally, it is used as a noninvasive neuromodulation approach, in conjunction with modalities used in physical therapy. It often serves as an alternative or prelude to more invasive interventions. Ostensibly, it is by far the most common application of peripheral neuromodulation in contemporary medical practice.

Recent reviews have analyzed the strength of evidence in the application of TENS to the treatment of neuropathic pain [7] and cancer pain [8]. Additionally, acupuncture-like application of TENS has also been reviewed in detail of late [9]. Outside of pain practice, posterior tibial nerve stimulation for the treatment of overactive bladder [10] and fecal incontinence [11] are the most commonly used TENS indications in patients. This modality has also been applied to stimulation of the phrenic and vagus nerves in the treatment of persistent hiccups [12] and seizures [13], and stimulation of the trigeminal nerve in treatment of epilepsy [14] and depression [15]. Trigeminal TENS has also been tried for treatment of trigeminal neuralgia [16]. In the mid-1970s, several groups used TENS for selection of candidates to undergo permanent PNS implants; however, no difference was found in the long-term success rate among those who did and those who did not respond to TENS prior to PNS procedure [17, 18].

Percutaneous Electrical Nerve Stimulation

PENS treatment is a technique performed with bipolar needle-like temporary electrodes, which are inserted into the tissues (as opposed to TENS where electrical stimulation is delivered through the skin) and then removed at the end of the session. This relatively noninvasive neuromodulation approach has been used in the treatment of a variety of painful conditions including low back pain, sciatica, diabetic neuropathy, acute herpetic pain, and headaches (for detailed review see PENS section in [4]).

PENS treatment is not an accepted means of PNS screening. It may have value for the treatment of cancer related pain, whereby permanent implantation is not possible [19] or in some cases of facial pain, whereby trigeminal neuropathy does not respond to medical treatment [20]. PENS equipment has recently become commercially available (NeuroStimulator PENS therapy, Algotec Ltd., West Sussex, UK) but to this date, has not been approved for clinical use in the USA. Interestingly, the original illustration of the "gate-control" theory of pain came from Drs. Wall and Sweet, who used PENS to suppress pain sensation by inserting stimulating electrodes into their own infraorbital foramina [21].

Peripheral Nerve Stimulation

PNS requires implantation of an electrode lead across or along a nerve trunk to provide stimulation-induced paresthesias. When originally approved by the US Food and Drug Administration (FDA), this old modality was defined as a way to electrically stimulate a peripheral nerve in patients to relieve severe intractable pain. The FDA used the following definition for PNS devices: "An implanted peripheral nerve stimulator for pain relief is a device that is used to electrically stimulate a peripheral nerve in a patient to relieve severe intractable pain" [22]. This definition later added the following statement: "The stimulator consists of an implanted (sic) receiver with electrodes that are placed around a peripheral nerve and an external transmitter for transmitting the stimulating pulses across the patient's skin to the implanted receiver" [22], which referred to the radiofrequency (RF) coupled systems that were used in the past, including the original report of White and Sweet [2].

By limiting approved PNS devices to RF-coupled systems, current FDA approval effectively excludes all currently used implantable pulse generators [23] (these include prime-cell and rechargeable generators by Medtronic, Minneapolis, Minn.; St. Jude Medical, St. Paul, Minn.; and rechargeable generators by Boston Scientific, Natick, Mass.) In a surprising twist of technological development, a new, non-RF-coupled device, which satisfies FDA requirements, was recently introduced (StimRouter, Bioness, Valencia, Calif.) specifically for PNS applications [24].

The first decade of the twenty-first century has witnessed a dramatic increase in the use of PNS, not just for the treatment of chronic, intractable pain but also for the treatment of refractory epilepsy [25], treatment-resistant depression with vagal nerve stimulation [26] (VNS Pulse and Demipulse, Cyberonics, Houston, Tex.), diaphragmatic pacing by phrenic nerve stimulation for respiratory failure treatment [27] (Breathing Pacemaker System, Avery Biomedical Devices, Comack., N.Y.), reduction in apnea with implantable hypoglossal nerve stimulation systems [28] (Inspire II, Inspire Medical, Maple Grove, Minn.; HGNS, Apnex

Medical Inc., St Paul, Minn.; and Aura6000, ImThera Medical, San Diego, Calif.), somatic nerve stimulation of the extremities in patients after stroke [29] (NESS L300, Bioness; ActiGait, Neurodan, Aalborg, Denmark), and finally autonomic stimulation for urinary and gastrointestinal disorders [30] (InterStim, Medtronic).

A renewed interest in PNS treatment modality has been supported by ongoing technological advances in the field as well as adoption of minimally invasive neuromodulation techniques by non-neurosurgical colleagues, including interventional pain physicians.

PNS/PNFS Techniques

Two peripheral neuromodulation techniques are used by physicians for various types of neuropathic pain: (1) PNS, whereby leads are implanted in the subcutaneous tissue near a specific nerve, which has sensory distribution over the painful area; (2) PNFS, whereby leads are implanted within an area of pain perception [1, 31]. The aim of PNS is to produce paresthesias along the territory of the stimulated nerve, while the aim of PNFS is to distribute paresthesias in an electrical field around the lead's active electrodes, without achieving a clearly defined nerve distribution. Generally, this results in concentric stimulation-induced sensation in a specific area of precise painful zone, without radiation.

Implantation of a peripheral nerve stimulator is performed in two stages, which are similar to spinal cord stimulation. During the first stage, an electrode lead is inserted in the vicinity of the targeted nerve branch. This is followed by a trial of stimulation that lasts several days or weeks. If the trial is successful, the second stage of surgery involves insertion of a permanent electrode, which is anchored in place, usually to the underlying fascia, with subsequent tunneling of the electrode lead or an appropriate extension cable to an implantable pulse generator (IPG).

Indications and Patient Selection

Patient selection in PNS is generally consistent with guidelines used in the family of neuromodulation procedures. PNS is indicated for cases of chronic, severe, disabling neuropathic pain that has been refractory to medical treatments, which is associated with a clear diagnostic impression, and which occurs in the absence of correctable pathology. Additionally, patients are expected to be familiar with the modality and willing to use it, have a favorable neuropsychological profile, and respond positively to a trial of PNS before the permanent device is implanted. The usual contraindications, such as short life expectancy, active infection, uncorrectable coagulopathy or thrombocytopenia, and generally poor medical condition, which would preclude patients from undergoing elective surgery and/or anesthesia, should all be taken into consideration.

The most common indications for PNS in the extremities are chronic pain due to peripheral nerve injury, persistent pain from compressive neuropathy (following adequate decompression), complex regional pain syndromes (CRPS) type 1 (formerly known as reflex sympathetic dystrophy) and type 2 (formerly known as causalgia), and painful peripheral neuropathy. For PNS (of PNFS) of the chest wall, abdomen, neck, upper and lower back, groin area, and other parts of the trunk, the most common indications are postsurgical neuropathic pain, post-infectious (particularly post-herpetic) pain, and posttraumatic neuropathy.

In the last few years, most patients undergoing PNS below the head and face carried the diagnosis of failed back surgery syndrome (FBSS). At one point, this category of patients was dominated by pain from peripheral nerve injury and CRPS. This shift reflects the growing prevalence of back pain in the general population and is also likely secondary to recent growth in the number of spinal interventions, as well as the general ineffectiveness of other treatment modalities, including SCS, in management of axial back pain or paraspinal lumbar pain.

For extremity pain, patients with pain limited to the distribution of a single nerve are better candidates for PNS, whereas patients with pain in the trunk, chest, abdomen, generally respond better to PNS/PNFS. Pure sensory nerves tend to be better targets for PNS than mixed motor/sensory or pure motor nerves, whereby stimulation may also provoke undesired motor phenomena.

Neuropathic Limb Pain

Traditionally, complex regional pain syndromes from to an injury to a nerve (CRPS Type 2) or to a tissue (CRPS Type 1) have been the main indications for use of PNS in a limb [32]. Selection of PNS for patients with CRPS depends on chronicity as well as severity of pain, failure of less invasive treatment approaches, and mediation of pain by primary sensory nerves, since mixed and predominantly motor nerves may not tolerate stimulation [33]. Historically, PNS electrode lead implantation in the limbs was done by an open surgical approach due to the proximity of nerves to vessels and the deep course of nerves in the soft tissues. However, the risk of perineural scarring made the open approach less attractive. At the same time, introduction of ultrasound guidance has gained acceptance, as it allows one to use minimal access techniques for percutaneous electrode insertion [34, 35]. The variable course and depth of the nerves to be stimulated, as well as proximity to vessels, makes ultrasound guidance particularly helpful. Well documented class III evidence from two studies on limb neuropathic pain suggests that PNS could provide good relief for CRPS, which is limited to the distribution of one major nerve in 60 % of patients [32, 36].

Neuropathic Facial Pain

Post herpetic neuropathy, incidental trauma, and iatrogenic injury to the face are major causes of trigeminal neuropathic pain (TNP). PNS in the face is indicated for the management of TNP with clear anatomic distribution within one or several of the trigeminal branches. PNS of supraorbital, infraorbital, and mandibular branches of the fifth cranial nerve, alone or in combination, has been published [37–39]. In one recent case series, TNP was successfully treated with PNS with up to a 2 years follow-up [40].

Neuropathic Trunk Pain

Case reports and small series have documented successful application of PNS and PFNS to chronic neuropathic pains of the neck [41], chest wall [42], abdominal wall [43, 44], and low back [45–48]. Post-herpetic neuralgia and postoperative pain due to thoracic and abdominal surgeries were the common etiologies of neuropathic pain in these patients. Among newly introduced developments are the "cross talk" concept [49, 50] for low back PNS as well as "hybrid" stimulation concept that combines spinal cord stimulation with PNFS [51–55].

The largest PNFS series was based on an Austrian nationwide retrospective study, which analyzed 111 patients with non-cancer pain with successful trial and subsequent implantation with a permanent neurostimulation system [56]. Of these, 97 had pain in the trunk (lower back, neck, chest wall) with an impressive reduction in the average pain intensity, measured by the numerical rating scale before and after the implantation. This difference was particularly significant in patients with low back pain and failed back surgery syndrome [56] ($P < 0.0001$). Out of 111 patients, 27 (24 %) developed complications, including 7 infections (6 %), 14 lead migrations (13 %), and 6 (5 %) lead fractures; all of these developed within 6 months after implantation [56].

Another recent study showed that peripheral neuromodulation is a safe and effective treatment option for intractable chronic pain conditions. Results of a prospective, observational Australian study of 100 consecutive patients receiving PNFS for the treatment of chronic craniofacial, thoracic, lumbosacral, abdominal, pelvic, and groin pain conditions included 16 adverse events without any report of long term complications [57]. The frequency of adverse events were as follows: lead infection—1, hardware erosion—7, hardware migration—2, leads too superficial—3, leads too tight—1, hardware failure—2, with a total rate of complications reaching 14 %, with some patients having more than one complication [57]. The greatest reduction in pain was observed in the abdominal PNFS group, in which there was an average drop of 7.0 ± 1.0 pain scale points ($P < 0.007$). A statistically significant reduction in pain was observed in the lumbosacral group, with a reduction of 3.3 ± 2.3 pain scale points ($P < 0.000$) [57].

With ongoing accumulation of clinical and research data in the field of PNS, more in-depth understanding on the mechanisms of action, technical details, and complications will become available for review [58]. Further research in PNS will allow new indications, new targets, and new devices. For example, development of a dedicated PNS system for post-amputation pain with special cuff-like electrodes is now undergoing clinical trials [59] (Electrical Nerve Block, Neuros Medical, Willoughby, Ohio). A single piece ultra-compact electrode/generator combination (BION, Boston Scientific) is currently under evaluation for the effectiveness for chronic cluster headache [60]. In a very different approach, intramuscular nerve stimulation with a dedicated device (IMN, SPR Therapeutics, Cleveland, Ohio) is being tested for stimulation of the deltoid muscle for refractory shoulder pain in hemiplegic patients [61]. There are multiple recent reports of pioneering PNS applications including the use of splanchnic nerve PNS for chronic pancreatitis pain [62, 63], paravertebral plexus PNS for thoracic neuropathic pain [64], inguinal and genitofemoral PNS for postoperative testicular pain [65], and vagus nerve stimulation for migraines [66].

With recent regulatory approval of PNS in Europe for the treatment of chronic lower back pain and intractable chronic migraines, clinical interest in this modality will continue to grow and is expected to stimulate accrual of objective evidence in terms of safety, efficacy, best indications, and optimal stimulation parameters. All of these will be necessary for regulatory approval worldwide and for greater benefit to the patients who are still suffering from chronic neuropathic pain.

Peripheral Nerve Field Stimulation of the C2 Nerve

Electrical stimulation of the occipital branch of the C2 nerve takes a special place in PNFS, because of its seemingly widespread effects, most of which are not fully explained, even though hypotheses have been proposed of its hypothetical working mechanism [67].

The greater occipital nerve is a branch of the second cervical spinal nerve which leaves the spinal cord at the level of the second cervical vertebral body. It provides sensory innervation of occipital area of the scalp up to the vertex of the head. The main branches of the nerve arise in the subcutaneous tissue in a small area just underneath the occipital protuberance [68]. It usually has medial and lateral branches which spread and divide into smaller branches in the subcutaneous area from this point on. The greater occipital nerve afferents enter the C2 segment of the spinal cord at the level of the nucleus caudalis of the trigeminal nerve forming the trigeminocervical complex [69]. The nucleus caudalis projects to the thalamus, which relays sensory input to the cortex. Furthermore, animal studies have shown connections between neurons of the C2 spinal cord and the hypothalamus [70], the thalamus [71], the periaqueductal grey [71], the amygdala [70], anterior cingulate cortex [72], and posterior insula [72]. Thus, the C2 neurons in the spinal cord are directly connected to most areas of the pain matrix, and both to the medial and lateral spinothalamic pain pathways. C2 PNFS can thus theoretically modulate both the discriminatory (pain intensity, localization, etc.) and affective (attention to pain, unpleasantness, distress, etc.) components of the pain. This was also demonstrated in a recent fMRI study, showing that depending on the stimulation pattern (burst vs. tonic) and frequency, different brain areas are modulated [73]. For example burst stimulation exerts a BOLD activation of the dorsal anterior cingulate cortex, an activity which is related to unpleasantness, whereas tonic stimulation seems to exert a BOLD deactivation in a healthy volunteer [73]. But it also influences the thalamus, somatosensory cortex, and periaqueductal grey in a different way depending on the stimulation design [73]. PET scans performed during C2 stimulation in patients revealed significant changes in the regional cerebral blood flow in the dorsal rostral pons, anterior cingulate cortex, and the cuneus, correlated to pain scores. Changes in the anterior cingulate cortex and the left pulvinar correlated to paresthesia scores [74]. As these structures are well known to be involved in the brain pain matrix, these data might suggest that stimulation of the greater occipital nerve results in a modulation of brain activity in pain related cortical and subcortical structures.

Indications for C2 PNFS

Headache

Introduction of percutaneous insertion technique in the field of PNS allowed treatment of the craniofacial region [31]. PNS of occipital nerves has been successfully used for treatment of chronic headaches due to occipital neuralgia, cluster headache, and migraine [58]. In addition, occipital PNS was recently reportedly successful in the management of chronic headaches [75] as well as a complicated case of occipital neuralgia [76].

Headache: Occipital Neuralgia

Occipital neuralgia, or Arnold's neuralgia, has been one of the first clinical indications in which greater occipital nerve stimulation has been used. In this pathology, patients suffer from an aching, burning pain at the occipital nerve area which can be triggered by neck movements and touching trigger points at the occipital scalp. PNFS seemed to have a strong effect in pain reduction in this syndrome [17]. Further publications confirmed these results in a group of 17 patients with a follow-up of 1.5–6 years. Percutaneous cylindrical leads were placed on a horizontal line at the level of the occipital protuberance. Approximately two-third of the patients experienced a pain relief described as excellent and one-third described as good [5]. A more recent publication describes similar results in a group of 14 patients; however, 4 patients did not pass the trial phase of their study [77]. However, the results seem to be reproducible in various studies [78–82] (see Table 3.1 for overview).

Headaches: Chronic Migraine

The main developments in occipital PNS came from its use in migraine headaches. Despite disappointing results of the first two multicenter prospective randomized studies investigating occipital PNS in patients with intractable migraines [93, 95], the third multicenter double-blind, controlled study aimed to assess safety and efficacy of occipital PNFS for the management of chronic migraine. This sponsored study showed a significant difference between the active and control groups in essentially every monitored indicator [92], including a decrease in days of headache (22.5 vs. 3.4), improvement in MIDAS scores (64.6 vs. 20.4), improvement in Zung Pain and Distress Scales (13.3 vs. 5.5), improvement in visual analogue scale of pain severity (14.1 vs. 7.0) and improvement in quality-of-life measures. Furthermore, there was only a 1 % rate of serious device and procedure-related events in the entire cohort of 157 patients [92]. Based on these results, the authors concluded that occipital PNS is safe and effective in treatment of headache pain and disability associated with chronic migraine [92].

These studies were initiated after some evidence derived from smaller scale studies suggesting C2 PNFS could benefit migraine patients. In a publication of Oh et al. patients were included suffering from both occipital neuralgia and transformed migraine. The results were positive in nine out of ten patients at 6 months. Pain relief was rated as good to excellent [79]. Other studies achieved similar results [74, 84, 91]. A recent review by Young et al. provides an overview of these results [96] (see Table 3.1).

Simultaneous neuromodulation of occipital and supraorbital [97] or occipital and auriculotemporal nerve [98] has been used for challenging cases of severe migraine. PNFS of occipital nerves alleviates headache by acting on the trigeminocervical nucleus complex in the brainstem. In a multicenter retrospective study of 31 patients with various type of headache, 56 % had no headache after 1 year of peripheral neuromodulation, and 47 % stopped taking medication [99]. These results indicate that this treatment might have beneficial effects on the overall quality of life in

Table 3.1 Occipital nerve stimulation for headache syndromes

Study	Indication	Responders	Effect
Melvin et al. (2007) [83]	Occipital headache (n = 11)	11/11	67 %
Popeney et al. (2003) [84]	Migraine (n = 25)	20/25	88.7 % improvement MIDAS
Oh et al. (2004) [79]	Occipital neuralgia (n = 20)	18/20	90 %
Weiner et al. (1999) [5]	Occipital neuralgia (n = 13)	13/13	100 % good to perfect
Matharu et al.(2004) [74]	Migraine (n = 8)	8/8	100 % good to perfect
Kapural et al. (2005) [80]	Cervicogenic headache (n = 6)	6/6	70 %
Rodrigo-Royo et al. (2005) [82]	Occipital neuralgia (n = 4)	4/4	100 %
Slavin et al. (2006) [77]	Occipital neuralgia (n = 10)	10/10	>50 %
Magis et al. (2007) [85]	Cluster headache (n = 8)	7/8	50 %
Schwedt et al. (2007) [86]	Cluster headache (n = 3)	15/19	52 %
	Hemicrania (n = 6)		
	Migraine (n = 8)		
	Post-trauma (n = 2)		
Burns et al. (2007) [87]	Cluster headache (n = 8)	6/8	64 %
Picaza et al. (1977) [17]	Occipital neuralgia (n = 6)	3/6	100 % good to perfect
Schwedt et al. (2006) [88]	Hemicrania Continua (n = 2)	1/2	70 %
Ghaemi et al. (2008) [89]	Post cervical fusion pain (n = 1)	1/1	90 %
Amin et al. (2008) [90]	Supraorbital neuralgia (n = 10)	10/10	77 %
Brewer et al. (2012) [91]	Migraine (n = 12), Cluster headache (n = 5), Miscellaneous headaches (n = 8)	5/10, 4/5, 5/8	18 % decrease of headache, 27 % decrease in severity and 50 % decrease in MIDAS
Silberstein et al. (2012) [92]	Chronic Migraine (n = 105)	NA	22.5 % decrease in headache days, 64.6 % decrease in MIDAS scores, 14.1 % improvement in VAS of pain severity
Saper et al. (2011) [93]	Chronic migraine (n = 110)	43/110	>50 % decrease in headache days or/plus 3 or more points decrease in VAS
Burns et al. (2009) [94]	Cluster headache (n = 14)	10/14	52 %

chronic migraine patients and that the onset of beneficial effects can be expected after a period of 3 months of stimulation.

Headaches: Cluster Headache

Recently, a group from Belgium presented results of long-term follow-up (mean 36.82 months) of 15 chronic cluster headache patients, who were resistant to drug treatment, implanted with occipital stimulators [100]. This approach resulted in sustained disability reduction. Results indicated that 60 % became pain-free for prolonged periods [100]. PNS of occipital nerves in patients with cluster headache appears to stimulate metabolic normalization in the pain neuro-matrix, seen on PET scan [101]. Frequency, duration and severity of the cluster attacks were reduced in 90 % of the patients with refractory chronic cluster headache in a different series of ten patients [102]. Refractory cases of cluster headache may require trigeminal peripheral neuromodulation in addition to occipital PNS [97].

Burns et al. published their results on eight patients, with a 26 months follow-up period with an improvement in severity and frequency in six out of eight patients in the Lancet [87, 103]. Magis et al. describe similar results and a difference in the nociceptive blink reflex after stimulation [85, 104]. These studies teach us that the clinical beneficial effect starts after weeks, as well as the wash-out of the beneficial effects of stimulation after switching of the stimulator.

Fibromyalgia

Fibromyalgia is a disease which consists of chronic pain in all four limbs of the body, without any abnormalities on clinical, physical, and technical examinations. The syndrome is accompanied by other symptoms like fatigue, sleeping disorders, irritable bowel syndrome, and headaches [105, 106]. It has a prevalence of up to 4 % and the socioeconomic burden is high. Berger et al. report a mean total healthcare cost of $ 9,573 per patient per year in the USA [107, 108].

Thimineur and De Ridder published results on a group of 12 patients suffering from chronic migraine and fibromyalgia, treated with PNFS of the occipital branch of the C2 nerve. They implanted percutaneous cylindrical leads at a horizontal line underneath the occipital protuberance. Patients reported a reduction in the visual analogue scale for bodily pain of approximately 60 %. Besides these findings the authors report a decrease in fatigue and depressive mood as well as an increase in life quality [109]. Plazier et al. describe their results in a group of 11 patients, implanted with a cylindrical lead at the occipital nerve area. A double-blinded placebo controlled crossover design was applied for 10 weeks. A significant decrease in pain could be reported between the active stimulation scores and the sham stimulation (approximately 40 %). At 6 months these results remained stable. Besides the decrease in visual analogue scale a significant decrease in pain catastrophizing behavior could be found [110].

Pain catastrophizing behavior defines the emotional aspects of the total pain experience. As these scores get higher, patients get more distressed, worried, and occupied by their pain. Negative correlations between pain catastrophizing and life quality have been described [111, 112]. This might suggest that the overall beneficial effects of this form of stimulation on fibromyalgia might partially be caused by decreasing pain catastrophizing behavior.

The various functional imaging as well as source localized EEG studies (Plazier et al., unpublished data) reveal activity changes in various brain regions involved in catastrophizing behavior [73, 74, 101, 113–116].

In an ongoing sponsored trial the effects of this form of stimulation on the symptoms of fibromyalgia are being evaluated. Ad interim analysis reveals similar findings to the previously mentioned studies (Plazier et al., unpublished data).

Peripheral Pain

A case report shows that C2 PNFS might be capable of suppressing neuropathic pain in the setting of failed back surgery syndrome (FBSS) [117]. In summary, a subcutaneous C2 electrode was inserted under local anesthesia, and attached to an external pulse generator in a patient with FBSS. Classical tonic stimulation, consisting of 40 Hz stimulation, a placebo and a burst stimulation, consisting of 40 Hz burst mode, with five spikes delivered at 500 Hz at 1,000 μsec pulse width and 1,000 μsec interspike interval were tested. All stimulations were performed subthreshold for paresthesias. Burst mode was superior to placebo and tonic mode, and she received a fully implanted C2 electrode connected to an IPG via an extension wire. The burst design was capable of both suppressing the least and worst pain effectively, and she has remained almost pain-free for over 3 years.

Its mechanism is unclear but has been suggested to be related to similar mechanisms involved in fibromyalgia related pain suppression by ONS.

C1–C3 cells represent 45 % of all spinothalamic neurons and relay information from all levels of the cord to periaqueductal grey and/or thalamus [118] via a calbindin positive pathway [119]. C1–C3 spinothalamic tract neurons process sensory information from widespread regions of the body [120]. Upper spinal cord stimulation at C1–C3 modifies firing rate of >90 % of lumbosacral spinothalamic cells [121], and may therefore modulate transmission of noxious stimuli from lumbosacral origin, analogous to what has been proposed for the modulation of widespread bodily pain in fibromyalgia [67, 109].

Tinnitus

C2 nerve stimulation has been performed for suppressing tinnitus, using both TENS [122] and implanted electrodes [123]. The concept is based on well described somatosensory–auditory interactions [124]. Several studies have demonstrated the interactions between the somatosensory and auditory system, either at the dorsal cochlear nucleus (DCN) or at the inferior colliculus [125]. The aim of somatosensory stimulations is to decrease dorsal cochlear nucleus activity, as increased DCN activity has been implicated in tinnitus [126, 127]. The DCN receives auditory input from the cochlear nerve and somatosensory input, directly from the ipsilateral dorsal column and spinal trigeminal nuclei [128–130] or indirectly via the dorsal raphe and locus coeruleus [131]. The pinna and the neck are innervated by the upper cervical nerves (C1–C3), which project to spinal trigeminal nuclei [132–134]. C2 electrical stimulation produces a pattern of inhibition and excitation, of the principal cells [135] in the ventral and dorsal division of the cochlear nucleus [136–138], and can hereby suppress or enhance responses to sound [136, 137]. Not only C2 electrical stimulation can modulate the DCN. Electrical stimulation in the cat spinal trigeminal nuclei also yields strong inhibition and weak excitation of DCN principal cells [138, 139]. Thus both C2 and trigeminal stimulation can be proposed as treatments for tinnitus. For C2 electrical stimulation, noninvasive electrical stimulations using TENS have shown that it is possible to change the tinnitus percept [140, 141]. In a large study of 240 patients, only 17.9 % ($N = 43$) of the patients with tinnitus responded to C2 TENS. They had an improvement of 42.92 %, and only 6 of 240 patients had a reduction of 100 %. The first uncontrolled data do also show that similar results can be obtained by implanting wire electrodes subcutaneously in the C2 dermatome, as can implants on the spinal cord at the C2 level [123]. It can be expected that only very few people will respond to implants of the C2 or trigeminal dermatome, analogous to the amount of responders to TENS. A recent fMRI study demonstrated that subthreshold and suprathreshold stimulations are possible and evoke similar BOLD activation patterns in the brain [73], suggesting that placebo-controlled studies are feasible.

Device Choice

Traditionally, equipment used in PNS was originally designed for SCS. There was a wrap-around design of initial custom made electrode leads used in PNS for phrenic and vagal nerve stimulation for the treatment of diaphragmatic palsy, epilepsy, and depression. Subsequent introduction of the "multi-button" electrode design for PNS never went into mass production. These were designed to specifically stimulate separate fascicles of a large mixed nerve, such as sciatic, but for variety of reasons, the standard paddle electrodes already available for SCS applications became the preferred PNS delivery device. To overcome formation of scar tissue between the nerve and the electrode, paddles were then modified by attaching an integrated Dacron mesh, which could be wrapped around the nerve [142]. However, the open surgical approach with nerve exploration required for implantation of these electrodes meant this technique was mostly abandoned with the advent of percutaneous PNS techniques.

Although percutaneous placement now dominates the field of PNS, some neuromodulators still use paddle leads for PNS because of several important benefits of paddle leads. First, modern paddles have several rows of electrode contacts (between 1 and 5 rows), separated by a preset distance. This facilitates multiple stimulation paradigms in the longitudinal, transverse and oblique directions, with electrode contact configuration that matches the course of sensory fibers inside the nerve trunk. Second, the paddle structure ensures unidirectional stimulation, whereby electrical energy gets directed toward the nerve, while the surrounding tissue gets shielded by the insulation of the paddle's backing. Thereby, paddle leads consume less energy to produce the desired effect and may be associated with longer implantable pulse generator (IPG) battery life. Third, the use of paddle electrodes in PNS, similarly to SCS experience, is associated with a lower migration rate.

The invasiveness of paddle insertion and need for highly refined surgical skills to expose peripheral nerves were among the reasons for the lack of widespread acceptance of paddle-based PNS. Additionally, there have been multiple reports of perineural fibrosis following long-term PNS with paddle leads, which has raised concern about their safety and appropriateness, even though this phenomenon occurred in a very small percentage of patients. Nevertheless, percutaneous lead insertion for PNS/PNFS application has become so widespread that, by some estimates, this application accounts for between 25 and 50 % of the devices implanted in the USA in 2011.

Currently, percutaneous electrode leads are generally chosen when the nerve of interest is located in a predictable area, when stimulation may be delivered without direct contact with the nerve, and whenever the painful area may require coverage with one or more leads, whereby stimulating paresthesias are concordant with the pain distribution. Additionally, insertion of percutaneous PNS leads may be facilitated by the use of ultrasound guidance, which helps in localizing the nerve pathway and depth while avoiding adjacent vascular structures.

The choice of power source for PNS is usually determined by stimulation energy requirement. In the past (and even now in the USA), the only approved devices for PNS applications were radiofrequency (RF)-coupled systems. In such systems, the power source is external and delivers energy by means of a RF link between a transmitting antenna and an implanted receiver, which is connected to the electrode-leads either directly or via extensions. Once popular, these RF-coupled systems are rarely, if ever used today.

Initial IPGs were powered by a prime cell battery, which meant that the entire device had to be replaced when the battery became depleted. Such depletion could occur within a year after implantation, if high power settings were used in stimulation, or if stimulation was used continuously. The need for frequent IPG replacement was eliminated by the introduction of rechargeable technology. Today, rechargeable IPG devices dominate the neuromodulation marketplace. However, in some parts of the world, this technology is not available due to a lack of regulatory approval or the high cost of rechargeable IPGs. In PNS applications, use of rechargeable technology makes great sense since the low profile and smaller size of rechargeable IPG leads to less discomfort and better cosmoses for this patient population.

Of interest, several old PNS designs, including wrap-around electrode leads and RF-coupled power sources have been reincarnated with modern PNS applications. Two new companies have put their main focus on PNS-oriented devices. One company uses specially designed coil-like electrode leads, which are designed to be wrapped around peripheral nerves while delivering high-frequency electrical stimulation to eliminate pain of amputation neuroma [59]. Another company developed an RF-coupled implantable system whereby the electrode lead itself serves as an antenna linked to an external miniature power source, which is taped to the skin above it [24].

Procedural Details

Techniques used for PNS implantation depend on both the stimulation target and the choice of hardware. For direct stimulation of a specific peripheral nerve, the electrode lead may be implanted through open exploration of the nerve segment or by percutaneous placement in the vicinity of the nerve. In both scenarios, anatomical knowledge of the nerve course is important.

For percutaneous placement, electrode insertion may be facilitated by fluoroscopy (to define known skeletal landmarks) or ultrasound (to directly visualize the nerve and adjacent vascular bundle). Identification of the surgically accessible segment of the nerve, where branching is minimal, is important. Additionally, it is critical to plan electrode lead position, entry, and tunneling path in advance, to avoid major joints, since repetitive movement of the lead or extension cable may result in material fatigue or fracture. Furthermore, constant manipulation of metal wires and external plastic insulation may damage the equipment. Surgical experience is essential for implanting paddle electrodes for PNS, as is a great familiarity with intraoperative ultrasound, for PNS targeting.

Conversely, detailed knowledge of peripheral nerve anatomy is not as essential for PNFS applications. Here, the electrode leads are implanted either in the middle of the painful area, or on its edges. Traditionally, it was thought that one cylindrical electrode could cover an area the size of a business card (or a credit card) if the electrode was placed medially. Any larger treatment area, within a 10–12 cm limit, should be treated with two leads placed on the periphery of the painful region. More recently, this initial placement paradigm has evolved subsequent to the introduction of the "cross talk" approach, which postulates that very large areas can be covered with separate electrode leads placed far from each other [50]. This approach has been validated with theoretical modeling and in small clinical series, but thus far has not received widespread acceptance.

For both PNS and PNFS applications, the ideal depth of the electrode is just above the deep subcutaneous fascia. Placing leads in the epifascial plane has limited the development of muscle spasms, which would occur when the electrode was placed too deep. Additionally, this has limited the risk of lead erosion, which would occur if the lead were placed too superficially.

Depth of electrode placement is important in selection of an appropriate anchoring device. Some commercially available anchors have a high profile, which may lead to discomfort or visible deformation of the skin, and in turn, may lead to erosion over time. Anchoring electrode lead(s) in place is an important step in device implantation given the high mobility of soft tissues in PNS/PNFS applications. Improper anchoring may result in even higher migration rate than seen in SCS, where leads are relatively immobile in the epidural space or in DBS, where leads are skull mounted.

Whichever anchor or anchoring technique is used, it is generally recommended to use non-absorbable sutures and to fix the lead to a hard tissue, such as thick deep fascia. Additionally, it is recommended to use "strain relief" loops, which are intended to minimize lead displacement during the patient's body movement. These loops should be placed, if possible, next to the anchor (between the anchor and the generator) and next to the IPG, minimizing the chance of electrode migration and/or fracture.

The location and depth of IPG implantation should also be preplanned. Position of the IPG in PNS cases is usually dependent on the location of pain and electrode leads. Placing the IPG over bony prominences (edge of the rib cage, iliac crest, scapula, etc.), or too close to the midline, should be avoided to prevent patient discomfort. Placing the IPG too deep in the soft tissues may interfere with the ability to recharge the device. Alternatively, placing the IPG too superficially, immediately under the dermis increases the risk of poor wound healing, device erosion, and implant site pain.

Occipital Nerve Stimulation Techniques

The implantation and trial and permanent implantation phase of occipital nerve stimulation does not, technically, differ from the above mentioned. The electrode(s) are normally located in an area just underneath the occipital protuberance. This is the region where the main branches of the greater occipital nerve can be found [68]. Both techniques with paddle leads and percutaneous leads have been published [143]. Weiner et al. published their technique with introduction of the lead with a Tuohy needle [5] The lead is positioned in the subcutaneous tissue in a horizontal line between the two pinnae of the ears. If the lead is placed to low or to deep, it might stimulate the cervical muscle tissue. This will cause undesirable effects [144].

The lead can be anchored to the muscle fascia, or periosteum tissue, or be tunneled in a steep angle to prevent lead migration. Trial can be performed by connecting the lead to an extension cable and externalize the contacts of this cable. After successful stimulation, the extension cable can be removed and a full system can be implanted with the IPG at the desired site of the body. In some indications where the onset of effects might take long periods, like chronic migraine, the IPG can be implanted directly.

PNS Complications

Complications of all neuromodulation techniques are generally divided into ten main groups [145]. Some occur primarily with intrathecal pumps and other means of chemical neuromodulation; some others are specific to the central nervous system and apply to the electrical stimulation of spinal and cerebral structures. Several categories, however, are applicable to PNS including infection, hemorrhage, injury to nervous tissue, placement of device in the wrong compartment, hardware migration, erosion, and device malfunction, which includes lead fracture and disconnection.

Through advancement in technology, many initial PNS complications are rarely seen today, while others remain essentially unchanged.

In the early stages of PNS practice, electrodes were custom-made. Some wrap-around electrodes had Silastic backing [146] with platinum wires facing the nerve being stimulated. In some circumstances, this backing accumulated a significant amount of fluid, which subsequently affected electrical impedance, leading to loss of electrical conductivity [146]. Later, as cuff electrodes were designed to be more biocompatible, the principal complication was nerve injury secondary to development of fibrosis and possible ischemia, which was caused by electrodes strangling the nerve within the soft tissues. Reporting of multiple incidents of this complication significantly contributed to abandonment of this device [18, 33, 147]. Furthermore, despite meticulous dissection and secure anchoring, some cuff electrodes became displaced, necessitating electrode revision.

The migration incidence increased with introduction of the percutaneous PNS technique, whereby tissue friction is minimal and the only thing that holds the electrode in place is the anchor and the so-called "strain relief loop," which is commonly placed next to the anchoring site. Most surgeons who have revised percutaneous PNS electrode would agree that these electrodes easily migrate, and the tissue reaction around them is minimal. Migration is unlikely to happen in lateral (relative to the electrode axis) electrode placement. Most commonly, migration occurs secondary to the electrode pulling out from its original lead position. Sometimes, if the anchor is completely incompetent, or if the patient presents with hypermobility over the electrode path, migration can be dramatic. In addition to this "pull-out" phenomenon, the electrode lead may also migrate "in", shifting more distally along the electrode path. If migration is suspected, simple plain films compared to original images at time of electrode placement can help to differentiate. Thereby, it is important to obtain and save radiographic images of initial electrode lead position at time of original implantation. Incidence of migrations is variable, and ranges from 0 to 100 % depending on series [143, 148, 149]. Revision of malpositioned or migrated electrodes, which are still functioning, is relatively easy. A simple technique allows for repositioning without reopening the generator pocket [150, 151]. However, it is important to have the generator pocket prepped and ready for exploration should the electrode lead turn out to be damaged or otherwise unsuitable for reinsertion.

Electrode leads may break at any time after implantation. Breakage (fracture) is usually secondary to kinking in the electrode's lead insulation. The lead insulation of internal wires may break due to repetitive movement that involves repetitive stretch or compression of the device, resulting in material fatigue and eventual failure. This issue should be considered when choosing the path of electrode lead placement and generator location. Crossing large joints and tunneling greater distances is associated with higher rate of fractures and migrations.

Both infection and hemorrhage have occurred with PNS devices, but incidence is rare. Since most devices are placed in superficial locations, hemostasis is generally obtainable and hematoma formation is rarely symptomatic. Infection, on the other hand, may occur soon or late post-implantation. Surgical infection may result from poor surgical technique or insufficient dissection of anchors and connectors, resulting in excessive tissue tension, which prevents wound healing. In our series of 40 patients with PNS implants that were followed for longer than 30 months, there were two infections [23]; in each case, the device had to be removed. Infection was managed with systemic antibiotics specific to antibiotic sensitivities, once established. PNS systems may be reimplanted several months after infection is eradicated, as long as the cause of infection is understood and addressed.

Placement of the PNS device in the wrong compartment is a theoretical concern, since most PNS electrodes are inserted in a subcutaneous epifascial plane. However, since the proximity of electrode lead to the nerve being stimulated is extremely important in obtaining adequate paresthesias and maintaining stimulation parameters within reasonable range, various techniques have been suggested to improve the placement accuracy. Most PNS implanters rely on use of fluoroscopy for localization [152], but now multiple reports suggest ease of use of intraoperative ultrasound for localization of the nerve trunk and the surrounding structures [6, 153, 154]. Insertion of electrodes too deep into soft tissues can cause unpleasant muscle spasms during stimulation [144]; insertion too superficially may result in lead tip erosion [155].

Overall, most PNS complications are minor and rarely, if ever, require hospitalization. Recently, we analyzed our institutional experience with PNS. Among nearly 100 PNS cases since April 2000, we identified 40 patients who underwent original PNS trial at our institution, who were then followed up for 30 months or longer [23]. The remaining patients had either shorter follow-up, or had their initial surgery at another institution. Out of 40 patients, 8 did not sufficiently improve during the trial and 32 proceeded with permanent implantation. In a long-term follow-up series, 27/32 patients underwent subsequent operations (including 12 battery replacements) but only 1/32 had an infection requiring hospital admission. Out of 15 reoperations, there were 6 revisions (1 for electrode erosion 4 weeks after implantation, 4 for electrode migration at 1, 3, 5, and 9 months after original implantation, 1 for device disconnection), and 9 device removals (2 from infections at 1 and 49 months, due to a loss of effectiveness at 9, 10, and 25 months, and 4 due to improvement of symptoms at 13, 17, 21, and 56 months after original implantation) [23]. This experience illustrates the well-known observation about the high rate of complications but relatively minor morbidity associated with PNS [143, 149].

Outcomes

The long-term outcome of more recently introduced PNFS is still unknown. The large series from Australia and Europe, some of which were used for getting regulatory approval on these continents, discussed outcomes of 3 months in a heterogeneous cohort of 111 patients (the Austrian multicenter study [56]) and 7 months in 13 patients (the Australian experience [156]). All published studies documented consistently observed more than 50 % reduction in pain level in every group of PNS/PNFS patients.

In traditional PNS cases, much longer follow-up has been summarized in multiple publications. An average follow-up of more than 10 years in a combined German–Israeli experience of Dr. Waisbrod showed that among 46 implanted PNS patients, good results were observed in 22/30 (73 %) of lower extremity implants and in 10/12 (83 %) of upper extremity implants [157]. The patients with postsurgical nerve injury and entrapment neuropathy exhibited significant improvement in >80 % of cases, while those with pain after traumatic injections had 50 % success rate, and those with pain after nerve graft—0 %. Even longer follow-up (more than 20 years) was reported in the Belgian study of Drs. Van Calenbergh and Gybels where patients implanted in the 1980s continued to enjoy >50 % improvement in pain intensity when using their PNS devices [158].

Conclusions

The peripheral neuromodulation approach includes the following three modalities: (1) PNS, which requires implantation of stimulating electrode leads over the affected peripheral nerves; (2) percutaneous PNS, which involves insertion of stimulating electrode leads in the vicinity of the nerve with proper guidance; (3) PNFS that stimulates smaller nerves and nerve endings in the region of pain. Peripheral neuromodulation is an effective way to control chronic, disabling, neuropathic pain of various etiologies, which is refractory to medical treatment. Peripheral neuromodulation is expected to be more widely accepted (and properly covered by regulatory agencies and payers) once there is more prospective data showing long-term clinical efficacy and cost-effectiveness.

Although commonly used in clinical practice, peripheral nerve stimulation (PNS) for treatment of chronic neuropathic pain is mostly performed using devices developed and marketed for spinal cord stimulation applications. This may be one reason why PNS is marked by a relatively high complication rate, since the anatomy of peripheral nerves and surrounding soft tissues is quite different from the epidural spinal space, for which the current devices are designed. Based on literature data and analysis of the authors' experience with PNS, despite the high rate of complications, morbidity associated with the PNS approach is low, and most problems may be resolved with simple revision surgeries performed on an outpatient basis. Reduction in the complication rate is expected to occur when the hardware used in PNS procedures is appropriately adapted and designed for PNS applications. Introduction of dedicated PNS/PNFS devices will not only reduce complication rates, but will also likely improve reliability and sustainability of optimal outcomes. Based on the authors' observations and expectations, the next decade will bring both technical advances and clinical experience in the PNS/PNFS arena.

References

1. Abejon D, Perez-Cajaraville J. Peripheral nerve stimulation: definition. Prog Neurol Surg. 2011;24:203–9.
2. White JC, Sweet WH. Pain and the neurosurgeon. A forty-year experience. Springfield, IL: Thomas; 1969. p. 894–9.
3. Melzack RA, Wall PD. Pain mechanisms: a new theory. Science. 1965;150:971–9.
4. Slavin KV. History of peripheral nerve stimulation. Prog Neurol Surg. 2011;24:1–15.
5. Weiner RL, Reed KL. Peripheral neurostimulation for control of intractable occipital neuralgia. Neuromodulation. 1999;2:217–21.
6. Huntoon MA, Burgher AH. Ultrasound-guided permanent implantation of peripheral nerve stimulation (PNS) system for neuropathic pain of the extremities: original cases and outcomes. Pain Med. 2009;10:1369–77.
7. Johnson MI, Bjordal JM. Transcutaneous electrical nerve stimulation for the management of painful conditions: focus on neuropathic pain. Expert Rev Neurother. 2011;11:735–53.
8. Hurlow A, Bennett MI, Robb KA, Johnson MI, Simpson KH, Oxberry SG. Transcutaneous electric nerve stimulation (TENS) for cancer pain in adults. Cochrane Database Syst Rev. 2012;3: CD006276. doi:10.1002/14651858.CD006276.pub3.
9. Francis RP, Johnson MI. The characteristics of acupuncture-like transcutaneous electrical nerve stimulation (acupuncture-like TENS): a literature review. Acupunct Electrother Res. 2011;36:231–58.
10. Levin PJ, Wu JM, Kawasaki A, Weidner AC, Amundsen CL. The efficacy of posterior tibial nerve stimulation for the treatment of overactive bladder in women: a systematic review. Int Urogynecol J. 2012;23:1591–7.
11. Findlay JM, Maxwell-Armstrong C. Posterior tibial nerve stimulation and faecal incontinence: a review. Int J Colorectal Dis. 2011;26:265–73.
12. Schulz-Stubner S, Kehl F. Treatment of persistent hiccups with transcutaneous phrenic and vagal nerve stimulation. Intensive Care Med. 2011;37:1048–9.
13. Stefan H, et al. Transcutaneous vagus nerve stimulation (t-VNS) in pharmacoresistant epilepsies: a proof of concept trial. Epilepsia. 2012;53(7):e115–8.

14. Pop J, Murray D, Markovic D, DeGiorgio CM. Acute and long term safety of external trigeminal nerve stimulation for drug resistant epilepsy. Epilepsy Behav. 2011;22:574–6.
15. Schrader LM, Cool IA, Miller PR, Maremont ER, DeGiorgio CM. Trigeminal nerve stimulation in major depressive disorder: first proof of concept in an open pilot trial. Epilepsy Behav. 2011;22:475–8.
16. Singla S, Prabhakar V, Singla RK. Role of transcutaneous electrical nerve stimulation in the management of trigeminal neuralgia. J Neurosci Rural Pract. 2011;2:150–2.
17. Picaza JA, Hunter SE, Cannon BW. Pain suppression by peripheral nerve stimulation: chronic effects of implanted devices. Appl Neurophysiol. 1977–1978;40:223–34.
18. Kirsch WM, Lewis JA, Simon RH. Experiences with electrical stimulation devices for the control of chronic pain. Med Instrum. 1975;9:217–20.
19. Bhaskar A, White A, Patel K. Percutaneous electrical stimulation (PENS) therapy for management of focal neuropathic pain: a case series of 42 cancer patients. Neuromodulation. 2011;14:558. (abstract of the 10th INS conference)
20. Bhaskar A, Patel K, White A. Trigeminal field stimulation using percutaneous electrical nerve stimulation (PENS) therapy – preliminary case series of 8 patients. Neuromodulation. 2011;14:558. (abstract of the 10th INS conference)
21. Wall PD, Sweet WH. Temporary abolition of pain in man. Science. 1967;155:108–9.
22. U.S. Food and Drug Administration: Code of Federal Regulations. Title 21, Volume 8, 21CFR882.5870. http://www.gpo.gov/fdsys/pkg/CFR-2011-title21-vol8/pdf/CFR-2011-title21-vol8-sec882-5870.pdf
23. Slavin KV. Technical aspects of peripheral nerve stimulation: hardware and complications. Prog Neurol Surg. 2011;24:189–202.
24. Deer TR, Levy RM, Rosenfeld EL. Prospective clinical study of a new implantable peripheral nerve stimulation device to treat chronic pain. Clin J Pain. 2010;26:359–72.
25. Kotagal P. Neurostimulation: vagus nerve stimulation and beyond. Semin Pediatr Neurol. 2011;18:186–94.
26. Daban C, Martinez-Aran A, Cruz N, Vieta E. Safety and efficacy of vagus nerve stimulation in treatment-resistant depression. A systematic review. J Affect Disord. 2008;110:1–15.
27. DiMarco AF. Phrenic nerve stimulation in patients with spinal cord injury. Respir Physiol Neurobiol. 2009;169:200–9.
28. Oliven A. Treating obstructive sleep apnea with hypoglossal nerve stimulation. Current Opin Pulm Med. 2011;17:419–24.
29. Van Swigchem R, Weerdesteyn V, van Duijnhoven HJ, den Boer J, Beems T, Geurts AC. Near-normal gait pattern with peroneal electrical stimulation as a neuroprosthesis in the chronic phase of stroke: a case report. Arch Phys Med Rehabil. 2011;92:320–4.
30. Norderval S, Rydningen M, Lindsetmo RO, Lein D, Vonen B. Sacral nerve stimulation. Tidsskr Nor Laegefore. 2011;131:1190–3.
31. Levy RM. Differentiating the leaves from the branches in the tree of neuromodulation: the state of peripheral nerve field stimulation. Neuromodulation. 2011;14:201–5.
32. Hassenbusch SJ, Stanton-Hicks M, Schoppa D, Walsh JG, Covington EC. Long-term results of peripheral nerve stimulation for reflex sympathetic dystrophy. J Neurosurg. 1996;84:415–23.
33. Nashold Jr BS, Goldner JL, Mullen JB, Bright DS. Long-term pain control by direct peripheral-nerve stimulation. J Bone Joint Surg Am. 1982;64:1–10.
34. Kent M, Upp J, Spevak C, Shanon C, Buckenmaier C. Ultrasound-guided peripheral nerve stimulator placement in two soldiers with acute battlefield neuropathic pain. Anesth Analg. 2012;114:875–8.
35. Bouche B, Eisenberg E, Meigner M, Durand S, Papaniaou M, Suarez A, Verlysen M, Lemarie J. Facilitation of diagnostic and percutaneous trial lead placement with ultrasound guidance for peripheral subcutaneous field stimulation on infrapatellar branches of saphenous nerve. Neuromodulation. 2011;14:564.
36. Mobbs RJ, Nair S, Blum P. Peripheral nerve stimulation for the treatment of chronic pain. J Clin Neurosci. 2007;14:216–21.
37. Reverberi C, Dario A. The treatment of trigeminal neuralgia and atypical facial pain with peripheral nerve field stimulation (PNFS): a clinical case report. Neuromodulation. 2011;14:552.
38. Yakovlev A, Karasev SA, Resch BE, Yakovleva V, Strutsenko A. Treatment of atypical facial pain using peripheral nerve stimulation. Neuromodulation. 2011;14:553.
39. Deogaonkar M. Peripheral nerve/field stimulation for post-intervention trigeminal neuropathic pain. Neuromodulation. 2011;14:555.
40. Stidd DA, Wuollet A, Bowden K, Price T, Patwardhan A, Barker S, Weinand ME, Annabi J, Annabi E. Peripheral nerve stimulation for trigeminal neuropathic pain. Pain Physician. 2012;15:27–33.
41. De Carolis G, Paroli M, Psy Ciaramela A, Tollapi L, Paolo P. A case of successful treatment of post herpetic neuralgia using subcutaneous targeted neuromodulation. Neuromodulation. 2011;14:555.
42. Desai M, Sayal P, Leiphart J. Immediate outcomes of peripheral field nerve stimulation trials for thoracic neuropathic pain: a case series. Neuromodulation. 2011;14:559.
43. Bouche B, Eisenberg E, Meigner M, Durand S, Papaniaou M, Suarez A, Verlysen M, Dixneuf V, Lemarie J. Facilitation of diagnostic and percutaneous trial lead placement with ultrasound guidance for peripheral nerve stimulation on ilioinguinal neuralgia. Neuromodulation. 2011;14:563.
44. Bouche B, Eisenberg E, Meigner M, Durand S, Papaniaou M, Suarez A, Verlysen M, Lemarie J. Facilitation of diagnostic and percutaneous trial lead placement with ultrasound guidance for peripheral nerve stimulation on lateral cutaneous nerve. Neuromodulation. 2011;14:565.
45. Yakovlev AE, Resch BE, Yakovleva VE. Peripheral nerve field stimulation in the treatment of postlaminectomy syndrome after multilevel spinal surgeries. Neuromodulation. 2011;14:534–8.
46. Courtney P. Superior and middle cluneal nerves: an important target for stimulation in the treatment of failed back surgery syndrome (FBSS). Neuromodulation. 2011;14:552.
47. Djian MC, Page P, Viala A, Cherroun C, Roux FX. Successful back pain relief with peripheral nerve stimulation: case series of 3 patients. Neuromodulation. 2011;14:554.
48. Perruchoud C, Durrer A, Bovy M, Rutschmann B, Koeppel C, Kirchhofer E, Leberre J, Buchser E. Subcutaneous field stimulation for low-back pain: a 96-month follow-up. Neuromodulation. 2011;14:557.
49. Burgher A, Huntoon M, Turley TW, Doust MW, Stearns LJ. Subcutaneous peripheral nerve stimulation with inter-lead stimulation for axial neck and low back pain: case series and review of the literature. Neuromodulation. 2012;15:100–7.
50. Falco FJ, Berger J, Vrable A, Onyewu O, Zhu J. Cross talk: a new method for peripheral nerve stimulation. An observational report with cadaveric verification. Pain Physician. 2009;12:965–83.
51. Salmon J. Neuromodulation for refractory, truncal or diffuse neuropathic pain states. Clinical experience with subcutaneous (including C2 area) and combined subcutaneous and spinal cord stimulation treatment. Neuromodulation. 2011;14:550.
52. Reverberi C. The treatment of complex pain with combination of spinal cord stimulation (SCS) and peripheral nerve field stimulation (PNFS): our experience. Neuromodulation. 2011;14: 551.
53. Hamm-Faber TE, Aukes HA, de Loos F, Gultuna I. Subcutaneous stimulation as an additional therapy to spinal cord stimulation for the treatment of lower limb pain and/or back pain. Neuromodulation. 2011;14:553.
54. Cioni B, Tufo T, Conforti G, De Simone C, Meglio M. Combined spinal cord and peripheral subcutaneous filed stimulation. Neuromodulation. 2011;14:560.

55. Barolat G, Wolkowitz RM, Meyer J, McRoberts P, Lipov EG, Joshi J, Davis B, Cairns KD. A randomized controlled feasibility trial to evaluate peripheral nerve field stimulation (PNFS) using subcutaneous placement of neurostimulation leads in the management of localized chronic intractable pain of the back. Neuromodulation. 2011;14:562.
56. Sator-Katzenschlager S, Fiala K, Kress HG, Kofler A, Neuhold J, Kloimstein H, Ilias W, Mozes-Balla EM, Pinter M, Loining N, Fuchs W, Heinze G, Likar R. Subcutaneous target stimulation (STS) in chronic noncancer pain: a nationwide retrospective study. Pain Pract. 2010;10:279–86.
57. Verrills P, Vivian D, Mitchell B, Barnard A. Peripheral nerve field stimulation for chronic pain: 100 cases and review of the literature. Pain Med. 2011;12:1395–405.
58. Slavin KV, editor. Peripheral nerve stimulation. Basel: Karger; 2011.
59. Soin A, Kilgore K, Bhadra N, Fang ZP. Feasibility study on high-frequency electrical nerve block for amputation pain. Neuromodulation. 2011;14:561.
60. Strand NH, Trentman TL, Vargas BB, Dodick DW. Occipital nerve stimulation with the Bion microstimulator for the treatment of medically refractory chronic cluster headache. Pain Physician. 2011;14:435–40.
61. Chae J, Wilson RD, Bennet ME, Lechman TE, Stager KW. Single-lead percutaneous peripheral nerve stimulation for the treatment of hemiplegic shoulder pain: a case series. Pain Pract. 2013;13:59–67.
62. Goroszeniuk T, Khan R. Permanent percutaneous splanchnic nerve neuromodulation for management of pain due to chronic pancreatitis: a case report. Neuromodulation. 2011;14:253–7.
63. Atallah J, Davidov M, Davila V. Feasibility of placement of peripheral nerve stimulator in the splanchnic nerves for treatment of chronic abdominal pain, cadaveric study. Neuromodulation. 2011;14:556.
64. Hegarty D, Goroszeniuk T. Peripheral nerve stimulation of the thoracic paravertebral plexus for chronic neuropathic pain. Pain Physician. 2011;14:295–300.
65. Rosendal F, Moir L, de Pennington N, Green AL, Aziz TZ. Successful treatment of testicular pain with peripheral nerve stimulation of the cutaneous branch of the ilioinguinal and genital branch of the genitofemoral nerves. Neuromodulation. 2012;16:121–4.
66. Jenkins B, Tepper SJ. Neurostimulation for primary headache disorders: part 2, review of central neurostimulators for primary headache, overall therapeutic efficacy, safety, cost, patient selection, and future research in headache neuromodulation. Headache. 2011;51:1408–18.
67. Plazier M, et al. Peripheral nerve stimulation for fibromyalgia. Prog Neurol Surg. 2011;24:133–46.
68. Bovim G, et al. Topographic variations in the peripheral course of the greater occipital nerve. Autopsy study with clinical correlations. Spine. 1991;16(4):475–8.
69. Pfaller K, Arvidsson J. Central distribution of trigeminal and upper cervical primary afferents in the rat studied by anterograde transport of horseradish peroxidase conjugated to wheat germ agglutinin. J Comp Neurol. 1988;268(1):91–108.
70. Newman HM, Stevens RT, Apkarian AV. Direct spinal projections to limbic and striatal areas: anterograde transport studies from the upper cervical spinal cord and the cervical enlargement in squirrel monkey and rat. J Comp Neurol. 1996;365(4):640–58.
71. Edvinsson L. Tracing neural connections to pain pathways with relevance to primary headaches. Cephalalgia. 2011;31(6):737–47.
72. Keizer K, Kuypers HG. Distribution of corticospinal neurons with collaterals to the lower brain stem reticular formation in monkey (Macaca fascicularis). Exp Brain Res. 1989;74(2):311–8.
73. Kovacs S, et al. Central effects of occipital nerve electrical stimulation studied by functional magnetic resonance imaging. Neuromodulation. 2011;14(1):46–55. discussion 56-7.
74. Matharu MS, et al. Central neuromodulation in chronic migraine patients with suboccipital stimulators: a PET study. Brain. 2004;127(Pt 1):220–30.
75. Shin JH, Kim YC, Jang IK, Kim JH, Park SY, Lee SC. Occipital nerve stimulation in a patient with an intractable chronic headache - a case repot. Korean J Anesthesiol. 2011;60:298–301.
76. Skaribas I, Calvillo O, Delikanaki-Skaribas E. Occipital peripheral nerve stimulation in the management of chronic intractable occipital neuralgia in a patient with neurofibromatosis type 1: a case report. J Med Case Reports. 2011;5:174.
77. Slavin KV, Nersesyan H, Wess C. Peripheral neurostimulation for treatment of intractable occipital neuralgia. Neurosurgery. 2006;58(1):112–9. discussion 112-9.
78. Hammer M, Doleys DM. Perineuromal stimulation in the treatment of occipital neuralgia: a case study. Neuromodulation. 2001;4(2):47–51.
79. Oh MY, et al. Peripheral nerve stimulation for the treatment of occipital neuralgia and transformed migraine using a C1-2-3 subcutaneous paddle style electrode: a technical report. Neuromodulation. 2004;7(2):103–12.
80. Kapural L, et al. Occipital nerve electrical stimulation via the midline approach and subcutaneous surgical leads for treatment of severe occipital neuralgia: a pilot study. Anesth Analg. 2005;101(1):171–4.
81. Johnstone CS, Sundaraj R. Occipital nerve stimulation for the treatment of occipital neuralgia-eight case studies. Neuromodulation. 2006;9(1):41–7.
82. Rodrigo-Royo MD, et al. Peripheral neurostimulation in the management of cervicogenic headache: four case reports. Neuromodulation. 2005;8(4):241–8.
83. Melvin Jr EA, Jordan FR, Weiner RL, Primm D. Using peripheral stimulation to reduce the pain of C2-mediated occipital headaches: a preliminary report. Pain Physician. 2007;10:453–60.
84. Popeney CA, Alo KM. Peripheral neurostimulation for the treatment of chronic, disabling, transformed migraine. Headache. 2003;43:369–75.
85. Magis D, et al. Occipital nerve stimulation for drug-resistant chronic cluster headache: a prospective pilot study. Lancet Neurol. 2007;6(4):314–21.
86. Schwedt TJ, Dodick DW, Hentz J, Trentman TL, Zimmerman RS. Occipital nerve stimulation for chronic headache: long-term safety and efficacy. Cephalalgia. 2007;27:153–7.
87. Burns B, Watkins L, Goadsby PJ. Treatment of medically intractable cluster headache by occipital nerve stimulation: long-term follow-up of eight patients. Lancet. 2007;369(9567):1099–106.
88. Schwedt TJ, Dodick DW, Trentman TL, Zimmerman RS. Occipital nerve stimulation for chronic cluster headache and hemicrania continua: pain relief and persistence of autonomic features. Cephalalgia. 2006;26:1025–7.
89. Ghaemi K, Capelle HH, Kinfe TM, Krauss JK. Occipital nerve stimulation for refractory occipital pain after occipitocervical fusion: expanding indications. Stereotact Funct Neurosurg. 2008;86:391–3.
90. Amin S, Buvanendran A, Park KS, Kroin JS, Moric M. Peripheral nerve stimulator for the treatment of supraorbital neuralgia: a retrospective case series. Cephalalgia. 2008;28:355–9.
91. Brewer AC, et al. Long-term outcome in occipital nerve stimulation patients with medically intractable primary headache disorders. Neuromodulation. 2012;16:557.
92. Silberstein SD, Dodick DW, Saper J, Huh B, Slavin KV, Sharan A, Reed K, Narouze S, Mogilner A, Goldstein J, Trentman T, Vaisma J, Ordia J, Weber P, Deer T, Levy R, Diaz RL, Washburn SN, Mekhail N. Safety and efficacy

of peripheral nerve stimulation of the occipital nerves for the management of chronic migraine: results from a randomized, multicenter, double-blinded, controlled study. Cephalalgia. 2012;32:1165–79.
93. Saper JR, Dodick DW, Silberstein SD, McCarville S, Sun M, Goadsby PJ. ONSTIM Investigators: occipital nerve stimulation for the treatment of intractable chronic migraine headache: ONSTIM feasibility study. Cephalalgia. 2011;31:271–85.
94. Burns B, Watkins L, Goadsby PJ. Treatment of intractable chronic cluster headache by occipital nerve stimulation in 14 patients. Neurology. 2009;72:341–5.
95. Lipton RB, Goadsby PJ, Cady RK, Aurora SK, Grosberg BM, Freitag FG, Silbersteon SD, Whiten DM, Jaax KN. PRISM study: occipital nerve stimulation for treatment-refractory migraine. Cephalalgia. 2009;29 Suppl 1:30.
96. Young WB, Silberstein SD. Occipital nerve stimulation for primary headaches. J Neurosurg Sci. 2012;56(4):307–12.
97. Royster EI, Crumbley K. Initial experience with implanted peripheral nerve stimulation for the treatment of refractory cephalgia. Ochsner J. 2011;11:147–50.
98. Deshpande KK, Wininger KL. Feasibility of combined epicranial temporal and occipital neurostimulation: treatment of a challenging case of headache. Pain Physician. 2011;14:37–44.
99. Abejon D, Calvo R, Arranz J, Perez-Cajaraville J, del Saz J, Aguierre-Jaime A. Peripheral nerve stimulation in the treatment of various types of headache. Rev Esp Anesthesiol Reanim. 2011;58:589–94.
100. Magis D, Gerardy PY, Remacle JM, Schoenen J. Sustained effectiveness of occipital nerve stimulation in drug-resistant chronic cluster headache. Headache. 2011;51:1191–201.
101. Magis D, Bruno MA, Fumal A, Gérardy PY, Hustinx R, Laureys S, Schoenen J. Central modulation in cluster headache patients treated with occipital nerve stimulation: an FDG-PET study. BMC Neurol. 2011;11:25.
102. Mammis A, Gudesblatt M, Mogilner AY. Peripheral neurostimulation for the treatment of refractory cluster headache, long-term follow-up: case report. Neuromodulation. 2011;14:432–5.
103. Burns B, Watkins L, Goadsby PJ. Treatment of hemicrania continua by occipital nerve stimulation with a bion device: long-term follow-up of a crossover study. Lancet Neurol. 2008;7 (11):1001–12.
104. Magis D, Schoenen J. Neurostimulation in chronic cluster headache. Curr Pain Headache Rep. 2008;12(2):145–53.
105. Salaffi F, Sarzi-Puttini P. Old and new criteria for the classification and diagnosis of fibromyalgia: comparison and evaluation. Clin Exp Rheumatol. 2012;30(6 Suppl 74):3–9.
106. Fitzcharles MA, et al. The 2010 American college of rheumatology fibromyalgia survey diagnostic criteria and symptom severity scale is a valid and reliable tool in a French speaking fibromyalgia cohort. BMC Musculoskelet Disord. 2012;13:179.
107. Bennett RM, et al. An internet survey of 2,596 people with fibromyalgia. BMC Musculoskelet Disord. 2007;8:27.
108. Berger A, et al. Characteristics and patterns of healthcare utilization of patients with fibromyalgia in general practitioner settings in Germany. Curr Med Res Opin. 2008;24(9):2489–99.
109. Thimineur M, De Ridder D. C2 area neurostimulation: a surgical treatment for fibromyalgia. Pain Med. 2007;8(8):639–46.
110. Plazier M, Dekelver I, Vanneste S, Stassijns G, Menovsky T, Thimineur M, De Ridder D. Occipital nerve stimulation in fibromyalgia: a double-blind placebo-controlled pilot study with a six-month follow-up. Neuromodulation. 2014;17:256.
111. Velly AM, et al. The effect of catastrophizing and depression on chronic pain–a prospective cohort study of temporomandibular muscle and joint pain disorders. Pain. 2011;152(10):2377–83.
112. Arnow BA, et al. Catastrophizing, depression and pain-related disability. Gen Hosp Psychiatry. 2011;33(2):150–6.
113. Vanneste S, et al. The neural correlates of tinnitus-related distress. Neuroimage. 2010;52(2):470–80.
114. Gracely RH, Ambrose KR. Neuroimaging of fibromyalgia. Best Pract Res Clin Rheumatol. 2011;25(2):271–84.
115. Nebel MB, Gracely RH. Neuroimaging of fibromyalgia. Rheum Dis Clin North Am. 2009;35(2):313–27.
116. Gracely RH, et al. Pain catastrophizing and neural responses to pain among persons with fibromyalgia. Brain. 2004;127(Pt 4):835–43.
117. De Ridder D, Plazier M, Menovsky T, Kamerling N, Vanneste S. C2 subcutaneous stimulation for failed back surgery syndrome: a case report. Neuromodulation. 2013;16:610.
118. Mouton LJ, Klop EM, Holstege G. C1-C3 spinal cord projections to periaqueductal gray and thalamus: a quantitative retrograde tracing study in cat. Brain Res. 2005;1043(1–2):87–94.
119. Craig AD, Zhang ET, Blomqvist A. Association of spinothalamic lamina I neurons and their ascending axons with calbindin-immunoreactivity in monkey and human. Pain. 2002;97 (1–2):105–15.
120. Chandler MJ, Zhang J, Foreman RD. Vagal, sympathetic and somatic sensory inputs to upper cervical (C1-C3) spinothalamic tract neurons in monkeys. J Neurophysiol. 1996;76(4):2555–67.
121. Djouhri L, Brown AG, Short AD. Effects of upper cervical spinal cord stimulation on neurons in the lumbosacral enlargement of the cat: spinothalamic tract neurons. Neuroscience. 1995;68 (4):1237–46.
122. Vanneste S, De Ridder D. Noninvasive and invasive neuromodulation for the treatment of tinnitus: an overview. Neuromodulation. 2012;15(4):350–60.
123. De Ridder D, et al. Surgical brain modulation for tinnitus: the past, present and future. J Neurosurg Sci. 2012;56(4):323–40.
124. Shore SE, Zhou J. Somatosensory influence on the cochlear nucleus and beyond. Hear Res. 2006;216–217:90–9.
125. Szczepaniak WS, Moller AR. Interaction between auditory and somatosensory systems: a study of evoked potentials in the inferior colliculus. Electroencephalogr Clin Neurophysiol. 1993;88 (6):508–15.
126. Kaltenbach JA. The dorsal cochlear nucleus as a contributor to tinnitus: mechanisms underlying the induction of hyperactivity. Prog Brain Res. 2007;166:89–106.
127. Kaltenbach JA. Summary of evidence pointing to a role of the dorsal cochlear nucleus in the etiology of tinnitus. Acta Otolaryngol Suppl. 2006;556:20–6.
128. Wright DD, Ryugo DK. Mossy fiber projections from the cuneate nucleus to the cochlear nucleus in the rat. J Comp Neurol. 1996;365(1):159–72.
129. Itoh K, et al. Direct projections from the dorsal column nuclei and the spinal trigeminal nuclei to the cochlear nuclei in the cat. Brain Res. 1987;400(1):145–50.
130. Weinberg RJ, Rustioni A. A cuneocochlear pathway in the rat. Neuroscience. 1987;20(1):209–19.
131. Zhang J, Guan Z. Pathways involved in somatosensory electrical modulation of dorsal cochlear nucleus activity. Brain Res. 2007;1184:121–31.
132. Abrahams VC, Lynn B, Richmond FJ. Organization and sensory properties of small myelinated fibres in the dorsal cervical rami of the cat. J Physiol. 1984;347:177–87.
133. Hekmatpanah J. Organization of tactile dermatomes, C1 through L4, in cat. J Neurophysiol. 1961;24:129–40.
134. Abrahams VC, Richmond FJ, Keane J. Projections from C2 and C3 nerves supplying muscles and skin of the cat neck: a study using transganglionic transport of horseradish peroxidase. J Comp Neurol. 1984;230(1):142–54.
135. Kanold PO, Young ED. Proprioceptive information from the pinna provides somatosensory input to cat dorsal cochlear nucleus. J Neurosci. 2001;21(19):7848–58.

136. Shore SE. Multisensory integration in the dorsal cochlear nucleus: unit responses to acoustic and trigeminal ganglion stimulation. Eur J Neurosci. 2005;21(12):3334–48.
137. Shore SE, El Kashlan H, Lu J. Effects of trigeminal ganglion stimulation on unit activity of ventral cochlear nucleus neurons. Neuroscience. 2003;119(4):1085–101.
138. Young ED, Nelken I, Conley RA. Somatosensory effects on neurons in dorsal cochlear nucleus. J Neurophysiol. 1995;73 (2):743–65.
139. Davis KA, Miller RL, Young ED. Effects of somatosensory and parallel-fiber stimulation on neurons in dorsal cochlear nucleus. J Neurophysiol. 1996;76(5):3012–24.
140. Vanneste S, et al. Transcutaneous electrical nerve stimulation (TENS) of upper cervical nerve (C2) for the treatment of somatic tinnitus. Exp Brain Res. 2010;204(2):283–7.
141. Herraiz C, Toledano A, Diges I. Trans-electrical nerve stimulation (TENS) for somatic tinnitus. Prog Brain Res. 2007;166:389–94.
142. Mobbs RJ, Blum P, Rossato R. Mesh electrode for peripheral nerve stimulation. J Clin Neurosci. 2003;10:476–7.
143. Jasper J, Hayek S. Implanted occipital nerve stimulators. Pain Physician. 2008;11:187–200.
144. Hayek SM, Jasper JF, Deep DR, Narouze SN. Occipital neurostimulation-induced muscle spasms: implications for lead placement. Pain Physician. 2009;12:867–76.
145. Slavin KV. Placing neuromodulation in the human body: limiting morbidity. In: Arle JA, Shils JL, editors. Essential neuromodulation. Philadelphia, PA: Elsevier; 2011. p. 301–20.
146. Shelden CH, Paul F, Jacques DB, Pudenz RH. Electrical stimulation of the nervous system. Surg Neurol. 1975;4:127–32.
147. Nielson KD, Watts C, Clark WK. Peripheral nerve injury from implantation of chronic stimulating electrodes for pain control. Surg Neurol. 1976;5:51–3.
148. Franzini A, Messina G, Leone M, Broggi G. Occipital nerve stimulation (ONS). Surgical technique and prevention of late electrode migration. Acta Neurochir (Wien). 2009;151: 861–5.
149. Falowski S, Wang D, Sabesan A, Sharan A. Occipital nerve stimulator systems: review of complications and surgical techniques. Neuromodulation. 2010;13:121–5.
150. Slavin KV, Vannemreddy PSSV. Repositioning of supraorbital nerve stimulation electrode using retrograde needle insertion: a technical note. Neuromodulation. 2011;14:160–3.
151. Mammis A, Mogilner AY. A technique of distal to proximal revision of peripheral neurostimulator leads: technical note. Stereotact Funct Neurosurg. 2011;89:65–9.
152. Trentman TL, Zimmerman RS. Occipital nerve stimulation: technical and surgical aspects of implantation. Headache. 2008;48:319–27.
153. Carayannopoulos A, Beasley R, Sites B. Facilitation of percutaneous trial lead placement with ultrasound guidance for peripheral nerve stimulation trial of ilioinguinal neuralgia: a technical note. Neuromodulation. 2009;12:296–301.
154. Skaribas I, Aló K. Ultrasound imaging and occipital nerve stimulation. Neuromodulation. 2010;13:126–30.
155. Trentman TL, Dodick DW, Zimmerman RS, Birch BD. Percutaneous occipital stimulator tip erosion: report of 2 cases. Pain Physician. 2008;11:253–6.
156. Verrills P, Mitchell B, Vivian D, Sinclair C. Peripheral nerve stimulation; a treatment for chronic low back pain and failed back surgery syndrome? Neuromodulation. 2009;12:68–75.
157. Eisenberg E, Waisbrod H, Gerbershagen HU. Long-term peripheral nerve stimulation for painful nerve injuries. Clin J Pain. 2004;20:143–6.
158. Van Calenbergh F, Gybels J, Van Laere K, Dupont P, Plaghki L, Depreitere B, Kupers R. Long term clinical outcome of peripheral nerve stimulation in patients with chronic peripheral neuropathic pain. Surg Neurol. 2009;72:330–5.

Spinal Cord Stimulation

4

Kliment Gatzinsky

Introduction

Spinal cord stimulation (SCS) uses modern implantable technology to deliver long-term electric stimulation to the nervous system and reflects a transition away from ablative procedures towards reversible neuromodulation for pain treatment. Electrodes are implanted into the epidural space of the spinal column (lying outside the dura mater) for stimulation and activation of the dorsal columns of the spinal cord in order to block transmission of painful stimuli via the spinothalamic tracts to the brain. SCS is today the most commonly used interventional neuromodulation technique with estimated more than 30,000 stimulators implanted annually. The therapy reflects major advances in neuromodulation technology and methodology and is fully reversible. SCS does not cure chronic pain, but it can provide effective pain relief, either alone or in addition to medication and other treatments.

Mechanisms of Action of Spinal Cord Stimulation

Spinal cord stimulation as a treatment option for pain was first introduced by Norman Shealy in 1967 [1]. It was a spin-off of the gate control theory presented by Ron Melzack and Patrick Wall in the early 1960s, in which it was suggested that physical pain is not a direct result of activation of pain receptor neurons, but rather its perception is modulated by interaction between different neurons [2]. The experience of pain, according to the gate control theory, depends on a complex interplay between the peripheral and central nervous system (PNS and CNS) as they each process pain signals. Upon injury, pain messages originate in nerves associated with the damaged tissue and flow along the peripheral nerves to the spinal cord and on up to the brain where the pain is perceived. Before reaching the brain these pain messages encounter "nerve gates" in the spinal cord that open or close depending upon a number of factors (possibly including instructions coming down from the brain). When the gates are opening, pain messages "get through" more or less easily and pain can be intense. When the gates close, pain messages are prevented from reaching the brain, and may not even be experienced. In the original theory on how SCS acts to reduce pain it was proposed that electric stimulation of A-beta fibers in the dorsal columns of the spinal cord modulates the dorsal horn "gate," thereby reducing the input of pain signals from the periphery via A-delta and C-fibers. The therapy has therefore often been called dorsal column stimulation.

The exact neurophysiologic mechanisms of action of SCS have, however, proven to be more complex than initially suggested and are still not well understood [3]. The gate control theory does not explain the mechanisms of action of SCS accurately, as SCS principally modulates neuropathic pain without having an adequate effect on nociceptive pain. Current knowledge of SCS mode of action is predominantly derived from experimental animal models [4–6]. Data from these studies indicate that possible mechanisms, except for the gate control, include:

- Orthodromic supraspinal impulses that may activate descending inhibitory tracts [7].
- Modulation of the sympathetic nervous system [8].
- Upregulation and downregulation of neuromodulators and neurotransmitters [3].

More recent data suggest that it might be appropriate to use a more level-based approach when classifying the mechanisms by which SCS exerts its effects in pain relief. Three main levels emerge:

- Local effects at the spinal level
- Central effects at cerebral level
- Peripheral effects on vasculature in organs and tissue affected by ischemia

K. Gatzinsky (✉)
Department of Neurosurgery, Sahlgrenska University Hospital, 413 45 Gothenburg, Sweden
e-mail: kliment.gatzinsky@neuro.gu.se

H. Knotkova and D. Rasche (eds.), *Textbook of Neuromodulation*,
DOI 10.1007/978-1-4939-1408-1_4,

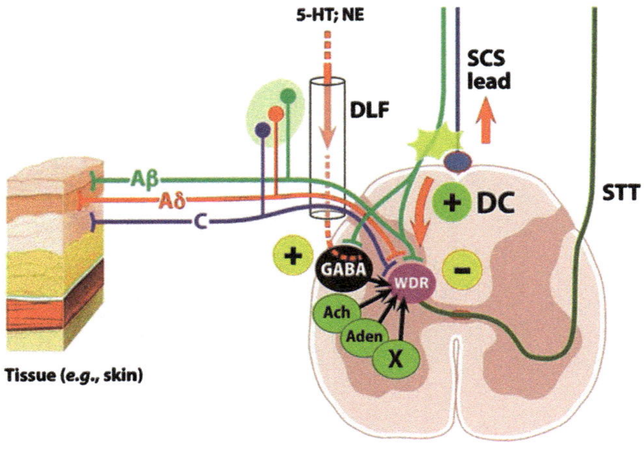

Fig. 4.1 Schematic presentation of spinal mechanisms and transmitters possibly involved in the spinal cord stimulation (SCS) effect in neuropathic pain based on current knowledge derived predominantly from experimental animal (rat) models of mononeuropathy. Antidromic activation of dorsal columns (DC) is, via collaterals, destined to the dorsal horns, establishing contact with a multitude of neurons, among them wide dynamic range (WDR) neurons and GABAergic interneurons. A stimulation induced release of gamma-aminobutyric acid (GABA), binding preferentially to GABA B receptors, may result in a decreased release of glutamate. Additional effects involve increased release of acetylcholine (Ach) binding to muscarinic M4 receptors and adenosine (Aden) binding to A1 receptors. These changes induce an attenuation of the hyperexcitability of predominantly WDR neurons, which are involved in transmission of pain signals. An additional important mechanism is activation of descending controls via serotonergic (5-HT) and noradrenergic (NE) pathways contained in the dorsolateral funiculus (DLF) originating in supraspinal, brainstem centers. Many of the mechanisms of action are still unknown (X). NE = norepinephrine; STT = spinothalamic tract (Adapted from Meyerson and Linderoth [4])

Local Effects at the Spinal Level

In neuropathic pain states, recent experimental data strongly suggests that SCS alters the neurochemistry locally at the segmental level in the dorsal horn where injured nerve fibers enter the spinal cord [9, 10]. This change induces an attenuation of the hyperexcitability of predominantly wide dynamic range (WDR) neurons, which are involved in transmission of pain signals [11, 12]. Specifically, there is some evidence for increased release of gamma-aminobutyric acid (GABA), acetylcholine, and serotonin (5-hydroxytryptamine [5-HT]) [13–17], and suppression of levels of some excitatory amino acids, including glutamate and aspartate [18]. Both antidromic and orthodromic signals are involved in the activation of the segmental modulating circuits. Possible mechanisms of action of SCS on neuropathic pain at the spinal level are summarized schematically in Fig. 4.1.

Caution is, however, warranted in uncritical translation of animal data to the bedside situation, because some behavioral signs interpreted as "pain" in animal models may be misleading [4]. We still need animal studies to generate basic data, but these findings should ideally also be confirmed in humans.

Effects at Cerebral Level

In addition to the demonstrated local spinal mechanisms involved in SCS-induced pain relief, investigation of possible functional alteration at supraspinal levels has attracted increasing interest during the last few years. Brain activation/attenuation during and after SCS treatment has been analyzed by means of positron emission tomography (PET) [19] and functional magnetic resonance imaging (fMRI) [20, 21]. $H_2{}^{15}O$ PET investigation of patients with various types of neuropathic pain disorders has shown significant increase in regional cerebral blood flow after SCS treatment which induces pain reduction [19]. These changes were identified in: (a) the thalamus contralateral to the painful limb and in the bilateral parietal association area which would regulate the pain threshold; (b) the anterior cingulated cortex and prefrontal areas which would control the emotional aspects of intractable pain. Similarly, fMRI in patients with failed back surgery syndrome (FBSS) presenting with chronic neuropathic pain (see Sect. "FBSS") has shown that pain relief obtained by short-term SCS correlated with deactivation of the cerebello-thalamocortical circuit which is supposed to function as an integrator of afferent input within a distributed network of pain processing [22]. These findings suggest an important role of central effects on the "pain matrix" in response to SCS.

Peripheral Effects on Vasculature

SCS is not only effective in reducing neuropathic pain but may also relieve pain resulting from ischemia in the extremities, as well as from cardiac ischemic disease which paradoxically are conditions of nociceptive nature [23]. The mechanisms involved in SCS-induced alleviation of ischemic pain are fundamentally different from those active in neuropathic pain with effects mainly on the peripheral vasculature with vasodilation and increased blood flow in the affected tissue. Possible mechanisms involved in the effect of SCS on pain of ischemic origin are discussed in greater detail in Sect. "SCS for treatment of painful ischemic disorders."

Indications for Spinal Cord Stimulation

The primary purposes of SCS are to improve quality of life and physical function in the long term by reducing the severity of pain and its associated characteristics. The patient's diagnosis is the main determinant for the appropriateness of SCS. Careful selection of indicated patients is, therefore, a key component of treatment success for SCS [24–26]. Based on clinical experience and available evidence of effectiveness, indications that are particularly suitable include:

- Chronic radiating neuropathic pain of peripheral origin including FBSS
- Pain in complex regional pain syndrome (CRPS)
- Ischemic pain conditions due to occlusive or vasospastic arterial disease, such as in lower extremity claudication and intractable, refractory angina pectoris

Spinal Cord Stimulation for Treatment of Peripheral Neuropathic Pain

The main indications for SCS are various forms of neuropathic pain and "mixed pain conditions" with a significant neuropathic component. Currently there is no "gold standard" for defining and classifying neuropathic pain [27–29]. According to the recent update in pain terminology from 2011, the International Association for the Study of Pain (IASP) defines neuropathic pain as "pain caused by a primary lesion or disease of the somatosensory nervous system." Neuropathic pain is a clinical description and not a diagnosis. It is mediated by *N*-methyl-D-aspartate (NMDA) and other neurotransmitting receptors [30]. Although the IASP definition does not specify type of lesion, it is generally understood that the lesion must involve the somatosensory pathways with damage to small fibers in peripheral nerves or to the spinothalamocortical system in the CNS. Current classifications are based on underlying disease (such as diabetic neuropathy or multiple sclerosis) or site of lesion (such as peripheral nerve or spinal cord). Recent advances in the understanding of the mechanisms involved in neuropathic pain have, however, fuelled interest in the development of a more mechanism-based classification [31]. Although not without difficulties, such an approach in the future is desirable, as it has potential for optimizing the management of patients with neuropathic pain. According to the mechanism-based approach [32], peripheral and central sensitization plays an important role in the generation of neuropathic pain.

Characterization of Neuropathic Pain

- Positive (e.g., spontaneous pain, allodynia, hyperalgesia) and negative (e.g., hypoalgesia) sensory symptoms and signs
- Typically described by terms like burning, tingling, shooting, and electric
- After-sensations—after a normally painful/non-painful stimulus
- Motor symptoms and signs may also be present, depending on the etiology

The accumulated knowledge and experience has shown that SCS is effective for treatment of neuropathic pain of PNS origin but generally not for pain emanating from the CNS. Consequently, SCS is not effective in post-stroke pain or pain after complete, transverse spinal cord injury (although SCS sometimes can be beneficial in partial injuries with segmental pain) or due to multiple sclerosis. The most common indications are painful radiculopathy with or without axial pain, e.g., FBSS, and pain after peripheral nerve injury, e.g., CRPS type II (see below). Other indications include phantom/stump pain [33] and painful diabetic neuropathy [34]. Indications for SCS in treatment of neuropathic pain depend on defined patient selection criteria based on a body of clinical evidence and recommendations. Multidisciplinary clinical evaluation plays a fundamental role in patient selection. Selection criteria include:

- Confirmed diagnosis of neuropathic pain
  - Pain localized in an area, e.g., along a dermatome, without major sensory deafferentation (large myelinated fibers largely intact)
  - Decrease in success rate in cases where there is sensory loss. In patients with a marked deafferentation it is sometimes impossible to produce adequate stimulation and SCS is then invariably ineffective [35]. Examples are the pain syndromes after total brachial plexus avulsion and complete transverse spinal cord injury.
  - Pain as a direct consequence of peripheral nerve injury
  - Lemniscal pathway must be preserved so that SCS can induce paresthesia covering the painful region.
- Chronic (>6 months)
- Unresponsive to conventional treatment (i.e., failure of first- and second-line treatment and/or unacceptable side effects)
- Absence of contraindications
  - Sepsis/ongoing infection
  - Drug abuse
  - Pain due to nociception (e.g., pain related only to physical activity or certain movements)
  - Major cognitive, psychiatric and personality disorders
  - Patients who have not received an adequate course of optimum conservative care
  - Coagulopathy
  - Active malignancy
  - Problems in understanding the technical aspects of the stimulation—insufficient compliance with the therapy
  - Inadequate resources for appropriate aftercare

Each patient considered a candidate for SCS must be screened and evaluated individually. The fundaments for patient selection are:

- Patient history
  - Pain history, including detailed drawing of pain distribution
  - Treatment history
  - General medical and psychological history
  - Patient questionnaires
- Neurological examination
  - Bedside examination with a focus on somatosensory functions
- Laboratory tests
- Psychological evaluation by a psychologist or a pain-oriented psychiatrist

Additional neurophysiological testing can be performed if considered necessary for adequate diagnosis of neuropathic pain.

Failed Back Surgery Syndrome

Patients diagnosed with FBSS constitute the largest group which may present with neuropathic pain considered for SCS treatment. This is actually not a syndrome but rather a misnomer that describes a subset of patients who have new or persistent pain after spinal surgery. The condition may better be included in the wider designation chronic back and leg pain (CBLP) which also comprises conditions such as degenerative disk disease, epidural fibrosis, and arachnoiditis in patients without previous spinal surgery [36, 37]. The incidence of FBSS varies widely among different studies, ranging from 10 to 40 % of spinal surgery patients [37]. The likelihood for developing the condition is considered greater with repeated surgery, and it is more prevalent in regions where spinal surgery is more common. Since the pain is usually of both nociceptive and neuropathic origin, problems are often encountered in finding an adequate therapy for treating patients diagnosed with FBSS. Despite previous anatomically successful spinal surgery, many of these patients show persistent or recurrent dermatome-based neuropathic pain (radiculopathy) down the legs with or without back pain. If considered not being candidates for additional spinal surgery and being refractory to physiotherapy, pharmacotherapy, or noninvasive peripheral stimulation therapies, such as transcutaneous electrical nerve stimulation (TENS), patients with predominantly radiculopathy symptoms may be referred for SCS. Patients presenting with a predominant or isolated back pain are usually not good candidates for SCS since these patients mainly present with nociceptive pain, which responds poorly to traditional SCS.

Spinal Cord Stimulation for Treatment of Complex Regional Pain Syndrome

Complex regional pain syndrome is a chronic systemic disease characterized by severe pain, swelling and changes in the skin following an injury which initially often appears regionally in an arm or a leg [38, 39]. The symptoms worsen over time and often spread to other parts of the body. The abnormal clinical findings associated with CRPS usually exceed the expected clinical course of the inciting event (often a relatively mild trauma or minor surgery) in both magnitude and duration [40]. Vasomotor dysfunction and impairment of motor function are often seen. IASP has proposed dividing CRPS into two types based on the nature of the inciting event, i.e., the absence or presence of a nerve lesion following the injury [41]:

- Type I, formerly known as reflex sympathetic dystrophy, Sudeck's atrophy, or algoneurodystrophy, does not have demonstrable nerve lesions and consequently does not fulfill the strict criteria for classification as neuropathic pain. The majority of patients diagnosed with CRPS are being of this type.
- Type II, formerly known as causalgia, has evidence of nerve damage. Type II CRPS tends towards the more painful and difficult to treat aspects of CRPS. Although the "cause" of the syndrome is the known or obvious injury, the mechanisms behind the development of CRPS Type II are as unknown as the mechanisms of type I.

CRPS is a multifactorial disorder associated with dysregulation of both CNS and the autonomic nervous sys tem resulting in multiple functional loss, impairment, and disability [42, 43]. Although some studies have suggested that dysfunction of the sympathetic nervous system is involved in the pathophysiology [44, 45], more recent data indicate that wind-up (the increased sensation of pain with time) and CNS sensitization are key processes that appear to be involved in the induction and maintenance of CRPS [46, 47].

No specific test is available for diagnosis of CRPS. The condition is diagnosed primarily through clinical observation of the symptoms that are shared by both types of the disorder (see above). However, thermography, sweat testing, X-rays, electrodiagnostics, and sympathetic blocks can be used to help building up a picture of the disease in addition to the typical clinical findings [48]. A delay in diagnosis and/or treatment can result in severe physical and psychological problems. Although some patients improve without treatment, early recognition and prompt treatment provide the greatest opportunity for recovery. The general strategy in CRPS treatment is multidisciplinary, with the use of different types of medications combined with distinct physical, psychosocial, and behavioral therapies [49]. If these treatment strategies do not work, patients can be referred for SCS which by large has replaced ablative surgical, chemical, or radiofrequency sympathectomy as second line therapy for this disorder [50]. Exclusion criteria include evidence of active, uncontrolled psychiatric disorder or inability to comply with the therapy [51].

Spinal Cord Stimulation for Treatment of Painful Ischemic Disorders

Spinal cord stimulation as a therapy in ischemic disorders started in Europe in the 1970s. While using SCS in a patient with painful ischemic ulcers in the lower extremities, Cook et al. in 1976 noted that following the application of SCS, the patient's pain was alleviated [52]. In addition, the perfusion to the lower extremities improved noticeably and the patient's ulcers began to heal. This observation led the authors to postulate a direct effect on peripheral vascular tone by SCS, which laid the basis for the use of SCS as a treatment option in ischemic conditions. In several European countries, SCS is frequently used to treat patients with painful ischemic disorders that are therapeutically refractory to standard treatment intended to decrease metabolic demand or following revascularization procedures. The most common indications are peripheral occlusive arterial disease and refractory angina pectoris [53–55]. Other indications include Raynaud's syndrome [56] and syndrome X [57].

Despite its use for more than 30 years, the mechanisms of SCS in painful ischemic disorders are yet not fully understood. It is evident that several different mechanisms are active when SCS is used to treat pain conditions of varying causes [3]. The active mechanisms in ischemic pain therapy seem to differ fundamentally from those relevant for the suppression of neuropathic pain. The postulated beneficial effects of SCS in peripheral occlusive arterial disease, which clinically mainly presents as painful, atherosclerotic critical ischemia in the legs, could be attributed to an improvement in the microcirculatory status of the limb [8]. The exact mechanisms of these circulatory changes are not known but seem to involve both an inhibitory modulation on the sympathetic nervous system as well as antidromic vasodilation mechanisms, thereby augmenting blood flow in the limbs [8].

In addition to its use in peripheral vascular disease, SCS has been reported to be successful in reducing pain due to myocardial ischemia. The use of SCS for chronic intractable anginal pain (refractory angina) was first described in 1987 [58] and has been shown to decrease anginal episodes, sublingual nitroglycerine consumption and signs of ischemia on the electrocardiogram [59–61]. The effect of SCS seems to involve a mutual interaction of decreased pain, decreased sympathetic tone, and redistribution of myocardial blood flow to ischemic regions [8, 62]. Similar to neuropathic pain conditions, SCS modulation of pain transmission in refractory angina has been suggested in part to be mediated by stimulation of intermediate neurons in the dorsal horns of the spinal columns, which blocks pain signals carried out by nociceptive afferent cardiac fibers [63, 64]. The mechanisms by which the therapy may improve myocardial ischemia and heart function are not well understood. It has been hypothesized that SCS exerts its beneficial effects by decreasing both pain and sympathetic tone, the result of which is decreased myocardial oxygen demand and consumption along with an improved myocardial microcirculatory blood flow [8, 65–68]. It has also been shown that SCS reduces the increased activity induced by myocardial ischemia in neurons of the intrinsic cardiac nervous system, which includes sympathetic and parasympathetic efferents, sensory afferents and interconnecting local circuit neurons [69]. This effect can result in a greater resistance of the heart to ischemia as shown in animal models [70, 71].

Spinal cord stimulation is not the first-line therapy for painful ischemic disorders but should be considered after optimal conventional medical and operative/interventional revascularization therapies have failed. Patients that suffer from inoperable chronic critical leg ischemia with pain at rest and/or ulcers may ultimately face amputation of the leg. These patients can be candidates for interventional management with SCS that is aimed at pain reduction and cure of the ulcers in order to prevent amputation. For selection of patients with refractory angina pectoris, a positive TENS test is highly predictive of successful SCS trial and should be tested preoperatively [72].

Irrespective of indication, patients selected for SCS should be adequately informed about the therapy. Preoperative discussions should include describing the procedure, possible outcomes and risks, and surgical expectations. It is important that the patient's expectations on the outcome should not be unrealistic since complete pain alleviation can generally not be expected. After the procedure has been planned and discussed, preoperative laboratory testing provides objective data to help reconfirm the patient's condition and identify contraindications, due to comorbidities, for surgery or anesthesia prior to SCS trialling. One also has to take into account possible technical contraindications. It is important to note that SCS can interact with diathermy, pacemakers, MRI and therapeutic ultrasound which can result in unexpected changes in stimulation, failure of the device, and in worst case scenario patient injury [73]. Caution is warranted for patients that have a pacemaker or implantable cardioverter defibrillator (ICD) due to a preexisting cardiac disease. If SCS is considered in these patients, proper evaluation should be performed and the patient should be cleared by a cardiologist prior to a permanent SCS implant. The coexistence of a cardiac pacemaker

Patient selection for SCS

⇩

Lead placement and intra-operative test stimulation

⇩

Trial stimulation period

⇩

Complete system implantation
(or removal of leads)

Fig. 4.2 Summary of spinal cord stimulation procedure

or ICD and a SCS device, previously thought to be a contra-indication, is now considered to be a factor in decision making, but not an absolute negating factor [74].

Spinal Cord Stimulation Stem Components and Implantation Technique

The procedure for SCS trialling and implantation is summarized in Fig. 4.2.

Several manufacturers supply commercially available devices for SCS. The components of the SCS system include the IPG, with its own battery, which is connected either directly or by an extension wire to a lead with one or several arrays of electrodes (Fig. 4.3).

Leads with up to 20 electrodes are available. Through the electrodes of the lead, which is implanted in the dorsal epidural space of the spinal canal, the IPG delivers mild electrical impulses to the dorsal aspects of the spinal cord. Lead placement is performed under local, spinal, or general anesthesia depending on type of lead that is used. Wire-like (percutaneous) leads are inserted under local anesthesia into the epidural space via Touhy needle using loss-of-resistance technique with air or saline (Fig. 4.4). Single or dual-lead implantation can be performed (Fig. 4.5). Plate (surgical) leads (Fig. 4.6) require surgical placement by a small laminectomy and usually under general anesthesia. Both percutaneous and surgical lead implantation requires access to biplane fluoroscopy (Fig. 4.7).

Preoperative preparation for the SCS trial, including patient positioning, draping and adherence to aseptic technique, are critical aspects of patient care. Available plain film x-rays, MRI or CT scanning may be helpful to define spinal anatomy preoperatively. The exact distribution of the stimulation-induced paresthesia is crucial for achieving optimal pain-relieving effect in SCS and therefore the ability to test an awake and cooperative patient yields the best results. Percutaneous technique is, accordingly, often used as first approach. This procedure is also less invasive as compared to implantation of surgical leads. Patient position is prone (most common) with flexion of the back (Fig. 4.8), sitting, or (rarely) lateral.

A paramedian Touhy needle approach is used which involves careful placement of the lead in the epidural space using C-arm fluoroscopic guidance (see Fig. 4.4). The needle is inserted with as shallow an angle (as nearly parallel to the

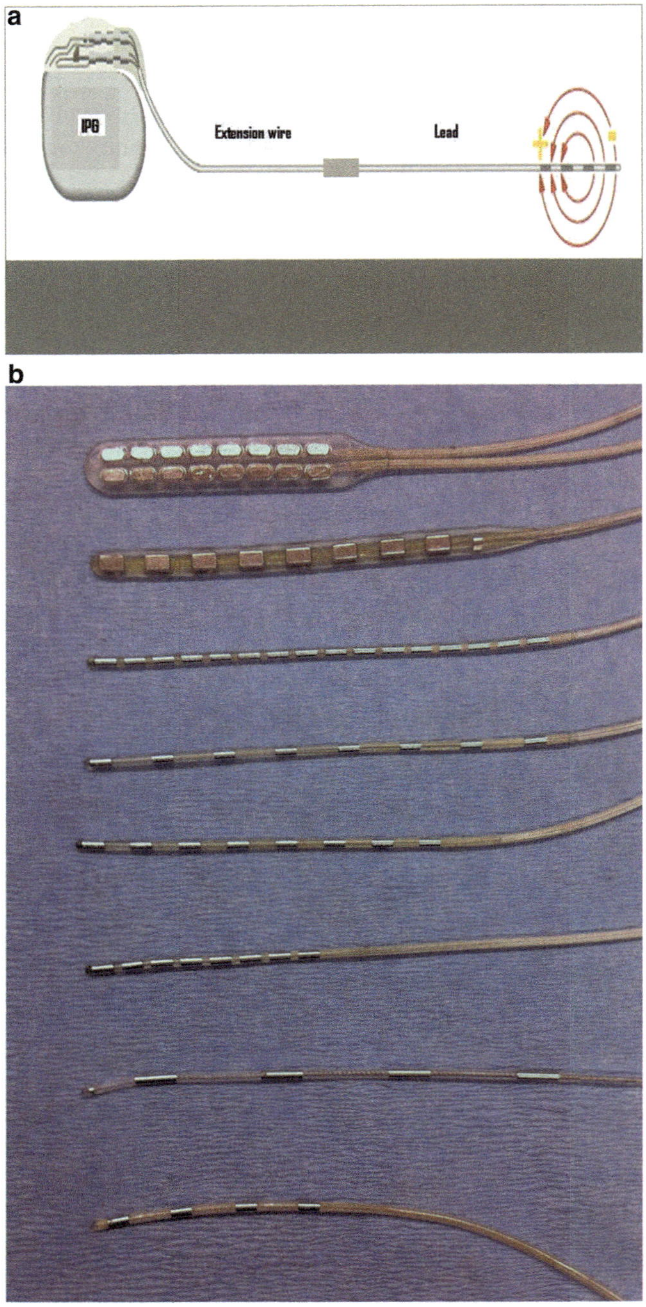

Fig. 4.3 (**a**) Schematic drawing of the components of the SCS system. IPG = Implantable pulse generator. (**b**) Some types of currently available percutaneous and surgical (plate) leads with 4–16 electrodes

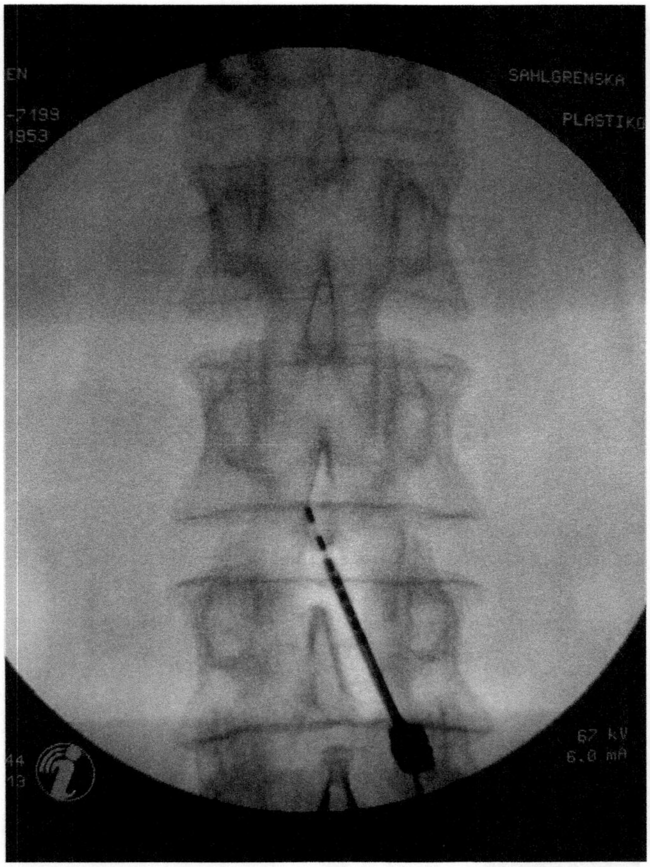

Fig. 4.4 Fluoroscopic image showing a percutaneous lead being inserted into the lumbar epidural space through a Touhy needle using a paramedian approach

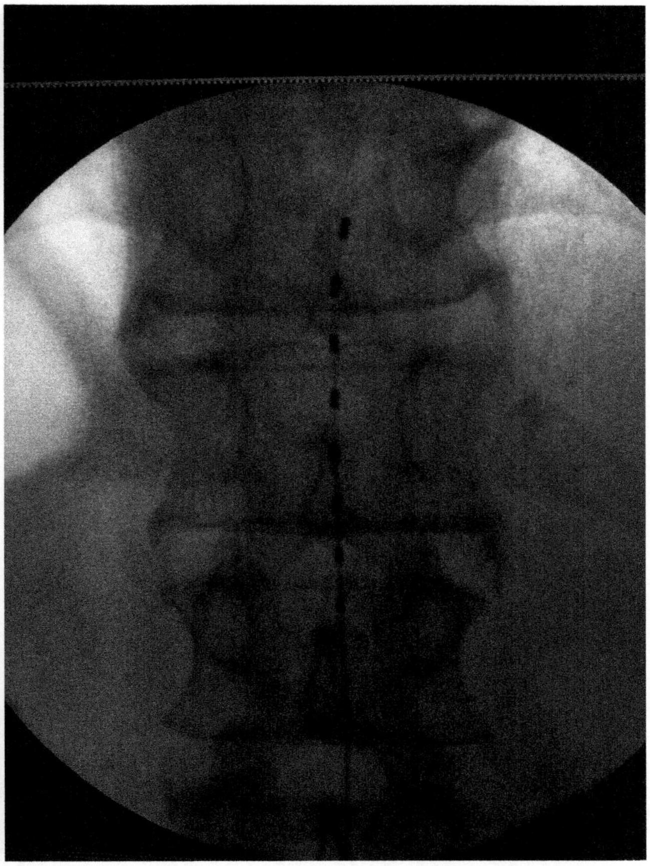

Fig. 4.5 An 8-electrode percutaneous lead placed epidurally with the tip at the T11 level for stimulation of the right leg

spinal canal) as possible because it facilitates the subsequent insertion and control of the lead in the epidural space (Fig. 4.9).

Upon needle insertion, the implanting physician must be aware of the varying angulation of the spinal processes at the different spine levels. Selection of leads depends on which arrangement will give the best paresthesia coverage to the painful area. Ideally, at least 15–20 cm of the lead should lie within the epidural space to assure maximal lead stability and minimize unwanted displacement. A patient could have one or two leads, which can be placed parallel to each other or at two different vertical sites (see Fig. 4.5). Leads with four to sixteen electrodes can be used. Today, octapolar leads with eight electrodes are mainly used. Single-lead stimulation is often used for simple pain patterns (e.g., unilateral radicular pain) and may not provide adequate paresthesia coverage for more complex pain patterns. In addition, positioning and maintaining a single lead in midline may be difficult. Dual-lead stimulation provides more programming options, enabling additional possibilities for more advanced stimulation patterns between the arrays of electrodes. Lead positioning for optimal paresthesiae coverage in different parts of the body are shown in Table 4.1. Intraoperative test stimulation is performed to create an appropriate field of pleasant paresthesias covering as much as possible of patient's pain area (Fig. 4.10).

After satisfactory coverage is obtained (>80 % of the painful area), the lead is fixed to the muscle fascia by a specially designed anchor and connected to an external pulse generator via an extension wire, which is tunnelled subcutaneously and externalized through the skin at least 20 cm from the insertion point of the lead into the epidural space.

A percutaneous lead retains a greater potential to migrate which can reduce or eliminate pain–paresthesia overlap. Surgical lead implantation (prone position) usually is reserved for second implantation in case of dislocation/migration of percutaneous leads or for patients in whom the predicted target area is in the area of scar tissue from prior surgery. Because of its shape, a surgical plate/paddle lead resists migration once it is encapsulated in fibrous tissue, and, if it has multiple columns of electrodes, these are fixed in position with respect to one another (see Fig. 4.6). Some centers prefer surgical leads as first approach since these leads resist migration better and appear to be

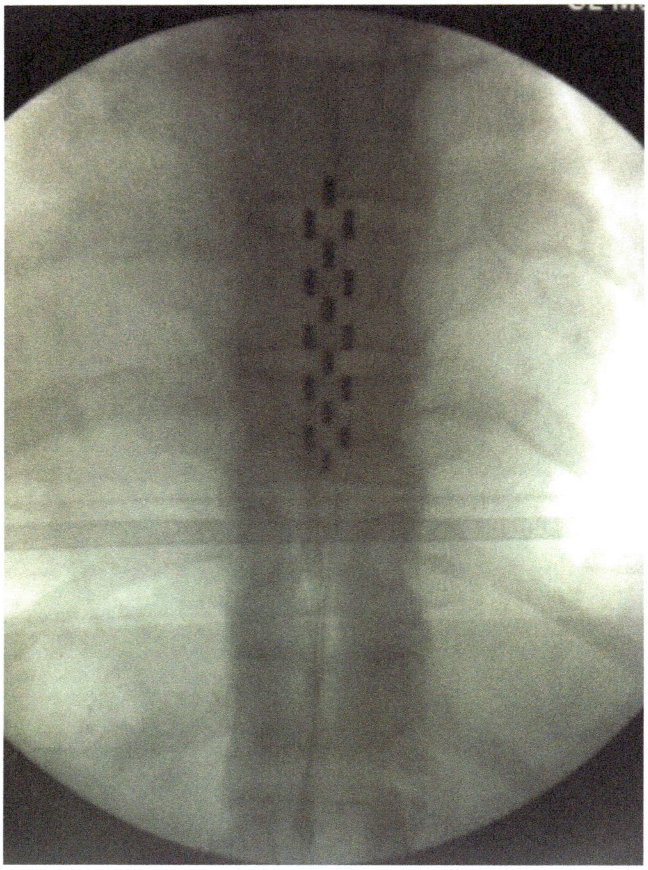

Fig. 4.6 A surgical plate lead with 16 electrodes arranged in 3 arrays in the epidural space covering the T9 and T10 vertebrae for stimulation of the low back (Courtesy of Dr. Philippe Rigoard)

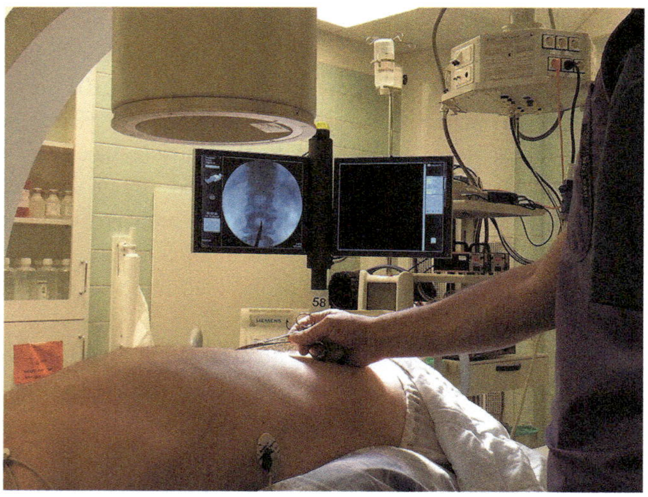

Fig. 4.7 Fluoroscopic guidance is used for indicating the appropriate level for epidural lead insertion

associated with better long-term effectiveness than leads placed percutaneously [75, 76]. A surgical lead generally also requires less power than a percutaneous lead with the same contact areas and spacing, thus increasing the time

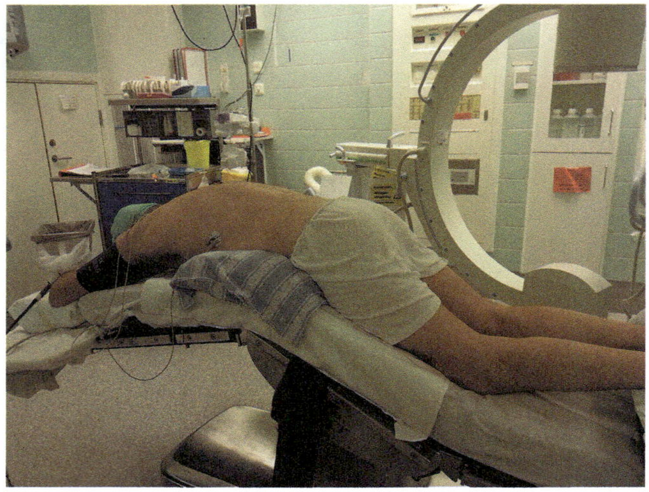

Fig. 4.8 Patient in prone position with flexion of the back in order to facilitate insertion of the Touhy needle into the epidural space

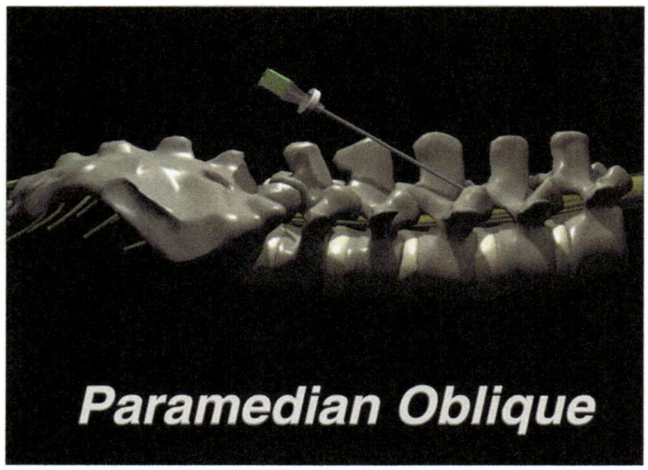

Fig. 4.9 Paramedian oblique technique for insertion of the Touhy needle epidurally (Courtesy of Dr. Jean-Pierre Van Buyten)

before surgical battery replacement or recharging is required [77]. However, using a surgical lead as first choice usually is associated with lower success rates for optimal paresthesia coverage and pain relief since intraoperative identification of appropriate paresthesias during the test stimulation is not possible in patients under general anesthesia. Since both the insertion and, if needed, removal of a surgical lead usually require open surgery, pain associated with the procedure is generally greater than that experienced after insertion of a percutaneous lead. In addition, the scarring that occurs after lead implantation is greater for surgical than for percutaneous leads which can present a greater problem if the lead requires a revision. Recently, placement under local anesthesia of a narrow paddle lead via a minimally invasive method using a Seldinger-guided percutaneous approach was introduced [78, 79]. This technique may minimize some of the problems encountered with conventional

Table 4.1 Lead positioning

Pain location	Tip of the lead
Neck	C1–C2 (difficult to stimulate)
Shoulder	C2–C4
Arm	C4–C7
Hand	C5–C7, T1
Upper chest (for refractory angina)	T1–T2
Lower chest (for abdominal pain)	T5–T6 (difficult to stimulate)
Lower back	T8–T10
Groin	T11–L1
Thigh and knee	T10–T12
Leg and ankle	T11–T12
Foot	T12–L1

The desired location of the tip of the lead for sensory responses to SCS in different parts of the body. The definitive location varies between patients

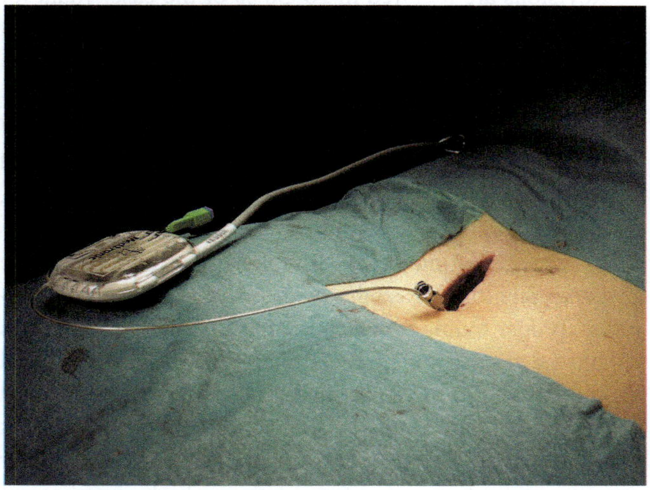

Fig. 4.10 Intraoperative test stimulation with a percutaneous lead connected to an extension cable

surgical paddle leads, keeping the benefits which these leads have compared to percutaneous ones.

There is no consensus regarding the use of prophylactic antibiotics during the intra-operative trial, although administration of systemic antibiotics immediately prior to the lead insertion is considered standard procedure for both percutaneous and surgical leads. In many centers, a 3-dose regimen for intravenous administration of antibiotics preoperatively and postoperatively is used.

After appropriate placement of the lead which either can be a temporary or a permanent one, a trial stimulation period is generally performed, which can last up to 4 weeks depending on reimbursement requirements. The test trial is normally carried out at home under prophylactic treatment with oral antibiotics. The purpose of the trial is to assess the efficacy of SCS and to increase the cost-effectiveness of the method by making proper patient selection. The patient uses the external pulse generator with one or several preset electrode combinations to achieve the best result in terms of paresthesia coverage and pain relief. Evaluation is performed using standard rating methods, such as Visual Analogue Scale (VAS) and function. Criteria for successful trial are:

- Comfortable stimulation covering at least 80 % of the painful area
- Patient should report a substantial level of pain reduction (>50 %) and improvement in function in terms of daily life activities
  - The pain relieving effect should be sustained for a period of at least 30–60 min after the stimulation has been turned off
  - Patient should consider the possibility of reducing concomitant pharmacotherapy

In case of doubt, the trial may be prolonged or reevaluated after a period of interruption.

If the results of pain relieving are satisfactory in the trial period, the patient receives a fully implantable SCS system. Otherwise the lead is removed. If a permanent lead has been used during the first-stage operation, and only subcutaneous tunneling and IPG placement are planned, patient participation is not needed, and general anesthesia may be applied. IPGs are of different sizes and capacity and are available as non-rechargeable or rechargeable devices. Multi-program IPGs are mainly used today. The IPG usually is implanted in the subcutaneous tissue infraclavicular (cervical leads), or in the lateral abdominal area or the superior gluteal region. It should be in a location that patients can access with their dominant hand for adjustment of the stimulation with their patient programmer (remote control). Stimulation parameters are amplitude (strength of pulse), pulse width (duration of each pulse), and frequency (number of pulses per second). IPG programming after full SCS system implantation involves selecting the best electrode stimulating configuration and adjusting the amplitude, pulse width, and frequency of electrical pulses for optimal pain relief and comfort for the patient. The electrical current is delivered in volts (0–10.5) or milliamperes (0–25.5) depending on the system used and must be set above the perception threshold and as close as possible below the discomfort level. Pulse width usually varies from 100–500 μs. Widening the pulse width will broaden the area of paresthesia. Frequency of pulse wave is typically between 20 and 120 Hz. It is an individual preference, some patients choose low-frequency buzzing sensation whereas others prefer high-frequency tingling. The patient programmer features are on/off and adjustment within limits considering amplitude, pulse width and frequency of the stimulation. Patterns of use vary widely. The stimulation regimen is decided by physician/patient and can vary between continuous and cycling. Selection of lowest possible setting on all parameters is important in conserving battery life in non-rechargeable IPG models. Changing of stimulation parameters and reprogramming may have to be undertaken during the course of therapy and follow-up.

Implant-to-trial ratios (responders to SCS) of 70–80 % on average have been reported in the literature [80]. It is important to remember that a successful stimulation trial not always equates with long-term success. Some patients with successful trials may experience failure of the therapy with time. These patients often experience a greater failure because they have undergone the potential morbidity and the expense of implantation of a device. In addition to continuing conventional pain treatment, they can be helped further to cope with the persisting pain through participation in pain management programs, such as cognitive behavioral therapy.

The procedure for SCS implantation in patients with refractory angina pectoris differs from that for other indications, provided that the patient has responded positively to TENS treatment preoperatively. In these patients the complete SCS system can be implanted in one session, without any trial evaluation, since a beneficial response to TENS is predictive for high success rate for SCS [72].

Safety Profile of Spinal Cord Stimulation

Spinal cord stimulation is generally considered to be a very safe therapy with exceedingly few serious complications primarily because it is a minimally invasive and reversible procedure. The risks associated with the surgery are presumably higher with surgical than with percutaneously inserted leads, though no study has compared these two techniques in a systematic or prospective trial. Patients should be fully informed of the benefits, burdens and complications of SCS before lead implantation and should receive specific outcome and complication rates relating to the unit where the procedure is being performed. It is important that SCS-related complications should be kept to a minimum to ensure continued long-term high success rates. In addition, these complications pose an added expense to the already high cost of the therapy. Although the incidence of adverse events associated with SCS has been shown to be quite high, the rate of serious complications is low. Data, which is more or less exclusively based on the use of the older 4-electrode type leads and single or double channel IPGs, has shown a great variety of complication rates (0–81 %) depending on duration of follow-up period [81–85]. The panorama of complications can be divided into three main categories:

- Technical (hardware-related) complications: most common [86]
  - Occur more frequently in the first 2 years following implantation of the device than in the long term [87].
  - Most frequent complication is lead movement with possible loss of paresthesia and efficacy.
  - Electrode fracture.
  - Hardware malfunction: lead insulation failure, IPG failure.
- Biological complications
  - More prevalent within the first 3 months after implantation [87].
  - Infection (2–5 %), mostly superficial and affecting the IPG pocket [88].
  - Spinal fluid leakage
  - Hemorrhage in IPG pocket.
  - Epidural hematomas are extremely rare and have mainly occurred in the setting of surgical leads [89].
- Post-procedure complications
  - Undesirable stimulation or pain at implant site.

Revisions are required in 20–30 % of the cases (data for quadripolar, 4-electrode leads) and do not generally affect patients' acceptance of treatment [87]. Recent advances in anchoring of wire leads and new technology with the introduction of rechargeable IPGs and leads with a minimum of eight electrodes appear to be reducing complications and need for revisions in general. No systematic analyses are, however, available on this subject.

In order to minimize complications and operative revisions and to increase the success rate of effective stimulation, proper training on technique is important. Implanters should be trained in interventional pain management and should be able to recognize and treat hardware-related and biological complications, as well as recognize the benefits and pitfalls of various commercial lead types and their specific indications. Centers with a high number of implantations generally have higher success rates and fewer complications. Clinicians performing SCS should, consequently, implant a sufficient number of leads to achieve and maintain competence. The implanter should be comfortable with troubleshooting during the implantation procedure, and with methods and techniques to achieve proper stimulation while maintaining safety. Guidelines have been published to help avoid complications and improve outcomes [87, 90].

Evidence-Based Support for Efficacy of Spinal Cord Stimulation

In today's clinical practice it is required that the use of treatments and existing devices firmly rests on medical evidence. Interventional pain management techniques, including SCS, have gradually become integrated into the treatment plan of patients suffering from chronic pain. Consequently, evidence-based guidelines based on target specific techniques have come to play an important role in optimizing treatment success [91–93]. Some indications for SCS are well established and as the evidence base evolves new indications are emerging. Well-designed, randomized controlled trials (RCTs) provide varying evidence of the benefit of SCS over comparative therapies for treatment of FBSS, CRPS type I, peripheral vascular disease/critical limb ischemia with pain and refractory angina pectoris. There are also numerous systematic reviews, meta-analyses, and Health Technology Assessment analyses that, in addition to RCT evidence, support the view that SCS is a safe and effective therapy for a variety of chronic pain conditions (for a comprehensive, regularly updated record, see www.inahta.org).

The available literature supplies good evidence for efficacy of SCS in the treatment of FBSS with painful radiculopathy [94–96]. In one prospective RCT it was shown that SCS was more successful than reoperation in FBSS patients during a 3-year follow up period [97]. In addition to a better outcome considering pain relief and patient satisfaction, rate of crossover from reoperation to SCS was consistently higher than from SCS to reoperation. Patients randomized to reoperation also required increased opiate analgesics significantly more often than those randomized to SCS. In an additional, prospective multicenter RCT (the Prospective Randomized Controlled Multicenter Trial of the Effectiveness of Spinal Cord Stimulation [PROCESS] study), SCS was compared with conventional medical management for a 24-month follow-up in FBSS patients with predominantly leg pain [98, 99]. It was shown that patients treated with a combination of SCS and conventional medical management reported significantly improved leg pain, quality of life, and functional capacity as compared with patients receiving medical treatment alone.

Early treatment with SCS provides best results in patients diagnosed with FBSS. A striking relationship emerges suggesting that the longer the duration of time between the first surgery and SCS, the poorer the response to SCS [100, 101]. The success rate can be as high as 85 % for patients with a delay less than 2 years and only 9 % for patients with 15-year delay [100]. When possible, SCS should be performed within 5 years of the onset of symptoms [101].

Efficacy and safety of SCS has also been demonstrated for CRPS and then mainly type I. Treatment algorithms for this disorder invariably include SCS [95, 102–105]. Several studies have shown reduced pain and allodynia, improved limb function and quality of life and lessened depression in patients with CRPS [106–108]. In one prospective RCT with 5-year follow-up, SCS and physical therapy were compared to physical therapy alone in patients with CRPS type I [109–112]. It was shown that SCS provides significant long-term pain relief, improves global perceived effect and improves quality of life in these patients. In the longest reported follow-up of SCS treated patients with CRPS to date, Kumar at al. showed that best results are associated with early stage 1 CRPS type I, patients younger than 40 years, and SCS treatment within a year of CRPS onset [108]. It has also been recommended that SCS should be started within 12–16 weeks if conventional therapy fails [106]. Earlier treatment aims to avoid permanent dystrophic changes. Accordingly, the treatment algorithm should be flexible and allow SCS earlier if rehabilitation fails to rapidly progress [50, 104].

SCS is frequently used in Europe to treat ischemic conditions refractory to conventional conservative and operative therapy. Although technically still an off-label indication in the USA, this practice is supported by several published studies. A Cochrane review on the effectiveness of SCS for treatment of nonreconstructable chronic critical ischemia compared to conservative treatment alone has been published [113]. In total, five randomized trials and one nonrandomized controlled clinical trial with a total of 444 patients were found to be of relevance. One of the studies was a randomized controlled trial in which it was shown that SCS, as compared with analgesic treatment alone, may reduce amputation levels in patients with severe refractory leg ischemia and be most effective in patients without arterial hypertension [114]. In the Cochrane review, the conclusion was drawn that SCS, compared to conservative treatment alone, may reduce amputation rate and pain in selected patients refractory to conservative and reconstructive surgical treatment [113]. Transcutaneous oxygen pressure ($tcPo_2$) measurements have been indicated to be useful in selecting the most respondent patients to SCS, particularly those having a moderately compromised peripheral circulation with foot $tcPo_2$ between 10 and 30 mmHg [115–118]. Based on available data and international expert opinion, SCS could merit being included as a second-line option, after conservative, pharmacological therapy, in the treatment algorithm for refractory chronic critical leg ischemia with pain (see, however, [95], [119]). Due to its nondestructive character for modulation of the nervous system, SCS may be considered before ablative sympathectomy, which presents with more undesirable and serious long-term complications. Well-designed RCTs with clear inclusion criteria are, however, needed to further elucidate which patients can benefit from SCS therapy and more firmly strengthen the evidence for SCS as an integral part in the treatment of refractory chronic pain due to peripheral vascular disease [113].

In addition to numerous observational studies, a number of RCTs have been performed to evaluate treatment of refractory angina pectoris with SCS. Most RCTs compare SCS stimulation (SCS ON) to either subthreshold or no SCS stimulation (SCS OFF) which is associated with a high risk of bias [120]. Compared to a no-stimulation control, there is some evidence from observational studies of improvement in all outcome measures following SCS implantation, with gains observed in pooled exercise capacity, short-acting nitrate consumption and health-related quality of life [121]. In two prospective RCTs, SCS was compared with an alternative therapy, coronary artery bypass grafting (CABG) and percutaneous laser myocardial revascularization (PMR) [122–125]. Long-term outcomes were similar when directly compared to either CABG or PMR. Fewer severe adverse events were seen for SCS when compared to CABG. Based on the accumulated evidence from RCTs, systematic reviews, and meta-analyses, there is sufficient evidence that SCS gives rise to symptomatic benefits (decrease in anginal attacks), improved quality of life and can improve the functional status of patients with severe angina [60, 61, 126–128]. Despite its effectiveness in preventing angina attacks and hospital admissions, SCS does not mask serious ischemic symptoms, which may lead to silent infarction [129, 130]. Accordingly, SCS is recommended both in the European (European Society for Cardiology) and US (American Heart Association/American College of Cardiology) guidelines for treatment of refractory angina.

The use of SCS for pain relief has also been evaluated for a variety of other pain conditions without any convincing proof of long-term efficacy (see Sect. "New Technology, Techniques and Indications"). Although the therapy may be useful for many of these indications, it still has an undetermined validity due to lack of RCTs and well-designed clinical studies.

In summary, there is sufficient evidence for SCS being a safe and effective therapy for a number of conditions involving neuropathic and ischemic pain. Due to the type of intervention and the presence of paresthesia, however, blinding patients and investigators is problematic. More methodologically rigorous studies, including the addition of objective data, are needed to provide definitive, solid proof regarding improvement in pain and function in the long term. The recent introduction of paresthesia-free, high frequency SCS may add new possibilities in this context (see Sect. "New Technology, Techniques and Indications").

Cost-Effectiveness of Spinal Cord Stimulation

Spinal cord stimulation has been shown to be cost-effective, despite the initial high costs of the implantable devices. However, cost-effectiveness is highly sensitive to the device selection, exact prices and longevity [95]. The cost-effectiveness of SCS in the treatment of FBSS patients, compared with best medical treatment/conventional pain therapy (control group), was evaluated by Kumar et al. [131]. They examined 104 patients, of which 60 were implanted with a spinal cord stimulator. The actual mean cumulative cost for SCS therapy for a 5-year period was CAD 29.123 per patient, compared with CAD 38.029 for conventional pain therapy. The cost of treatment for the SCS group was greater than that for the control group in the first 2.5 years but became less than for conventional pain therapy after that period and remained so during the rest of the follow-up. The higher costs in the non-stimulator group were in the categories of medications, emergency center visits, x-rays, and ongoing physician visits. In addition, 15 % of SCS-treated patients were able to return to work versus 0 % in the control group. Later systematic reviews of the literature and analyses examining specifically the cost-effectiveness of SCS for FBSS have confirmed that SCS is less costly than other options in the long term ([95, 132–136], cf. [137]). Based on extrapolation from RCTs and cost-effectiveness model analysis, some evidence has also been presented for the cost-effectiveness of SCS for the management of patients with CRPS type I [103, 138] and refractory angina pectoris [61, 139]. The foremost reason to the cost-effectiveness of SCS for angina, where "break-even" is seen after approximately 15–16 months, seems to be due to decreased hospital admissions [61]. It has also been pointed out that, despite their initial increased expense, rechargeable IPGs should be considered when IPG longevity is likely to be short [135, 138].

New Technology, Techniques, and Indications

The use of SCS has rapidly expanded during the last few years due to increased clinical experience and better evidence-based support for the therapy. Despite varying levels of success in the literature, approximately 40–50 % of patients treated with traditional SCS for neuropathic pain disorders will not receive adequate, long-term pain relief [97, 99, 110]. Therefore, technical SCS system refinements, as well as new techniques have emerged [140]. Being evolved from simple monopole and bipole configurations, complicated electrode arrays are available today. In conjunction with improved IPG technology, using multiple programming options and position adaptive stimulation to further optimize desired paresthesia capture and patient comfort, these technical refinements have the potential to increase the success rate of the therapy. In addition, new treatment modalities based on traditional SCS technology have appeared to further optimize the outcome for certain painful conditions. Emerging therapies include:

- Peripheral nerve stimulation with needle-delivered wire leads placed subcutaneously in the vicinity of a supposedly injured nerve, such as the greater occipital nerve in patients with occipital neuralgia [141, 142]. Percutaneous occipital nerve stimulation has recently also been introduced for treatment of refractory migraine and cluster headache [143].

- Peripheral nerve field stimulation in which one or several leads are placed subcutaneously in a pain area where the innervation is undetermined, e.g., in the axial low back for FBSS [144] or chest for refractory angina pectoris [145].
- Novel targets for stimulation, such as the dorsal root ganglion (DRG), the medial branch of the dorsal ramus or the cluneal nerve. Due to minimal CSF layer near neural target, DRG stimulation uses lower amplitudes (<5 % of conventional SCS) to more specifically treat pain in areas that have been hard to reach with traditional SCS [146, 147]. This therapy offers new possibilities in treating conditions like postoperative neuropathic groin pain, isolated foot pain and postamputation pain.
- High-frequency stimulation (up to 10,000 Hz) offering paresthesia-free therapy mainly for axial low back pain, e.g., in FBSS patients [148].
- Burst stimulation in which closely spaced, high-frequency paresthesia-free stimuli are delivered to the spinal cord for suppression of limb and back pain [149].

Several of these therapies have shown promising preliminary results in terms of efficacy and safety and have been approved in Europe and Australia for clinical use. The best indications for most new approaches are, however, still subject of intense study being in various preclinical and clinical phases, why no firm conclusions can be drawn currently considering long-term efficacy.

New indications for SCS, including several that do not involve classical neuropathic or ischemic pain, have emerged which elucidates the need to better define the appropriate use of the therapy. Indications, for which SCS has been applied without obtaining any conclusive evidence of effectiveness, include human immunodeficiency virus (HIV) neuropathy, fibromyalgia, chronic visceral pain, non-radicular focal bone pain, chest wall pain syndromes, congestive heart failure, and cerebral vasospasm. Limited data, often presented as case reports and small case series, have indicated clinical improvements for these indications when using SCS. While many of the reports suggest beneficial effects concerning pain relief, caution is warranted for the use of SCS for most of these conditions on a more regular basis until a more systematic validation has been performed considering long-term responsiveness to the therapy. However, some conditions are at present being investigated more actively and merit mentioning in terms of putative good responders to SCS. One is painful diabetic neuropathy. This pervasive and costly symptom is present in up to 50 % of all diabetic patients with long duration of the disease and poses major treatment challenges [150]. Since drug therapies are ineffective in many patients, interest in the use of SCS as a treatment option has increased in the past decade. The available literature, including a systematic review [34], indicates that SCS seems to be an efficacious and feasible treatment for intractable painful diabetic neuropathy [151–153]. A large-scale, prospective RCT has recently been initiated in order to provide definitive high-quality proof of the short- and long-term beneficial effects of SCS in this condition [154]. In addition, painful conditions with peripheral vasospasm, such as Raynaud's disease and Buerger's disease, seem to have a good potential for responding positively to SCS based on their underlying pathophysiological mechanisms, which are similar to those behind peripheral ischemic disorders with pain [56, 155].

The axial low back pain component in patients with FBSS has posed a major treatment challenge [156]. Because of its resistance to conventional therapies, including traditional SCS, several new treatment options, involving refinement and further development of the SCS technique, have evolved in order to find a solution to this problem. Recent reports on the use of 16-electrode, multiarray surgical leads [157], peripheral nerve field stimulation in combination with SCS [144, 158, 159] and high-frequency stimulation [148] have all presented with good outcomes for the treatment of axial low back pain in small cohorts of FBSS patients. Systematic and randomized prospective controlled trials are still missing and need to be conducted to evaluate these initial data and the significance in the long term of these therapies for low-back pain treatment.

The Future

The technical revolution in SCS that has taken place during the last decade is continuing [160]. Future visions and ongoing technical research in order to further improve outcome include:

- Continuing development in IPG technology with smaller devices with prolonged battery life, improved programming options and evolution of stimulators that can switch between ampere and voltage for current deliverance. The sensing technology for position-adaptive stimulation that has recently been introduced for amplitude in order to avoid unpleasant, jolting stimulation as a result of posture changes [161], has the potential to be extended to involve automatic, posture adaptive switching also between programs for maximal patient comfort. In addition, the new patient diary for position registration included in this new type of IPG can help to integrate objective data into clinical practice and further strengthen the evidence for the efficacy of the therapy.
- Further development of MRI-compatible leads and IPGs for full body scan also in 3-T scanners. The recently

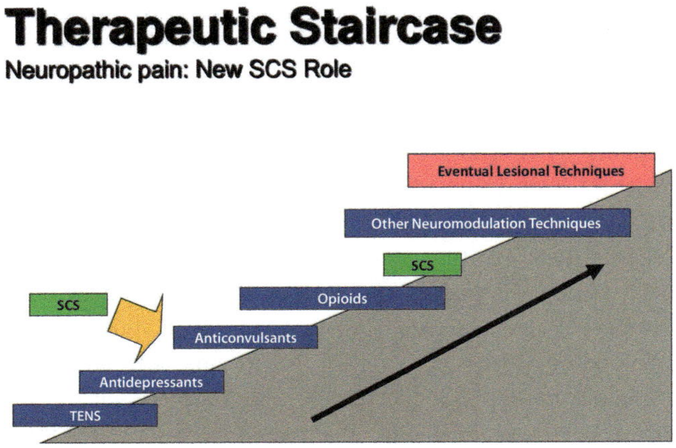

Fig. 4.11 Therapeutic staircase for treating neuropathic pain: Proposed new role for SCS ahead of opioid treatment (Courtesy of Dr. Bengt Linderoth)

introduced MRI-compatible devices can only be used in 1.5-T scanners.

- Telemetry for adjustment of stimulation parameters via Internet or secured online connections between the clinical department or practice and the patient.
- Global registries for collection of target specific data on implantation technique, complications and efficacy of SCS in order to optimize the outcome of the therapy.

Since SCS has proven to be a safe and effective therapy for a variety of chronic pain conditions, its use earlier in the treatment algorithm for several of these conditions has been urged, although this issue is still controversial [50, 162, 163]. This is mainly valid for FBSS and CRPS type I where SCS has been shown to have a better outcome if used early in the course of the disease process (see above). SCS and related stimulation techniques may offer a better alternative to chronic opioid administration for conditions with chronic neuropathic pain, especially with hyperalgesia. High-dose opioid medication is often associated with severe side effects, such as hormonal dysfunction, weight gain, obstipation, hyperalgesia, development of tolerance with time, and the potential for dependence, abuse, and addiction [164–166]. In addition to the side effects of high-dose opioids, outcome data examining their long-term efficacy in treatment of chronic nonmalignant pain are lacking. Unlike opioid administration, SCS also remains under physician control. Therefore, SCS could deserve to be put ahead of opioids in the treatment algorithm for conditions with chronic neuropathic pain (Fig. 4.11). With further strengthening of the evidence-based support for the therapy, SCS may have the potential to compete also with other pharmacological therapies in the analgesic treatment ladder for chronic pain conditions responsive to SCS.

References

1. Shealy CN, Mortimer JT, Reswick JB. Electrical inhibition of pain by stimulation of the dorsal columns: preliminary clinical report. Anesth Analg. 1967;46:489–91.
2. Melzack R, Wall PD. Pain mechanisms: a new theory. Science. 1965;150:971–9.
3. Foreman RD, Linderoth B. Neural mechanisms of spinal cord stimulation. Int Rev Neurobiol. 2012;107:87–119.
4. Meyerson BA, Linderoth B. Mode of action of spinal cord stimulation in neuropathic pain. J Pain Symptom Manage. 2006;31(4 Suppl):S6–12.
5. Guan Y. Spinal cord stimulation: neurophysiological and neurochemical mechanisms of action. Curr Pain Headache Rep. 2012;16:217–25.
6. Smits H, van Kleef M, Holsheimer J, Joosten EA. Experimental spinal cord stimulation and neuropathic pain: mechanism of action, technical aspects, and effectiveness. Pain Pract. 2013;13:154–68.
7. El-Khoury C, Hawwa N, Baliki M, Atweh SF, Jabbur SJ, Saadé NE. Attenuation of neuropathic pain by segmental and supraspinal activation of the dorsal column system in awake rats. Neuroscience. 2002;112:541–53.
8. Wu M, Linderoth B, Foreman RD. Putative mechanisms behind effects of spinal cord stimulation on vascular diseases: a review of experimental studies. Auton Neurosci. 2008;138:9–23.
9. Smits H, Kleef MV, Honig W, Gerver J, Gobrecht P, Joosten EA. Spinal cord stimulation induces c-Fos expression in the dorsal horn in rats with neuropathic pain after partial sciatic nerve injury. Neurosci Lett. 2009;450:70–3.
10. Smits H, van Kleef M, Joosten EA. Spinal cord stimulation of dorsal columns in a rat model of neuropathic pain: evidence for a segmental spinal mechanism of pain relief. Pain. 2012;153:177–83.
11. Yakhnitsa V, Linderoth B, Meyerson BA. Spinal cord stimulation attenuates dorsal horn neuronal hyperexcitability in a rat model of mononeuropathy. Pain. 1999;79:223–33.
12. Guan Y, Wacnik PW, Yang F, Carteret AF, Chung CY, Meyer RA, et al. Spinal cord stimulation-induced analgesia: electrical stimulation of dorsal column and dorsal roots attenuates dorsal horn neuronal excitability in neuropathic rats. Anesthesiology. 2010;113:1392–405.
13. Linderoth B, Gazelius B, Franck J, Brodin E. Dorsal column stimulation induces release of serotonin and substance P in the cat dorsal horn. Neurosurgery. 1992;31:289–96.
14. Cui JG, Linderoth B, Meyerson BA. Effects of spinal cord stimulation on touch-evoked allodynia involve GABAergic mechanisms. An experimental study in the mononeuropathic rat. Pain. 1996;66:287–95.
15. Schechtmann G, Song Z, Ultenius C, Meyerson BA, Linderoth B. Cholinergic mechanisms involved in the pain relieving effect of spinal cord stimulation in a model of neuropathy. Pain. 2008;139:136–45.
16. Song Z, Ultenius C, Meyerson BA, Linderoth B. Pain relief by spinal cord stimulation involves serotonergic mechanisms: an experimental study in a rat model of mononeuropathy. Pain. 2009;147:2418.
17. Ultenius C, Song Z, Lin P, Meyerson BA, Linderoth B. Spinal GABAergic mechanisms in the effects of spinal cord stimulation in a rodent model of neuropathic pain: is GABA synthesis involved? Neuromodulation. 2013;16:114–20.
18. Cui JG, O'Connor WT, Ungerstedt U, Linderoth B, Meyerson BA. Spinal cord stimulation attenuates augmented dorsal horn release

of excitatory amino acids in mononeuropathy via a GABAergic mechanism. Pain. 1997;73:87–95.
19. Kishima H, Saitoh Y, Oshino S, Hosomi K, Ali M, Maruo T, et al. Modulation of neuronal activity after spinal cord stimulation for neuropathic pain; H(2)15O PET study. Neuroimage. 2010;49:2564–9.
20. Rasche D, Siebert S, Stippich C, Kress B, Nennig E, Sartor K, et al. Spinal cord stimulation in Failed-Back-Surgery-Syndrome. preliminary study for the evaluation of therapy by functional magnetic resonance imaging (fMRI). Schmerz. 2005;19 (497–500):502–5.
21. Stancák A, Kozák J, Vrba I, Tintera J, Vrána J, Polácek H, Stancák M. Functional magnetic resonance imaging of cerebral activation during spinal cord stimulation in failed back surgery syndrome patients. Eur J Pain. 2008;12:137–48.
22. Moens M, Sunaert S, Mariën P, Brouns R, De Smedt A, Droogmans S, et al. Spinal cord stimulation modulates cerebral function: an fMRI study. Neuroradiology. 2012;54:1399–407.
23. Linderoth B, Meyerson B. Spinal cord stimulation. Techniques, indications and outcome. In: Lozano AM, Gildenberg PL, Tasker RR, editors. Textbook of stereotactic and functional neurosurgery. Berlin: Springer; 2009. p. 2305–30.
24. Atkinson L, Sundaraj SR, Brooker C, O'Callaghan J, Teddy P, Salmon J, et al. Recommendations for patient selection in spinal cord stimulation. J Clin Neurosci. 2011;18:1295–302.
25. Williams KA, Gonzalez-Fernandez M, Hamzehzadeh S, Wilkinson I, Erdek MA, Plunkett A, et al. A multi-center analysis evaluating factors associated with spinal cord stimulation outcome in chronic pain patients. Pain Med. 2011;12:1142–53.
26. Yampolsky C, Hem S, Bendersky D. Dorsal column stimulator applications. Surg Neurol Int. 2012;3 Suppl 4:S275–89.
27. Treede RD, Jensen TS, Campbell JN, Cruccu G, Dostrovsky JO, Griffin JW, et al. Neuropathic pain: redefinition and a grading system for clinical and research purposes. Neurology. 2008;70:1630–5.
28. Cruccu G, Sommer C, Anand P, Attal N, Baron R, Garcia-Larrea L, et al. EFNS guidelines on neuropathic pain assessment: revised 2009. Eur J Neurol. 2010;17:1010–8.
29. Haanpää M, Attal N, Backonja M, Baron R, Bennett M, Bouhassira D, et al. NeuPSIG guidelines on neuropathic pain assessment. Pain. 2011;152:14–27.
30. Collins S, Sigtermans MJ, Dahan A, Zuurmond WW, Perez RS. NMDA receptor antagonists for the treatment of neuropathic pain. Pain Med. 2010;11:1726–42.
31. Baron R. Neuropathic pain: a clinical perspective. Handb Exp Pharmacol. 2009;194:3–30.
32. Jensen TS, Hansson PT. Classification of neuropathic pain syndromes based on symptoms and signs. In: Cervero F, Jensen TS, editors. Handbook of clinical neurology, vol. 81 (3rd series). Amsterdam: Elsevier; 2006. p. 517–26.
33. Knotkova H, Cruciani RA, Tronnier VM, Rasche D. Current and future options for the management of phantom-limb pain. J Pain Res. 2012;5:39–49.
34. Pluijms WA, Slangen RA, Joosten EA, Kessels AG, Merkies IS, Schaper NC, et al. Electrical spinal cord stimulation in painful diabetic polyneuropathy, a systematic review on treatment efficacy and safety. Eur J Pain. 2011;15:783–8.
35. Cioni B, Meglio M, Pentimalli L, Visocchi M. Spinal cord stimulation in the treatment of paraplegic pain. J Neurosurg. 1995;82:35–9.
36. Slipman CW, Shin CH, Patel RK, Isaac Z, Huston CW, Lipetz JS, et al. Etiologies of failed back surgery syndrome. Pain Med. 2002;3:200–14.
37. Chan CW, Peng P. Failed back surgery syndrome. Pain Med. 2011;12:577–606.
38. Turner-Stokes L, Goebel A, Guideline Development Group. Complex regional pain syndrome in adults: concise guidance. Clin Med. 2011;11:596–600.
39. Harden RN, Oaklander AL, Burton AW, Perez RS, Richardson K, Swan M, et al. Complex regional pain syndrome: practical diagnostic and treatment guidelines, 4th edition. Pain Med. 2013;14:180–229.
40. Stanton-Hicks M, Jänig W, Hassenbusch S, Haddox JD, Boas R, Wilson P. Reflex sympathetic dystrophy: changing concepts and taxonomy. Pain. 1995;63:127–33.
41. Bruehl S, Harden RN, Galer BS, Saltz S, Bertram M, Backonja M, et al. External validation of IASP diagnostic criteria for Complex Regional Pain Syndrome and proposed research diagnostic criteria. International Association for the Study of Pain. Pain. 1999;81:147–54.
42. Bruehl S. An update on the pathophysiology of complex regional pain syndrome. Anesthesiology. 2010;113:713–25.
43. Marinus J, Moseley GL, Birklein F, Baron R, Maihöfner C, Kingery WS, et al. Clinical features and pathophysiology of complex regional pain syndrome. Lancet Neurol. 2011;10:637–48.
44. Ali Z, Raja SN, Wesselmann U, Fuchs PN, Meyer RA, Campbell JN. Intradermal injection of norepinephrine evokes pain in patients with sympathetically maintained pain. Pain. 2000;88:161–8.
45. Baron R, Schattschneider J, Binder A, Siebrecht D, Wasner G. Relation between sympathetic vasoconstrictor activity and pain and hyperalgesia in complex regional pain syndromes: a case-control study. Lancet. 2002;359:1655–60.
46. Correll GE, Maleki J, Gracely EJ, Muir JJ, Harbut RE. Subanesthetic ketamine infusion therapy: a retrospective analysis of a novel therapeutic approach to complex regional pain syndrome. Pain Med. 2004;5:263–75.
47. Vartiainen NV, Kirveskari E, Forss N. Central processing of tactile and nociceptive stimuli in complex regional pain syndrome. Clin Neurophysiol. 2008;119:2380–8.
48. Harden RN. Objectification of the diagnostic criteria for CRPS. Pain Med. 2010;11:1212–5.
49. Albazaz R, Wong YT, Homer-Vanniasinkam S. Complex regional pain syndrome: a review. Ann Vasc Surg. 2008;22:297–306.
50. Poree L, Krames E, Pope J, Deer TR, Levy R, Schultz L. Spinal cord stimulation as treatment for complex regional pain syndrome should be considered earlier than last resort therapy. Neuromodulation. 2013;16:125–41.
51. Campbell CM, Jamison RN, Edwards RR. Psychological screening/phenotyping as predictors for spinal cord stimulation. Curr Pain Headache Rep. 2013;17:307.
52. Cook AW, Oygar A, Baggenstos P, Pacheco S, Kleriga E. Vascular disease of extremities. Electric stimulation of spinal cord and posterior roots. N Y State J Med. 1976;76:366–8.
53. Deer TR, Raso LJ. Spinal cord stimulation for refractory angina pectoris and peripheral vascular disease. Pain Physician. 2006;9:347–52.
54. Deer TR. Spinal cord stimulation for the treatment of angina and peripheral vascular disease. Curr Pain Headache Rep. 2009;13:18–23.
55. Mekhail NA, Cheng J, Narouze S, Kapural L, Mekhail MN, Deer T. Clinical applications of neurostimulation: forty years later. Pain Pract. 2010;10:103–12.
56. Francaviglia N, Silvestro C, Maiello M, Bragazzi R, Bernucci C. Spinal cord stimulation for the treatment of progressive systematic sclerosis and Raynaud's syndrome. Br J Neurosurg. 1994;8:567–71.
57. Sgueglia GA, Sestito A, Spinelli A, Cioni B, Infusino F, Papacci F, et al. Long-term follow-up of patients with cardiac syndrome X treated by spinal cord stimulation. Heart. 2007;93:591–7.

58. Murphy DF, Giles KE. Dorsal column stimulation for pain relief from intractable angina pectoris. Pain. 1987;28:365–8.
59. Buchser E, Durrer A, Albrecht E. Spinal cord stimulation for the management of refractory angina pectoris. J Pain Symptom Manage. 2006;31(Suppl):S36–42.
60. van Kleef M, Staats P, Mekhail N, Huygen F. 24. Chronic refractory angina pectoris. Pain Pract. 2011;11:476–82.
61. Börjesson M, Andréll P, Mannheimer C. Spinal cord stimulation for long-term treatment of severe angina pectoris: what does the evidence say? Future Cardiol. 2011;7:825–33.
62. Latif OA, Nedeljkovic SS, Stevenson LW. Spinal cord stimulation for chronic intractable angina pectoris: a unified theory on its mechanism. Clin Cardiol. 2001;24:533–41.
63. Foreman RD, Linderoth B, Ardell JL, Barron KW, Chandler MJ, Hull Jr SS, et al. Modulation of intrinsic cardiac neurons by spinal cord stimulation: implications for its therapeutic use in angina pectoris. Cardiovasc Res. 2000;47:367–75.
64. Ardell JL, Cardinal R, Vermeulen M, Armour JA. Dorsal spinal cord stimulation obtunds the capacity of intrathoracic extracardiac neurons to transduce myocardial ischemia. Am J Physiol Regul Integr Comp Physiol. 2009;297:R470–7.
65. Mannheimer C, Eliasson T, Andersson B, Bergh CH, Augustinsson LE, Emanuelsson H, et al. Effects of spinal cord stimulation in angina pectoris induced by pacing and possible mechanisms of action. BMJ. 1993;307:477–80.
66. Hautvast RW, Blanksma PK, DeJongste MJ, Pruim J, van der Wall EE, Vaalburg W, et al. Effect of spinal cord stimulation on myocardial blood flow assessed by positron emission tomography in patients with refractory angina pectoris. Am J Cardiol. 1996;77:462–7.
67. Linderoth B, Foreman RD. Physiology of spinal cord stimulation: review and update. Neuromodulation. 1999;2:150–64.
68. Jessurun GA, Hautvast RW, Tio RA, DeJongste MJ. Electrical neuromodulation improves myocardial perfusion and ameliorates refractory angina pectoris in patients with syndrome X: fad or future? Eur J Pain. 2003;7:507–12.
69. Armour JA. Myocardial ischaemia and the cardiac nervous system. Cardiovasc Res. 1999;41:41–54.
70. Cardinal R, Page P, Vermeulen M, Bouchard C, Ardell JL, Foreman RD, Armour JA. Spinal cord stimulation suppresses bradycardias and atrial tachyarrhythmias induced by mediastinal nerve stimulation in dogs. Am J Physiol Regul Integr Comp Physiol. 2006;291:R1369–75.
71. Linderoth B, Foreman RD. Mechanisms of spinal cord stimulation in painful syndromes: role of animal models. Pain Med. 2006;7:S14–26.
72. Börjesson M, Eriksson P, Dellborg M, Eliasson T, Mannheimer C. Transcutaneous electrical nerve stimulation in unstable angina pectoris. Coron Artery Dis. 1997;8:543–50.
73. Kunnumpurath S, Srinivasagopalan R, Vadivelu N. Spinal cord stimulation: principles of past, present and future practice: a review. J Clin Monit Comput. 2009;23:333–9.
74. Ooi YC, Falowski S, Wang D, Jallo J, Ho RT, Sharan A. Simultaneous use of neurostimulators in patients with a preexisting cardiovascular implantable electronic device. Neuromodulation. 2011;14:20–5.
75. Villavicencio AT, Leveque JC, Rubin L, Bulsara K, Gorecki JP. Laminectomy versus percutaneous electrode placement for spinal cord stimulation. Neurosurgery. 2000;46:399–405.
76. North RB, Kidd DH, Petrucci L, Dorsi MJ. Spinal cord stimulation electrode design: a prospective, randomized, controlled trial comparing percutaneous with laminectomy electrodes: part II–clinical outcomes. Neurosurgery. 2005;57:990–6.
77. North RB, Kidd DH, Olin JC, Sieracki JM. Spinal cord stimulation electrode design: prospective, randomized, controlled trial comparing percutaneous and laminectomy electrodes-part I: technical outcomes. Neurosurgery. 2002;51:381–9.
78. Logé D, De Coster O, Pollet W, Vancamp T. A novel percutaneous technique to implant plate-type electrodes. Minim Invasive Neurosurg. 2011;54:219–22.
79. Deer T, Bowman R, Schocket SM, Kim C, Ranson M, Amirdelfan K, et al. The prospective evaluation of safety and success of a new method of introducing percutaneous paddle leads and complex arrays with an epidural access system. Neuromodulation. 2012;15:21–9.
80. Mekhail NA, Mathews M, Nageeb F, Guirguis M, Mekhail MN, Cheng J. Retrospective review of 707 cases of spinal cord stimulation: indications and complications. Pain Pract. 2011;11:148–53.
81. Cameron T. Safety and efficacy of spinal cord stimulation for the treatment of chronic pain: a 20-year literature review. Safety and efficacy of spinal cord stimulation for the treatment of chronic pain: a 20-year literature review. J Neurosurg. 2004;100(3 Suppl Spine):254–67.
82. Turner JA, Loeser JD, Deyo RA, Sanders SB. Spinal cord stimulation for patients with failed back surgery syndrome or complex regional pain syndrome: a systematic review of effectiveness and complications. Pain. 2004;108:137–47.
83. Taylor RS, Van Buyten JP, Buchser E. Spinal cord stimulation for chronic back and leg pain and failed back surgery syndrome: a systematic review and analysis of prognostic factors. Spine. 2005;30:152–60.
84. Kumar K, Wilson JR, Taylor RS, Gupta S. Complications of spinal cord stimulation, suggestions to improve outcome, and financial impact. J Neurosurg Spine. 2006;5:191–203.
85. Kumar K, Wilson JR. Factors affecting spinal cord stimulation outcome in chronic benign pain with suggestions to improve success rate. Acta Neurochir Suppl. 2007;97(Pt 1):91–9.
86. Rainov NG, Heidecke V. Hardware failures in spinal cord stimulation (SCS) for chronic benign pain of spinal origin. Acta Neurochir Suppl. 2007;97(Pt 1):101–4.
87. Kumar K, Buchser E, Linderoth B, Meglio M, Van Buyten JP. Avoiding complications from spinal cord stimulation: practical recommendations from an international panel of experts. Neuromodulation. 2007;10:24–33.
88. Rathmell JP, Lake T, Ramundo MB. Infectious risks of chronic pain treatments: injection therapy, surgical implants, and intradiscal techniques. Reg Anesth Pain Med. 2006;31:346–52.
89. Levy R, Henderson J, Slavin K, Simpson BA, Barolat G, Shipley J, et al. Incidence and avoidance of neurologic complications with paddle type spinal cord stimulation leads. Neuromodulation. 2011;14:412–22.
90. Deer T, Stewart D. Complications of spinal cord stimulation: identification, treatment and prevention. Pain Med. 2008;9(S1): S93–101.
91. Boswell MV, Trescot AM, Datta S, Schultz DM, Hansen HC, Abdi S, et al. Interventional techniques: evidence-based practice guidelines in the management of chronic spinal pain. Pain Physician. 2007;10:627–50.
92. American Society of Anesthesiologists Task Force on Chronic Pain Management and the Society of Regional Anesthesia and Pain Medicine. Practice guidelines for chronic pain management: an updated report by the American Society of Anesthesiologists Task Force on Chronic Pain Management and the Society of Regional Anesthesia and Pain Medicine. Anesthesiology. 2010;112:810–33.
93. Van Zundert J, Hartrick C, Patijn J, Huygen F, Mekhail N, van Kleef M. Evidence-based interventional pain medicine according to clinical diagnoses. Pain Pract. 2013;11:423–9.
94. Frey ME, Manchikanti L, Benyamin RM, Schultz DM, Smith HS, Cohen SP. Spinal cord stimulation for patients with failed back surgery syndrome: a systematic review. Pain Physician. 2009;12:379–97.
95. Simpson EL, Duenas A, Holmes MW, Papaioannou D, Chilcott J. Spinal cord stimulation for chronic pain of neuropathic or

ischaemic origin: systematic review and economic evaluation. Health Technol Assess. 2009;13:1–154.
96. Van Boxem K, Cheng J, Patijn J, van Kleef M, Lataster A, Mekhail N, Van Zundert J. Evidence-based interventional pain medicine according to clinical diagnoses. 11. Lumbosacral radicular pain. Pain Pract. 2010;10:339–58.
97. North RB, Kidd DH, Farrokhi F, Piantadosi SA. Spinal cord stimulation versus repeated lumbosacral spine surgery for chronic pain: a randomized, controlled trial. Neurosurgery. 2005;56:98–106.
98. Kumar K, Taylor RS, Jacques L, Eldabe S, Meglio M, Molet J, et al. Spinal cord stimulation versus conventional medical management for neuropathic pain: a multicentre randomised controlled trial in patients with failed back surgery syndrome. Pain. 2007;132:179–88.
99. Kumar K, Taylor RS, Jacques L, Eldabe S, Meglio M, Molet J, et al. The effects of spinal cord stimulation in neuropathic pain are sustained: a 24-month follow-up of the prospective randomized controlled multicenter trial of the effectiveness of spinal cord stimulation. Neurosurgery. 2008;63:762–70.
100. Kumar K, Hunter G, Demeria D. Spinal cord stimulation in treatment of chronic benign pain: challenges in treatment planning and present status, a 22-year experience. Neurosurgery. 2006;58:481–96.
101. Van Buyten JP. Neurostimulation for chronic neuropathic back pain in failed back surgery syndrome. J Pain Symptom Manage. 2006;31 Suppl 4:S25–9.
102. Grabow TS, Tella PK, Raja SN. Spinal cord stimulation for complex regional pain syndrome: an evidence-based medicine review of the literature. Clin J Pain. 2003;19:371–83.
103. Taylor RS, Van Buyten JP, Buchser E. Spinal cord stimulation for complex regional pain syndrome: a systematic review of the clinical and cost-effectiveness literature and assessment of prognostic factors. Eur J Pain. 2006;10:91–101.
104. van Eijs F, Stanton-Hicks M, Van Zundert J, Faber CG, Lubenow TR, Mekhail N, van Kleef M, Huygen F. Evidence-based interventional pain medicine according to clinical diagnoses. 16. Complex regional pain syndrome. Pain Pract. 2011;11:70–87.
105. Cossins L, Okell RW, Cameron H, Simpson B, Poole HM, Goebel A. Treatment of complex regional pain syndrome in adults: a systematic review of randomized controlled trials published from June 2000 to February 2012. Eur J Pain. 2013;17:158–73.
106. Stanton-Hicks M. Complex regional pain syndrome: manifestations and the role of neurostimulation in its management. J Pain Symptom Manage. 2006;31 Suppl 4:S20–4.
107. Taylor RS. Spinal cord stimulation in complex regional pain syndrome and refractory neuropathic back and leg pain/failed back surgery syndrome: results of a systematic review and meta-analysis. J Pain Symptom Manage. 2006;31 Suppl 4:S13–9.
108. Kumar K, Rizvi S, Bnurs SB. Spinal cord stimulation is effective in management of complex regional pain syndrome I: fact or fiction. Neurosurgery. 2011;69:566–78.
109. Kemler MA, Barendse GA, van Kleef M, de Vet HC, Rijks CP, Furnée CA, et al. Spinal cord stimulation in patients with chronic reflex sympathetic dystrophy. N Engl J Med. 2000;343:618–24.
110. Kemler MA, De Vet HC, Barendse GA, Van Den Wildenberg FA, Van Kleef M. The effect of spinal cord stimulation in patients with chronic reflex sympathetic dystrophy: two years' follow-up of the randomized controlled trial. Ann Neurol. 2004;55:13–8.
111. Kemler MA, de Vet HC, Barendse GA, van den Wildenberg FA, van Kleef M. Spinal cord stimulation for chronic reflex sympathetic dystrophy–five-year follow-up. N Engl J Med. 2006;354:2394–6.
112. Kemler MA, de Vet HC, Barendse GA, van den Wildenberg FA, van Kleef M. Effect of spinal cord stimulation for chronic complex regional pain syndrome Type I: five-year final follow-up of patients in a randomized controlled trial. J Neurosurg. 2008;108:292–8.
113. Ubbink DT, Vermeulen H. Spinal cord stimulation for non-reconstructable chronic critical leg ischemia. Cochrane Database of Systematic Reviews 2009, (1)
114. Jivegård LE, Augustinsson LE, Holm J, Risberg B, Ortenwall P. Effects of spinal cord stimulation (SCS) in patients with inoperable severe lower limb ischaemia: a prospective randomised controlled study. Eur J Vasc Endovasc Surg. 1995;9:421–5.
115. Claeys LG, Horsch S. Transcutaneous oxygen pressure as predictive parameter for ulcer healing in endstage vascular patients treated with spinal cord stimulation. Int J Angiol. 1996;15:344–9.
116. Spincemaille GH, de Vet HC, Ubbink DT, Jacobs MJ. The results of spinal cord stimulation in critical limb ischaemia: a review. Eur J Vasc Endovasc Surg. 2001;21:99–105.
117. Amann W, Berg P, Gersbach P, Gamain J, Raphael JH, Ubbink DT. Spinal cord stimulation in the treatment of non-reconstructable stable critical leg ischaemia: results of the European peripheral vascular disease outcomes study (SCS-EPOS). Eur J Vasc Endovasc Surg. 2003;26:280–6.
118. Ubbink DT, Gersbach PA, Berg P, Amann W, Gamain J. The best TcpO(2) parameters to predict the efficacy of spinal cord stimulation to improve limb salvage in patients with inoperable critical leg ischemia. Int Angiol. 2003;22:356–63.
119. Devulder J, van Suijlekom H, van Dongen R, Diwan S, Mekhail N, van Kleef M, et al. Evidence-based interventional pain medicine according to clinical diagnoses. 25. Ischemic pain in the extremities and Rayanaud's phenomenon. Pain Pract. 2011;11:483–91.
120. Zipes DP, Svorkdal N, Berman D, Boortz-Marx R, Henry T, Lerman A, et al. Spinal cord stimulation therapy for patients with refractory angina who are not candidates for revascularization. Neuromodulation. 2012;15:550–8.
121. Lanza GA, Barone L, Di Monaco A. Effect of spinal cord stimulation in patients with refractory angina: evidence from observational studies. Neuromodulation. 2012;15:542–9.
122. Mannheimer C, Eliasson T, Augustinsson LE, Blomstrand C, Emanuelsson H, Larsson S, et al. Electrical stimulation versus coronary artery bypass surgery in severe angina pectoris: the ESBY study. Circulation. 1998;97:1157–63.
123. Ekre O, Eliasson T, Norrsell H, Währborg P, Mannheimer C. Electrical stimulation versus coronary artery bypass surgery in severe angina pectoris. Long-term effects of spinal cord stimulation and coronary artery bypass grafting on quality of life and survival in the ESBY study. Eur Heart J. 2002;23:1938–45.
124. McNab D, Khan SN, Sharples LD, Ryan JY, Freeman C, Caine N, et al. An open label, single-centre, randomized trial of spinal cord stimulation vs. percutaneous myocardial laser revascularization in patients with refractory angina pectoris: the SPiRiT trial. Eur Heart J. 2006;27:1048–53.
125. Dyer MT, Goldsmith KA, Khan SN, Sharples LD, Freeman C, Hardy I, et al. Clinical and cost-effectiveness analysis of an open label, single-centre, randomised trial of spinal cord stimulation (SCS) versus percutaneous myocardial laser revascularisation (PMR) in patients with refractory angina pectoris: the SPiRiT trial. Trials. 2008;9:40.
126. Börjesson M, Andrell P, Lundberg D, Mannheimer C. Spinal cord stimulation in severe angina pectoris–a systematic review based on the Swedish Council on Technology assessment in health care report on long-standing pain. Pain. 2008;140:501–8.
127. Taylor RS, De Vries J, Buchser E, Dejongste MJ. Spinal cord stimulation in the treatment of refractory angina: systematic review and meta-analysis of randomised controlled trials. BMC Cardiovasc Disord. 2009;9:13.

128. De Decker K, Beese U, Staal MJ, Dejongste MJ. Electrical neuromodulation for patients with cardiac diseases. Neth Heart J. 2013;21:91–4.
129. Murray S, Carson KG, Ewings PD, Collins PD, James MA. Spinal cord stimulation significantly decreases the need for acute hospital admission for chest pain in patients with refractory angina pectoris. Heart. 1999;82:89–92.
130. Andersen C, Hole P, Oxhøj H. Does pain relief with spinal cord stimulation for angina conceal myocardial infarction? Br Heart J. 1994;71:419–21.
131. Kumar K, Malik S, Demeria D. Treatment of chronic pain with spinal cord stimulation versus alternative therapies: cost-effectiveness analysis. Neurosurgery. 2002;51:106–15.
132. Manca A, Kumar K, Taylor RS, Jacques L, Eldabe S, Meglio M, et al. Quality of life, resource consumption and costs of spinal cord stimulation versus conventional medical management in neuropathic pain patients with failed back surgery syndrome (PROCESS trial). Eur J Pain. 2008;12:1047–58.
133. North RB, Kidd D, Shipley J, Taylor RS. Spinal cord stimulation versus reoperation for failed back surgery syndrome: a cost effectiveness and cost utility analysis based on a randomized, controlled trial. Neurosurgery. 2007;61:361–8.
134. Bala MM, Riemsma RP, Nixon J, Kleijnen J. Systematic review of the cost-effectiveness of spinal cord stimulation for people with failed back surgery syndrome. Clin J Pain. 2008;24:741–56.
135. Taylor RS, Ryan J, O'Donnell R, Eldabe S, Kumar K, North RB. The cost-effectiveness of spinal cord stimulation in the treatment of failed back surgery syndrome. Clin J Pain. 2010;26:463–9.
136. Mekhail N, Wentzel DL, Freeman R, Quadri H. Counting the costs: case management implications of spinal cord stimulation treatment for failed back surgery syndrome. Prof Case Manag. 2011;16:27–36.
137. Hollingworth W, Turner JA, Welton NJ, Comstock BA, Deyo RA. Costs and cost-effectiveness of spinal cord stimulation (SCS) for failed back surgery syndrome: an observational study in a workers' compensation population. Spine. 2011;36:2076–83.
138. Kemler MA, Raphael JH, Bentley A, Taylor RS. The cost-effectiveness of spinal cord stimulation for complex regional pain syndrome. Value Health. 2010;13:735–42.
139. Andréll P, Ekre O, Eliasson T, Blomstrand C, Börjesson M, Nilsson M, et al. Cost-effectiveness of spinal cord stimulation versus coronary artery bypass grafting in patients with severe angina pectoris—long-term results from the ESBY study. Cardiology. 2003;99:20–4.
140. Foletti A, Durrer A, Buchser E. Neurostimulation technology for the treatment of chronic pain: a focus on spinal cord stimulation. Expert Rev Med Devices. 2007;4:201–14.
141. Weiner RL, Reed KL. Peripheral neurostimulation for control of intractable occipital neuralgia. Neuromodulation. 1999;2:217–21.
142. Aló KM, Abramova MV, Richter EO. Percutaneous peripheral nerve stimulation. Prog Neurol Surg. 2011;24:41–57.
143. Young WB, Silberstein SD. Occipital nerve stimulation for primary headaches. Neurosurg Sci. 2012;56:307–12.
144. Mironer YE, Hutcheson JK, Satterthwaite JR, LaTourette PC. Prospective, two-part study of the interaction between spinal cord stimulation and peripheral nerve field stimulation in patients with low back pain: development of a new spinal-peripheral neurostimulation method. Neuromodulation. 2011;14:151–4.
145. Buiten MS, DeJongste MJ, Beese U, Kliphuis C, Durenkamp A, Staal MJ. Subcutaneous electrical nerve stimulation: a feasible and new method for the treatment of patients with refractory angina. Neuromodulation. 2011;14:258–65.
146. Koopmeiners AS, Mueller S, Kramer J, Hogan QH. Effect of electrical field stimulation on dorsal root ganglion neuronal function. Neuromodulation. 2013;16:304–11.
147. Deer TR, Grigsby E, Weiner RL, Wilcosky B, Kramer JM. A prospective study of dorsal root ganglion stimulation for the relief of chronic pain. Neuromodulation. 2013;16:67–71.
148. Van Buyten JP, Al-Kaisy A, Smet I, Palmisani S, Smith T. High-frequency spinal cord stimulation for the treatment of chronic back pain patients: results of a prospective multicenter European clinical study. Neuromodulation. 2013;16:59–65.
149. De Ridder D, Vanneste S, Plazier M, van der Loo E, Menovsky T. Burst spinal cord stimulation: toward paresthesia-free pain suppression. Neurosurgery. 2010;66:986–90.
150. Tesfaye S, Vileikyte L, Rayman G, Sindrup S, Perkins B, Baconja M, et al. Painful diabetic peripheral neuropathy: consensus recommendations on diagnosis, assessment and management. Diabetes Metab Res Rev. 2011;27:629–38.
151. Tesfaye S, Watt J, Benbow SJ, Pang KA, Miles J, MacFarlane IA, et al. Electrical spinal cord-stimulation for painful diabetic peripheral neuropathy. Lancet. 1996;348:1698–701.
152. Daousi C, Benbow SJ, MacFarlane IA. Electrical spinal cord stimulation in the long-term treatment of chronic painful diabetic neuropathy. Diabet Med. 2005;22:393–8.
153. de Vos CC, Rajan V, Steenbergen W, van der Aa HE, Buschman HP. Effect and safety of spinal cord stimulation for treatment of chronic pain caused by diabetic neuropathy. J Diabetes Complicat. 2009;23:40–5.
154. Pluijms WA, Slangen R, Bakkers M, Faber CG, Merkies IS, Kessels AG, et al. Pain relief and quality-of-life improvement after spinal cord stimulation in painful diabetic polyneuropathy: a pilot study. Br J Anaesth. 2012;109:623–9.
155. Raso AM. Results of electrostimulation of the spinal cord in Raynaud's disease and syndrome. J Mal Vasc. 1989;14:52–4. French.
156. North RB. Neurostimulation for pain of spinal origin. Clin Neurosurg. 2006;53:272–8.
157. Rigoard P, Delmotte A, D'Houtaud S, Misbert L, Diallo B, Roy-Moreau A, et al. Back pain: a real target for spinal cord stimulation? Neurosurgery. 2012;70:574–84.
158. Burgher AH, Huntoon MA, Turley TW, Doust MW, Stearns LJ. Subcutaneous peripheral nerve stimulation with inter-lead stimulation for axial neck and low back pain: case series and review of the literature. Neuromodulation. 2012;15:100–6.
159. Reverberi C, Dario A, Barolat G. Spinal cord stimulation (SCS) in conjunction with peripheral nerve field stimulation (PNfS) for the treatment of complex pain in failed back surgery syndrome (FBSS). Neuromodulation. 2013;16:78–82.
160. Levy RM. Spinal cord stimulation in 2020. Neuromodulation. 2013;16:93–6.
161. Schultz DM, Webster L, Kosek P, Dar U, Tan Y, Sun M. Sensor-driven position-adaptive spinal cord stimulation for chronic pain. Pain Physician. 2012;15:1–12.
162. Krames E, Poree L, Deer T, Levy R. Implementing the SAFE principles for the development of pain medicine therapeutic algorithms that include neuromodulation techniques. Neuromodulation. 2009;12:104–13.
163. Krames ES, Monis S, Poree L, Deer T, Levy R. Using the SAFE principles when evaluating electrical stimulation therapies for the pain of failed back surgery syndrome. Neuromodulation. 2011;14:299–311.
164. Eisenberg E, McNicol ED, Carr DB. Efficacy and safety of opioid agonists in the treatment of neuropathic pain of nonmalignant origin: systematic review and meta-analysis of randomized controlled trials. JAMA. 2005;293:3043–52.
165. Pohl M, Smith L. Chronic pain and addiction: challenging co-occurring disorders. J Psychoactive Drugs. 2012;44:119–24.
166. de Leon-Casasola OA. Opioids for chronic pain: new evidence, new strategies, safe prescribing. Am J Med. 2013;126(3 Suppl 1): S3–11.

Dorsal Root Ganglion Stimulation: A Target for Neuromodulation Therapies

5

A. Liong Liem, Imre Poldino Krabbenbos, and Jeffery Kramer

Role of the Dorsal Root Ganglion in Chronic Pain

Embryologically stemming from the neural crest, the primary sensory neuron (PSN) begins as a pseudounipolar cell (a single soma with 2 axons) and forms into its final anatomical phenotype as a pseudounipolar neuron. The primary sensory neurons form a ganglion located within the epidural space in the spine known as the spinal ganglion or more commonly referred to as the dorsal root ganglion (DRG) [1]. The somas of the PSNs are housed within the DRG. Other support cells such as satellite glia are also present to provide metabolic and trophic support. Also supporting the relatively high metabolic rate of cells in the DRG is a vast microvasculature complex [2].

Anatomically, the location of the dorsal root ganglion is within the spinal canal (typically within the neural foramina) [3, 4]. In general, the ganglion is located within the medial and lateral borders of the spinal pedicles—just inferior to the superior pedicle. Some authors have noted that the ganglion was overwhelmingly located between these anatomical boarders. Rarely the ganglion could be just slightly adjacent to these. Moreover, the ganglia have been noted to assume not just an oblong morphology but also bi- and tri-ganglionic shapes.

A single DRG is located bilaterally at each spinal level, and the neurons within the ganglia innervate specific regions of the body. The area of the dermis which is innervated by a specific ganglion is known as a dermatome. Origins and first work on the sensory dermatomes date back to the eighteenth century when "loss-of-function" techniques were used to determine how sensory input was organized at the spinal level [5]. Classic dermatome maps are now currently used to track sensory input to particular spinal levels—and this helps physicians target interventional therapies. Neurosurgical interventions complemented these early experiments and added information about the divergence of sensory inputs from peripheral structures. Often in cases where dorsal root ganglionectomies or dorsal root rhizotomies were performed, multiple levels would need to be targeted at the same time in order to reliably cover a painful region. However, the treatment would often fail to provide long-term relief as the nervous system was significantly altered, and secondary physiologic mechanisms would provide a platform for the return of pain (Fig. 5.1).

Phylogenetically, the formation of ganglia, including spinal dorsal root ganglia (DRG), peripheral ganglia and also the brain as a large ganglion, was also recognized as an important integrative development which allowed cells to form complex connections within a discrete location.

The role of the dorsal root ganglion in the development and maintenance of chronic pain has been a topic of investigation for some time and in the last decade has become a "hot topic" [1, 6, 7]. In general, both the early and later stages of injury or neuroinflammatory activation are characterized by several pathophysiologic alterations in PSN function. Alterations in sodium channel expression and function and increased production of neuroinflammatory intermediates all have an impact on the basic membrane excitability of the PSNs. As these cells become hyperexcitable, the threshold for generating action potentials is lowered which in turn produces a heightened "painful" input into the spinal cord. Neurons in the DRG also have been shown to produce ectopic, or spontaneous, action potentials that are generally not observed in healthy conditions. The secondary ramifications of this overactivity and increased action potential generation are manifested at the first synapse in the dorsal horn of the spinal cord.

A.L. Liem (✉) • I.P. Krabbenbos
Department of Anaesthesiology, Intensive Care and Pain Medicine, St. Antonius Hospital Nieuwegein, Koekoekslaan 1, 3435 CM, Nieuwegein, The Netherlands
e-mail: l.liem@antoniusziekenhuis.nl

J. Kramer
Spinal Modulation Inc., Menlo Park, CA, USA

College of Medicine, University of Illinois, Peoria, IL, USA

H. Knotkova and D. Rasche (eds.), *Textbook of Neuromodulation*,
DOI 10.1007/978-1-4939-1408-1_5, © Springer Science+Business Media, LLC 2015

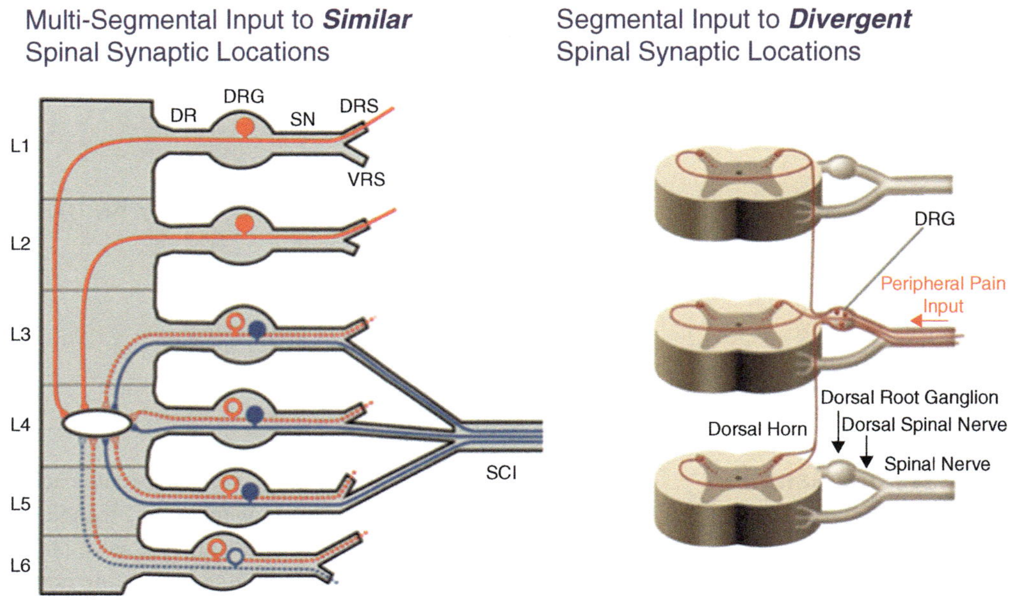

Fig. 5.1 Both divergent and convergence of sensory input have been documented. *Left* figure demonstrated the convergence of sensory input into the CNS. Ganglionectomies performed in the 1970s and 1980s documented this associated with multilevel sensory input. *Right panel* depicts the divergence of sensory input from a single level then synapsing at multiple spinal levels within the dorsal horn

Increased excitatory amino acid release, neuropeptide release, and a host of other secondary neuroinflammatory cascades result from the effects on the DRG. Thus, the PSNs in the DRG contribute both to the development and maintenance of chronic pain conditions.

Interventional Techniques Targeting the DRG

As the dorsal root ganglion has long been recognized as playing a critical role in the transfer of sensory information (including nociceptive neural signals), it is not surprising that previous therapies have and continue to focus on this neural structure. Several reviews have been published on the role of ganglionectomy [8, 9] as well as radiofrequency and pulsed radiofrequency [10–15]. Although transforaminal drug delivery is still consistently utilized, it is unclear what direct effect the agents are having on cells in the DRG and given the amount of spread into the epidural space could possibly compound effects on other structures.

While various techniques have been safely and effectively used to target the DRG, the effects of these treatments are often relatively short lived and in many patients require repeated administration. Repeated therapies may show a reduction in effectiveness over time. A longer-term solution is to provide a technique that provides sustained or prolonged effect on the DRG. Recent work by Koopermeiners et al. have demonstrated that neurostimulation of PSNs provides distinct alterations in membrane function [16]. Reduction of membrane excitability and alteration of the filtering function of the "T-junction" are potential mechanisms of action explaining how neurostimulation may provide pain relief. Although data are lacking it is likely that there are also effects at the DRG in addition to the upstream and downstream effects previously documented for other neurostimulation modalities [17, 18].

One possible technique is to use electrical stimulation to modulate PSN function. Within the central nervous system (CNS), this strategy is used to target different neural tissues including cortices in the brain, deeper brain structures, dorsal columns in the spine, and sacral spinal nerves. Very few case reports have previously been published regarding stimulation of the DRG in the treatment of chronic pain. There are conflicting reports on the effectiveness of the therapy, and this is likely due partly to differences in implantation techniques and also due to the fact that the equipment being used was not designed to target the DRG. On the whole, the stimulation leads used in earlier reports were designed for an epidural midline approach and for targeting the dorsal columns. The contact size and spacing are inappropriate for the smaller target—this is important to remember when considering the potential limitations of earlier work in this area.

Recently, a new system was created which is specifically designed for stimulating the DRG. This system comprises a delivery system, a temporary neurostimulator, and a fully implantable pulse generator. Similar to previous systems, leads are placed through a 14 g needle. Leads are then placed into the epidural space and guided toward the lateral recesses and to the neural foramen. Multiple needle approaches are

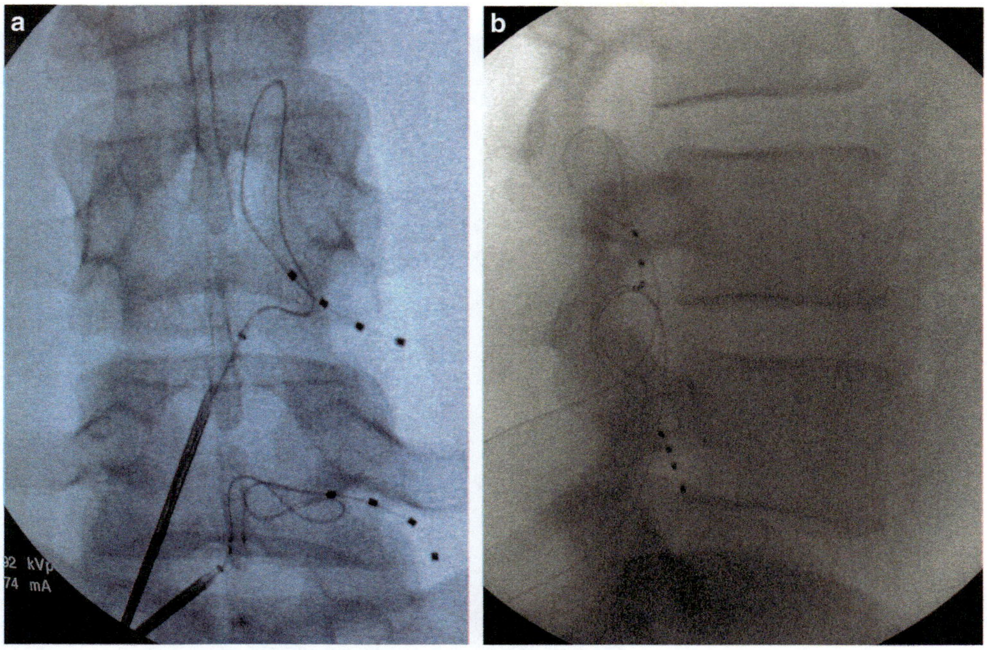

Fig. 5.2 X-rays of implanted neurostimulation system for SCS of the DRG. (**a**) Anterior and (**b**) lateral views

available for delivering leads including a classic paramedian approach as well as a contralateral approach. Both of these techniques allow for accurate lead delivery while providing flexibility in the approach methodology in individual patients. The quadripolar leads are comprised of four contacts enabling configuration of individual contact polarities as well as configuration of typical pulse parameters including pulse width, pulse amplitude, and pulse frequency (Fig. 5.2).

Case 1: Neuropathic Groin Pain

A 44-year-old patient suffered severe neuropathic pain in his left groin following a surgical procedure to release a torsed testicle. He was unable to continue his work as a manual laborer due to persistent pain, depressed mood, and reduced quality of life. After numerous treatment failures, he received a SCS device with initial satisfactory pain alleviation. However, 4 years later reimplantation had to be performed because of lead breakage. Unfortunately this did not result in adequate long-term pain relief due to the inability of reaching the target area. Finally, a single L2 lead for SCS of the left DRG was placed epidurally. After successful trial stimulation, he was implanted with a permanent device (Fig. 5.3). Induced paresthesia covered 100 % of the painful area. Within the first week, he reported an 88 % reduction in VAS pain intensity. During follow-up he reported excellent pain relief and did not feel the paresthesia since the stimulation was subthreshold. His sleep quality improved significantly and he is currently planning to return to work.

Case 2: Postamputation Pain

A 45-year-old female experienced cruciate ligament rupture after a horse riding accident. Her recovery was complicated with the development of muscular atrophy and therapy-resistant pain of the left leg. Progressive severe wound infection of the left foot and multiple treatment failures eventually led to amputation of the lower limb. She subsequently underwent several surgical interventions because of postamputation pain due to neuroma formation. Despite this, severe neuropathic stump pain continued to be a problem. Determined a candidate for SCS, a device was implanted which provided satisfactory pain relief. Despite initially promising results, clinical effects declined over time. SCS leads were placed epidurally at the left L3 and L4 DRGs (Fig. 5.4). SCS of the L3 and L4 DRG provided excellent paresthesia coverage and almost complete pain relief. The patient was able to resume activities of daily life at home.

The largest pilot study conducted and published on stimulation of the DRG in the treatment of chronic pain offered evidence of significant pain relief [19]. This initial study demonstrated that 7/9 subjects patients receiving a stimulation system would have gone on to have the fully implantable system if it had been available at that time. Average overall pain relief was 70 %, with subjects obtaining excellent pain relief in a variety of anatomical locations including the leg, foot, and lower back. Anecdotal observations were made as well. Firstly, 2/4 subjects described excellent pain relief despite the fact that they had previously failed traditional spinal cord stimulation.

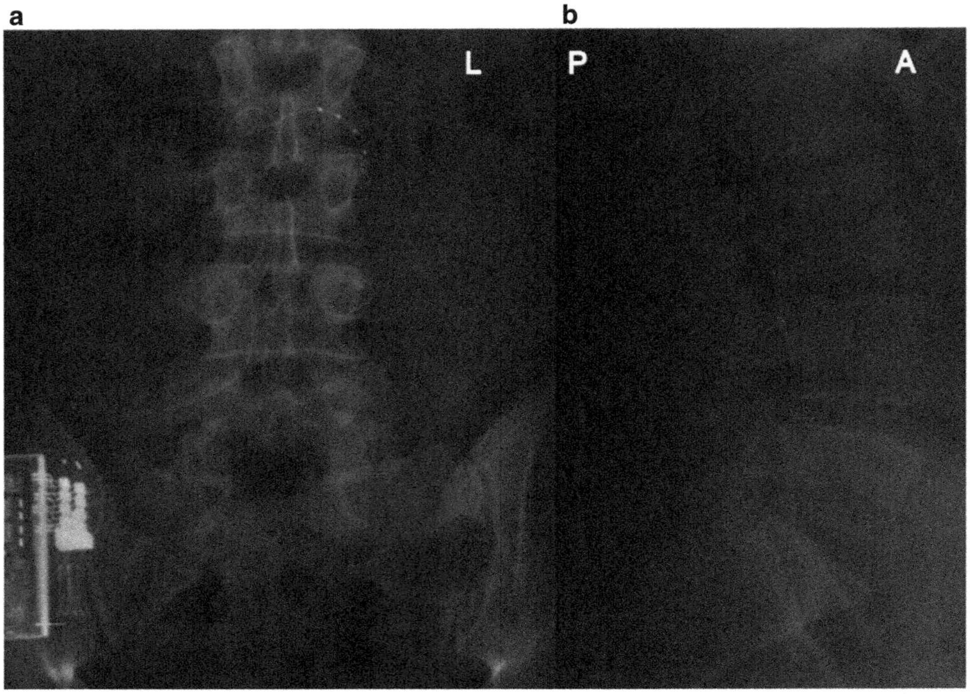

Fig. 5.3 Anterior (**a**) and (**b**) lateral X-ray views

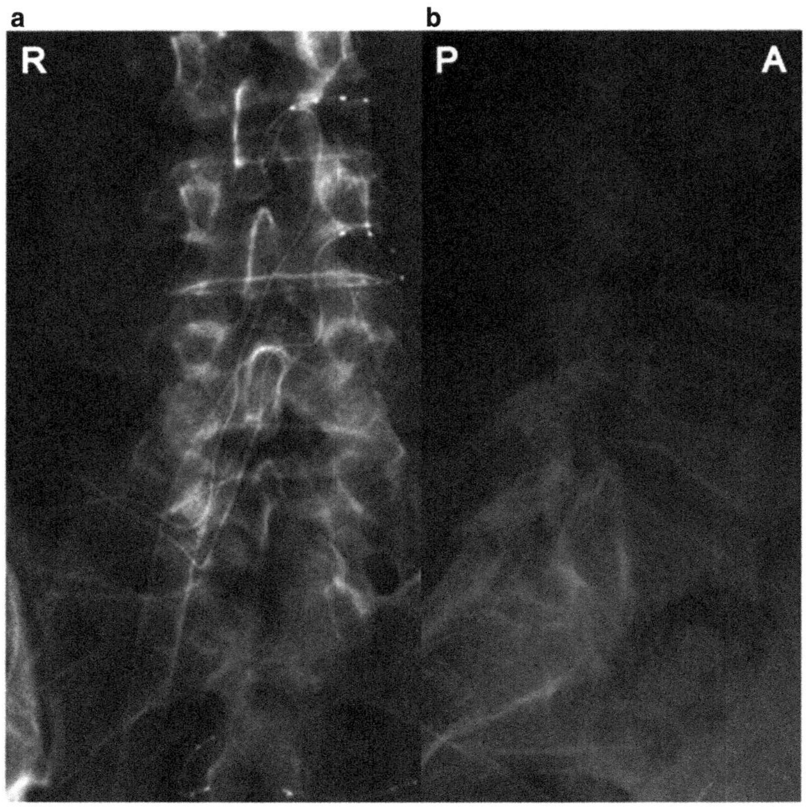

Fig. 5.4 Anterior (**a**) and lateral (**b**) X-ray views

Secondly, little to no postural effects were observed. That is, if the patient moved from an upright to recumbent position, there was little change in stimulation intensity. Thirdly, very discrete anatomical regions of therapy delivery could be achieved by stimulating the dorsal root ganglia. These findings were attributed to the fact that the leads were near the individual ganglion thus permitting precise targeting of the painful anatomical location and also because the electrical fields could be shaped around the ganglia in such a way as to produce subdermatomal specificity.

Table 5.1 Subject by subject results from the first prospective pilot study utilizing technology described in the text

Subject	Diagnosis	#Leads	Lead positions	% Pain relief
1	Discogenic LBP with lower extremity radiculopathy	3	L4–L5, L5–S1	100
2	LBP with lower extremity radiculopathy	2	L4–L5, L5–S1	100
3	LBP with lower extremity radiculopathy	4	L3, L4, L5	99
4	Diabetic peripheral neuropathy (foot)	2	L4, L5	80
5	Discogenic LBP with left leg radiculopathy	3	L4–L5, L5–S1, S1	67
6	Discogenic LBP with lower extremity radiculopathy	4	L4–L5, L5–S1	67
7	LBP with right leg radiculopathy	2	L4–L5, L5–S1	32
8	Peripheral neuropathy (foot, ankle)	2	L4–L5, L5–S1	17
9	Postherpetic neuralgia (chest, back)	3	T2–T3, T3, T6	*
10	Neuropathic chest pain	3	T12, T10, T8	**

*Did not complete all follow-up visits
**Did not complete baseline visual analog scale

Larger prospective, multicenter trials are currently being conducted to strengthen the levels of evidence available for this therapy.

The ganglia, as previously mentioned, are located within the spinal canal. As the dorsal nerve root extends laterally, a nerve root sheath extends over and around the DRG that eventually becomes the spinal nerve epineurium. Because the amount of cerebrospinal fluid (CSF) that circulates around the DRG is minimal compared to the level of CSF that is present within the midline spinal canal, a significant source of energy sink is eliminated. This coupled with the fact that the electrodes are closer to the anatomical target explains why stimulation settings are relatively low (Table 5.1).

Case 3: Complex Regional Pain Syndrome

A 66-year-old male developed CRPS type I with intractable neuropathic pain after knee replacement surgery. The pain was localized in the area of the left knee and lower leg. He received multiple unsuccessful treatments including a SCS system, but the induced paresthesia did not reach the target area and produced unacceptable postural effects. The patient was determined a candidate for SCS of the DRG. Two leads were successfully placed at the level of the left L4 and L5 DRG (Fig. 5.5). Prior to this, the patient experienced considerable sleep disturbance and chronic daily fatigue. The treatment resulted in complete pain relief and substantially improved sleep.

Case 4: Failed Back Surgery Syndrome

A 38-year-old patient reported a 16-year history of pain in his lower back and right leg following surgical treatment of an L4–L5 herniated nucleus pulposus (HNP). Subsequent epidural injections only provided temporary relief. Overall VAS pain intensity score pretreatment was 80 mm. Determined a candidate for SCS of the DRG, two leads were placed epidurally to stimulate the left and right L2 DRGs (Fig. 5.6) two levels above the back surgery site (surgery site at L4–L5). No complications were noted. Stimulation resulted in 100 % coverage of his pain area with minimal extraneous stimulation in non-painful areas. The patient did not experience significant changes in perceived stimulation level while standing up and/or lying down and at his 1-month follow-up visit reported an overall pain reduction of 97.5 %.

Conclusions

Our understanding of the role of the primary sensory neurons in the development and maintenance of chronic pain—of varying diagnoses and etiologies—has significantly increased over the past decade. The membrane properties of these cells are altered which in turn results in an enhanced state of excitability involving multiple ion channels, second messenger systems, and other physiological changes. These membrane alterations provide a fundamental opportunity to direct the delivery of therapy to a specific region of pathology as opposed to an upstream or downstream area as is so often the case in palliative neuromodulation techniques.

Previous techniques targeting the DRG have yielded excellent results demonstrating not only the safety of targeting the DRG but also the potential opportunity for developing techniques that can provide longer-lasting pain relief. Preliminary results from completed and ongoing prospective studies suggest that DRG stimulation can provide good pain relief while avoiding the unwanted side effects of current neurostimulation techniques. Several ongoing prospective studies will contribute to elucidating the potential mechanisms of action and the clinical implications of neurostimulation of the DRG. Clinical experience with the administration of DRG stimulation in the elderly is limited. However,

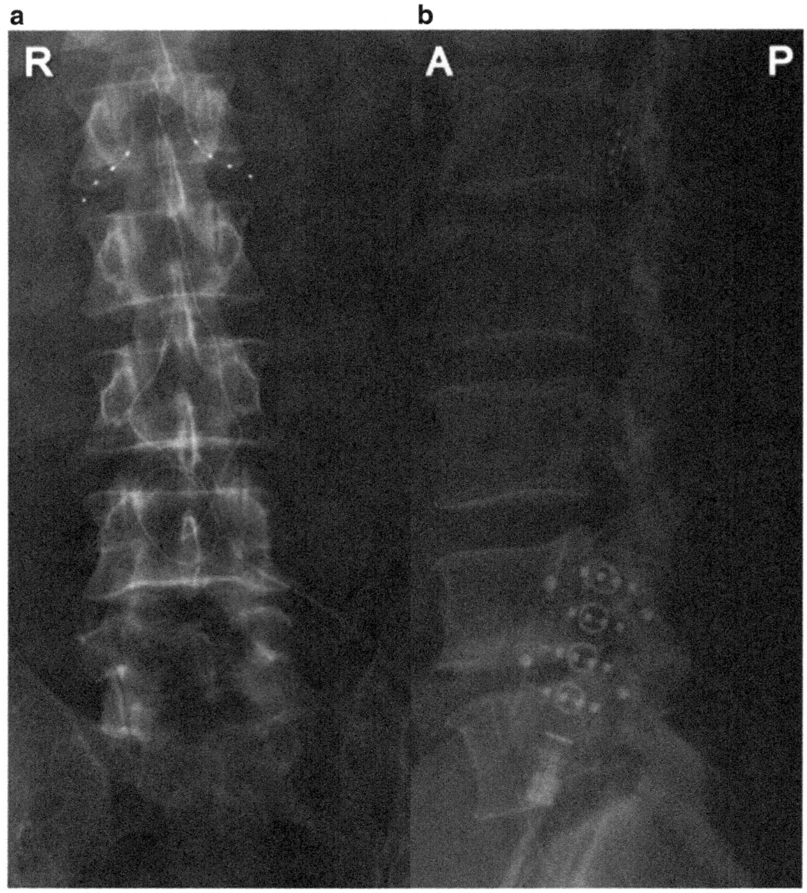

Fig. 5.5 Anterior (**a**) and (**b**) lateral X-ray views

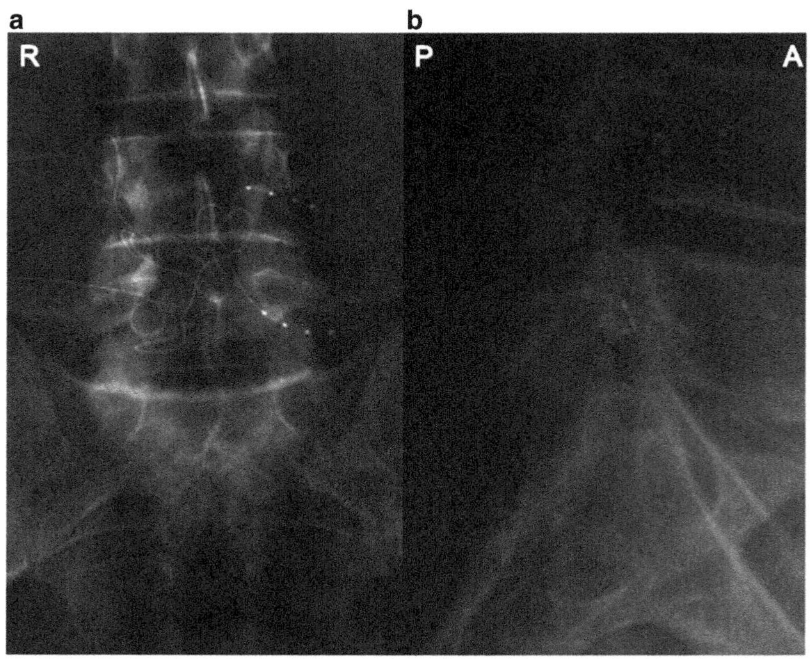

Fig. 5.6 Anterior (**a**) and (**b**) lateral X-ray views

neuromodulation treatments are of particular interest to the management of pain in geriatric patients. DRG stimulation has the potential to reduce the need for heavy medication use and thereby minimize unwanted side effects associated with larger drug doses.

References

1. Hogan QH. Labat lecture: the primary sensory neuron: where it is, what it does, and why it matters. Reg Anesth Pain Med. 2010;35 (3):306–11.
2. Kobayashi S, Mwaka ES, Baba H, et al. Microvascular system of the lumbar dorsal root ganglia in rats. Part I: a 3D analysis with scanning electron microscopy of vascular corrosion casts. J Neurosurg Spine. 2010;12(2):197–202.
3. Hasegawa T, Mikawa Y, Watanabe R, An HS. Morphometric analysis of the lumbosacral nerve roots and dorsal root ganglia by magnetic resonance imaging. Spine. 1996;21(9):1005–9.
4. Shen J, Wang HY, Chen JY, Liang BL. Morphologic analysis of normal human lumbar dorsal root ganglion by 3D MR imaging. AJNR. 2006;27(10):2098–103.
5. Greenberg SA. The history of dermatome mapping. Arch Neurol. 2003;60(1):126–31.
6. Waxman SG. The molecular pathophysiology of pain: abnormal expression of sodium channel genes and its contributions to hyperexcitability of primary sensory neurons. Pain. 1999;82(S1): S133–40.
7. Sapunar D, Kostic S, Banozic A, Puljak L. Dorsal root ganglion – a potential new therapeutic target for neuropathic pain. J Pain Res. 2012;5:31–8.
8. Cetas JS, Saedi T, Burchiel KJ. Destructive procedures for the treatment of nonmalignant pain: a structured literature review. J Neurosurg. 2008;109(3):389–404.
9. Wilkinson HA, Chan AS. Sensory ganglionectomy: theory, technical aspects, and clinical experience. J Neurosurg. 2001;95(1):61–6.
10. Van Boxem K, Cheng J, Patijn J, et al. 11. Lumbosacral radicular pain. Pain Pract. 2010;10(4):339–58.
11. Nagda JV, Davis CW, Bajwa ZH, Simopoulos TT. Retrospective review of the efficacy and safety of repeated pulsed and continuous radiofrequency lesioning of the dorsal root ganglion/ segmental nerve for lumbar radicular pain. Pain Physician. 2011;14 (4):371–6.
12. Chua NH, Vissers KC, Sluijter ME. Pulsed radiofrequency treatment in interventional pain management: mechanisms and potential indications-a review. Acta Neurochir. 2011;153(4):763–71.
13. Van Zundert J, Huntoon M, Patijn J, Lataster A, Mekhail N, van Kleef M. 4. Cervical radicular pain. Pain Pract. 2010;10(1):1–17.
14. van Boxem K, van Eerd M, Brinkhuizen T, Patijn J, van Kleef M, van Zundert J. Radiofrequency and pulsed radiofrequency treatment of chronic pain syndromes: the available evidence. Pain Pract. 2008;8(5):385–93.
15. Malik K, Benzon HT. Radiofrequency applications to dorsal root ganglia: a literature review. Anesthesiology. 2008;109(3):527–42.
16. Koopmeiners AS, Mueller S, Kramer J, Hogan QH. Effect of electrical field stimulation on dorsal root ganglion neuronal function. Neuromodulation. 2013;16(4):304–11.
17. Linderoth B, Foreman RD. Physiology of spinal cord stimulation: review and update. Neuromodulation. 1999;2(3):150–64.
18. Wu M, Linderoth B, Foreman RD. Putative mechanisms behind effects of spinal cord stimulation on vascular diseases: a review of experimental studies. Auton Neurosci. 2008;138(1–2):9–23.
19. Deer TR, Grigsby E, Weiner RL, Wilcosky B, Kramer JM. A prospective study of dorsal root ganglion stimulation for the relief of chronic pain. Neuromodulation. 2013;16(1):67–71. discussion 71-62.

Deep Brain Stimulation

6

Volker M. Tronnier and Dirk Rasche

Introduction

While deep brain stimulation (DBS) is meanwhile an established therapy treating different forms of movement disorders as Parkinson's disease, dystonias, or tremor, it has to be stressed that originally about 60 years ago, DBS was performed to treat otherwise intractable pain syndromes [1–3], even before the so-called gate control theory [4] was created which lead to the development of more peripheral stimulation techniques as spinal cord or peripheral nerve stimulation. At about the same time, based on the studies by Albe-Fessard, Krüger [5–7] and others, Mazars described the stimulation of the neospinothalamic pathway at its termination in the somatosensory thalamus [8]. Animal research in the late 60ies lead to the concept of "stimulation analgesia" [9] and to the initial trials with stimulation in the periaqueductal (PAG) or periventricular grey (PVG) [10, 11]. In 1970s and 1980s of the last century many uncontrolled studies were performed with DBS either in the lateral somatosensory thalamus and/or the medial periventricular structures [12]. A meta-analysis about the published studies until then, performed in 1991, summarizing the clinical results and critically evaluating the selection and outcome criteria [13] as well as the result of two multicenter studies demonstrating either no long-term reproducible pain relief or had to be closed early because of slow enrollment and high drop-outs [14], finally lead to a missing approval by the FDA and to a marked decrease of usage of this technique. Only few centers in the US or Europe continued to offer DBS for the treatment of chronic pain thereafter [15–17]. However, the success of DBS for movement disorders, epilepsy, and psychiatric disorders as well as the better understanding of pain pathophysiology leads to a renewed interest of this technique for the treatment of intractable pain.

V.M. Tronnier (✉)
Department of Neurological Surgery, University Hospital Lübeck, Ratzeburger Allee 160, Lübeck D-23538, Germany
e-mail: volker.tronnier@uksh.de

D. Rasche
Department of Neurosurgery, University of Lübeck, University Hospital of Schleswig-Holstein, Campus Lübeck, Lübeck, Germany

Mechanism of Action

Stimulation of the Lateral Somatosensory Thalamus

The somatosensory thalamus (VPL = nucl. Ventropostero-lateralis and VPM = nucl. ventroposteromedialis) is the major terminal of the neospinothalamic tract and is considered the important relay for pain processing to areas 3b/1 of the cortex. It is proposed that neurons in the lateral thalamus receive input from nociceptive specific neurons in lamina I of the dorsal horn as well as wide dynamic range neurons (WDR) of lamina V, which send gradually increased signals depending on the activity of primary nociceptive or non-nociceptive afferents. Therefore, these thalamocortical relay neurons signal either acute pain or generate symptoms of central pain syndromes due to alterations in their activity. Increased neuronal bursting activity has been found in pain due to deafferentation or central pain syndromes [18–28]. This increased neuronal firing parallels the clinical findings in central pain syndromes with lesions in the somatosensory pathways and the occurrence of spontaneous and evoked pain to noxious (hyperalgesia) and innocuous (allodynia) stimuli [29]. It was demonstrated that after lesioning this pathway a somatotopic reorganization in the somatosensory thalamus takes place and that a mismatch between receptive fields and projection fields evoked by microstimulation develops [30]. Stimulation of VPL inhibits spinothalamic tract neurons in the dorsal horn of monkeys [31, 32] and is able to reduce mechanical allodynia in an animal model using a partial nerve injury [33].

H. Knotkova and D. Rasche (eds.), *Textbook of Neuromodulation*,
DOI 10.1007/978-1-4939-1408-1_6, © Springer Science+Business Media, LLC 2015

Stimulation of the Periventricular or Periaqueductal Grey

The mechanism of pain modulation with PAG/PVG stimulation is mainly related to an opioid dependent pathway, although also nonopioid dependent mechanisms are involved [34, 35]. A detailed review of the descending inhibitory control mechanisms for the suppression of pain is given by Millan in 2002 [36]. From animal research, the phenomenon of "stimulation produced analgesia" (SPA) was originally coined by Reynolds in 1969 [9]. Further studies revealed that SPA was at least partially reversed by the opiate antagonist naloxone and a cross-tolerance between exogenously given opiates and PAG stimulation could be demonstrated [37, 38]. Elevation of endogenous opioids, such as ß-endorphin and met-enkephalin, has been found in patients after PAG and PVG stimulation but not after VPL stimulation [39–43, 86]. SPA was proven to be effective in acute and chronic pain states in humans [10, 11, 44–46]. The neural substrates of this endogenous analgesia pathway include the PVG, parts of the PAG (sending projections to the rostroventral medulla), the nucleus raphe magnus and the magnocellular part of the nucleus reticularis gigantocellularis [37, 47, 87]. Stimulation of this pathway is able to inhibit spinothalamic tract neurons in the dorsal horn [48–50] mainly via serotoninergic descending inhibition. Sectioning of this pathway in the dorsolateral funiculus in the rat has shown to increase the response to noxious stimuli [51]. Our group was able to demonstrate that stimulation of the PVG could inhibit neuronal activity in VPL neurons in humans [34].

Stimulation of CM-PF Thalamic Nuclei

The nomenclature of the centre median -parafascicular complex of the thalamus is derived from Jules Bernard Luys [52] and Oskar and Cecile Vogt [53]. This complex is integrated to the intralaminar thalamic nuclei and was considered as a surgical target for lesioning [54] and stimulation [12, 55].

While the neospinothalamic pathways primarily aim towards the lateral somatosensory thalamus, the paleospinothalamic pathways have several relay stations within the brainstem and the diencephalon before reaching the associative and limbic cortex (insula, cingulum) [56–58]. At least in the medial and intralaminar nuclei spontaneous hyperactivity due to deafferentation was demonstrated [59–61] and nociceptive neurons were described [5, 62]. Newer binding studies with calbindin and parvalbumin did not confirm a single specialized nucleus (Vmpo) which exclusively yields terminations of nociceptive and thermoceptive fibers [63–65]. Somatosensory thalamic stimulation in rat has been shown to inhibit neuronal activity in CM-PF complex [66, 67].

Stimulation of the Posteromedial Hypothalamus

The rationale for stimulation of the posteromedial hypothalamus for the treatment of trigeminoautonomic headaches (chronic cluster headache, shortlasting unilateral neualgiform headache with conjunctival injection and tearing [SUNCT]) originates from functional neuroimaging and volumetric studies during cluster attacks [68–71], although this target was already much earlier considered for the treatment of intractable pain [72, 73]. It is hypothesized that descending antinociceptive activation of the trigeminocervical complex and the PAG leads to changes in the pain matrix [74–76].

Operative Technique

The implantation of permanent electrodes for the treatment of chronic pain follows in general the most recent recommendations for DBS for movement disorders [77] in 19 steps. However, a testing trial for 7–14 days is strongly recommended. The advantage of subthreshold stimulation and blinding the patient and even the physician/nurse who calls up the different pain scales makes it possible to markedly rule out placebo effects as false-positive responders.

Step 1: Preoperative Imaging (Without Frame)

A preoperative MRI whenever possible should be performed before surgery. In cases with implanted cardiac pacemakers, a CT scan can be performed. This imaging information is necessary to rule out structural changes of the patients' brain (tumor, arterio-venous [AV] malformation, ventriculomegaly). In cases with post-stroke pain, the intended target could be involved in the lesion.

Step 2: Stereotactic Frame Placement

The frame can be applied either in the operating room (OR) in anesthesia stand-by or local anesthesia or in the radiological unit. Having anesthesia in the magnetic resonance (MR) environment usually prolongs the procedure. It has been demonstrated that two occipital (n. occipitalis major and minor) as well as supraorbital blocks before starting the procedure are advantageous [78]. If necessary, additional local anesthetics can be applied around the pins of the frame (mixture of short and long acting local anesthetic). The frame should be placed parallel to the orbitomeatal line. The commercial software programs are usually able to correct any tilts but only to a certain amount.

Table 6.1 Target coordinates

Target	*X*-coordinate	*Y*-coordinate	*Z*-coordinate	Comments
VPL	16–18 mm laterally	3–5 mm in front of PC	0–2 mm below AC-PC line	Arm more medial than leg
VPM	10–12 mm laterally	3–5 mm in front of PC	0–2 mm below AC-PC line	
CM-PF	7–8 mm lateral	8–9 mm behind mid.AC-PC	At AC-PC line	
PVG	2 mm laterally. ventricular wall	2–3 mm in front of PC	2 mm above—2 mm below AC-PC line	Below often ocular symptoms
PAG	2–3 mm laterally	2 mm behind PC	2–4 mm below AC-PC line	Diplopia
Post. Hypothal.	2 mm laterally ventricular wall	2–3 mm post mid AC-PC	5 mm below AC-PC line	

Step 3: Magnetic Resonance Imaging with Frame

This is nowadays performed with a 1.5T or 3T MR scanner. Usually, a three-dimensional (3D) T1-weighted with contrast enhancement is carried out. A double dose of contrast media allows also the delineation of small vessels, especially in the hypothalamic area. Unfortunately, a delineation of the different thalamic nuclei is not possible with these field strengths. First promising results of parcellation of the thalamus are yielded with 7T-MRI [79].

Step 4: Presurgical Target Planning

This is either performed at the MRI console or with the available planning system. Depending on the type and localization of pain the targets are planned and "visionalized" on the screen. Usually, the reference is still the anterior commissure-posterior commissure (AC-PC) line or the mid AC-PC point, because, in contrast to other structures as the STN or GPI, the desired targets are not "directly" visible (see above).

Step 5: Presurgical Trajectory Planning

Planning the trajectory makes planning of the entry point necessary. This is much easier with a center of arc system (e.g., Leksell, ZD, CRW). The software system allows a stepwise visionalization of the trajectory to rule out any traversing larger vessels and to avoid the ventricular wall.

Step 6: Prepare the Patient for the OR

In our experience it is beneficial to give the patient prior to surgery 20 mg dexamethasone and iv. antibiotics. Also continuous blood pressure measuring is recommended. The hair is carefully shaved and the skin prepared with antiseptics. Local anesthesia is applied around the intended skin incision and the outlet of the temporary percutaneous extensions. The draping is performed in order to keep eye contact with the patient. Oxygen supply is optional.

Step 7: Stereotactic Arc Fixation

The calculated target coordinates are transferred and set with the frame, always double checked by attending and resident (Target coordinates: Table 6.1).

Step 8: Incision and Making the Burrhole

The incision is usually carried out semicircularly and precoronarly to avoid scar tissue above the burrhole device. The size of the burrhole depends on the number of electrodes placed, the use of a burrhole fixating device, the performance of microrecordings or not. Sometimes extra drilling is necessary to prevent extreme bending of the electrodes or to fit in the lead fixation device. The dura is incised and coagulated. At this step already it should be checked, whether the opening is large enough to perform microrecordings with five electrodes if necessary.

Step 9: Attachment of Lead Fixation Device on Burrhole

This step is highly variable and depends on several factors such as thickness of skin, baldness, reimbursement of special devices, etc. If a device is used it should be rigidly be fixed to the skull.

Step 10: Stereotactic Arc Fixation

Depending on whether microrecordings are used all attachments should be calibrated to the lengths of guiding cannulas, micro- and macroelectrodes. Again all settings should be double checked.

Step 11: Physiological Confirmation of Anatomical Target

In general, microelectrode recordings are not useful for target delineation in chronic pain, they are rather used for scientific reasons. In the thalamus rhythmic or randomly bursting cells are detected which have the typical characteristics of low-threshold calcium spike bursts [80–82]. Especially in patients with large areas of deafferentation (i.e., paraplegia) cells in the representation of the anesthetic body part have no receptive fields [30]. In other patients we found a distortion of the receptive and projection fields (i.e., face instead of the amputated arm 16 mm lateral) as described by Lenz [83]. Microrecording of the hypothalamus displayed low frequency random spikes with an average frequency of 18 Hz.

Step 12: Intraoperative Testing with Microelectrode Recording System

If microelectrode recording (MER) is used, microstimulation usually up to 10 mA can be carried out. This is rather helpful to determine the threshold for side effects than to cause clinical effects (pain relief). We recommend testing the efficacy and side effects with the permanent electrode.

Step 13: DBS Lead Placement

Depending on the type of fixation additional X-ray should be used to be certain that the permanent electrode is located in the right place (same as chosen microelectrode path).

Step 14: Intraoperative Clinical Testing with DBS Lead

Stimulation in the PVG creates a feeling of warmth, floating, and dizziness at threshold stimulation with frequencies of 50 Hz and a pulse width of 210 μs. At higher intensities anxiety or even panic is reported by the patients. Below the intercommissural line diplopia, gaze deviation or gaze paralysis can be elicited. Further posterior sometimes paresthesias in the contralateral body without somatotopy are reported caused by current spread to the medial lemniscus. Very helpful are reproducible elevations of the blood pressure and heart rate at threshold stimulation in PVG [17, 84] or

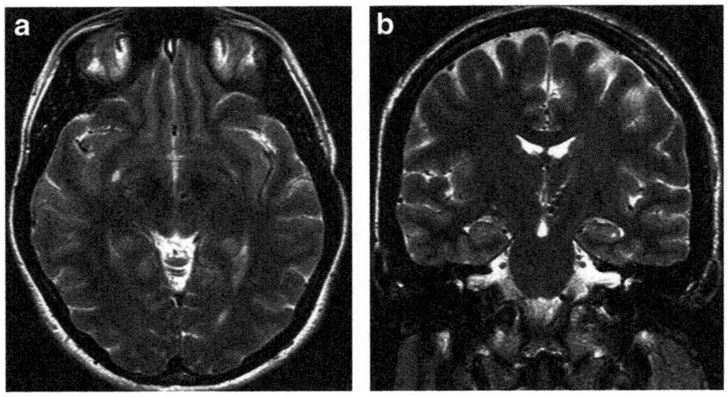

Fig. 6.1 Cluster and hypothalamic stimulation

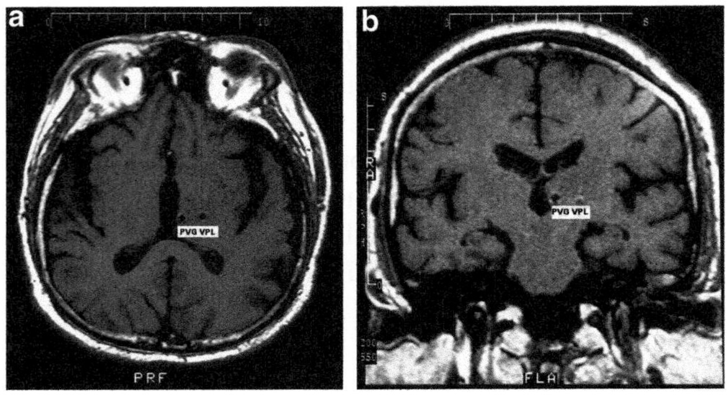

Fig. 6.2 PVG/VPL Stim

hypothalamus. Interestingly these effects fade with chronic stimulation (Figs. 6.1 and 6.2).

Stimulation of the lateral thalamus elicits paresthesias in different body areas according to the laterality of the placed electrode. We can confirm the results of Lenz and others that there is a mismatch of receptive field and projection field, especially in patients with phantom pain or central pain syndromes. In patients with thalamic pain or paraplegia only very few cells have receptive fields at all. Especially in patients with thalamic pain suprathreshold stimulation is reported painful by the patients. In one of our patients with phantom pain just placing the macroelectrode caused immense pain in the phantom. Dystonic movements of the extremities are caused by stimulation of the internal capsule. In those cases the electrode has to be moved more medially.

Step 15: DBS Lead Fixation

The lead has to be securely fixed with the fixation device without damaging the lead or bending it above the bony edge.

Step 16: Intraoperative Final Lead Confirmation

Intraoperative X-ray is helpful to prevent final dislocation (especially with the available cup, which often pushes the lead 1–2 mm more down). Also a final stimulation testing is recommended (same threshold for effects and side effects as before).

Step 17: Dismantle Equipment and Suturing Incision

Rinsing with a local antibiotic is recommended. The extension outlet is sutured and covered with iodine cream.

Step 18: Postoperative Final Lead Confirmation

This can be done with CT or MRI. These images can then be fused with the preoperative images. Also postoperative complications can be ruled out.

Step 19: IPG Placement

In chronic pain patients a blinded testing trial is recommended before the IPG is placed. The second procedure is generally performed in general anesthesia.

Clinical Results

No randomized controlled study exists up to now for deep brain stimulation for neuropathic pain. One study with a short-term randomized phase exists for the treatment of chronic cluster headache [85]. According to the criteria of evidence-based medicine, there are usually level 4 or 5, i.e., historic case-control studies, published. Only a few papers used a disinterested third party for evaluation of the results. There are in general no standardized selection and evaluation criteria in those studies besides in the cluster studies where always the IHS (International Headache Society) criteria were used. Especially no blinded stimulation was carried out, which is possible in contrast to spinal cord stimulation, where paresthesias have to mask the painful area. In DBS especially subthreshold stimulation proved to be beneficial, while suprathreshold stimulation sometimes is rather experienced unpleasant. A summary of more recently published studies is given in Tables 6.2, 6.3, and 6.4.

Most series include patients with different etiologies of peripheral and central neuropathic pain syndromes. Older studies also included patients with Failed Back Surgery Syndrome after more conservative treatments (as spinal cord stimulation) had failed. Interestingly these patients showed in general satisfying results over years. More conflicting are the results in neuropathic pain. From the review of the literature it seems that more circumscribed, well-localized pain responds better to either lateral or thalamic or periventricular pain, than below the level pain in spinal cord injury or post-stroke pain. Patients with pure nociceptive or cancer pain are no candidates for DBS.

In chronic cluster headache more rigid selection criteria were chosen and usually a psychological or psychiatric examination had been performed. In general, the long-term results demonstrate a success in 50 % of the implanted patients of which 50 % were pain free and the remaining had a significant drop in frequency of attacks as well as duration and intensity of their pain.

The fear that hypothalamic stimulation causes long-term autonomic side effects could be ruled out (Figs. 6.3 and 6.4).

The most serious complications in functional stereotactic neurosurgery are intracranial hemorrhages. The incidence in major series ranged between 1.9 and 4.1 % and permanent neurologic complications were reported in about 2 %. In some cases just the insertion of the electrodes can cause neurologic deficits (e.g., diplopia in PAG stimulation) without visible hemorrhage on postoperative imaging.

Some patients developed compulsion stimulation behavior with stimulation in the lateral somatosensory thalamus. In our series this happened in two patients with the lowest electrode contacts probably stimulating hypothalamic fibers.

The risk of infection ranged between 3 and 12 %. In our series infection occurred in 1 patient with a purulent otitis media and diabetes (2 %). Prophylactic oral antibiotics during the trial stimulation are now routinely administered. The connector between the electrode and the extension cable should be placed over the parietal skull and not behind the ear. The latter position increases the risk of disconnection, and breakage of the connecting cables. New extension cables with smaller connectors were developed and reduce the risk of scalp erosion.

Table 6.2 Summary of patient series with somatosensory thalamic stimulation or combined stimulation

Reference	Year	Target	Pain	Follow-up	Outcome	Measurement of pain	Level
Hosobuchi et al. [47]	1986	Lat. Thal.	Thalamic pain	2–14 years	6 Successful	Successful = pain reduction + no narcotics anymore	5
			Anesthesia dolorosa		4 Successful		
			Postherpetic		2 Successful		
			Plexus avulsion		2 Successful		
			Postcordotomiedys]		8 Successful		
			Lumbar radiculopathy		19 Successful		
			Paraplegia		2 Successful		
Levy et al. [89]	1987	Lat. Thal	Thalamic pain	80 months	24 % Long-term success	Verbal, questionnaire; third disinterested party	4
			Periph. neuropathy		50 % Long-term success		
			Anesthesia dolor		18 % Long-term success		
			Paraplegia		0 % Long-term success		
			Postchordotomicdys		40 % Long-term success		
			Phantom pain		20 % Long-term success		
Siegfried [92]	1987	Lat. Thal.	Postherpetic (VI) pain <2 years	67 % Excellent, 14 % good	VAS, use of narcotics; pain profile; ADL		
			Anesthesia dolorosa	39 % Excellent, 44 % good			
			Thalamic pain	42 % Excellent, 29 % good			
			Plexus avulsion	36 % Excellent, 36 % good			
			Phantom/stump	50 % Excellent, 20 % good			
			Paraplegia	50 % Excellent, 20 % good			
			Paraplegia	50 % Excellent, 50 % good			
Tsubokawa et al. [93]	1986	Lat. Thal.	Periph. neuropathy	?	4 Excellent, 2 good	Verbal, exz. = > 80 %; pain reduction: exc. = > 80 %; good = 60 %–80 %, fair = <60 %	
			Central pain		2 Excellent, 3 good, 3 fair		
			Carcinoma pain		3 Excellent, 1 good, 6 fair		
Kumar et al. [90]	1990	Lat. Thal	Thalamic pain	6–70 months	No long-term success		5
			Phantom pain		No long-term success		
Gybels et al. [33]	1993	VPL/VPM, Caps. interna	Thalamic pain	4 years	1 Good	?	5

			Anesthesia dolorosa		2 Good		
			Root avulsion		3 Good		
			Phantom pain		1 Good		
			Spinal cord lesion		2 Good		
			Postherpetic		0 Good		
Rasche et al. [16]	2006	VPL/ VPM + PVG	Failed back surgery	3–5 years	4 Excellent, 5 good, 1 fair, 3 failures	Excellent = 75 %–100 % pain reduction; good = 50 %–75 %; fair = 25 %–50 %	4
			Phantom		1 Excellent, 1 fair, 2 failures		
			Central pain (SCI)		1 Excellent, 1 fair; 10 failures		
			Dysesthesia dol		2 Excellent, 1 good, 1 fair, 1 failure		
			CRPS II		2 Excellent, 2 good, 2 failures		
			Thalamic pain		1 Good, 1 fair, 9 failures		
			Postherpetic		1 Excellent, 1 failure		
Boccard et al. [15]	2013		Phantom	4 years	89 % patients with 53 % improvement on VAS* at 3 months	Prospective, VAS, MPQ, SF-36, EQ-5D, statistical evaluation with $P < 0.5$ significance*	3
			Poststroke		70 % Patients with 38 % improvement		
			SCI		57 % Patients with 69 % improvement		
			Plexus avulsion		50 % with 44 % improvement (only PVG)		
			Cephalgia		55 % with 62 % improvement		

Table 6.3 Stimulation in periaqueductal/periventricular grey or medial thalamus (CM-PF)

Author	Year	Target	Type of pain	Follow-up	Outcome	Pain measurement	Level
Plotkin [95]	1982	PVG	Postdiscectomy	3 years	80 % success	Verbal response, preoperatively; morphine test	5
Andy [94]	1983	CM-PF	CRPS II	?	1 Good, 1 excellent	4-Point scale	5
			Thalamic pain		1 Good, 1 excellent		
			Migraine		Good		
Young et al. [97]	1985	PAG/PVG	Postdiscectomy	2–60 months	9 Excellent, 5 partially	Verbal, morphine test	5
		+ Combinations	Carcinoma		3 Excellent, 3 partially		
			Paraplegia		1 Excellent, 3 partially		
			Anesthesia dolorosa (4		2 Partially, 2 poor		5
			Root avulsion		2 Partially, 2 poor		
			Postherpetic		2 Partially		
Hosobuchi et al. [98]	1986	PAG	Carcinoma	2–14 years	5 Successful	Successful = pain relief + no narcotics; preoperative morphine test	
			Failed back		39 Successful		
			Nociceptive pain		6 Successful		
Hosobuchi et al. [96]	1987	Dors. PAG	Head/neck—carcinoma	?	2 Good, 5 failure	Verbal	5
Levy et al. [89]	1987	PVG	Failed back	80 months	32 % Long-term success	Verbal, questionnaire, disinterested third party	4
			Carcinoma		33 % Long-term success	Disinterested third party	
Kumar et al. [90]	1990	PVG	Failed back	6–118 months	73 % Long-term success	Success = good to excellent pain relief + no narcotics; preop psychol testing	5
Krauss et al. [55]	2001	CM-PF	Neuropathic pain	?	10 Patients good relief		5

Table 6.4 Selective patient series with posteromedial hypothalamic stimulation for cluster headache (w/o abstracts)

Author/year	Patients, n	Patients improved	Benefit complete/partial	Follow-up, y
Schoenen et al. [49]/2005	6	3	2/1	4
Starr et al. [100]/2007	4	2	0/2	1
Bartsch et al. [91]/2008	6	3	2/1	1.4
Fontaine et al. [85]/2010	11	6	3/3	1
Leone et al. [101]/2013	19	12	6/6	8.7

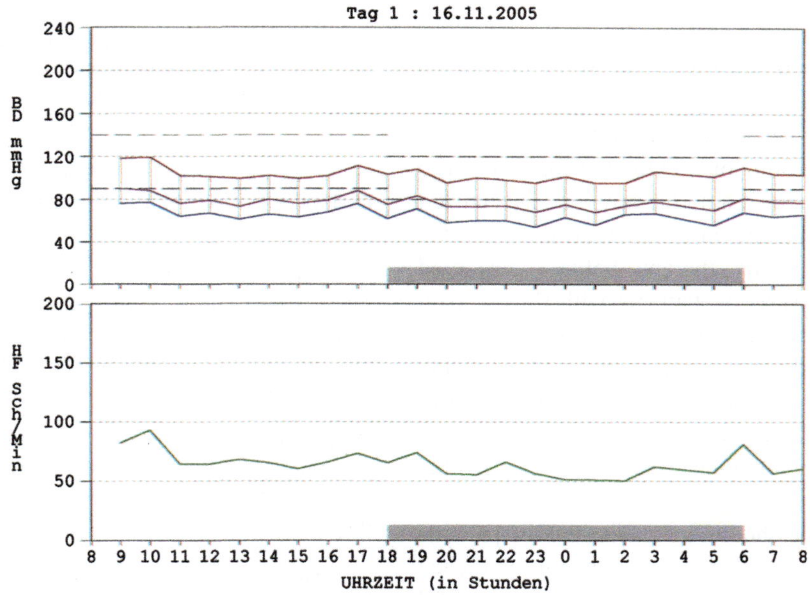

Fig. 6.3 24 h blood pressure recording 3 months following hypothalamic DBS does not show RR changes with stimulation (*gray bar*)

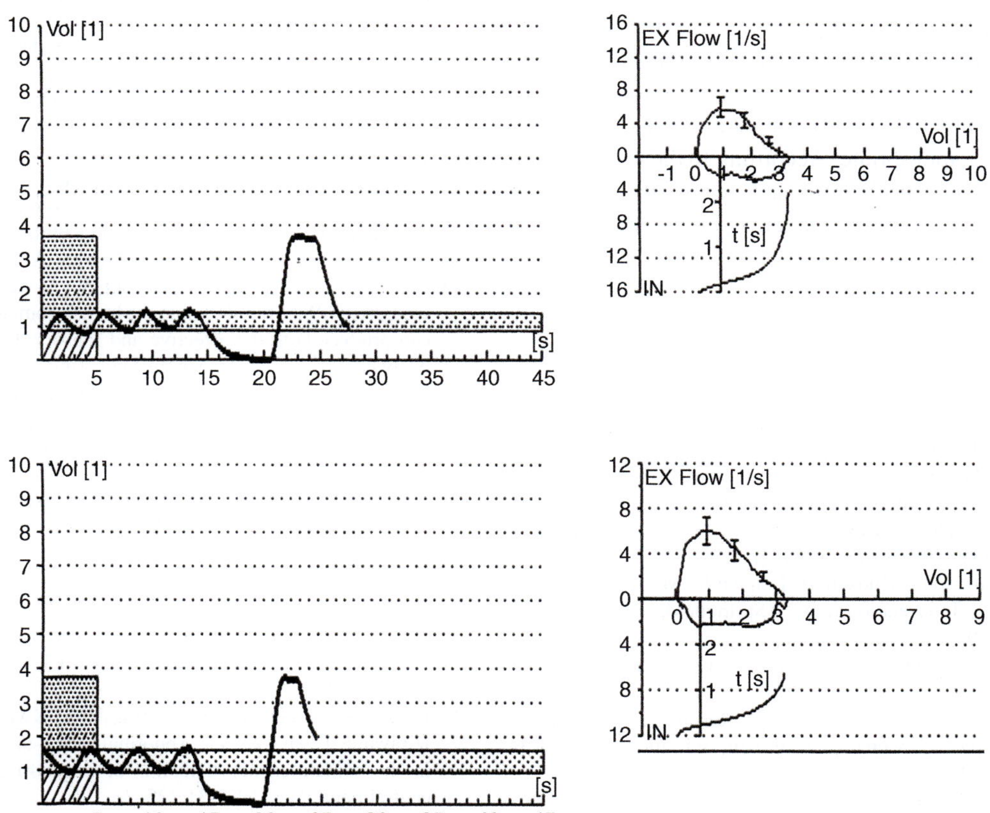

Fig. 6.4 No changes in tidal volume, inspiratory ventilation capacity, inspiratory and expiratory respiratory volume, and forced expiratory volume without (above) or with (below) hypothalamic stimulation

Conclusion

Deep brain stimulation is a treatment option in patients not responding to less invasive or more conventional therapeutic measures. A neural substrate for the origin of the pain should be obvious. Patients should undergo always a multi-modal pain therapy in specialized departments with concomitant psychological/psychiatric evaluation and eventually therapy before considered candidates for DBS surgery. Patients with diffuse pain states without detectable reason for the underlying cause of pain should be excluded. Also pain states in the rectal, genital, or perineal region do not respond to DBS according to our experience. One reason might be the small representation of those midline areas in the thalamic somatotopy.

Medical treatment should be exhausted in patients considered for brain stimulation, either due to inefficacy or due to intolerable side effects. However, a careful patient history should be taken to rule out inefficient dosages or side effects due to missing co-medication. Especially patients with neuropathic pain should be treated for a sufficient amount of time with tricyclic antidepressants (i.e., amitriptyline), anticonvulsants (i.e., carbamazepine and gabapentine), and other medications (i.e., mexiletine, baclofen, etc.). Pain of peripheral origin should be treated first with spinal cord or peripheral nerve stimulation, if appropriate. According to the results in this review, DBS can be helpful and add to the quality of life in highly selected patients with chronic pain syndromes.

References

1. Ervin FR, Brown CE, Mark VH. Striatal influence on facial pain. Confin Neurol. 1966;27:75–86.
2. Heath RG, Mickle WA. Evaluation of 7 years' experience with depth electrode studies in human patients. In: Ramsey ER, O'Doherty DS, editors. Electrical studies on the unanaesthetized brain. New York: PB Hoeber; 1960. p. 214–47.
3. Pool JL, Clark WD, Hudson P, Lombardo M. Hypothalamus-hypophyseal Interrelationships. Springfield, IL: Charles C. Thomas; 1956.
4. Melzack R, Wall PD. Pain mechanisms: a new theory. Science. 1965;150:971–9.
5. Albe-Fessard D, Berkley KJ, Kruger L, Ralston 3rd HJ, Willis Jr WD. Diencephalic mechanisms of pain sensation. Brain Res. 1985;356:217–96.
6. Albe-Fessard D, Rougeul A. Thalamic relays of somato-sensory afferent fibers ending in certain localized regions of the associative cortex of the cat. J Physiol. 1956;48:370–4. Article in French.
7. Kruger L, Albe-Fessard D. Distribution of responses to somatic afferent stimuli in the diencephalon of the cat under chloralose anesthesia. Exp Neurol. 1960;2:442–67.
8. Mazars G, Ruge R, Mazars Y. Résultats de la stimulation du faisceau spino-thalamique et leur incidence sur la pathophysiologie de la douleur. Rev Neurol. 1960;103:136–8.
9. Reynolds DV. Surgery in the rat during electrical analgesia induced by focal brain stimulation. Science. 1969;164:444–5.
10. Adams JE. Naloxone reversal of analgesia produced by brain stimulation in human. Pain. 1976;2:161–6.
11. Hosobuchi Y, Adams JE, Linchitz R. Pain relief by electrical stimulation of the central gray matter in human and its reversal by naloxone. Science. 1977;197:183–6.
12. Thoden U, Doerr M, Dieckmann G, Krainick JU. Medial thalamic permanent electrodes for pain control in man: an electrophysiological and clinical study. Electroenc Clin Neurophysiol. 1979;47:582–91.
13. Duncan GH, Bushnell MC, Marchand S. Deep brain stimulation: a review of basic research and clinical studies. Pain. 1991;45:49–59.
14. Coffey RJ. Deep brain stimulation for chronic pain: results of two multicenter trials and a structured review. Pain Med. 2000;2:183–92.
15. Boccard SGJ, Pereira EAC, Moir L, Aziz TZ, Green AL. Long-term outcomes of deep brain stimulation for neuropathic pain. Neurosurgery. 2013;72:221–31.
16. Rasche D, Rinaldi PC, Young RF, Tronnier VM. Deep brain stimulation for the treatment of various chronic pain syndromes. Neurosurg Focus. 2006;21(6):E8.
17. Young RF, Rinaldi PC. Brain stimulation in pain. In: North RB, editor. Neurosurgical management of pain. New York: Springer; 1997.
18. Chung JM, Lee KH, Surmeier DJ, Sorkin LS, Kim J, Willis WD. Response characteristics of neurons in the ventral posterior lateral nucleus of the monkey thalamus. J Neurophysiol. 1986;56:370–90.
19. Gorecki J, Hirayama T, Dostrovsky JO, Tasker RR, Lenz FA. Thalamic stimulation and recording in patients with deafferentation and central pain. Stereotact Funct Neurosurg. 1989;52:219–26.
20. Hirayama T, Dostrovsky JO, Gorecki J, Tasker RR, Lenz FA. Recordings of abnormal activity in patients with deafferentation and central pain. Stereotact Funct Neurosurg. 1989;52:120–6.
21. Lenz FA. The ventral posterior nucleus of thalamus is involved in the generation of central pain syndromes. APS J. 1992;1:42–51.
22. Lenz FA, Gracely RH, Romanoski AJ, Hope EJ, Rowland LH, Dougherty PM. Stimulation in the human somatosensory thalamus can produce both the affective and sensory dimensions of previously experienced pain. Nature Med. 1995;1:910–3.
23. Lenz FA, Gracely RH, Rowland LH, Dougherty PM. A population of cells in the human thalamic principal sensory nucleus respond to painful mechanical stimuli. Neurosci Lett. 1994;180:46–50.
24. Lenz FA, Seike M, Lin YC, Baker FH, Rowland LH, Gracely RH, Richardson RT. Neurons in the area of human thalamic nucleus ventralis caudalis respond to painful heat stimuli. Brain Res. 1993;623:235–40.
25. Lenz FA, Seike M, Richardson RT, Lin YC, Baker FH, Khoja I, et al. Thermal and pain sensations evoked by microstimulation in the area of human ventrocaudal nucleus. J Neurophysiol. 1993;70:200–12.
26. Lenz FA, Tasker RR, Dostrowsky JO, Kwan HC, Gorecki J, Hirayama T, Murphy JT. Abnormal single-unit activity recorded in the somatosensory thalamus of a quadriplegic patient with central pain. Pain. 1987;31:225–36.
27. Weng HR, Lee JI, Lenz FA, Schwartz A, Vierck C, Rowland L, Dougherty PM. Functional plasticity in primate somatosensory thalamus following chronic lesion of the ventral lateral spinal cord. Neuroscience. 2000;101:393–401.
28. Yamashiro K, Tomiyama N, Ishida A, Terada Y, Mukawa J, Yoshii Y, et al. Characteristics of neurons with high-frequency discharge in the central nervous system and their relationship to chronic pain. Stereotact Funct Neurosurg. 1997;68:149–54.

29. Cassinari V, Pagni P. Central pain: a neurosurgical survey. Cambridge, MA: Harvard University Press; 1969.
30. Lenz FA, Kwan HC, Martin R, Tasker R, Richardson T, Dostrovsky JO. Characteristics of somatotopic organization and spontaneous neuronal activity in the region of the thalamic principal sensory nucleus in patients with spinal cord transsection. J Neurophysiol. 1994;72:1570–87.
31. Gerhart KD, Yezierski RP, Wilcox TK, Grossman AE, Willis WD. Inhibition of primate spinothalamic tract neurons by stimulation in ipsilateral or contralateral ventral posterior lateral (VPLC) thalamic nucleus. Brain Res. 1981;229:514–9.
32. Gerhart KD, Yezierski RP, Fang ZR, Willis WD. Inhibition of spinothalamic tract neurons by stimulation in ventral posterior lateral (VPL) thalamic nuclei. J Neurophysiol. 1983;49:406–23.
33. Gybels J, Kupers R, Nuttin B. What can the neurosurgeon offer in peripheral neuropathic pain? Acta Neurochir Suppl. 1993;58:136–40.
34. Rinaldi PC, Young RF, Tronnier VM. Bursting activity of thalamic neurons from chronic pain patients is modified by electrical stimulation in PVG. Soc Neurosci Abstr. 1991;17:1560.
35. Young RF, Chambi I. Pain relief by electrical stimulation of the periaqueductal and periventricular grey matter. J Neurosurg. 1987;66:364–77.
36. Millan MJ. Descending control of pain. Prog Neurobiol. 2002;66:355–474.
37. Basbaum AI, Fields HL. Endogenous pain control mechanism: review and hypothesis. Ann Neurol. 1987;4:451–62.
38. Mayer DJ, Hayes RL. Stimulation produced analgesia: development of tolerance and cross-tolerance to morphine. Science. 1975;188:941–3.
39. Akil H, Richardson DE, Barchas JD, Li CH. Appearance of beta-endorphin-like immunoreactivity in human ventricular cerebrospinal fluid upon analgesic electrical stimulation. Proc Natl Acad Sci U S A. 1978;75:5170–2.
40. Akil H, Richardson DE, Hughes J, Barchas JD. Enkephalin-like material elevated in ventricular cerebrospinal fluid of pain patients after analgetic focal stimulation. Science. 1978;201:463–5.
41. Besson JM, Dickenson AH, Le Bars D, Oliveras JL. Opiate analgesia: the physiology and pharmacology of the spinal pain system. In: Dumont C, editor. Advances in pharmacology and therapeutics. New York: Pergamon Press; 1978. p. 61–81.
42. Hosobuchi Y, Rossier J, Bloom FE. Stimulation of human periaqueductal gray for pain relief increases immunoreactive beta-endorphin in ventricular fluid. Science. 1979;203:279–81.
43. Young RF, Bach FW, Van Norman AS, Yaksh TL. Release of beta-endorphin and met-enkephalin into cerebrospinal fluid during deep brain stimulation for chronic pain. Effects of stimulation locus and site of sampling. J Neurosurg. 1993;79:816–25.
44. Meyerson BA, Boethius J, Carlsson AM. Alleviation of malignant pain by electrical stimulation in the periventricular-periaqueductal region. Pain relief as related to stimulation sites. In: Albe-Fessard D, editor. Advances in pain research and therapy, vol. 3. New York: Raven; 1979. p. 525–33.
45. Richardson DE, Akil H. Pain reduction by electrical brain stimulation in man. I. Acute administration in periaqueductal and periventricular sites. J Neurosurg. 1977;47:178–83.
46. Richardson DE, Akil H. Pain reduction by electrical stimulation in man: part II: chronic selfadministration in the periventricular grey matter. J Neurosurg. 1977;47:184–94.
47. Hosobuchi Y. Current issues regarding subcortical electrical stimulation for pain control in humans. Prog Brain Res. 1988;77:189–92.
48. Gerhart KD, Yezierski RP, Wilcox TK, Willis WD. Inhibition of primate spinothalamic tract neurons by stimulation in periaqueductal gray or adjacent midbrain reticular formation. J Neurophysiol. 1984;51:450–66.
49. Schoenen J, Di Clemente L, Vandenheede M, Fumal A, De Pasqua V, Mouchamps M, et al. Hypothalamic stimulation in chronic cluster headache: a pilot study of efficacy and mode of action. Brain. 2005;128:940–7.
50. Yezierski RP, Wilcox TK, Willis WD. The effects of serotonin antagonists on the inhibition of primate spinothalamic tract cells produced by stimulation of the nucleus raphe magnus or periaqueductal gray. J Pharmacol Exper Ther. 1982;220:266–77.
51. Li HS, Monhemius R, Simpson BA, Roberts MHT. Supraspinal inhibition of nociceptive dorsal horn neurones in the anaesthetized rat: tonic or dynamic? J Physiol. 1998;506:459–69.
52. Luys JB. Reserches sur la systéme nerveux cerebrospinal: sa structure, ses functions, et ses maladies. Paris: Ballière; 1865.
53. Vogt C, Vogt O. Das Griseum centrale centrum medianum: in: thalamusstudien I-III. J Psychol Neurol. 1941;50:32–154.
54. Hécaen H, Talairach J, David M, Dell MB. Coagulations limitèe du thalamus dans les algies du syndrome thalamique. Rev Neurol. 1949;81:917–31.
55. Krauss JK, Pohle T, Weigel R, Kalbarczyk A. Somatosensory thalamic stimulation versus center median-parafascicular complex stimulation in 11 patients with neuropathic pain. Stereotact Funct Neurosurg. 2001;77:194.
56. Apkarian AV, Hodge CJ. Primate spinothalamic pathways. III. Thalamic terminations of the dorsolateral and ventral spinothalamic pathways. J Comp Neurol. 1989;288:493–511.
57. Mantyh PW. The spinothalamic tract in primate: a reexamination using wheatgerm agglutinine conjugated with horse radish peroxidase. Neuroscience. 1983;9:847–63.
58. Ralston III HJ, Ralston D. The primate dorsal spinothalamic tract: evidence for a specific termination in the posterior nuclei (Po/SG) of the thalamus. Pain. 1992;48:107–18.
59. Jeanmonod D, Magnin M, Morel A. Thalamus and neurogenic pain: physiological, anatomical and clinical data. Neuroreport. 1993;4:475–8.
60. Liz-Planells M, Tronnier V, Rinaldi PC. Neural activity of medial and lateral thalamus in a deafferentation model. Soc Neurosci Abstr. 1992;18:288.
61. Rinaldi PC, Young RF, Albe-Fessard D, Chodakiewitz J. Spontaneous neuronal hyperactivity in the medial and intralaminar thalamic nuclei of patients with deafferentation pain. J Neurosurg. 1991;74:415–21.
62. Ishijima B, Yoshimasu N, Fukushima T, Hori T, Sekino H, Sano K. Nociceptive neurons in the human thalamus. Confinia Neurol. 1975;37:99–106.
63. Blomquist A, Zhang ET, Craig J. Cytoarchitectonic and immunohistochemical characterization of a specific pain and temperature relay, the posterior portion of the ventral medial nucleus in the human thalamus. Brain. 2000;123:601–19.
64. Craig AD, Bushnell MC, Zhang ET, Blomqvist A. A thalamic nucleus specific for pain and temperature sensation. Nature. 1994;372:770–3.
65. Jones EG, Lensky KM, Chan VH. Delineation of thalamic nuclei immunoreactive for calcium-binding proteins in and around the posterior pole of the ventral posterior complex. Thalamus Related Syst. 2001;1:213–24.
66. Benabid AL, Henriksen SJ, McGinty JF, Bloom FE. Thalamic nucleus ventroposterolateralis inhibits nucleus parafascicularis response to noxious stimuli through a non-opioid pathway. Brain Res. 1983;280:217–31.
67. Cesaro P, Amsallem B, Pollin B, Nguyen-Legros J, Moretti JL. Organization of the median and intralaminar nuclei of the thalamus: hypotheses on their role in the onset of certain central pain. Rev Neurol. 1986;142:297–302.
68. May A, Ashburner J, Büchel C, McConigle DJ, Friston KJ, Frackowiak RS, Goadsby PJ. Correlation between structural and

functional changes in brain in an idiopathic headache syndrome. Nat Med. 1999;5(7):836–8.
69. May A, Bahra A, Büchel C, Frackowiak RS, Goadsby PJ. Hypothalamic activation in cluster headache attacks. Lancet. 1998;352:275–8.
70. May A, Bahra A, Büchel C, Turner R, Goadsby PJ. Functional magnetic resonance imaging in spontaneous attacks of SUNCT (shortlasting unilateral neuralgiform headache with conjunctival injection and tearing). Ann Neurol. 1999;46:791–4.
71. Sprenger T, Boecker H, Tölle TR, Bussone G, May A, Leone M. Specific hypothalamic activation during a spontaneous cluster attack. Neurology. 2004;62:516–7.
72. Sano K, Mayanagi Y, Sekino H, Ogashiwa M, Ishijima B. Results of stimulation and destruction of the posterior hypothalamus in man. J Neurosurg. 1970;33:689–707.
73. Sano K, Sekino H, Hashimoto I, Amano K, Sugiyama H. Posteromedial hypothalamotomy in the treatment of intractable pain. Confin Neurol. 1975;37:285–90.
74. Bartsch T, Levy MJ, Knight YE, Goadsby PJ. Inhibition of nociceptive dural input in the trigeminal nucleus caudalis by somatostatin receptor blockade in the posterior hypothalamus. Pain. 2005;117:30–9.
75. Holstege G. Some anatomical observations on the projections from the hypothalamus to brain stem and spinal cord: an HRP and autoradiographiv tracing study in the cat. J Comp Neurol. 1987;260:98–126.
76. May A, Leone M, Boecker H, Sprenger T, Juergens T, Bussone G, Tölle TR. Hypothalamic deep brain stimulation in positron emission tomography. J Neurosci. 2006;26:3589–93.
77. Abosch A, Timmermann L, Bartley S, Rietkerk HG, Whithing D, Conolly PJ, et al. An international survey of deep brain stimulation procedural steps. Stereotact Funct Neurosurg. 2013;91:1–11.
78. Kocuj F, Epple J, Polarz H, Tronnier VM, Martin E. Nerve blocks in stereotactic neurosurgery. Stereotact Funct Neurosurg. 2002;78:29–38.
79. Lenglet C, Abosch A, Yacoub E, De Martino F, Sapiro G, Harel N. Comprehensive in vivo mapping of the human basal ganglia and thalamic connectome in individuals using 7T MRI. PLoS One. 2012;7:e29153. doi:10.1371/journal.pone.0029153.
80. Jeanmonod D, Magnin M, Morel A. Low-threshold calcium spike bursts in the human thalamus. Common physiopathology for sensory, motor and limbic positive symptoms. Brain. 1996;119:363–75.
81. Jeanmonod D, Magnin M, Morel A, Siegemund M, Cancro R, Lanz M, et al. Thalamocortical dysrhythmia II. Clinical and surgical aspects. Thalamus Related Syst. 2001;1:245–54.
82. Zirh TA, Lenz FA, Reich SG, Dougherty PM. Patterns of bursting occurring in thalamic cells during Parkinsonian tremor. Neuroscience. 1998;83:107–21.
83. Lenz FA, Zirh TA, Garonzik IM, Dougherty PM. Neuronal activity in the region of the principle sensory nucleus of the human thalamus (ventralis caudalis) in patients with pain following amputations. Neuroscience. 1998;86:1065–81.
84. Hyam JA, Kringelbach ML, Silburn PA, Aziz TZ, Green AL. The autonomic effects of deep brain stimulation: a therapeutic opportunity. Nat Rev Neurol. 2012;8:391–400.
85. Fontaine D, Lazorthes Y, Mertens P, Blond S, Géraud G, Fabre N, et al. Safety and efficacy of deep brain stimulation in refractory cluster headache: a randomized placebo-controlled double-blind trial followed by a 1-year open extension. J Headache Pain. 2010;11:23–31.
86. Richardson DE. Analgesia produced by stimulation of various sites in the human beta-endorphin system. Appl Neurophysiol. 1982;45:116–22.
87. Sandkühler J, Fu QG, Zimmermann M. Spinal pathways mediating tonic or stimulation-produced descending inhibition from the periaqueductal gray or nucleus raphe magnus are separate in cat. J Neurophysiol. 1987;58:327–41.
88. Albe-Fessard D, Kruger L. Duality of unity discharges from cat centrum medianum in response to natural and electrical stimulation. J Neurophysiol. 1962;25:3–20.
89. Levy R, Lamb S, Adams JE. Treatment of chronic pain by deep brain stimulation: long-term follow-up and review of the literature. Neurosurgery. 1987;6:885–93.
90. Kumar K, Wyant GM, North R. Deep brain stimulation for control of intractable pain in humans, present and future. 17 year follow-up. Neurosurgery. 1990;26:744–82.
91. Bartsch T, Pinsker MO, Rasche D, Kinfe T, Hertel F, Diener HC, et al. Hypothalamic deep brain stimulation for cluster headache from a new multicase series. Cephalalgia. 2008;28:285–95.
92. Siegfried J. Sensory thalamic neurostimulation for chronic pain. Pacing Clin Electrophsiol. 1987;10:209–12.
93. Tsubokawa T, Katayama Y, Yamamoto T, Hirayama T. Deafferentiation pain and stimulation of the thalamic sensory relay nucleus: clinical and experimental study. Appl Neurophysiol. 1985;48:166–71.
94. Andy OJ. Thalamic stimulation for chronic pain. Appl Neurophysiol. 1983;46:116–23.
95. Plotkin R. Results in 60 cases of deep brain stimulation for chronic intractable pain. Appl Neurophysiol. 1982;4:173–8.
96. Hosobuchi Y. Dorsal periaqueductal gray matter stimulation in humans. Pacing Clin Electrophysiol. 1987;10:213–6.
97. Young RF, Kroening R, Fulton W, Feldman RA, Chambi I. Electrical stimulation of the brain in treatment of chronic pain. J Neurosurg. 1985;62:389–96.
98. Hosobuchi Y. Subcortical electrical stimulation for control of intractable pain in humans. J Neurosurg. 1986;64:543–53.
99. Lenz FA, Gracely RH, Hope EJ, Baker FH, Rowland LH, Dougherty PM, Richardson RT. The sensation of angina can be evoked by stimulation of the human thalamus. Pain. 1994;59:119–25.
100. Starr PA, Barbaro NM, Raskin NH, Ostrem JL. Chronic stimulation of the posterior hypothalamic region for cluster headache: technique and 1-year results in four patients. J Neurosurg. 2007;106:999–1005.
101. Leone M, Franzini A, Cecchini AP, Bussone G. Success, failure, and putative mechanisms in hypothalamic stimulation for drug-resistant chronic cluster headache. Pain. 2013;154:89–94.

Motor Cortex Stimulation

7

Dirk Rasche and Volker M. Tronnier

Introduction and History of Invasive Cortical Stimulation

Invasive and surgical procedures for the treatment of different pathological conditions and diseases are as old as human history. In accordance to this one can assume that the treatment of pain, which is a specific evolutionary function of the nervous system, is also an ongoing problem of millenniums. The treatment of chronic pain syndromes is often frustrating and a certain percentage of patients are refractory to any multimodal, pharmacological, psychological or conservative treatment [1, 2]. A lot of these patients suffer from neuropathic pain, which is defined by the International Association for the Study of Pain as "a pain caused by a lesion or disease of the somatosensory system" (www.iasp-pain.org/resources/painDefinition; [1]). Therefore the perception and cognition of chronic pain is an individual function of the human brain. In these selected, refractory cases invasive treatment options at all levels of the nervous system were performed for many centuries [3–5]. Mainly neurodestructive procedures like neurotomies, chordotomies, corticotomies and lesions of deep brain structures but also limb amputations were conducted [4]. Despite initial pain reduction follow-up observation revealed poor results regarding pain control and complications [4, 5].

The development of neuromodulation techniques with electrical stimulation of nervous tissue lead to a significant change and improvement of therapy. This is mainly based on the work and experience of Penfield and Rasmussen with functional mapping of the cortical surface, in detail the motor strip and central region [6]. These data lead to a well-known and accepted landscape of the cortical surface, the so-called "homunculus" of the precentral gyrus. To date this cortical representation is the background for functional targeting of the somatotopic correlate of the affected, painful part of the body.

Since the 1980s, direct epi- or subdural motor cortex stimulation (MCS) is offered to patients with post-stroke pain (PSP), trigeminal neuropathic pain (TNP) or deafferentation pain of the upper or lower extremities [7–31].

Until today more than 75 publications and several reviews regarding MCS and chronic pain exist and one can assume that more than 700 patients worldwide were treated with this neuromodulation therapy [4, 22, 30, 32–40]. Only a few prospective randomised controlled studies with small patient numbers were performed [15, 26, 28, 29, 41]. Neither consent nor guidelines exist concerning indications for surgery, site of stimulation, stimulation parameters or even the implantation materials. Besides chronic pain syndromes the indication list expanded to other refractory syndromes and also different stimulation sites on the cortical surface with the aim to modulate dysfunctional activities of motor or sensory systems [42–57].

In the future on the one hand the lack of understanding of human brain function must be resolved and may lead to the development of modern, specific or individual non-invasive or invasive techniques. On the other hand a level of evidence regarding patient selection, indications and implantation techniques must be acquired to establish an algorithm for the efficacy and clinical significance of invasive cortical stimulation (ICS).

Mode of Action

To date, the specific pathophysiological mode of action of MCS is still unknown. Several experimental studies for pain are published to evaluate the theoretical mode of action of cortical stimulation, either on the precentral gyrus or on other cortical structures [16, 18, 23, 26, 58–70]. These include animal models of acute and chronic pain and cortical

D. Rasche (✉) • V.M. Tronnier
Department of Neurosurgery, University Hospital of Schleswig-Holstein, University of Lübeck, Campus Lübeck, Ratzeburger Allee 160, 23538 Lübeck, Germany
e-mail: dirk.rasche@uksh.de

H. Knotkova and D. Rasche (eds.), *Textbook of Neuromodulation*,
DOI 10.1007/978-1-4939-1408-1_7, © Springer Science+Business Media, LLC 2015

stimulation but also human experiments with different imaging techniques like functional MRI, positron emission tomography (PET) and single-photon emission computed tomography (SPECT). The most important studies using positron emission tomography (PET) and electrophysiology were performed by Garcia-Larrea et al. [60–62]. They demonstrated that subthreshold electrical stimulation of the motor area leads to modulation of pain-related areas like the ipsilateral thalamus, anterior cingulate gyrus, insula and upper brainstem [60, 61]. An antidromic activation of thalamocortical connections is postulated the most important effect of MCS. Furthermore, multiple "network effects" like the increased release of endogenous opioids, enhanced gamma-aminobutyric acid (GABA)-concentrations and descending modulation down to the dorsal horn of the spinal cord were evaluated [4, 16, 18, 26, 35, 38, 60–64, 66–70].

Patient Selection

The indication for MCS is restricted to the diagnosis of chronic refractory syndromes like treatment-resistant neuropathic pain syndromes as listed in Table 7.1. Certain contraindications need to be taken into account (see Tables 7.2 and 7.3). It was shown by Yamamoto et al. and Carroll et al. that severe motor weakness or paralysis in the area of pain with injury of the corticospinal tract is of negative predictive value for pain relief by MCS [11, 17]. This is mainly due to the missing thalamocortical connections to the motor strip and can be evaluated by MRI (Fig. 7.2), diffusion tensor imaging techniques and fibre tracking [12, 16, 20, 21, 59, 62–64, 71–73].

Clinical experience demonstrated that usually patients had a history of several years and multiple interdisciplinary treatments before evaluation of an invasive pain procedure [27]. Also pharmacological therapies, including different analgesics World Health Organisation (WHO) level 3, antiepileptics and coanalgesics, were proven to be ineffective or were accompanied by intolerable side effects. A concomitant psychological therapy by a pain-experienced psychologist is mandatory.

In neuropathic pain syndromes usually a specific nerve deficit, e.g. tactile hyp- or hyperaesthesia, or dysfunction like allodynia or dysaesthesia can be detected in the pain area [1, 2].

Patients should be informed about the procedure and the implanted hardware as an off-label use as an individual and experimental treatment option and written informed consent should be documented.

Nevertheless, patient selection criteria are very subjective and may vary among the experienced centres and publications [4, 8, 12, 15, 22, 27, 29, 30, 32–37, 40, 53].

Table 7.1 List of different indications for motor cortex stimulation (MCS)

MCS indication list
Trigeminal neuropathic pain incl. dys/anaesthesia dolorosa
Brachial plexus avulsion/cervical nerve root avulsion
CRPS I/II of the upper extremity
Central pain/post-stroke pain
Phantom limb pain
Movement disorders like Parkinson's disease and essential tremor
Post-stroke rehabilitation

Table 7.2 Contraindications for invasive cortical stimulation (ICS)

Contraindications for ICS
Severe paresis or paralysis in the pain area
Severe psychiatric disorders
Incompliance of the patient with alcohol or drug addiction/abuse
Refractory epilepsy
Coagulopathy
Contraindication for general anaesthesia or chronic infection
Cardiac pacemaker or cardioverter
Pregnancy

Table 7.3 Indications and cortical stimulation sites

Indication	Stimulation site
Chronic pain:	Precentral gyrus and sulcus centralis
Parkinson's disease:	Precentral gyrus and sulcus centralis
Stroke:	Precentral gyrus and sulcus centralis
Tinnitus:	Auditory cortex, Heschl gyrus (BA 41–42)
Depression:	Dorsolateral prefrontal cortex (BA 46)
Tremor:	BA 4

BA Brodmann area

Therefore this needs to be suspected to be a substantial bias in every prospective trial and reduces comparability of these investigations and results.

Perioperative Management

Today neuronavigation is a worldwide standard for many neurosurgical procedures of intracranial lesions. A morphological three-dimensional (3D) data set of the patient's brain should be implemented into modern neuronavigation systems, either as an MRI or a computed scan [4, 20, 21, 25, 27, 58, 59, 62, 63, 73–76]. In some patients with brachial plexus evulsion (BPA) and complete deafferentation due to cervical nerve root avulsion the authors were able to detect specific morphological changes and side differences of the detailed anatomy of the precentral gyrus in the area of the arm and hand representation as a consequence of denervation (see also Fig. 7.2). Cortical surface reconstruction is as

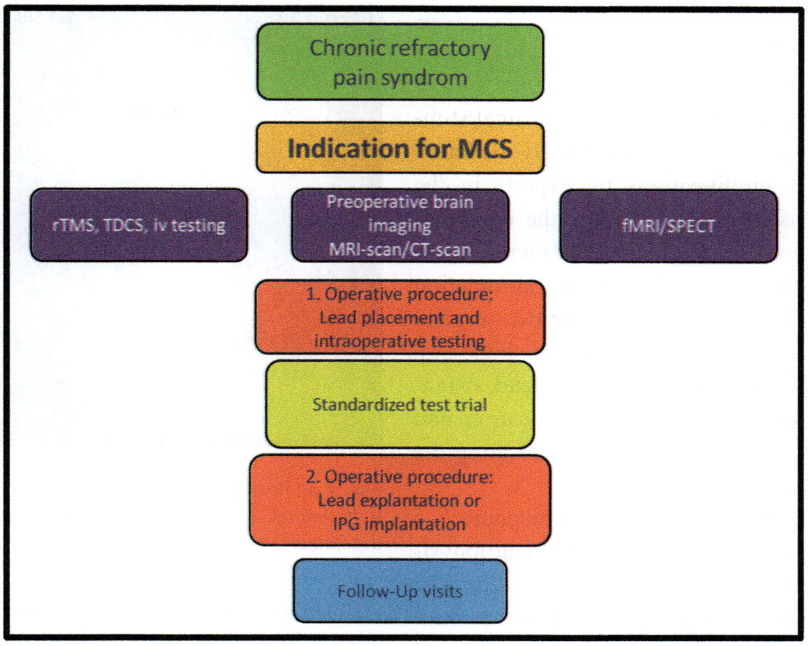

Fig. 7.1 Diagram showing the algorithm for MCS (pre/intra/post-operative) in chronic neuropathic pain syndromes

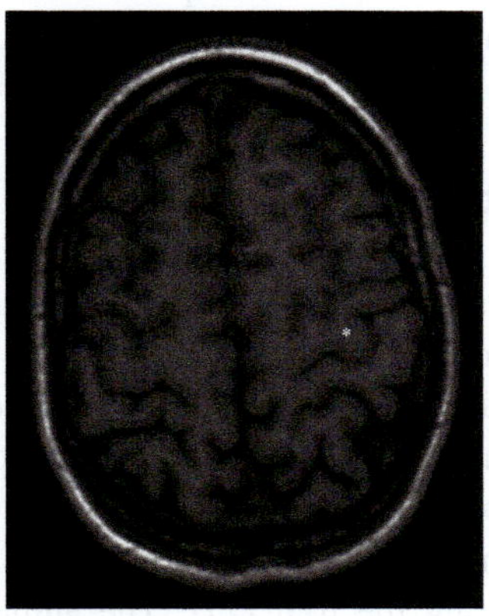

Fig. 7.2 Standard axial T1 MRI scan with identification of the left precentral gyrus and motor cortex for the upper limb (* = hand knob")

helpful as matching with functional data like BOLD-fMRI to identify the target structures of the painful areas and to achieve additional information regarding certain neuroplastic changes and cortical reorganisation [21, 63, 67, 70, 77, 78]. This information is essential regarding the correct and ideal position of the lead covering the motor area of the painful body part.

In addition to these morphological and functional data it should also be taken into account that in cases of brain atrophy and a large distance between the dura and the cortex, which means a significant cerebrospinal fluid (CSF) layer in the computed tomography (CT) or MRI scan, one should consider subdural direct cortical implantation of the leads [4, 27].

Also neurophysiological evaluation of somatosensory or motor-evoked potentials and even electromyographic recordings may be helpful to gain more information about central or peripheral nervous system abnormalities and possible modulations during lead placement and ongoing MCS [3, 4, 16, 18, 23, 26, 27, 42, 58, 62, 64, 68, 69, 73].

A few publications exist concerning the predictive value of pharmacological or electrophysiological testing of patients for MCS [11, 13, 14]. Comparison of the results of MCS with pharmacological testing in 39 patients with PSP was performed by Yamamoto [11]. Franzini et al. demonstrated a positive predictive effect of propofol in two patients with PSP [14]. Non-respondence to propofol has also been investigated as negative predictor for pain relief by MCS [13].

The same effect as epidural placement of an electrode can be achieved with repetitive transcranial magnetic cortical stimulation (rTMS) and transient pain relief is possible [40, 61, 65, 66, 79–81]. In a study with 60 patients with predominated unilateral pain in the face, upper or lower limb of different origin, Lefaucheur et al. [65] have shown that best pain relief with rTMS was achieved for facial pain. In this study the authors stress that the target point for stimulation can be different from the anatomical localisation and best pain relief for facial pain was observed stimulating over the hand cortical area. This may be due to the effects of neuroplasticity known from fMRI studies with phantom limb pain [77, 78]. Overall, negative response to rTMS is not considered as a contraindication or negative predictor for MCS response [65, 66, 80, 81].

Operative Procedure

The implantation of leads for sub- or epidural cortical stimulation has been performed in various, totally different techniques and ongoing modifications by experts in the field worldwide. No consent exists regarding the implantation technique, size or model of implanted leads with 4, 8 or more contacts, neurostimulation devices or stimulation parameters and settings. Most commonly one or two surgical leads with 4 or 8 electrodes are implanted (see Fig. 7.3). There is no legal approval for the usage of any lead, extension and neurostimulator for this specific indication and patient should sign informed consent clearly indicating the off-label use of the devices.

In all publications regarding these procedures a neuronavigation system and also intraoperative neurophysiological monitoring is recommended to identify the precentral gyrus and central sulcus opposite to the painful area. The procedure can be performed in local or general anaesthesia. In most cases the burr-hole technique is performed in local anaesthesia whereas the craniotomy or even subdural placement of the leads is mostly conducted in general anaesthesia. Nevertheless, also the subdural lead implantation and craniotomy is possible in local anaesthesia and mild sedation [4, 27, 35–37, 40].

Intraoperative testing includes recording of evoked potentials and also stimulation via the implanted leads. Identification of the pre- and postcentral gyrus can be performed by phase reversal of median or tibial nerve somatosensory-evoked potentials (SEP). Direct stimulation of the epi- or subdural leads is performed to identify the individual motor threshold and to detect motor responses of the affected body part. In low-frequency stimulation (<10 Hz) focal muscle tics and with higher frequencies (>50 Hz) dystonic muscle cramps can be observed with different stimulation intensities. Due to the direct cortical surface stimulation in cases of subdural lead placement one has to be aware of much lower stimulation intensities (about 10–30 % compared with epidural stimulation). In patients with phantom limb pain or cervical/brachial nerve root avulsion no direct muscle response can be evoked. The operative procedure can be terminated with percutaneous tunnelling of connected extensions for testing with an external stimulation device or consecutive implantation of a neurostimulation device in the infraclavicular or abdominal subcutaneous tissue as a one-stage procedure [4, 22, 32, 34, 38, 48, 51, 53, 57]. In the first scenario a testing trial up to several weeks is possible (increasing risk of infection of the percutaneous extensions) whereas in the other, the one-stage scenario, testing with the internal device can be conducted for several months to evaluate the effects and possible pain reduction. One must mention that performing a test trial and achieving a positive effect seems to be favourable before a definite device implantation is justified, also when looking at the negative aspects like reimbursement and MRI-compatibility.

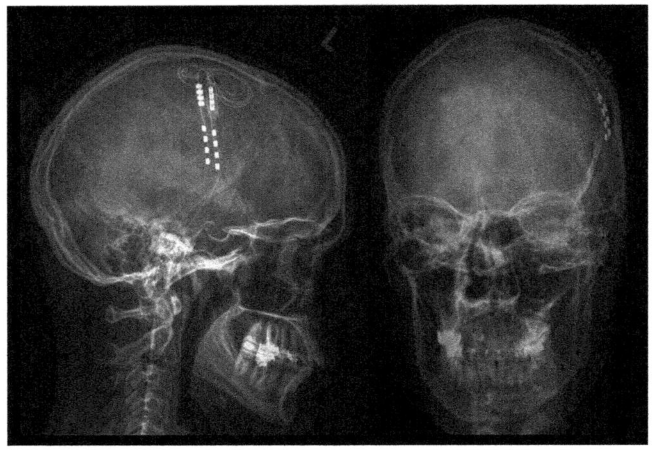

Fig. 7.3 Postoperative X-ray for documentation of the lead position (*left*: lateral, *right*: anterior-posterior) in a patient with right-sided trigeminal neuropathic pain

The author's standard protocol for this procedure performed as "burr-hole" technique and in local anaesthesia is shown in Table 7.4 and Fig. 7.1.

Post-operative Test Trial

In case of a test trial with an external stimulation device a standard protocol with different stimulation parameters and settings should be followed. Therefore at least 8 days are necessary; sometimes the test trial needs to be extended up to 2 weeks. Despite there is no evidence, the authors recommend the administration of a prophylactic oral antibiotic medication during the trial [27]. The authors also recommend a standard plane X-ray of the skull (anterior-posteriorly and laterally) to document the exact position of the lead (see Fig. 7.3). Also a computed scan of the head is performed to match these data with the preoperative MRI data set using image fusion techniques. This technique is also used to superimpose the position of the lead contacts, visualised as the centre of the metal artefact, on the preoperative MRI and three-dimensional cortical surface reconstructions (see Fig. 7.4).

During the test trial subthreshold stimulation with different electrode combinations and stimulation parameters using an external stimulation device is conducted. The stimulation intensity varies individually between 50 and 75 % of the intraoperative motor threshold [22, 16–18, 27, 37, 61, 64, 68, 69, 73]. This kind of subthreshold stimulation offers the possibilities of implementation of double-blinded and placebo stimulation settings during the test trial [4, 27, 40]. Programming can be performed by an individual, blinded

Table 7.4 Step-by-step protocol of the standard operative procedure (SOP) for ICS using the “burr-hole technique”

Standard operative procedure: “Burr-hole technique”
Head fixation in a 3-point pin holder in local anaesthesia
Calibration and adjustment of the neuronavigation data set
Identification of the precentral gyrus
Target planning and operative approach in local anaesthesia
Adjustment of intraoperative neuromonitoring
Parietal burr hole and epidural spacing
Navigation controlled epidural implantation of lead strips (2 × 4 contacts)
Intraoperative testing with SSEP/phase reversal recording and suprathreshold stimulation
Identification of the optimal lead position
Fixation of the leads
Percutaneous extensions in local anaesthesia
Wound closure and head clamp detachment

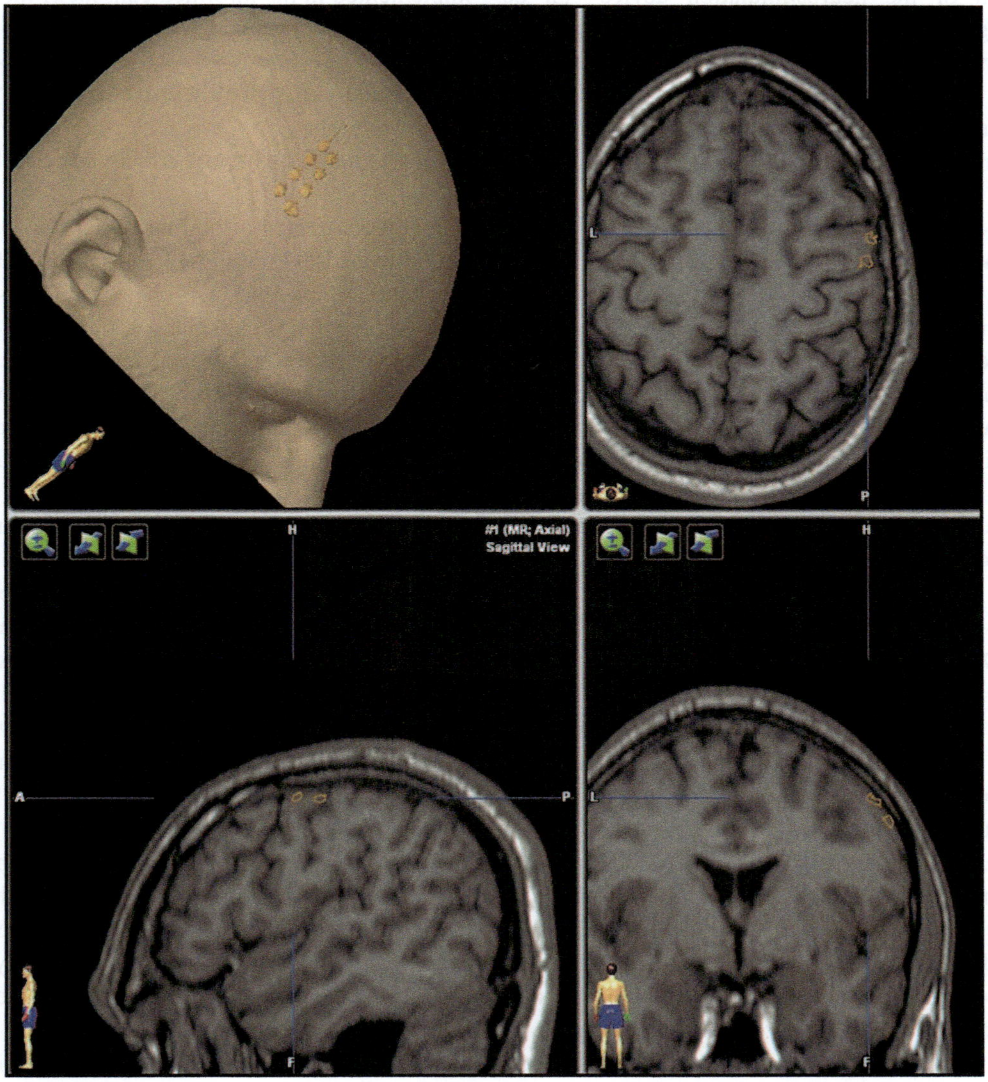

Fig. 7.4 Post-operative image fusion and matching of the lead position with the preoperative MRI data set using a neuronavigation system

physician and clinical documentation by specially trained nurses or physicians 6–8 times per day to complete a pain diary, document functional behaviour like mobility and subjective impressions, e.g. night's rest.

The test trial is terminated in case of positive effect with pain reduction of greater than 30 %, accompanied with reduction of analgesic medication. The importance and clinical significance of the placebo and double-blinded testing settings with identification of false-positive responders are underlined. In the patient sample of the authors 15 % (9/60) of the patients were identified as false-positive responders with reproducible pain reduction during placebo stimulation. This was considered to be a psychological or placebo effect and discussed with the patient. In these cases the leads were consecutively explanted.

Implantation of the neurostimulation device can be performed in general anaesthesia in the infraclavicular or abdominal subcutaneous tissue. The patient needs to be informed that, at the moment and with current knowledge, no MRI examination with the body-coil and these implanted devices is approved.

Follow-Up Visits

In all patients individual adaption and control of the stimulation parameters during follow-up are necessary. This may vary from stimulating 3 × 0.5 h/day up to continuous stimulation. The authors prefer a cyclic stimulation mode to avoid habituation [27]. Reprogramming is sometimes necessary every 3–6 months with change of polarity of the cathode and anode and impedance check to detect lead fracture, battery depletion, etc.

Complications

As in every surgical procedure a certain rate of complications can occur and the patient needs to sign an informed consent following a detailed preoperative discussion. On the one hand procedure-related complications like wound infections, bleeding or re-bleeding at the surgical sites can occur [3, 4, 22, 27, 37, 38, 40, 51, 55, 57]. The risk of wound infections might be increased in these cases with implanted materials. In case of the so-called burr-hole technique, the occurrence of an epidural bleeding is a much-feared complication [4, 27, 38, 40]. In the patient sample of the authors no epidural hematoma was detected by routine computed scan of the head performed on the first postoperative day [27].

Also epileptic seizures, either intraoperative or during follow-up, with or without neurological deficits and need of antiepileptic medication were reported.

In patients with MCS of the dominant hemisphere also speech disturbances with aphasia and speech arrest were observed and may be resolved in case of ongoing symptoms only by termination of MCS or explantation of the leads [4, 27, 48]. The problem of significantly increased complication rates in patients with subdural implants and therefore elevated risks of seizures, infection etc. cannot definitively been answered due to the small patient numbers and published case-reports.

On the other hand technical problems with the implanted materials like lead fracture or dislocations were observed in the published series. In this context one has to mention that all implanted materials, surgical leads, extensions and neurostimulation devices have no approval for this specific therapy and are used off-label. This also needs to be implemented in the informed consent of the patient.

Discussion and Review of the Literature

MCS in the Treatment of Chronic Pain

The authors treated a total number of 60 patients during a period from 1994 until 2013 and performed either epidural or subdural implantation of one or two leads over the motor cortex for the treatment of refractory chronic pain syndromes. In 36 of 60 (60 %) patients, pain reduction during the standardised test trial was evaluated and a permanent neurostimulator implanted. Pain reduction of at least 30 % of the initial visual analogue scale (VAS) ratings was considered acceptable and is in accordance with the current view of success rates in pharmacological pain therapies [82]. In detail, success rate was 17 of 25 in TNP (68 %), in PSP 38 % (6/16), in the BPA group 11/15 (73 %) and 2/4 of the patients with other indications. This was accompanied by identification of 9 false-positive responders (4 in the TNP and 5 in the PSP group) during placebo and double-blinded testing. At the last follow-up (mean: 4.5 years postoperatively) positive responders were evaluated in 14/17 patients with TNP (82 %), 4/6 of the PSP (67 %) and 8/11 in the BPA group (73 %).

The lowest success rate was found in the patients with PSP and central pain syndromes. This might be due to the fact that the pain origin and injury is located in the central pain transmission network itself. Also, it may be comparable with the bad results in other central neuropathic pain syndromes like postherpetic neuropathy. In contrast to this one can assume that the good results for pain in the face or upper limb might be due to the good representation on the convexity of the motor cortex and the multiple central connections to the "pain matrix". Therefore the authors favour and recommend MCS in cases with chronic neuropathic pain syndromes of the face or upper limb compared to

Table 7.5 List of relevant publications, number of patients, diagnosis, follow-up (months) and responders regarding MCS and chronic pain syndromes

Author	Year	Patient#	Diagnosis	Follow-up	Responder
Tsubokawa et al. [7]	1991	11	PSP	24	8
Meyerson et al. [9]	1993	5	TNP	28	5
Katayama et al. [89]	1994	3	Central pain	12	2
Migita et al. [79]	1995	15	PSP, spinal cord lesion pain	>24	11
Ebel et al. [10]	1996	6	TNP	24	3
Katayama et al. [12]	1998	31	PSP	>24	15
Garcia-Larrea et al. [61]	1999	10	PSP, plexus avulsion	6	5
Nguyen et al. [16]	1999	31	PSP, TNP, SCI, PHP	>24	7
Mertens et al. [15]	1999	23	Central neuropathic pain, SCI, BPA	74	11
Carroll et al. [17]	2000	10	PSP, phantom limb pain, traumatic neuralgia, brachialgia	>24	5
Saitoh et al. [19]	2000	8	PSP, peripheral deafferentation pain	26	6
Drouot et al. [64]	2002	31	Peripheral neuropathy and central lesions	18	21
Rainov et al. [24]	2003	2	TNP	18	2
Tirakotai et al. [25]	2004	5	Central pain	24	5
Brown et al. [26]	2005	10	Central and neuropathic facial pain	24	8
Nuti et al. [83]	2005	31	PSP, SCI	48	16
Cioni et Meglio [34]	2007	14	PSP, TNP, SCI	n.s.	3
Hosomi et al. [84]	2008	34	PSP, TNP, BPA, SCI, PLP	112	12
Velasco et al. [28]	2008	11	Central and peripheral neuropathic pain	12	8
Lefaucheur et al. [30]	2009	16	Peripheral neuropathic pain	12	9
Velasco et al. [29]	2009	5	CRPS	36–72	4
Nguyen et al. [4]	2011	100	PSP, TNP, BPA, SCI	89	64
Rasche et al. [27][a]	2013	60	TNP, PSP, BPA, peripheral pain	74	36

[a]Updated summary, published in part in 2006

other invasive procedures, e.g. deep brain stimulation [4, 27, 39, 57].

An overview concerning selected publications and reviews regarding MCS is given in Tables 7.5, 7.6 and 7.7.

The first operated patients with PSP were reported by Tsubokawa et al. in 1990, respectively 1991 (Tsubokawa, annual IASP congress in Adelaide 1990; [7]). In 1993 Tsubokawa et al. [8] reported an initial success rate of 73 % (8/11 patients) in PSP. After 2 years only five patients were still positive responders (45 %). Meyerson et al. reported the first patients with TNP and MCS in 1993 [9]. Initial positive effect of MCS was demonstrated in all cases with a follow-up of 4–28 months. Reporting positive MCS effect in 50 % (three of six) of the patients with TNP and a follow-up of 5–24 months was performed by Ebel et al. [10]. Pain relief by MCS in 7 of 12 (58 %) patients with TNP was reported by Nguyen et al. in 1999 [16]. Reporting a series of 20 patients with central neuropathic pain and a follow-up of more than 1 year, Mertens et al. [15] reported an excellent pain relief in 5 (25 %), good in 7 (35 %) and fair in 3 (15 %) patients. Five patients (25 %) were negative responders. The success rates reported for TNP and PSP are higher than in the patient sample of the authors. Brown and Pilitsis [26] reported the results of a prospective series of ten patients with central and neuropathic facial pain. In eight of ten cases (80 %), all patients with TNP, implantation of the stimulation device after successful trial was performed. Of the two patients without positive effect there was one case each with central pain after lateral medullary infarction and with pain of unknown origin. Positive effect of the MCS with improvement of facial weakness, sensory impairment and also dysarthria was also evaluated in three patients. All patients with implanted devices were able to reduce daily pain medication dose by more than 50 %. In these publications no hint is given about the clinical test trial after insertion of the lead and therefore it can be assumed that no double-blinded or placebo testing was performed.

Table 7.6 Relevant reviews regarding MCS

Authors (reference)	Year
Brown and Barbaro [22]	2003
Osenbach [33]	2006
Cioni and Meglio [34]	2007
Lazorthes et al. [35]	2007
Saitoh and Yoshimine [36]	2007
Arle and Shils [37]	2008
Lima and Fregni [38]	2008
Lefaucheur et al. [30]	2009
Nguyen et al. [4]	2011
Monsalve [40]	2012

Table 7.7 ICS complications

Complications	%
Wound infection/meningitis	≤10
Epileptic seizures	≤5
Technical failure	≤5
Sub/epidural haematoma	≤10
Neurological worsening	≤8

In contrast to other centres the burr-hole technique with epidural spacing for positioning of the lead was used in this series. A small craniotomy over the central sulcus is the preferred technique in other centres because of epidural bleeding during or after detachment of the dura [12, 14, 16, 32]. In our series no intra- or post-operative bleeding could be observed in routine cranial computed tomography on the first post-operative day [27]. It is obvious that a larger craniotomy over the central sulcus allows a more detailed monitoring and mapping of the pre- and postcentral area. It is discussable that placement of the lead via the burr-hole technique is not as precise as with the craniotomy technique and therefore, like in some patients of this series, the applied current for intra- and post-operative stimulation is higher because of the distance to the target. This disadvantage of the burr-hole technique can be a reason for a less favourable response rate compared with other centres. One has to mention that the success rate of patients with TNP is not much lower than in other centres. Targeting of the functional area of the primary pain site and not the craniotomy technique seems to be the major component of the procedure.

The authors prefer lead positioning over the convexity of the medial part of the precentral gyrus running perpendicular with the motor cortex from medially to laterally [27]. This is in contrast to other centres that prefer placing the lead over the post- and precentral gyrus crossing the central sulcus horizontally [14, 16]. fMRI studies revealed that the localisation of the cortical motor area can be highly variable [67, 77, 78] and discussion about the correct or ideal site of stimulation is still going on. Placing all contacts of the lead over the precentral gyrus was performed to cover most of the cortical area to improve stimulation effect to the primary pain site.

In 2005 Nuti et al. published the results of their patient sample with 31 patients and PSP or SCI [83]. A positive effect and pain relief was evaluated in 16 patients and it was stated that efficacy of MCS may be predicted in the first month of therapy. Less impressive were the results reported by Cioni and Meglio [34]. Only 2/14 patients experienced pain relief by chronic MCS. In contrast to these findings, Velasco reported positive effects of MCS in 8/11 patients with unilateral neuropathic pain of different origin in a randomised double-blind trial with postoperative follow-up of 12 months [28].

Direct stimulation of the cortical surface by implantation of the lead within the central sulcus and on the precentral gyrus was performed by Hosomi et al. [84]. Out of a collective of 34 patients 12 responded well to MCS. In detail, 10 of 12 patients experienced pain relief by direct stimulation within the central sulcus and in 4 of 10 patients positive effects maintained at follow-ups. The efficacy of direct lead positioning and electrical stimulation within the central sulcus needs to be evaluated and compared with MCS in a prospective randomised trial.

Concerning BPA only about 20 patients are reported in the literature [15, 84]. The first published patients by Mertens et al. suffered from chronic posttraumatic pain following brachial plexus avulsion [15]. In four cases a subdural or epidural lead was placed over the motor area of the upper limb and 2 patients were screened to achieve pain reduction by stimulation during a follow-up of about 2 years. Hosomi et al. reported the largest collective with seven patients suffering from chronic pain following brachial plexus avulsion [84]. In 6/7 patients a permanent neurostimulator was implanted. Pain reduction of the remaining patients varied from 10 to 90 %. After a follow-up from 9 to 112 months the lead was removed in two cases and one patient died after 36 months due to a cerebral hemorrhage. Only in one case the pain reduction achieved by subdural stimulation of the precentral gyrus was stable with 50 % over a follow-up of 50 months. In all other cases the effect diminished over time. The initial responder rate in the patient sample of the authors was 11/15 (73 %) in cases with BPA.

Until now about 14 patients with phantom limb pain and MCS are reported [5, 17, 19, 36, 38]. Two out of three patients published by Carroll et al. showed a benefit by MCS in phantom limb pain [17]. Saitoh et al. reported two patients with phantom limb pain and lasting positive effect over 6–20 months [5, 19, 36]. In 2001 Katayama et al. published five cases, but only one patient improved by this therapy with a follow-up of more than 24 months [85]. Four patients are reported in the patient series of Hosomi et al. [84]. Only in one patient a stable pain reduction of 90 % was achieved for 54 months. In the remaining three patients the system was removed during the first 6 post-operative months.

Only a small number of cases with chronic postherpetic pain are published. Recently Velasco et al. reported five patients with postherpetic neuralgia in a prospective randomised double-blind trial [28]. The pain distribution involved was cervical in two patients; the thoracic spine in two patients and only in one patient the first branch of the trigeminal nerve was affected. Two patients with postherpetic neuralgia of the spine and one with trigeminal pain improved by MCS and pain reduction of 56–80 % was achieved. The positive effect was stable over the follow-up period of 1 year.

In 2009 Velasco et al. published their results in five patients with MCS and complex regional pain syndrome type I and II (CRPS) [29]. In detail, three patients suffered from BPA, one patient each from pain due to hemangiectasis and dermatosclerosis neuropathy. Four/five patients responded to the MCS with pain reduction and improved sympathetic symptoms.

Several literature reviews regarding MCS and ICS are published (see Tables 7.6 and 7.7). The most recent review of one of the most experienced neurosurgeons summarises the efficacies and mechanisms of action of MCS [4]. In their review 100 patients out of their own sample were included and they evaluated 64 % responders. Looking at meta-analyses of MCS therapy it is found that 64 % [38], respectively 57 % [86] of treated patients responded to MCS. In 2012 Monsalve published a literature review of 126 relevant articles and a total of 118 patients with chronic facial neuropathic pain and MCS [40]. A responder rate of 84 % is reported.

Most of the published series represent a very inhomogeneous and mixed collective of pain patients (see Table 7.7). Also some cases of rare pain syndromes including both neuropathic and nociceptive pain were reported (e.g. stumb pain, neuroma, sclerodermia) with different results. Additionally, in most of the clinical trials no information is given about placebo or double-blinded testing. Therefore it can be assumed that in many studies no standard protocol with double-blinded or placebo testing was followed.

The scientific and clinical evidence of MCS in chronic pain treatment is insufficient. Only a few prospective randomised studies were found [4, 26, 28, 40, 86]. In 2005 Brown and Pilitsis reported ten patients with neuropathic pain treated by MCS [26]. In eight patients a permanent neurostimulator was implanted after a successful test trial. Another prospective study was reported by Velasco et al. [28]. Again 10 patients with different chronic pain syndromes were treated with MCS. In eight of the ten patients pain reduction was achieved. Randomisation procedure to "ON" or "OFF" stimulation was performed at day 60 or 90 after permanent implantation in a double-blinded fashion. It was demonstrated that randomisation to "OFF" stimulation led to significant increase of pain ($p < .05$) and that significant improvement of pain was induced by MCS ($p < .01$).

ICS in the Treatment of Non-painful Conditions/Syndromes

Parkinson's Disease and Movement Disorders

Nguyen et al. were the first in 1998 who published the chronic application of MCS in patients with Parkinson disease (PD) [43]. Woolsely already evaluated initial experience in 1979 [42]. Arle and Shils published an overview of the literature including four own patients with PD in 2008 [37]. With either subdural or epidural lead placement over the motor cortex short- and mid-term benefits were achieved but faded away after 12 months.

Moro et al. reported six patients with essential tremor and five patients with PD and unilateral subdural lead implantation over the motor cortex [50]. A significant improvement of contralateral hand tremor was evaluated at 3-month and 1-year follow-ups, but no significant effect was seen in the PD group. In contrast to these results Bentivoglio et al. published a series of nine patients with PD and also unilateral extradural MCS [52]. They demonstrated a moderate improvement of motor symptoms and quality of life at 12-month follow-up.

Therefore currently no clear recommendations can be stated regarding the clinical significance of MCS in PD and other movement disorders. In conclusion, MCS cannot be recommended as an alternative procedure, compared to DBS of the basal ganglia, for patients with severe PD or movement disorders.

Depression

In patients with treatment-resistant or major depression a lot of studies using non-invasive methods like rTMS or transcranial direct current stimulation (tDCS) are published (see Chap. 8). Only limited data are available for invasive cortical stimulation for this indication. A prospective randomised, single-blind, sham-controlled study with 11 patients and a follow-up period of 104 weeks was published in 2011 by Kopell et al. [49]. A single lead was placed over the left dorsolateral prefrontal cortex (Brodmann area 9/46) and continuous stimulation with 50 Hz, 150 μs and amplitude of 6.5 mA was delivered. Although there was no statistical significance between the active and sham stimulation, a trend towards efficacy with active stimulation was evaluated. Another case series including five patients with treatment-resistant depression was published by Nahas et al. in 2010 [47]. Leads were implanted bilaterally over the anterior frontal poles and midlateral prefrontal cortex. Stimulation paradigm varied in contrast to other series with cyclic stimulation mode. Stimulation was active from 8 a.m. until 10 p.m. with 30 min ON and 2.5 h OFF at 60 Hz and intensity from 2 to 4 V. At 7-month follow-up mean improvement was 54.9 % on the Hamilton Rating Scale for Depression and 60.1 % for the Inventory of Depressive Symptoms—Self Report. Three patients reached remission while in one case the left-sided leads were explanted due to infection.

In conclusion it has to be stated that these early results are promising but additional studies with larger patient samples need to be conducted. Currently it remains doubtful if these invasive procedures will play a significant role for the treatment algorithms of these patients compared to the variety and results of non-invasive techniques [54].

Tinnitus

In contrast to MCS the leads are placed over the auditory cortex, so called the Heschl gyrus or Brodmann area 41. De Ridder et al. in 2010, 2011 and an overview in 2012 published the greatest experience with this indication [46, 48, 55]. In a series with 43 implanted patients 33 % remained unaffected by the auditory cortex stimulation (ACS). 67 % (29/43) of the patients responded to either tonic ACS or bursts of high-frequency stimulation. It could be evaluated that ACS with burst stimulation was favourable for noise like tinnitus. Preoperative evaluation of the predictive effect of transcranial magnetic stimulation was negative. However, one must mention that the failure rate of 33 % of the patients as non-responders and the complication rate with epileptic seizures (3/43), intracranial bleeding and abscess in one case each following intradural lead implantation are remarkable.

Stroke

The improvement of motor function with reduction of spasticity, dystonia or myoclonus was observed in many studies using MCS in patients with PSP [4, 5, 7, 12, 14, 19, 27, 31]. The authors interpreted these findings as secondary effects of MCS.

In 2006 Brown et al. published a prospective multicentre safety study for the evaluation of the enhancement of recovery from stroke using MCS [87]. Although the patient sample was small, an improved outcome was documented for patients receiving MCS and rehabilitation than rehabilitation alone. Canavero et al published their experience with bilateral MCS in movement disorders in 2007 [88]. They found differential effects of ipsi- and contralateral MCS in the follow-up period of 1 year. Yamamoto et al. published a small case series of six patients with improvement of motor function at 6-month follow-up [31].

A recent review by Edwardson et al. summarises the results of the published series and demonstrates the lack of scientific data regarding the different results of the phase I and II in contrast to the phase III "EVEREST" trial [56]. Despite the initial good results of phase I and II no statistical significant improvement was found in the phase III trial with a larger cohort of patients. It is suspected that a bias remains regarding patient selection and the authors conclude that the number of intact corticothalamic or corticospinal tract fibres is essential for the efficacy of cortical stimulation.

Epilepsy

The implantation of leads, either sub- or epidural, is an invasive part of epilepsy surgery for many years. Usually these leads were used for recording of electrocortical activity to identify epileptogenic foci for detailed surgical mapping and resection control. The clinical use for cortical stimulation was first implemented only for patients with refractory epilepsy who were not candidates for respective epilepsy surgery [51, 53, 57]. In 2011 the results of a multicenter, double-blind, randomised controlled trial using responsive cortical stimulation with a closed-loop system for the treatment of medically refractory partial epilepsy were published [51]. This stimulation device combines a lead in the hippocampus for recording and a cortical lead on the ipsilateral inferior temporal lobe for on-demand stimulation. In a sample of 191 patients a significant reduction of partial seizure frequency and increase of quality of life was evaluated during the blinded and open-label period of 84 weeks. This is the only study, at the moment for ICS, reaching class of evidence level I.

Recently two reviews regarding brain stimulation for the treatment of epilepsy summarise the current significance of these invasive therapies [53, 57].

Conclusion

MCS is an alternative invasive procedure for a selected patient group with chronic neuropathic pain. Well-located neuropathic pain syndromes after nerve injury, like in cases with TNP, seem to respond more favourably than pain syndromes after lesion of the central pain pathways itself, like in patients with PSP or thalamic infarction. Until today neither standardised protocols nor guidelines for this procedure exist. The rating of efficacy is different and has a wide spectrum. MCS should be performed in an experienced centre of neurosurgical pain therapy following a standardised protocol including double-blinded or placebo testing. Undoubtedly, there is an urgent need for prospective randomised controlled trials of the experienced centres to gain a level of evidence and recommendations for the significance of MCS as an invasive pain therapy.

In contrast to this, the level of evidence for ICS is developing and best for refractory partial epilepsy with a significant positive effect demonstrated in a prospective, multicentre, randomised controlled, double-blind trial.

Overall, ICS can be considered as a safe and effective treatment option for highly selected patients with different chronic, treatment-resistant neuropathic pain syndromes, movement disorders, tinnitus, depression or epilepsy.

References

1. Jensen TS, Baron R, Haanpää M, Kalso E, Loeser JD, Rice ASC, Treede RD. A new definition of neuropathic pain. Pain. 2011;152:2204–5.
2. Finnerup NB, Scholz J, Attal N, Baron R, Haanpää M, Hansson P, Raja SN, Rice ASC, Rief W, Rowbotham MC, Simpson DM, Treede RD. Neuropathic pain needs systematic classification. Eur J Pain. 2013;17(7):953–6.
3. King RB, Schnell GR. Cortical localisation and monitoring during cerebral operations. J Neurosurg. 1987;67:210–9.
4. Nguyen JP, Nizard J, Keravel Y, Lefaucheur JP. Invasive brain stimulation for the treatment of neuropathic pain. Nat Rev Neurol. 2011;7:699–709.
5. Saitoh Y, Shibata M, Hirano SI, Kato A, Kishima H, Hirata M, Yamamoto K, Yoshimine T. Motor cortex stimulation for deafferentation pain. Neurosurg Focus. 2001;11:1–5.
6. Penfield W, Rasmussen T. The cerebral cortex of man. A clinical study of localization of function. New York: Macmillan; 1950.
7. Tsubokawa T, Katayama Y, Yamamoto T, Hirayama T, Koyama S. Chronic motor cortex stimulation for the treatment of central pain. Acta Neurochir Suppl (Wien). 1991;52:137–9.
8. Tsubokawa T, Katayama Y, Yamamoto T, Hirayama T, Koyama S. Chronic motor cortex stimulation in patients with thalamic pain. J Neurosurg. 1993;78:393–401.
9. Meyerson BA, Lindblom U, Linderoth B, Lind G, Herregodts P. Motor cortex stimulation as treatment of trigeminal neuropathic pain. Acta Neurochir Suppl (Wien). 1993;58:150–3.
10. Ebel H, Rust D, Tronnier V, Spies EH, Böker D, Kunze S. Chronic precentral stimulation in trigeminal neuropathic pain. Acta Neurochir. 1996;138:1300–6.
11. Yamamoto T, Katayama Y, Hirayama T, Tsubokawa T. Pharmacological classification of central post-stroke pain: comparison with the results of chronic motor cortex stimulation therapy. Pain. 1997;72:5–12.
12. Katayama Y, Fukaya C, Yamamoto T. Poststroke pain control by chronic motor cortex stimulation: neurological characteristics predicting a favourable response. J Neurosurg. 1998;89:585–91.
13. Canavero S, Bonicalzi V, Castellano G, Perozzo P, Massa-Micon B. Painful supernumerary phantom arm following motor cortex stimulation for central poststroke pain. Case report. J Neurosurg. 1999;91:121–3.
14. Franzini A, Dones I, Ferroli P, et al. (1999): La stimolazione corticale nel trattamento della distonia focale e del dolore centrale dell'arto superiore. In: Abstracts of the XLVIII Congresso Nazionale, Societa Italiana di Neurochirurgia, Copanello. 1999: 274
15. Mertens P, Nuti C, Sindou M, Guenot M, Peyron R, Garcia-Larrea LB. Precentral cortex stimulation for the treatment of central neuropathic pain: results of a prospective study in a 20-patient series. Stereotact Funct Neurosurg. 1999;73:122–5.
16. Nguyen JP, Lefaucheur JP, Decp P, Uchiyama T, Carpentier A, Fontaine D, Brugières P, Pollin B, Fève A, Rostaing S, Cesaro P, Keravel Y. Chronic motor cortex stimulation in the treatment of central and neuropathic pain. Correlations between clinical, electrophysiological and anatomical data. Pain. 1999;82:245–51.
17. Carroll D, Joint C, Maartens N, Shlugman D, Stein J, Aziz TZ. Motor cortex stimulation for chronic neuropathic pain: a preliminary study of 10 cases. Pain. 2000;84:431–7.
18. Kuroda R, Yamada Y, Kondo S. Electrical stimulation of the second somatosensory cortex for intractable pain: a case report and experimental study. Stereotact Funct Neurosurg. 2000;74:226.
19. Saitoh Y, Shibata M, Hirano SI, Hirata M, Moshimo T, Yoshimine T. Motor cortex stimulation for central and peripheral deafferentation pain. J Neurosurg. 2000;92:150–5.
20. Roux FE, Ibarrola D, Lazorthes Y, Berry I. Chronic motor cortex stimulation for phantom limb pain: a functional magnetic resonance imaging study: technical case report. Neurosurgery. 2001;48:681–8.
21. Sol JC, Casaux J, Roux FE, Lotterie JA, Bousquet P, Verdie JC, Mascott C, Lazorthes Y. Chronic motor cortex stimulation for phantom limb pain: correlations between pain relief and functional imaging studies. Stereotact Funct Neurosurg. 2001;77:172–6.
22. Brown JA, Barbaro NM. Motor cortex stimulation for central and neuropathic pain: current status. Pain. 2003;104:431–5.
23. Fukaya C, Katayama Y, Yamamoto T, Kobayashi K, Kasai M, Oshima H. Motor cortex stimulation in patients with post-stroke pain: conscious somatosensory response and pain control. Neurol Res. 2003;25(2):153–6.
24. Rainov NG, Heidecke V. Motor cortex stimulation for neuropathic facial pain. Neurol Res. 2003;25:157–61.
25. Tirakotai W, Riegel T, Sure U, Rohlfs J, Gharabaghi A, Bertalanffy H, Hellwig D. Image-guided motor cortex stimulation in patients with central pain. Minim Invasive Neurosurg. 2004;47:273–7.
26. Brown JA, Pilitsis JG. Motor cortex stimulation for central and neuropathic facial pain: a prospective study of 10 patients and observations of enhanced sensory and motor function during stimulation. Neurosurgery. 2005;56:290–7.
27. Rasche D, Ruppolt M, Stippch C, Unterberg A, Tronnier VM. Motor cortex stimulation for long-term relief of chronic neuropathic pain: a ten year experience. Pain. 2006;121:43–52.
28. Velasco F, Argüelles C, Carrillo-Ruiz JD, Castro G, Velasco AL, Jiménez F, Velasco M. Efficacy of motor cortex stimulation in the treatment of neuropathic pain: a randomized double-blind trial. J Neurosurg. 2008;108:698–706.
29. Velasco F, Carrillo-Ruiz JD, Castro G, Argüelles C, Velasco AL, Kassian A, Guevara U. Motor cortex electrical stimulation applied to patients with complex regional pain syndrome. Pain. 2009;147:91–8.
30. Lefaucheur JP, Drouot X, Cunin P, Bruckert R, Lepetit H, Créange A, Wolkenstein P, Maison P, Keravel Y, Nguyen JP. Motor cortex stimulation for the treatment of refractory peripheral neuropathic pain. Brain. 2009;132:1463–71.
31. Yamamoto T, Katayama Y, Watanabe M, Sumi K, Obuchi T, Kobayashi K, Oshima H, Fukaya C. Changes in motor function induced by chronic motor cortex stimulation in post-stroke pain patients. Stereotact Funct Neurosurg. 2011;89:381–9.
32. Canavero S, Bonicalzi V. Therapeutic extradural cortical stimulation for central and neuropathic pain: a review. Clin J Pain. 2002;18:48–55.
33. Osenbach RK. Motor cortex stimulation for intractable pain. Neurosurg Focus. 2006;21:E7.

34. Cioni B, Megglio M. Motor cortex stimulation for chronic non-malignant pain: current state and future prospects. Acta Neurochir Suppl. 2007;97(2):45–9.
35. Lazorthes Y, Sol JC, Fowo S, Roux FE, Verdié JC. Motor cortex stimulation for neuropathic pain. Acta Neurochir Suppl. 2007;97 (2):37–44.
36. Saitoh Y, Yoshimine T. Stimulation of primary motor cortex for intractable deafferentation pain. Acta Neurochir Suppl. 2007;97:51–6.
37. Arle JE, Shils JL. Motor cortex stimulation for pain and movement disorders. Neurotherapeutics. 2008;5:37–49.
38. Lima MC, Fregni F. Motor cortex stimulation for chronic pain: systematic review and meta-analysis of the literature. Neurology. 2008;70:2329–37.
39. Knotkova H, Cruciani RA, Tronnier VM, Rasche D. Current and future options for the management of phantom-limb pain. J Pain Res. 2012;5:39–49.
40. Monsalve GA. Motor cortex stimulation for facial chronic neuropathic pain: a review of the literature. Surg Neurol Int. 2012;3: S290–311.
41. Delavallée M, Abu-Serieh B, de Tourchaninoff M, Raftopoulos C. Subdural motor cortex stimulation for central and peripheral neuropathic pain: a long-term follow-up study in a series of eight patients. Neurosurgery. 2008;63:101–8.
42. Woolsely CN, Erickson TC, Gilson WE. Localization in somatic sensory and motor area of human cerebral cortex as determined by direct recording of evoked potentials and electrical stimulation. J Neurosurg. 1979;51:476–509.
43. Nguyen JP, Pollin B, Feve A, Geny C, Cesaro P. Improvement of action tremor by chronic cortical stimulation. Mov Disord. 1998;13:84–8.
44. Hantraye P, Palfi S. Functional recovery in a primate model of Parkinson's disease following motor cortex stimulation. Neuron. 2004;44(5):769–78.
45. Arle JE, Apetauerova D, Zani J, Deletis DV, Penney DL, Hoit D, Gould C, Shils JL. Motor cortex stimulation in patients with Parkinson disease: 12-month follow-up in 4 patients. J Neurosurg. 2008;109:133–9.
46. De Ridder D, Vanneste S, Van der Loo E, Plazier M, Menovsky T, Van de Heyning P. Burst stimulation of the auditory cortex: a new form of neurostimulation for noise-like tinnitus suppression. J Neurosurg. 2010;112:1289–94.
47. Nahas Z, Anderson BS, Borckardt J, Arana AB, George MS, Reeves ST, Takacs I. Bilateral epidural prefrontal cortical stimulation for treatment-resistant depression. Biol Psychiatry. 2010;67:101–9.
48. De Ridder D, Vanneste S, Kovacs S, Sunaert S, Menovsky T, van de Heyning P, Moller A. Transcranial magnetic stimulation and extradural electrodes implanted on secondary auditory cortex for tinnitus suppression. J Neurosurg. 2011;114:903–11.
49. Kopell BH, Halverson J, Butson CR, Dickinson M, Bobholz J, Harsch H, Rainey C, Kondziolka D, Howland R, Eskandar E, Evans KC, Dougherty DD. Epidural cortical stimulation of the left dorsolateral prefrontal cortex for refractory major depressive disorder. Neurosurgery. 2011;69:1015–29.
50. Moro E, Schwalb JM, Piboolnurak P, Poon YYW, Hamani C, Hung SW, Arenovich T, Lang AE, Chen R, Lozano AM. Unilateral subdural motor cortex stimulation improves essential tremor but not Parkinson's disease. Brain. 2011;134:2096–105.
51. Morrell MJ, RNS System in Epilepsy Study Group. Responsive cortical stimulation for the treatment of medically intractable partial epilepsy. Neurology. 2011;77:1295–304.
52. Bentivoglio AR, Fasano A, Piano C, Soleti F, Daniele A, Zinno M, Piccininni C, De Simone C, Policicchio D, Tufo T, Meglio M, Cioni B. Unilateral extradural motor cortex stimulation is safe and improves Parkinson disease at 1 year. Neurosurgery. 2012;71:815–25.
53. Fridley J, Thomas JG, Navarro JC, Yoshor D. Brain stimulation for the treatment of epilepsy. Neurosurg Focus. 2012;32:E13.
54. Holtzheimer PE, Mayberg HS. Neuromodulation for treatment-resistant depression. F1000 Med Rep. 2012;4:22.
55. Vanneste S, De Ridder D. Noninvasive and invasive neuromodulation for the treatment of tinnitus: an overview. Neuromodulation. 2012;15:350–60.
56. Edwardson MA, Lucas TH, Carey JR, Fetz EE. New modalities of brain stimulation for stroke rehabilitation. Exp Brain Res. 2013;224:335–58.
57. Wu C, Sharan AD. Neurostimulation for the treatment of epilepsy: a review of current surgical interventions. Neuromodulation. 2013;16:10–24.
58. Wood CC, Spencer DD, Allison T, McCarthy G, Williamson PD, Goff WR. Localization of human sensorimotor cortex during surgery by cortical surface recording of somatosensory evoked potentials. J Neurosurg. 1988;68:99–111.
59. Rao SM, Binder JR, Hammeke TA, Bandettini PA, Bobholz JA, Frost JA, Myklebust BM, Jacobson RD, Hyde JS. Somatotopic mapping of the human primary motor cortex with functional magnetic resonance imaging. Neurology. 1995;45:919–24.
60. Garcia-Larrea L, Peyron R, Mertens P, Gregoire MC, Lavenne F, Bonnefoi F, Convers P, Mauguiere F, Laurent B, Sindou M. Positron emission tomography during motor cortex stimulation for pain control. Stereotact Funct Neurosurg. 1997;68:141–8.
61. Garcia-Larrea L, Peyron R, Mertens P, Gregoire MC, Lavenne F, Lebars D, Convers P, Mauguiere F, Sindou M, Laurent B. Electrical stimulation of motor cortex for pain control: a combined PET-scan and electrophysiological study. Pain. 1999;83:259–73.
62. Garcia-Larrea L, Peyron R, Mertens P, Laurent B, Mauguiere F, Sindou M. Functional imaging and neurophysiological assessment of spinal and brain therapeutic modulation in humans. Arch Med Res. 2000;31:248–57.
63. Peyron R, Laurent B, Garcia-Larrea L. Functional imaging of brain responses to pain. A review and analysis. Neurophysiol Clin. 2000;30:263–88.
64. Drouot X, Nguyen JP, Peschanski M, Lefaucheur JP. The antalgic effect of chronic motor cortex stimulation is related to sensory changes in the painful zone. Brain. 2002;125:1660–4.
65. Lefaucheur JP, Drouot X, Menard-Lefaucheur I, Zerah F, Bendib B, Cesaro P, Keravel Y, Nguyen JP. Neurogenic pain relief by repetitive transcranial magnetic cortical stimulation depends on the origin and the site of pain. J Neurol Neurosurg Psychiatry. 2004;75:612–6.
66. Starafella AP, Vanderwerf Y, Sadikot AF. Transcranial magnetic stimulation of the human motor cortex influences the neuronal activity of subthalamic nucleus. Eur J Neurosci. 2004;20:2245–9.
67. Tinazzi M, Valeriani M, Moretto G, Rosso T, Nicolato A, Fiaschi A, Aglioti SM. Plastic interactions between hand and face cortical representation in patients with trigeminal neuralgia: a somatosensory-evoked potentials study. Neuroscience. 2004;127:769–76.
68. Cioni B, Meglio M, Perotti V, De Bonis P, Montano N. Neurophysiological aspects of chronic motor cortex stimulation. Neurophysiol Clin. 2007;37(6):441–7.
69. Holsheimer J, Nguyen JP, Lefaucheur JP, Manola L. Cathodal, anodal or bifocal stimulation of the motor cortex in the management of chronic pain? Acta Neurochir Suppl. 2007;97(2):57–66.
70. Pirotte B, Voordecker P, Brotchi J, Levivier M. Anatomical and physiological basis, clinical and surgical considerations, mechanisms underlying efficacy and future prospects of cortical stimulation for pain. Acta Neurochir Suppl. 2007;97(2):81–9.
71. Stippich C, Ochmann H, Sartor K. Somatotopic mapping of the human primary sensorimotor cortex during motor imagery and motor execution by functional magnetic resonance imaging. Neurosci Lett. 2002;331:50–4.

72. Stippich C, Kress B, Ochmann H, Tronnier V, Sartor K. Preoperative fMRI in patients with rolandic brain tumors: indication, investigation strategy, possibilities and limitations of clinical application. Fortsch Röntgenstr. 2003;175:1042–50.
73. Pirotte B, Voordecker P, Neugroschl C, Baleriaux D, Wikler D, Metens T, Denolin V, Joffroy A, Massager N, Brotchi J, Levivier M. Combination of functional magnetic resonance imaging-guided neuronavigation and intraoperative cortical brain mapping improves targeting of motor cortex stimulation in neuropathic pain. Neurosurgery. 2005;56:344–59.
74. Herregodts P, Stadnik T, De Ridder F, D'Haens J. Cortical stimulation for central neuropathic pain: 3-D surface MRI for easy determination of the motor cortex. Acta Neurochir Suppl. 1995;64:132–5.
75. Nguyen JP, Lefaucheur JP, Le Guerinel C, Fontanine D, Nakano N, Sakka L, Eizenbaum JF, Pollin B, Keravel Y. Treatment of central and neuropathic facial pain by chronic stimulation of the motor cortex: value of neuronavigation guidance for the localization of the motor cortex. Neurochirurgie. 2000;46:483–91.
76. Velasco M, Velasco F, Brito F, Velasco AL, Nguyen JP, Marquez I, Boleaga B, Keravel Y. Motor cortex stimulation in the treatment of deafferentation pain. I. Localisation of the motor cortex. Stereotact Funct Neurosurg. 2002;79:146–67.
77. Flor H, Elbert T, Mühlnickel W, Pantev C, Wienbruch C, Taub E. Cortical reorganization and phantom phenomena in congenital and traumatic upper-extremity amputees. Exp Brain Res. 1998;119:205–12.
78. Karl A, Birbaumer N, Lutzenberger W, Cohen LG, Flor H. Reorganization of motor and somatosensory cortex in upper extremity amputees with phantom limb pain. J Neurosci. 2001;21:3609–18.
79. Migita K, Uozumi T, Arita K, Monden S. Transcranial magnetic coil stimulation of the motor cortex in patients with central pain. Neurosurgery. 1995;36:1037–40.
80. Canavero S, Bonicalzi V, Dotta M, Vighetti S, Asteggiano G, Cocito D. Transcranial magnetic cortical stimulation relieves central pain. Stereotact Funct Neurosurg. 2002;78(3–4):192–6.
81. Lefaucheur JP, Drouot X, Menard-Lefaucheur I, Keravel Y, Nguyen JP. Motor cortex rTMS in chronic neuropathic pain: pain relief is associated with thermal sensory perception improvement. J Neurol Neurosurg Psychiatry. 2008;79(9):1044–9.
82. Farrar JT, Portenoy RK. Neuropathic cancer pain: the role of adjuvant analgesics. Oncology (Williston Park). 2001;15:1435–42.
83. Nuti C, Peyron R, Garcia-Larrea L, Brunon J, Laurent B, Sindou M, Mertens P. Motor cortex stimulation for refractory neuropathic pain: four year outcome and predictors of efficacy. Pain. 2005;118:43–52.
84. Hosomi K, Saitoh Y, Kishima H, Oshino S, Hirata M, Tani N, Shimokawa T, Yoshimine T. Electrical stimulation of primary motor cortex within central sulcus for intractable neuropathic pain. Clin Neurophysiol. 2008;119:993–1001.
85. Katayama Y, Yamamoto T, Kobayashi K, Kasai M, Oshima H, Fukaya C. Motor cortex stimulation for phantom limb pain: a comprehensive therapy with spinal cord and thalamic stimulation. Stereotact Funct Neurosurg. 2001;77:159–61.
86. Fontaine D, Hamani C, Lozano A. Efficacy and safety of motor cortex stimulation for chronic neuropathic pain: critical review of the literature. J Neurosurg. 2009;110:251–6.
87. Brown JA, Lutsep HL, Weinand M, Cramer SC. Motor cortex stimulation for the enhancement of recovery from stroke: a prospective, multicenter safety study. Neurosurgery. 2006;58:464–73.
88. Canavero S, Bonicalzi V. Extradural cortical stimulation for movement disorders. Acta Neurochir Suppl. 2007;97:223–32.
89. Katayama Y, Tsubokawa T, Yamamoto T. Chronic motor cortex stimulation for central deafferentation pain: experience with bulbar pain secondary to Wallenberg syndrome. Stereotact Funct Neurosurg. 1994;62:295–9.

Physiological Basis of Transcranial Magnetic Stimulation

8

Anne P. Caruso and Monica A. Perez

Introduction

Transcranial magnetic stimulation (TMS) has emerged as one of the most efficient ways to noninvasively stimulate the motor cortex in humans. Principles of electromagnetism were utilized to make it possible to stimulate the human brain with pulses generated by magnetic coils. The knowledge gained by studies using electrical stimulation of the motor cortex and principles of electromagnetism were combined to aid in the successful development of a non-painful, noninvasive method of brain stimulation (Barker et al. [1]). Neuronal elements that can be accessed through a magnetic pulse generated by TMS can be recorded through epidural recording from the spinal cord and surface electromyographic (EMG) recordings from limb muscles. Specifically, we address how TMS can be used to examine the contribution of both direct and indirect corticospinal pathways to spinal motoneurons. The origin of direct (D) and indirect (I) waves elicited by TMS stimulation over the motor cortex and recorded from epidural electrodes positioned over the spinal cord will be discussed. TMS methodology has evolved tremendously during the past 20 years. We describe the most common types of TMS coils used in experiments today and the types of waves elicited by different coil orientations. This includes the circular coil, figure-of-eight coil, double cone coil, and batwing coil. For each coil, we review the type of protocols for which it is used and the strength of the magnetic field that can be generated. We focus on the ability of a particular coil orientation to elicit D and I waves and how paired-pulse TMS protocols can be used to provide insight into the nature of the cortical circuitry that is activated by TMS. In the last section of our review, we examine the ways in which researchers are using TMS for therapeutic purposes; in particular, we look at the effects of repetitive TMS (rTMS) administered to patients with Parkinson's disease, stroke, dystonia, depression, and other conditions.

History of Motor Cortical Stimulation

Magnetic stimulation is based on the elements of electromagnetic induction, reported for the first time in 1831 by Michael Faraday [2]. In his experiment, he arranged two wires in a parallel configuration, and he passed an electrical current through one of them. The current flow in the first wire produced a current of equal magnitude and direction in the second wire. However, when the current in the first wire was stopped, a current of equal magnitude was induced in the second wire in the opposite direction. This effect could be described as a changing primary current in a loop of wire. Since each electric current has a magnetic field surrounding it, a changing primary electrical current produced a changing magnetic field. This changing magnetic field could *induce* a secondary current of opposite direction in a new second loop of wire. This effect is called magnetoelectric *induction.* This time-varying magnetic field induces an electric field whose magnitude is proportional to the time rate of change of the magnetic field, which in the case of TMS is determined by the rate of change of the current in the stimulating coil. Electric charge is stored in a capacitor and is discharged through the coil, producing a current pulse in the circuit that generates a magnetic field pulse in the vicinity of the coil. If the coil is held over a subject's head, the magnetic field penetrates the scalp and skull and induces an electric field in the brain [3].

Electrical pulses were used before magnetic pulses as a means by which the cortex could be stimulated. In 1876,

A.P. Caruso
Seton Hill University's Physician Assistant Program, Seton Hill University, Greensburg, PA, USA
e-mail: ap.caruso@setonhill.edu

M.A. Perez (✉)
Department of Physical Medicine and Rehabilitation, Center for the Neural Basis of Cognition, University of Pittsburgh, Pittsburgh, PA, USA
e-mail: perezmo@pitt.edu

H. Knotkova and D. Rasche (eds.), *Textbook of Neuromodulation*,
DOI 10.1007/978-1-4939-1408-1_8, © Springer Science+Business Media, LLC 2015

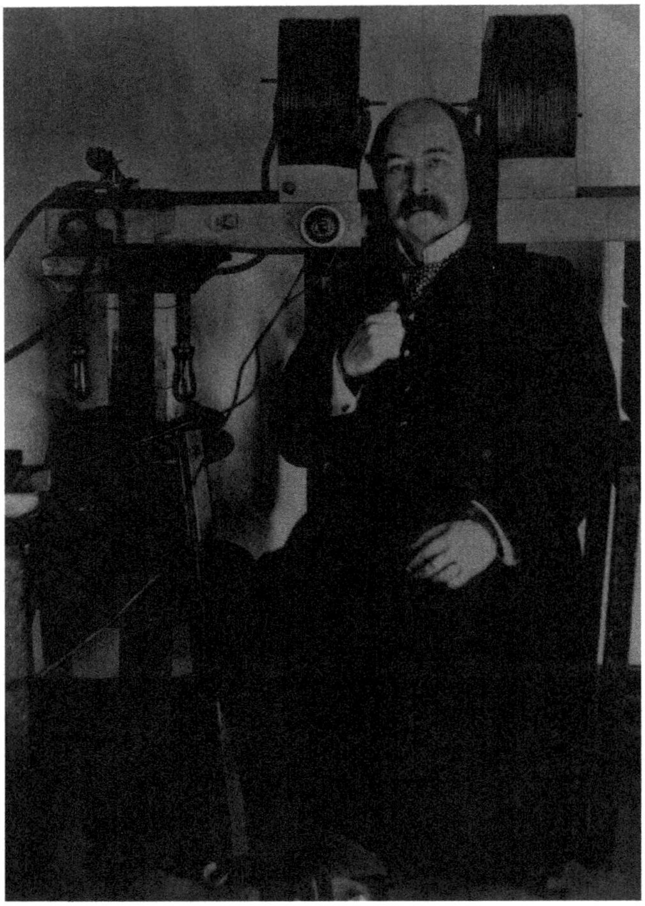

Fig. 8.1 Thompson SP (1910). Pictured with the apparatus that he used to stimulate the brain with electromagnetic pulses (Transcranial Magnentic Stimulation, Scholarpedia)

electrical stimulation of the exposed cortex was reported in monkeys [4]. It was demonstrated that certain areas stimulated in the cortex would elicit movements and that, by using electrical stimulation, it was possible to differentially activate muscles in the hindlimbs. When the superior or postero-parietal lobule was stimulated, the hindlimbs of the monkey would elicit walking movements, while stimulation on the upper extremity of the ascending parietal and adjoining portion of the ascending frontal convolution caused the hindlimbs to exert a scratching motion, as if the monkey was touching the abdomen. Similar experiments were conducted in dogs, jackals, cats, rats, rabbits, and guinea pigs.

In 1910, Silvanus P. Thompson stimulated the head in humans with a magnetic field (Fig. 8.1). For this purpose, a coil was constructed out of copper wire wound around a wooden cylinder. Later the cylinder was removed to allow the possibility of inserting the head in the middle of the coil. The main finding from this stimulation was what Thompson perceived as the appearance of flickering lights regardless of whether the eyes were open or closed [5].

A visual area of the cortex might have been stimulated in these experiments, but no motor responses from muscles in the periphery were reported. The efficacy of this type of stimulation on muscle responses was tested in 1965 by Bickford and Fremming [6], who applied this type of stimulation in the periphery. These authors used a stimulator built by the Westinghouse Corporation (a magnetic system that was capable of producing 20,000–30,000 G fields of 300 μs duration) that generated magnetic fields that were discharged through an electromagnet. Peripheral nerves were stimulated in rabbits, frogs, and humans. It was reported that with precise placement of the electromagnet, a muscle contraction could be achieved in different muscle groups in frogs and rabbits. In humans, a similar result was reported; stimulation of the ulnar nerve, the peroneal nerve, and the sciatic nerve resulted in contractions in muscles innervated by those specific nerves. Bickford and Fremming suggested that their results were consistent with the hypothesis that magnetic stimulation of peripheral nerves and subsequent contraction of muscles were caused by eddy currents generated by the stimulator that was in the area near the nerves.

Polson and colleagues [7] also applied electromagnetic stimulation to peripheral nerves, but they used a circular electromagnetic coil. In these experiments the median nerve was identified and then a coil of 35 mm diameter was placed tangential to the nerve. During the experiments, EMG activity was recorded by using surface electrodes placed over the thenar eminence. The thumb was observed to twitch upon triggering the stimulator attached to the coil, and an EMG response was observed on an oscilloscope. Subjects who were tested reported that magnetic stimulation produced a tingling sensation, whereas electrical stimulation produced a more intense stabbing sensation. Magnetic stimulation produced less of an artifact in the oscilloscope than electrical stimulation, which allowed better visualization of the responses. Merton and Morton [8] applied electrical stimulation to motor cortex in man through the scalp. They used electroencephalographic electrodes that were 1 cm wide over the scalp. One electrode was placed over the arm representation of the motor cortex, and the other electrode was placed 4 cm anterior. Stimulation of motor cortex with this electrode configuration produced action potentials in the muscles of the forearm. When the electrodes were placed over an area at the back of the head, Merton and Morton observed a similar result to Thompson's stimulation of the head; subjects saw bright bursts of light during stimulation. It was assumed that the appearance of visual patterns and shapes which subjects reported seeing were caused by stimulation of the visual cortex. Although this method was successful in evoking motor responses in arm muscles, it was still painful for subjects, and there was a need for an alternative method of cortical stimulation.

Table 8.1 Progression of research in both electrical and magnetic stimulations

Year	Group	Findings
1831	M. Faraday	Electromagnetic induction
1876	D. Ferrier	Stimulation of primate cortex. Elicited movements in limbs. Identified associations between cortical areas and muscle groups
1910	S.P. Thompson	Stimulation of head with electromagnetism, observation of flickering lights when head was placed in the middle of magnetic coil
1965	R.G. Bickford and B.D. Fremming	Electromagnetic stimulation of muscles
1980	P.A. Merton and H.B. Morton	Electrical stimulation of the motor cortex through the scalp with electroencephalogram electrodes
1982	M.J.R. Polson, A.T. Barker, and S. Gardiner	Stimulation of peripheral nerves with magnetic pulses. Targeted thenar eminence via stimulation of the median nerve. Used a circular coil

Five years later, Barker and colleagues [1] conducted the first published experiment in which the motor cortex of an awake human was stimulated with a magnetic pulse. This method of stimulation would eventually be called TMS. They used a round coil with an outside diameter of 100 mm. The coil was placed on the scalp over a region of the motor cortex. TMS stimulation caused those muscles contralateral to the stimulated motor cortex to contract. Motor-evoked potentials (MEPs) were observed in hand and leg muscles. Subject discomfort was greatly reduced during stimulation with TMS in comparison to the sensation felt with electrical stimulation over the motor cortex. It was easy to move the coil to a different location on the subject's head, and the field generated by the magnetic pulse was able to penetrate the skull and reach cortical structures, which further promoted its use in humans.

In summary, noninvasive stimulation of motor cortex has evolved from the most basic tenets of electromagnetic induction. Electrical stimulation of the cortex by Ferrier in monkeys, and later by Merton and Morton in humans, proved to be effective but painful, and therefore, a similarly successful method of stimulation was needed. Barker and colleagues used TMS to evoked painless responses in skeletal muscles of the limbs, building a foundation for subsequent experiments in cortical stimulation. A chronological summary of the progression from electromagnetic induction to cortical stimulation with magnetic pulses is presented in Table 8.1.

Neuronal Elements Activated by TMS

One of the key areas targeted by TMS is the motor cortex. Motor cortex is one of the major sources of descending pyramidal tract neurons originated in layer V. There are two types of corticospinal tract neurons. One type has axons terminating in the intermediate zone of the spinal cord, where they synapse with spinal interneurons. In turn, some of these interneurons make connections with spinal motoneurons and conduct the descending commands necessary for movement. The other group makes monosynaptic connections onto the spinal motoneurons, and these neurons are called corticomotoneuronal (CM) cells.

Previous studies have used tracers to study the distribution of corticospinal projections and their indirect versus direct connections with spinal motoneurons. For example, using retrograde transport of the rabies virus into the hand muscles of macaque monkeys, corticospinal cells that make monosynaptic and non-monosynaptic connections with the motoneurons of the injected muscle were investigated (Rathelot and Strick [9]). In this study, the authors examined the distribution of CM cells that project to motoneurons of three thumb and finger muscles. They found that the CM cells for these digit muscles were restricted to the caudal portion of motor cortex, which is located in the central sulcus. In this area of motor cortex, CM cells for one specific muscle showed a remarkably widespread distribution and extended to the mediolateral arm area. These authors also found that the cortical territories occupied by CM cells for different muscles overlapped extensively. It was concluded that the overlap and intermingling among the different populations of CM cells may be the neural substrate to create a wide variety of muscle synergies. More recently, these two types of corticospinal cells were identified in different regions in the motor cortex (Rathelot and Strick [10]). Retrograde transneuronal transport of rabies virus from single muscles of monkeys was used to identify CM cells in motor cortex that make monosynaptic connections with motoneurons innervating shoulder, elbow, and finger muscles. It was found that the motor cortex has two subdivisions. The first division was a rostral region which lacks CM cells and represents an "old" motor cortex. It is proposed that the descending commands mediated by corticospinal efferents from old motor cortex might use the integrative mechanisms of the spinal cord to generate motoneuron activity and motor output. Rathelot and Strick also identified a caudal region of motor cortex that contained shoulder, elbow, and finger CM cells. This region represents a "new" motor cortex that is present only in some higher primates and humans. It is possible that the direct access to motoneurons by CM cells enables the new motor cortex to bypass spinal cord mechanisms and shape novel patterns of motor output that are important for skilled behaviors. It is important to consider that both direct and indirect corticospinal projections to motoneurons could potentially be activated by a magnetic pulse from TMS.

In humans, electrophysiological studies support the view that TMS can be used to assess monosynaptic corticospinal connections by examining their effects on the probability of discharge of single motor units that are voluntarily preactivated (i.e., peristimulus time histograms (PSTHs); Palmer and Ashby [11]; Brouwer and Ashby [12]) and the amplitude of H-reflexes (Petersen et al. [13]). Palmer and Ashby [11] applied TMS over the motor cortex in humans, and PSTHs of the discharges of single motor units were used to record changes in the firing probability of individual spinal motoneurons of upper limb muscles. The authors reported that for the majority of motor units, the initial effect was short-latency facilitation. The estimated central conduction velocities and the rise times of the underlying excitatory postsynaptic potentials were compatible with monsynaptic facilitation by a fast corticospinal pathway. It was also reported that some units showed no statistically significant changes in firing probability. All sampled units of the first dorsal interosseous muscle showed short-latency facilitation, as well as the majority of units in the forearm and the biceps brachii. Interestingly, more than half of the sampled motor units of triceps brachii and deltoid either showed no effect or were inhibited. The authors concluded that the short-latency corticospinal projections to upper limb motoneurons in humans have a distinct pattern that is similar to that in other primates. Monosynaptic projections to motoneurons have also been seen for leg muscles, and a similar distribution of short-latency responses in PSTHs has been reported (Brouwer and Ashby [11]). Nielsen and Petersen [14] tested, in resting subjects, the effects of low-intensity TMS over the leg representation of the motor cortex on the size of the soleus H reflex at short latency at different conditioning-test intervals. It was reported that short- and long-latency facilitations, of different thresholds, were differently regulated during voluntary movement. The authors suggested that these responses were caused by activation by the magnetic stimulus of different monosynaptic and non-monosynaptic descending pathways.

Patton and Amassian [15] were the first to describe the responses elicited by electrical stimulation of the motor cortex that would later be assessed with TMS. In these experiments the motor cortex was stimulated and recordings were acquired from the bulbar pyramid in the cat and monkeys. It was observed that after cortical stimulation, there was a wave that was reproducible at progressively larger depths into the bulb. This wave was termed "D" or direct wave. In the more intact bulbar preparations, delayed waves that they called "I" or indirect waves were observed. It was concluded that D waves resulted from direct activation of pyramidal cells by cortical stimulation because of their short latency (0.4 ms after cortical stimulation). The latency indicated that there was not sufficient time for a synaptic impulse to be transmitted from a neuron in the cortex to the bulbar pyramid. Therefore, D waves were thought to originate from direct stimulation of pyramidal cell bodies or basal dendrites, while I waves were proposed to originate from indirect excitation of pyramidal neurons through cortical interneurons.

Several studies have demonstrated that TMS of the motor cortex can produce D waves at higher stimulus intensities (Day et al. [16]; Di Lazzaro et al. [17]). An explanation for this was proposed by Day and collaborators in 1989 [16]. These authors examined the effects of different forms of brain stimulation on the discharge pattern of single motor units by using the PSTH technique and by recording surface EMG responses in the first dorsal interosseous muscle. Electrical and magnetic methods were used to stimulate the brain through the intact scalp of intact subjects. Electrical stimuli were applied either with the anode over the lateral central scalp and cathode at the vertex (anodal stimulation) or with the anode at the vertex and the cathode lateral (cathodal stimulation). A circular 9 cm diameter TMS coil was used and centered at the vertex. It was reported that suprathreshold stimuli produced one or more narrow peaks of increased firing in the PSTHs of all units tested. Anodal stimulation always produced an early peak. The latencies of the peaks produced by the stimulation, including high intensities of anodal stimulation, were grouped into four time bands relative to this early peak, including intervals of −0.5 to 0.5, 1–2, 2.5–3.5, and 4–5.5 ms. The peaks reported within these intervals were referred to as P0 (the earliest anodal), P1, P2, and P3, respectively. At threshold intensity, anodal stimulation evoked only the P0 peak; at higher intensities, the P2 or, more commonly, the P3 peak, was recruited. It was hypothesized that the P0, P1, P2, and P3 peaks corresponded to arrival at spinal motoneurons of excitatory postsynaptic potentials generated by D, I1, I2, and I3 waves in the pyramidal tract. It has been suggested that different sets of neural elements that are presynaptic to the pyramidal neurons (Sakai et al. [18]) and oscillatory activity in intracortical neurons, which activates pyramidal tract neurons (Kernell and Wu [19]), might contribute to I wave generation. The first I wave (I1) is thought to be generated through the depolarization of an axon synapsing directly onto a corticospinal neuron (i.e., monosynaptically), and the following I waves (I2 and later) may require local polysynaptic circuits.

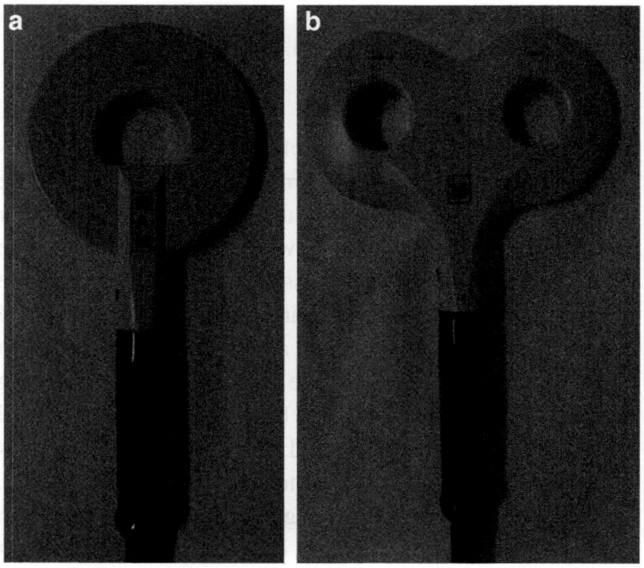

Fig. 8.2 Circular coil. Each side of the coil is marked with a different letter. (**a**) Side A has an *arrow* pointing in the anticlockwise direction, which means that the induced current in the brain with this side up is clockwise. (**b**) Side B has an *arrow* pointing in the clockwise direction, which means that the induced current in the brain with this side up is anticlockwise (From [71]; with permission)

TMS Methodology and Measurements

Coil Types

Since the experiments of Barker and colleagues [1], several TMS coils have been developed to serve various experimental purposes. Innovations in coil design and stimulation techniques have allowed the possibility of making more precise measurements and better understanding of motor cortical functions in humans.

Circular Coil

The circular coil was the first coil design used both in the periphery (Polson et al. [7]) and on the motor cortex (Barker et al. [1]). Circular coils are often labeled with letters that are assigned to the direction in which the current moves in the brain. For example, side A of a circular coil, shown in Fig. 8.2a, is marked with an arrow pointing in the anticlockwise direction when viewed from the top of the head, which means that current in the brain is flowing in the clockwise direction, and side B (Fig. 8.2b) is marked with an arrow pointing in the clockwise direction, which indicates that the induced current in the brain moves in the anticlockwise direction.

A circular coil oriented tangentially to the surface of the head with its center 10 mm above the vertex produced an electric field in the clockwise direction, as calculated by a mathematical model (Roth et al. [20]), but by placing the opposite surface of the coil against the scalp, the direction of the electric field can be changed to anticlockwise (Day et al. [21]). The directionality of the current is useful for producing responses of different latencies and thresholds, and it is also used to preferentially target one hemisphere or the other. For example, clockwise stimulation by a coil of 90 mm diameter placed over the vertex produced EMG responses in the right first dorsal interosseous muscle at a lower threshold and shorter latency than that of anticlockwise stimulation of the same cortical area (Day et al. [21]). Moving a circular coil posteriorly with respect to the vertex by 50 mm so that the edge of the coil was 10 mm above the vertex produced a charge distribution and decreased the size of the peak electric field under the coil (Roth et al. [20]). A circular coil with the B side facing upwards produced an anticlockwise current in the brain which targeted the right hemisphere of the motor cortex (Trompetto et al. [22]). It was shown in the results of this experiment that the intensity needed for motor threshold of an EMG response in the active right first dorsal interosseous muscle were lower when a clockwise current was produced in the brain than an anticlockwise current. This showed that preferential activation of one hemisphere (in this case, the left hemisphere) could occur when the current flowed from the back of the brain to the front across the targeted hemisphere. It should be noted that a circular coil produces loops of current, and stimulation can occur anywhere along these loops. Furthermore, the stimulation pulse is less focal when a large diameter coil is used.

Figure-of-Eight Coil

This design was first proposed in 1988 by Ueno and colleagues [23] in an effort to reduce the size of the area stimulated by the magnetic coil (Fig. 8.3a). These authors reported that a very focal pulse is more easily achieved with a figure-of-eight configuration than with a circular coil. A mathematical model was used to determine the magnetic field that would be generated by a figure-of-eight coil, which it was estimated to be more powerful at the point at which the two halves of the coil intersect. This effect is produced from an addition of currents from each of the circular halves that flow in opposite directions. This particular flow of current restricts the maximum level of stimulation to the current convergence point (Barker and Freeston [24]). A cumulative electric field is produced that is both larger and more focused than the field of other coils such as the circular coil (Roth et al. [20]). Furthermore, current density between two coils is two to three times greater at the point between two coils than at regions away from this point (Ueno et al. [23]). Changes in position of the figure-of-eight coil can target different areas of the cortex depending on the direction of current produced (Ueno et al. [25]). For example, a current that moves posterior-anterior with respect to the top

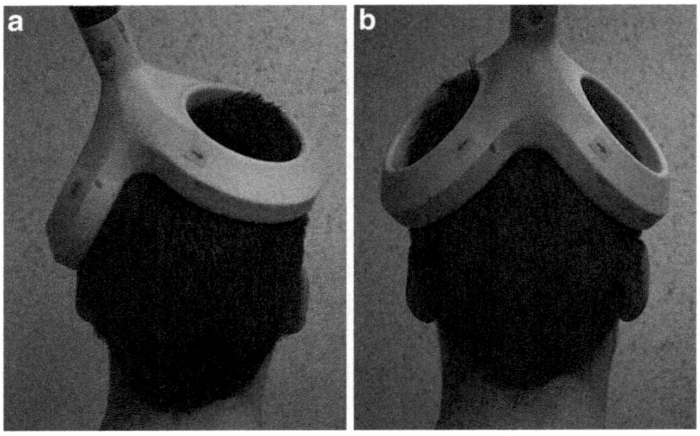

Fig. 8.3 Double-loop coils. (**a**) Figure-of-eight coil. The electric field generated by this coil is at its peak where the two halves of the coil intersect. Therefore, the center of the coil is placed over the target site. (**b**) Double cone coil. Internal diameter of 95 mm, external diameter of 123 mm, and magnetic field of 1.34 Tesla (T). As with the figure-of-eight coil, the area of greatest stimulus intensity is at the center of the coil at the intersection of the two loops. However, this coil can produce a much stronger and deeply penetrating pulse than that of a circular coil ((**a**) From [71], with permission. (**b**) From [72], with permission)

of the head could activate a mechanism mediated by one population of neurons in the cortex, while a current that moves in the lateromedial (LM) direction could target a slightly different mechanism (see below for a discussion of different coil orientations).

Double Cone Coil

This type of coil is composed of two curved circular rings that are situated next to each other, as in the figure-of-eight design (Fig. 8.3b). These two circles share a flattened central area, and they are angled inward with respect to the area of intersection. This design allows the coil to be placed on the subject's head in a way that it conforms to the natural curvature of the skull. Therefore, most of the magnetic flux passes through the brain and not out from the sides of the coil (Reza Jalinous, direct correspondence). Furthermore, the power of this coil and the depth to which its pulses can penetrate is 70 % greater in comparison with these same parameters for a circular coil because of the increased coupling of the magnetic fields of the two loops that are angled inward in the double cone coil. This type of coil has been used in protocols, for example, in which the motor representation of the lower limbs in the motor cortex (Stokić et al. [26]; Guzman-Lopez et al. [27]), the corticospinal axons at the cervicomedullary junction (Taylor and Gandevia [28]), and the cerebellum (Ugawa et al. [29]; Werhahn et al. [30]; Pinto and Chen [31]) are stimulated. This coil is typically used when other coil designs fail to evoke responses from target muscles or when an experimenter is attempting to access deeper structures. Also, if a subject has a very high threshold of stimulation, then it might be necessary to use the double cone coil because of its high output (Reza Jalinous, direct correspondence).

Batwing Coil

The batwing coil is composed of two loops angled towards their intersection with downturned ends. Like the double cone coil, it is also used to stimulate leg areas of the motor cortex (Nielsen et al.[14]). However, the coupling of the magnetic fields is not as great as it is with the double cone coil, so its depth of penetration and power is between that of a flat figure-of-eight coil and a double cone coil (Reza Jalinous, direct correspondence). In one study involving spinal cord-injured subjects, the batwing coil was employed for more focal stimulation, and the double cone coil was used only when a patient had a more severe injury (Roy et al. [32]). This is an example of the gradient of power and depth of penetration from the weakest coil, the flat figure-of-eight coil, to the double cone coil.

TMS Coil Orientations

The effects of changing the orientations of the figure-of-eight coil to stimulate motor cortex have been extensively studied in humans. Three main coil orientations will be discussed in this section: posteroanterior (PA), anteroposterior (AP), and lateromedial (LM) orientations.

PA Orientation

This orientation produces a current that flows from the back to the front of the head towards the nose (Fig. 8.4a). Several studies have examined the nature of the responses evoked by a figure-of-eight coil in this particular orientation. Di Lazzaro et al. [33] compared the effects of transcranial electric and magnetic stimulations of the human motor cortex. In the study, spinal volleys evoked by single transcranial magnetic or electric stimulation over the motor cortex were recorded from a bipolar electrode inserted into the cervical epidural space of two conscious subjects. These volleys were termed D and I waves according to their latency (see details in a previous section). Using active motor threshold intensity, magnetic stimulation with a figure-of-eight coil held over the motor cortex with the induced current flowing in a PA direction evoked pure I1 activity. Using magnetic stimulation with a PA-induced current, at stimulus intensity above the active motor threshold, a small D wave appeared in one but not in other subject. It was concluded that magnetic stimulation with PA-induced current, at threshold intensities, evokes preferentially I waves. Werhahn and colleagues [34] examined the effect of the orientation of a figure-of-eight coil on the latency of surface EMG responses and the firing pattern of single motor units evoked in the first dorsal interosseous muscle by TMS. Two coil positions were

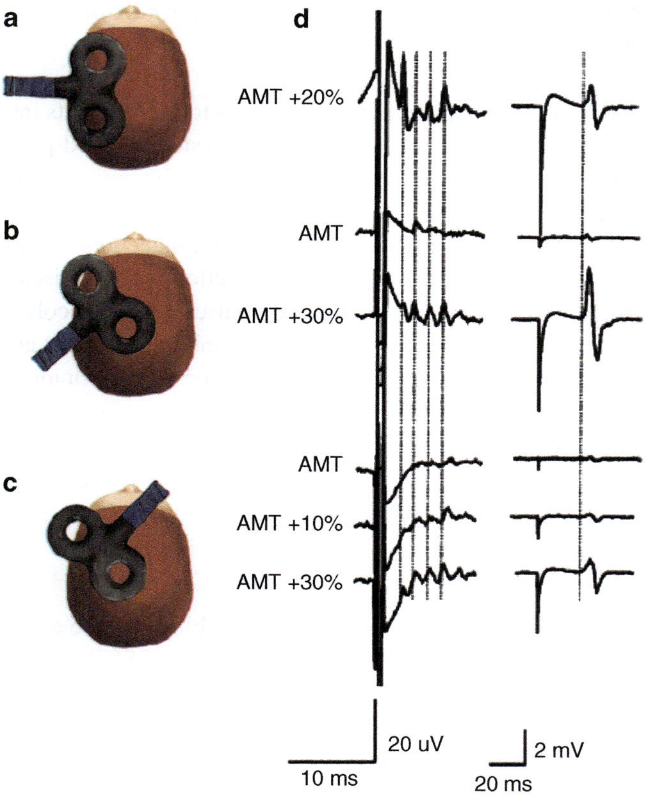

Fig. 8.4 Descending volleys recorded from the high cervical cord at the C1-C2 level in one representative subject. The diagrams show (**a**) lateromedial (LM), (**b**) posteroanterior (PA), and (**c**) anteroposterior (AP) coil orientations, and the corresponding epidural volleys (**d**, *left column*) and electromyographic (EMG) responses (**d**, *right column*) recorded for each of these orientations are to the right of each of the coil orientation diagrams. The *vertical dotted lines* indicate latencies of D, I1, I2, and I3 waves and the latency of the EMG response at threshold intensity for the PA configuration. The scale on the *left* is for the epidural responses, and the scale on the *right* is for EMG responses. AP stimulation at active motor threshold (AMT) evoked an epidural volley with a latency of 3.5 ms longer than the I1 wave evoked by PA stimulation. At 10 % of the maximal stimulator output (MSO) above AMT, this wave increases in amplitude, and at 30 % above AMT, this wave is replaced by four waves with latencies that are similar to D and I waves evoked by PA stimulation but 0.2 ms later. LM stimulation produced D waves and I waves at 20 % MSO above AMT that were equal to those produced by PA stimulation at 30 % MSO above AMT. EMG responses were shortest with LM stimulation at 20 % MSO above AMT and were longest with AP stimulation at AMT (Modified from Di Lazzaro et al. [33])

used: the coil held on a parasagittal line either with the induced current in the brain flowing in a PA direction or with the current flowing in the LM direction. PA stimulation produced surface and single unit responses that occurred 0–3 msec later than LM stimulation. It was found that responses evoked by PA stimulation were more affected by changes in motor cortical excitability (including cortico-cortical inhibition and transcallosal inhibition) than those to LM stimulation. The authors concluded that PA stimulation tends to activate corticospinal fibers *trans*-synaptically and not directly. In addition to determining which coil orientations produce D or I waves, some studies have used coil orientation to explore the mechanisms that produce the early and late I waves. Ni et al. [35] studied the neuronal mechanisms mediating I waves by examining the influence of short-latency afferent inhibition (SAI) on various I waves. SAI was tested with electrical stimulation of the median nerve at the wrist followed by TMS to the contralateral motor cortex at different current directions. Surface EMG and single motor units were recorded from the first dorsal interosseous muscle. SAI was weaker for the AP compared with that for the PA current direction, and SAI produced more inhibition of late I waves generated by PA than those generated by AP current direction. The authors concluded that although both current directions generate a series of I waves with comparable latencies, these waves are likely mediated by different mechanisms because sensory afferent inputs have different effects on the I waves generated by the two current directions. Similar to the work of Ni and colleagues, Sakai et al. [18] studied the effect of direction of stimulating current on the latencies of responses to TMS. The latencies were measured from surface EMG responses of the first dorsal interosseous muscle and the peaks of the PSTHs of single motor units from the same muscle. The coil was placed over the motor cortex, with eight different directions each separated by 45°. In the study the stimulus intensity was adjusted just above the motor threshold, while subjects made a weak tonic voluntary contraction. TMS with medially and anteriorly (PA orientation) directed currents in the brain produced more often responses or a peak that occurred around 1.5 ms later than those to anodal electrical stimulation. It was concluded that TMS with medially and anteriorly directed current in the brain readily elicits I1 waves. The finding by this group of the dependence of the preferentially activated I waves on the current direction in the brain suggests that different sets of cortical neurons are responsible for different I waves. Overall, most studies agree that TMS stimulation with the coil in the PA direction target preferentially I waves in human subjects.

LM Orientation

In this orientation, the coil is positioned with the handle pointing horizontally away from the head (Fig. 8.4b). When the coil is placed over the right or left motor cortex, the current flows from the lateral side of the head to the midline. Di Lazzaro et al. [17] observed that when an LM-induced current was used, magnetic stimulation evoked both D and I1 activities. Both the D and I1 waves increased in size as the intensity was increased. Werhahn et al. [34] also found short-latency responses from LM stimulation. It was reported that LM stimulation produced surface and single unit responses that occurred earlier than PA stimulation, and in many cases responses to LM stimulation had the same latency as those produced by anodal electrical stimulation. In addition, responses evoked by LM stimulation were less affected by changes in motor cortical excitability than those to PA stimulation. The authors suggested that LM stimulation can sometimes stimulate corticospinal fibers directly, at, or near the same site as anodal stimulation and that LM stimulation tends to produce either D or I1 wave firing. The tendency for LM magnetic stimulation to produce D wave activation of corticospinal fibers probably accounts for the reduced sensitivity of the evoked EMG responses to changes in the level of cortical excitability. Short-latency responses from LM stimulation were also reported in the first dorsal interosseous muscle by Ni and colleagues in 2011 [35].

AP Orientation

This coil orientation has an angle that is similar in magnitude to that of the PA configuration, but the induced current flows from the front of the head to the back and from a lateral position to a more medial location (Fig. 8.4c). Di Lazzaro et al. [36] found that descending volleys evoked by AP stimulation often had slightly different peak latencies and/or longer duration than those seen after PA stimulation. These volleys were recorded from a bipolar electrode inserted into the cervical epidural space of four conscious human subjects (Fig. 8.4d; Di Lazzaro et al. [36]). Additionally, in 1977 Sakai and colleagues [18] observed that TMS with laterally and posteriorly (AP orientation) directed current produced responses or a peak that occurred about 4.5 ms later than those to anodal electrical stimulation. This group concluded that laterally and posteriorly directed current preferentially elicits I3 waves. Further exploration has been made to elucidate more precise differences between PA and AP stimulation. As described above, SAI has been shown to be weaker for the AP compared with that for the PA current direction (Ni et al. [35]). The authors emphasized that MEP generated by the AP current direction in which more late I waves were produced were less inhibited compared with MEPs generated by the PA direction. This result indicated that the AP-directed current activated different neuronal populations of late I wave generating neurons that were less sensitive to SAI than those activated by the PA current direction.

In conclusion, coil orientation can greatly impact the nature of responses generated by TMS. Therefore, knowledge of the characteristics of responses generated by LM, PA, and AP stimulation can affect neural mechanisms contributing to modulate corticospinal output and needs to be carefully considered in experimental paradigms.

Neurophysiological Measurements Examined by TMS

TMS has been applied in multiple ways to gain insights into the physiology of the human motor system. Paired-pulse TMS protocols have provided insight into the nature of the cortical circuitry that is activated by TMS. A variety of different methods exist to examine the connections within and between motor cortices. In this section we will discuss two of the most widely used paired-pulse TMS protocols in humans: (a) short-interval intracortical inhibition (SICI) and (b) interhemispheric inhibition (IHI). For both techniques, direct recordings of the effects on descending volleys have not only confirmed the mechanisms of these effects but also revealed some degree of selectivity for different waves (D, I1, I2, etc.) of the response.

SICI

In humans, GABAergic intracortical inhibition can be examined using a paired-pulse TMS protocol named SICI (Kujirai et al. [37]). Here, a subthreshold, conditioning TMS pulse decreases the size of an MEP elicited by a later suprathreshold test stimulus when applied over M1. This effect can be observed at conditioning time intervals between 1 and 5 ms (Fig. 8.5).

The intensity of the conditioning stimulus was below the threshold for activating motoneurons; therefore, it was suggested that this effect was occurring at the cortical level. Later evidence (Di Lazzaro et al. [17]) confirmed the cortical origin of SICI demonstrating that a subthreshold conditioning stimulus which itself did not evoke motoneuronal activation produced a clear suppression of late I waves if the interval between the stimuli was between 1 and 5 ms. Subsequent studies have shown that administration of a single oral dose of GABAA agonists increases the amount of SICI and also increases the inhibition of later descending I waves (Reis et al. [38]). Furthermore, it was postulated that SICI might be mediated by GABAergic mechanisms as it has been shown that GABAA receptor agonists increase the effects of SICI (Ilic et al. [39]; Ziemann et al. [40]) and that a dose of lorazepam (a GABAA receptor agonist) can further inhibit late I waves (Di Lazzaro et al. [17]).

IHI

Earlier studies in monkeys demonstrated the existence of callosal connections between motor cortices, being more numerous between cortex representing proximal compared to distal forelimb representations (Pandya et al. [41]; Jenny

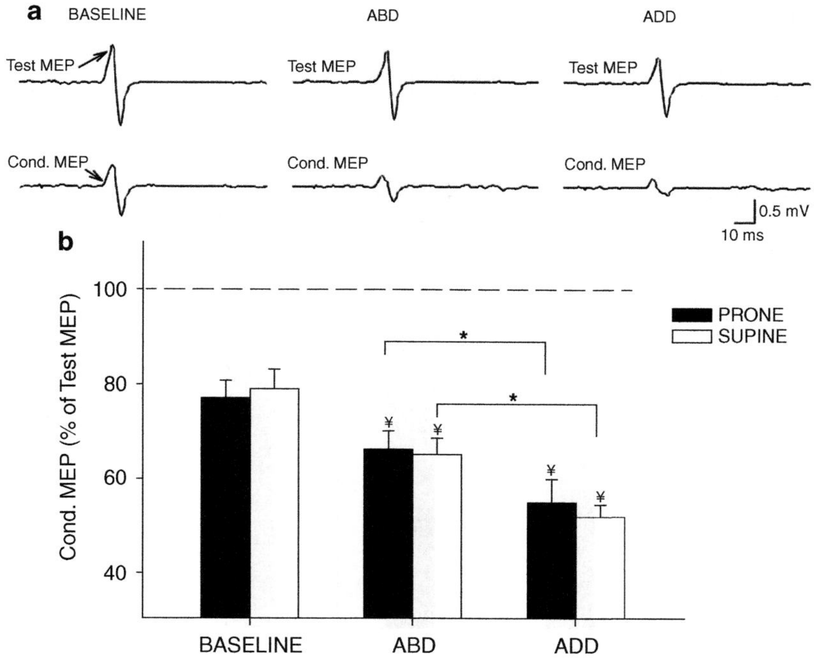

Fig. 8.5 Interhemispheric inhibition (IHI). (**a**) IHI recorded from the left first dorsal interosseous muscle of a representative subject during 10 % of left index finger abduction (ABD), whereas the right index finger remained at rest (*baseline*) or performed 30 % of ABD or adduction (ADD). The actions by the right index finger are indicated as *Baseline*, ABD, and ADD. In this example the right hand was positioned in prone posture. Test motor-evoked potential (MEP) and conditioned MEP (Cond. MEP) are indicated by *arrows*. (**b**) Group data ($n = 12$). The abscissa shows the conditions tested during the assessment of IHI contractions in prone (*black bars*) and supine (*white bars*) postures. The ordinate indicates the magnitude of the conditioned MEP expressed as a percentage of the Test MEP ((Cond. MEP*100)/(Test MEP)) during bilateral isometric forces. The *horizontal dashed line* represents the size of the Test MEP. Note that IHI was increased to a larger extent during ADD forces regardless of the right-hand posture. *Error bars* indicate SEs. *P 0.05. Also note that IHI was significantly increased with respect to the baseline in all conditions tested (¥ indicates significant difference with respect to baseline) (Modified from [73])

[42]; Pappas and Strick [43]; Rouiller et al., [44]). Studies also suggested the existence of intrinsic connections between different regions within the motor cortex forelimb representation (Gould et al. [45]; Huntley and Jones [46]), which might contribute to functional specialization of limb movements. The first extensive study that demonstrated interhemispheric interactions between motor cortices in intact human subjects by using TMS was published by Ferbert et al. [47]. The authors demonstrated that a TMS suprathreshold pulse applied over the motor cortex of one hemisphere can inhibit motor responses evoked in distal and proximal muscles by a magnetic stimulus given 6–30 ms later over the opposite hemisphere (Fig. 8.6).

It was suggested that the inhibition was produced at cortical level via a transcallosal route. Direct proof of the cortical origin of the inhibition was provided by Di Lazzaro et al. [48] who recorded descending volleys produced by the test MEP alone and with and without a prior conditioning stimulus to the contralateral motor cortex. In the spinal recordings it was demonstrated that the inhibitory effect was present in the later I3 waves. Two main phases of IHI have been reported: one at a short interval of 10 ms (IHI10) and another at a long interval of 40 ms (IHI40) (Chen et al. [49]). Significant differences exist between IHI10 and IHI40 (Chen et al. [49]; Kukaswadia et al. [50]; Lee et al. [51]; Ni et al. [52]), including that IHI40 is mediated by postsynaptic gamma-aminobutyric acid type B (GABAB) receptors. The transmitter system mediating IHI10 remains inconclusive (Irlbacher et al. [53]).

In addition, a single suprathreshold TMS pulse is also capable of inhibiting ongoing voluntary EMG activity when applied to the motor cortex ipsilateral to the contracting arm (i.e., ipsilateral silent period). This inhibition lasted for about 30 ms and began 10–15 ms after the minimum corticospinal conduction time to the muscle. It has been proposed that changes in the depth and area of the ipsilateral silent period reflect activity in fibers passing through the corpus callosum since the silent period was absent or delayed in patients with agenesis or lesions of the corpus callosum (Rothwell et al. [54]; Meyer et al. [55]) and conditioning TMS applied to M1 reduced MEPs evoked by stimulation over the other hemisphere by affecting primarily the I3 wave (Di Lazzaro et al. [48]).

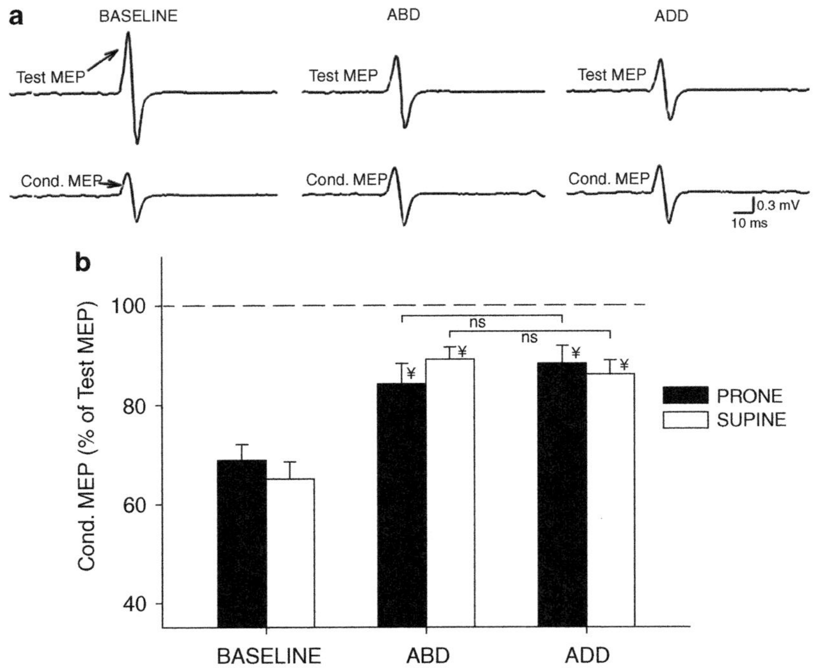

Fig. 8.6 Short-interval intracortical inhibition (SICI). (**a**) SICI recorded from the left first dorsal interosseous of a representative subject during 10 % of left abduction (ABD), whereas the right index finger remained at rest (*baseline*) or performed 30 % of ABD or adduction (ADD). The actions by the right index finger are indicated as *Baseline*, ABD, and ADD. In this example the right hand was positioned in prone posture. Test motor-evoked potential (MEP) and conditioned MEP (Cond. MEP) are indicated by *arrows*. (**b**) Group data ($n = 12$). The abscissa shows all conditions tested during the assessment of SICI in prone (*black bars*) and supine (*white bars*) postures. The ordinate indicates the magnitude of the conditioned MEP expressed as a percentage of the Test MEP ((Cond. MEP*100)/(Test MEP)) during bilateral activation. The *horizontal dashed line* represents the size of the Test MEP. Note that the magnitude of SICI was decreased to a similar extent during both bilateral forces in both right-hand postures. *Error bars* indicate SEs. *P 0.05. Also note that SICI was significantly decreased with respect to the baseline in all conditions tested (¥ indicates significant difference with respect to baseline) (Modified from [73])

Therapeutic Uses of TMS: Repetitive TMS

rTMS has been used to investigate possible therapeutic methods to improve function in parts of the brain that are functioning suboptimally after injury or in chronic central nervous system (CNS) diseases (Ridding and Rothwell [56]). For example, in stroke patients, it has been shown that three sessions of rTMS at 1 Hz frequency (600 pulses) at motor threshold intensity significantly decreased simple and choice reaction time and improved performance of the Purdue Pegboard tested with their affected hand after rTMS was administered to the unaffected hemisphere of the motor cortex (Mansur et al. [57]). Furthermore, stimulation at 1 Hz frequency at 90 % of resting motor threshold for 25 min with a figure-of-eight coil over the unaffected motor cortex reduced the transcallosal inhibition and improved motor function in the affected hand of stroke patients, suggesting that transcallosal inhibition from contralesional to ipsilesional motor cortex contributed to suppress the affected hand function (Takeuchi et al. [58]). Other studies have explored the results from stimulation of the affected motor cortex in stroke patients. Repetitive stimulation of the affected motor cortex with a train of 20 pulses at 10 Hz frequency and 80 % of resting motor threshold (defined as the lowest simulation intensity needed to elicit MEP of at least 50 μV peak-to-peak amplitude in five out of ten trials) repeated eight times with a 58 s intertrain interval with a figure-of-eight coil can produce a larger increase in corticospinal excitability than sham stimulation, and these changes in corticospinal excitability were associated with enhanced motor skill acquisition (Kim et al. [59]). In a longitudinal study with stroke patients, rTMS was applied at the same time every day for 10 days over the affected hemisphere in ten s trains of 3 Hz stimulation, while patients continued to receive their normal therapy (Khedr et al. [60]). This study showed that this intervention employed as an add-on intervention to normal physical and drug therapies improved immediate clinical outcome in early stroke patients. A high-frequency type of repetitive stimulation, theta burst stimulation (TBS), when given over the stroke hemisphere in bursts of three stimuli repeating at 50 Hz with the bursts repeating at 5 Hz at 80 % of active motor threshold, significantly improved motor behavior and physiological outcomes of the paretic hand (Talelli et al. [61]). Interestingly, Talelli and colleagues did not observe any behavioral effects on the paretic side when the non-affected hemisphere was stimulated, which is in contrast to the findings of Takeuchi et al. [58] and Mansur et al. [57].

In addition to its use in stroke patients, rTMS has been administered to motor cortex and supplementary and premotor areas to improve motor function in persons with motor deficits of various origins. Transient pain relief has been shown to be induced by rTMS at 10 Hz of the motor cortex in patients suffering from chronic neurogenic pain (Lefaucheur et al. [62]).

rTMS has also been used in patients with dystonia. Dystonia is a movement disorder characterized clinically by excessive and disorganized muscle contraction leading to abnormal posturing and writhing movements, which, at the spinal level, is commonly associated with abnormalities in the spinal reciprocal inhibitory pathways due to a mutation in the DYT1 gene. Previous evidence demonstrated that abnormalities in reciprocal inhibition in patients with dystonia could be ameliorated by using 20 min of 1 Hz rTMS over the premotor cortex (Huang et al. [63]). Furthermore, in patients with Parkinson disease (PD), rTMS applied over the supplementary motor area (SMA) also appears to contribute to modulate abnormal involuntary movements. These behavioral effects were largely dependent on the type of rTMS protocol utilized. For example, drug-induced dyskinesias were markedly reduced by 15 min of 1 Hz rTMS (total pulses 900) at 90 % of resting motor threshold (Koch et al. [64]). Conversely, in this same study, 18 trains of 5 Hz rTMS with a duration of 10 s (total pulses 900) for each train separated by 40 s of pause at 110 % of resting motor threshold were associated with only a slight, but not significant, increase of dyskinetic behavior in PD patients.

There are other cortical areas in addition to the motor cortex that TMS has been used to target, such as the prefrontal lobes of the cortex, which have been shown to function abnormally during episodes of clinical depression (George et al. [65]). Some review studies have examined in detail the utility of rTMS in alleviating the symptoms of depression (Couturier et al. [66]; Martin et al. [67]). Couturier and colleagues found in their review of 87 randomized controlled trials investigating that the use of high-frequency rTMS compared with sham therapy for the treatment of a major depressive episode was not more efficacious than sham therapy in treating depression. It was hypothesized that the lack of effectiveness of rTMS may be in part related to the stimulation parameters used in the study, such as frequency, intensity, duration of train of pulses, and days of treatment. Martin and colleagues found a similar result in their review of 14 randomized controlled trials that compared rTMS with sham rTMS in patients with depression. Here it was concluded that there is currently insufficient evidence to suggest that rTMS is effective in the treatment of depression. They noted, however, that the results do not exclude the possibility that the intervention (rTMS) may be of benefit. Despite the inconclusive results of these review studies, there have been individual studies conducted in which the symptoms of depression and other psychological deficits have been alleviated. For example, George et al. [68] showed that administration of rTMS (20 Hz for 20 min each morning at 80 % of motor threshold) on a daily basis for at least 1 week (5 days) to the left prefrontal cortex of six medication-resistant subjects with primary mood disorders (one unipolar, five bipolar disorder type II) resulted in significant improvements in mood, and some subjects showed a slight clinical antidepressant response. Similarly, in a study conducted with 17 patients who met diagnostic criteria for major depression, psychotic subtype (DSM-III-R), and had a history of relapsing unipolar major depression, rTMS (10 Hz at of 90 % of motor threshold) applied over the dorsolateral prefrontal cortex resulted in some behavioral improvements (Pascual-Leone et al. [69]).

All together, these studies demonstrate that the effects of rTMS protocols are complex and largely variable in individuals with motor disorders. Therefore, caution is needed in their use and interpretation. Recent evidence in intact humans suggested that the variability of the results after rTMS protocols might be, at least in part, related to the interneuronal circuits that are activated by rTMS (Hamada et al. [70]). This implies that the absence of effects of an rTMS protocol, in intact humans and in individuals with motor disorders, may not be related to altered synaptic plasticity in the cortex, but may reflect the efficiency of I wave recruitment.

Conclusions

At present, TMS is the most widely used technique that allows us to examine transmission in the corticospinal pathway, primary motor cortex, and cortical areas projecting to primary motor cortex noninvasively and with minimal discomfort in human subjects. A suprathreshold TMS stimulus results in multiple descending waves as recorded from epidural electrodes placed over the spinal cord. A short-latency direct wave (D wave) is followed by several longer latency indirect waves (I waves). The D wave is thought to result from direct depolarization of the initial axon segment of corticospinal neurons and is most effectively activated in human subjects by using high-intensity TMS or by using transcranial electrical stimulation. I waves are thought to be generated through the depolarization of an axon synapsing directly onto a corticospinal neuron (i.e., monosynaptically, I1), and the following I waves (I2 and later) may require local polysynaptic circuits. The use of different coil designs has expanded the range of TMS protocols, giving flexibility to administer more focal stimulation paradigms targeting different intracortical circuits (I waves). Furthermore, multiple pulse protocols have been used to examine the role of TMS as an adjunct therapy for individuals with various psychological and motor disorders. The results from these studies are still inconclusive, and the current data suggest that rTMS after effects are complex, and there is a need of a more in-depth characterization of the stimulation parameters used in individual patients. The development of tailored TMS and rTMS protocols in humans with and without motor disorders may represent an avenue to further improve the therapeutic use of this widely used neurophysiological tool in human subjects.

References

1. Barker AT, Jalinous R, Freeston IL. Non-invasive magnetic stimulation of human motor cortex. Lancet. 1985;1:1106–7.
2. Faraday M. The correspondence of Michael Faraday (Vol 1). In: James FAJL, editor. London: Institution of Electrical Engineers; 1991.
3. Rossi S, Hallett M, Rossini PM, Pascual-Leone A, The Safety of TMS Consensus Group. Safety, ethical considerations, and application guidelines for the use of transcranial magnetic stimulation in clinical practice and research. Clin Neurophysiol. 2009;120:2008–39.
4. Ferrier D. The functions of the brain. 2nd ed. New York, NY: G.P. Putnam's Sons; 1886.
5. Thompson SP. A physiological effect of an alternating magnetic field. Proc R Soc Lond B Biol Sci. 1910;82:396–8.
6. Bickford RG, Fremming BD. Neuronal stimulation by pulsed magnetic fields in animals and man. Dig. 6th Int. Conf. Med. Electron. & Biol. Eng. 1965;112:6–7.
7. Polson MJR, Barker AT, Freeston IL. Stimulation of nerve trunks with time-varying magnetic fields. Med Biol Eng Comput. 1982;20:243–4.
8. Merton PA, Morton HB. Stimulation of the cerebral cortex in the intact human subject. Nature. 1980;285:227.
9. Rathelot JA, Strick PL. Muscle representation in the macaque motor cortex: an anatomical perspective. Proc Natl Acad Sci U S A. 2006;103:8257–62.
10. Rathelot JA, Strick PL. Subdivisions of primary motor cortex based on cortico-motoneuronal cells. Proc Natl Acad Sci U S A. 2009;106:918–23.
11. Palmer E, Ashby P. Corticospinal projections to upper limb motoneurones in humans. J Physiol. 1992;448:397–412.
12. Brouwer B, Ashby P. Corticospinal projections to lower limb motoneurons in man. Exp Brain Res. 1992;89:649–54.
13. Petersen NT, Pyndt HS, Nielsen JB. Investigating human motor control by transcranial magnetic stimulation. Exp Brain Res. 2003;152:1–16.
14. Nielsen J, Petersen N, Ballegaard N. Latency of effects evoked by electrical and magnetic brain stimulation in lower limb motoneurons in man. J Physiol. 1995;484:791–802.
15. Patton HD, Amassian VE. Single and multiple-unit analysis of cortical stage of pyramidal tract activation. J Neurophysiol. 1954;17:345–63.
16. Day BL, Dressler D, Maertens de Noordhout A, Marsden CD, Nakashima K, Rothwell JC, et al. Electric and magnetic stimulation of human motor cortex: surface EMG and single motor unit responses. J Physiol. 1989;412:449–73.
17. Di Lazzaro V, Restuccia D, Oliviero A, Profice P, Ferrara L, Insola A, et al. Magnetic transcranial stimulation at intensities below active motor threshold activates intracortical inhibitory circuits. Exp Brain Res. 1998;119:265–8.
18. Sakai K, Ugawa Y, Terao Y, Hanajima R, Furubayashi T, Kanazawa I. Preferential activation of different I waves by transcranial magnetic stimulation with a figure-of-eight-shaped coil. Exp Brain Res. 1977;113:24–32.
19. Kernell D, Chien-Ping W. Responses of the pyramidal tract to stimulation of the baboon's motor cortex. J Physiol. 1967;191:653–72.
20. Roth BJ, Saypol JM, Hallett M, Cohen LG. A theoretical calculation of the electric field induced in the cortex during magnetic stimulation. Electroencephalogr Clin Neurophysiol. 1991;81:47–56.
21. Day BL, Dressler D, Maertens de Noordhout A, Marsden CD, Rothwell JC, Thompson PD. Magnetic stimulation of the human brain can activate different neuronal elements when magnetic field direction is reversed. J Physiol. 1988;401:46P.
22. Trompetto C, Assini A, Buccolieri A, Marchese R, Abbruzzese G. Intracortical inhibition after paired transcranial magnetic stimulation depends on the current flow direction. Clin Neurophysiol. 1999;110:1106–10.
23. Ueno S, Tashiro T, Harada K. Localized stimulation of neural tissues in the brain by means of a paired configuration of time varying magnetic fields. J Appl Phys. 1988;64:5862.
24. Barker AT, Freeston I. Transcranial magnetic stimulation. Scholarpedia. 2007;2:2936.
25. Ueno S, Matsuda T, Hiwaki O. Localized stimulation of the human brain and spinal cord by a pair of opposing pulsed magnetic fields. J Appl Phys. 1990;67:5838.
26. Stokić DS, McKay WB, Scott L, Sherwood AM, Dimitrijević MR. Intracortical inhibition of lower limb motor-evoked potentials after paired transcranial magnetic stimulation. Exp Brain Res. 1997;117:437–43.
27. Guzman-Lopez J, Costa J, Selvi A, Gonzalo B, Casanova-Molla J, Valls-Sole J. The effects of transcranial magnetic stimulation on vibratory-induced presynaptic inhibition of the soleus H reflex. Exp Brain Res. 2012;220:223–30.
28. Taylor JL, Gandevia SC. Noninvasive stimulation of the human corticospinal tract. J Appl Physiol. 1985;2004(96):1496–503.
29. Ugawa Y, Uesaka Y, Terao Y, Hanajima R, Kanazawa I. Magnetic stimulation over the cerebellum in humans. Ann Neurol. 1995;37:703–13.
30. Werhahn KJ, Taylor J, Ridding M, Meyer B-U, Rothwell JC. Effect of transcranial magnetic stimulation over the cerebellum on the excitability of human motor cortex. Electroencephalogr Clin Neurophysiol. 1996;101:58–66.
31. Pinto AD, Chen R. Suppression of the motor cortex by magnetic stimulation of the cerebellum. Exp Brain Res. 2001;140:505–10.
32. Roy FD, Yang JF, Gorassini MA. Afferent regulation of leg motor cortex excitability after incomplete spinal cord injury. J Neurophysiol. 2010;103:2222–33.
33. Di Lazzaro V, Oliviero A, Profice P, Saturno E, Pilato F, Insola A, et al. Comparison of descending volleys evoked by transcranial magnetic and electric stimulation in conscious humans. Electroencephalogr Clin Neurophysiol. 1998;109:397–401.
34. Werhahn KJ, Fong JK, Meyer BU, Priori A, Rothwell JC, Day BL, et al. The effect of magnetic coil orientation on the latency of surface EMG and single motor unit responses in the first dorsal interosseous muscle. Electroencephalogr Clin Neurophysiol. 1994;93:138–46.
35. Ni Z, Charab S, Gunraj C, Nelson AJ, Udupa K, Yeh I, et al. Transcranial magnetic stimulation in different current directions activates separate cortical circuits. J Neurophysiol. 2011;105:749–56.
36. Di Lazzaro V, Oliviero A, Saturno E, Pilato F, Insola A, Mazzone P, et al. The effect on corticospinal volleys of reversing the

direction of current induced in the motor cortex by transcranial magnetic stimulation. Exp Brain Res. 2001;138:268–73.
37. Kujirai T, Caramia MD, Rothwell JC, Day BL, Thompson PD, Ferbert A, et al. Corticocortical inhibition in human motor cortex. J Physiol. 1993;471:501–19.
38. Reis J, Swayne OB, Vandermeeren Y, Camus M, Dimyan MA, Harris-Love M, et al. Contribution of transcranial magnetic stimulation to the understanding of cortical mechanisms involved in motor control. J Physiol. 2008;586:325–51.
39. Ilic TV, Meintzschel F, Cleff U, Ruge D, Kessler KR, Ziemann U. Short-interval paired-pulse inhibition and facilitation of human motor cortex: the dimension of stimulus intensity. J Physiol. 2002;545:153–67.
40. Ziemann U, Lonnecker S, Steinhoff BJ, Paulus W. The effect of lorazepam on the motor cortical excitability in man. Exp Brain Res. 1996;109:127–35.
41. Pandya DN, Vignolo LA. Intra- and interhemispheric projections of the precentral, premotor and arcuate areas in the rhesus monkey. Brain Res. 1971;26:217–33.
42. Jenny AB. Commissural projections of the cortical hand motor area in monkeys. J Comp Neurol. 1979;188:137–45.
43. Pappas CL, Strick PL. Anatomical demonstration of multiple representation in the forelimb region of the cat motor cortex. J Comp Neurol. 1981;200:491–500.
44. Rouiller EM, Babalian A, Kazennikov O, Moret V, Yu XH, Wiesendanger M. Transcallosal connections of the distal forelimb representations of the primary and supplementary motor cortical areas in macaque monkeys. Exp Brain Res. 1994;102:227–43.
45. Gould 3rd HJ, Cusick CG, Pons TP, Kaas JH. The relationship of corpus callosum connections to electrical stimulation maps of motor, supplementary motor, and the frontal eye fields in owl monkeys. J Comp Neurol. 1986;247:297–325.
46. Huntley GW, Jones EG. Relationship of intrinsic connections to forelimb movement representations in monkey motor cortex: a correlative anatomic and physiological study. J Neurophysiol. 1991;66:390–413.
47. Ferbert A, Priori A, Rothwell JC, Day BL, Colebatch JG, Marsden CD. Interhemispheric inhibition of the human motor cortex. J Physiol. 1992;453:525–46.
48. Di Lazzaro V, Oliviero A, Profice P, Insola A, Mazzone P, Tonali P, et al. Direct demonstration of interhemispheric inhibition of the human motor cortex produced by transcranial magnetic stimulation. Exp Brain Res. 1999;124:520–4.
49. Chen R, Yung D, Li JY. Organization of ipsilateral excitatory and inhibitory pathways in the human motor cortex. J Neurophysiol. 2003;89:1256–64.
50. Kukaswadia S, Wagle-Shukla A, Morgante F, Gunraj C, Chen R. Interactions between long latency afferent inhibition and interhemispheric inhibitions in the human motor cortex. J Physiol. 2005;563:915–24.
51. Lee H, Gunraj C, Chen R. The effects of inhibitory and facilitatory intracortical circuits on interhemispheric inhibition in the human motor cortex. J Physiol. 2007;580:1021–32.
52. Ni Z, Gunraj C, Nelson AJ, Yeh IJ, Castillo G, Hoque T, et al. Two phases of interhemispheric inhibition between motor related cortical areas and the primary motor cortex in human. Cereb Cortex. 2009;19:1654–65.
53. Irlbacher K, Brocke J, Mechow JV, Brandt SA. Effects of GABA (A) and GABA(B) agonists on interhemispheric inhibition in man. Clin Neurophysiol. 2007;118:308–16.
54. Rothwell JC, Colebatch J, Britton TC, Priori A, Thompson PD, Day BL, et al. Physiological studies in a patient with mirror movements and agenesis of the corpus callosum. J Physiol. 1991;438:34P.
55. Meyer B-U, Roricht S, von Grafin EH, Kruggel F, Weindl A. Inhibitory and excitatory interhemispheric transfers between motor cortical areas in normal humans and patients with abnormalities of the corpus callosum. Brain. 1995;118:429–40.
56. Ridding MC, Rothwell JC. Is there a future for therapeutic use of transcranial magnetic stimulation? Nat Rev Neurosci. 2007;8:559–67.
57. Mansur CG, Fregni F, Boggio PS, Riberto M, Gallucci-Neto J, Santos CM, Wagner T, Rigonatti SP, Marcolin MA, Pascual-Leone A. A sham-stimulation controlled trial of rTMS of the unaffected hemisphere in stroke patients. Neurology. 2005;641802–4.
58. Takeuchi N, Chuma T, Matsuo Y, Watanabe I, Ikoma K. Repetitive transcranial magnetic stimulation of contralesional primary motor cortex improves hand function after stroke. Stroke. 2005;36:2681–6.
59. Kim YH, You SH, Ko MH, Park JW, Lee KH, Jang SH, Yoo WK, Hallett M. Repetitive transcranial magnetic stimulation-induced corticomotor excitability and associated motor skill acquisition in chronic stroke. Stroke. 2006;37:1471–6. Erratum in: Stroke. 2006;37:2861.
60. Khedr EM, Ahmed MA, Fathy N, Rothwell JC. Therapeutic trial of repetitive transcranial magnetic stimulation after acute ischemic stroke. Neurology. 2005;65:466–8.
61. Talelli P, Greenwood RJ, Rothwell JC. Exploring Theta Burst Stimulation as an intervention to improve motor recovery in chronic stroke. Clin Neurophysiol. 2007;118:333–42.
62. Lefaucheur JP, Drouot X, Keravel Y, Nguyen JP. Pain relief induced by repetitive transcranial magnetic stimulation of precentral cortex. Neuroreport. 2001;12:2963–5.
63. Huang YZ, Edwards MJ, Bhatia KP, Rothwell JC. One-Hz repetitive transcranial magnetic stimulation of the premotor cortex alters reciprocal inhibition in DYT1 dystonia. Mov Disord. 2004;19:54–9.
64. Koch G, Brusa L, Caltagirone C, Peppe A, Oliveri M, Stanzione P, Centonze D. rTMS of supplementary motor area modulates therapy-induced dyskinesias in Parkinson disease. Neurology. 2005;65(4):623–5.
65. George MS, Ketter TA, Post RM. Prefrontal cortex dysfunction in clinical depression. Depression. 1994;2:59–72.
66. Couturier JL. Efficacy of rapid-rate repetitive transcranial magnetic stimulation in the treatment of depression: a systematic review and meta-analysis. J Psychiatry Neurosci. 2005;30:83–90.
67. Martin JL, Barbanoj MJ, Schlaepfer TE, Thompson E, Pérez V, Kulisevsky J. Repetitive transcranial magnetic stimulation for the treatment of depression. Systematic review and meta-analysis. Br J Psychiatry. 2003;182:480–91.
68. George MS, Wassermann EM, Williams WA, Callahan A, Ketter TA, Basser P, Hallett M, Post RM. Daily repetitive transcranial magnetic stimulation (rTMS) improves mood in depression. Neuroreport. 1995;6:1853–6.
69. Pascual-Leone A, Rubio B, Pallardó F, Catalá MD. Rapid-rate transcranial magnetic stimulation of left dorsolateral prefrontal cortex in drug-resistant depression. Lancet. 1996;348:233–7.
70. Hamada M, Murase N, Hasan A, Balaratnam M, Rothwell JC. The role of interneuron networks in driving human motor cortical plasticity. Cereb Cortex. 2012;23(7):1593–605.
71. Maurits N. Spinal dysfunction, transcranial magnetic stimulation, and motor evoked potentials, Neurology to methodology and back. New York, NY: Springer; 2012.
72. Vanneste S, van der Loo E, Plazier M, De Ridder D. Parietal double-cone coil stimulation in tinnitus. Exp Brain Res. 2012;221:337–43.
73. Yedimenko JA, Perez MA. The effect of bilateral isometric forces in different directions on motor cortical function in humans. J Neurophysiol. 2010;104:2922–31.

Transcranial Direct Current Stimulation: Protocols and Physiological Mechanisms of Action

9

Michael A. Nitsche, Min-Fang Kuo, Walter Paulus, and Andrea Antal

Introduction

Brain stimulation techniques have generated renewed interest in recent decades as promising tools to explore human cortical functions and to treat neuropsychiatric diseases [1]. Apart from invasive stimulation paradigms such as deep brain and vagal nerve stimulation, noninvasive tools like repetitive transcranial magnetic stimulation (rTMS) and transcranial direct current stimulation (tDCS) are attractive for use in humans, because they permit painless modulation of cortical activity and excitability through the intact skull [1]. Brain stimulation via tonic application of direct currents, although a relatively old method in strict terms, has regained increasing interest as a potentially valuable tool for the induction and modulation of neuroplasticity. About 45 years ago it was demonstrated that in anesthetized rats direct currents, delivered by intracerebral or epidural electrodes, induced stimulation polarity-dependent activity and excitability alterations of the sensorimotor cortex, which can be stable for hours after the end of stimulation [2]. A few years later it was verified that also *transcranial* application of direct currents could induce an intracerebral current flow sufficiently large to achieve physiological and functional effects [3, 4]. It was also found that this kind of stimulation alters EEG patterns and evoked potentials at the cortical level in humans [5]. Apart from early clinical studies in which mainly depressive patients were treated with mixed results [6–9], tDCS was reported to optimize performance in a choice reaction time task in healthy subjects [10, 11]. In the following years, electrical stimulation of the human brain via transcranial application of direct currents as a tool to influence brain function was nearly forgotten. Nevertheless, in the last decade it has been reevaluated following the development of methods that allow probing its neurophysiological effects (e.g., transcranial magnetic stimulation [TMS], functional magnetic resonance imaging [fMRI], and positron emission tomography [PET]). tDCS developed into a technique that reliably induces and modulates neuroplasticity in the human cerebral cortex noninvasively, and painlessly in order to elicit prolonged—but yet reversible—shifts of cortical excitability [12–15]. This review offers an overview of tDCS protocols, and their physiological effects.

tDCS Protocols

For tDCS, direct currents are delivered via a pair of surface conductive rubber electrodes covered with saline-soaked sponges (size between 3.5 and 100 cm^2 in different studies). A medium NaCl concentration (between 15 and 140 mM) is optimally suited to minimize discomfort [16]. Alternatively the rubber electrodes can be spread with electrode cream and mounted directly on the head. The correct position of both electrodes is crucial for achieving the intended effects [12]. The electrodes are connected with a stimulator. Since applied current strength determines the effects of electrical stimulation on cerebral tissue, a stimulator delivering constant current is needed. The current strength delivered varies between 1 and 2 mA in most studies. The resulting current densities are sufficient to induce physiological, and cognitive or behavioral effects, and are considered to be safe, as shown by behavioral measures, electroencephalography (EEG), serum neurone-specific enolase concentration, diffusion-weighted and contrast-enhanced MRI measures, and missing severe side-effects in a multitude of studies conducted so far in laboratories worldwide in patients and healthy subjects, as well as results of animal experiments [13–15, 17–20]. However, electrode positions above cranial foraminae and fissures should be avoided because these could increase effective current density, and thus safety of stimulation may no longer be guaranteed. Most subjects will perceive a slight itching sensation at the beginning of stimulation, which then fades

M.A. Nitsche (✉) • M.-F. Kuo • W. Paulus • A. Antal
Department of Clinical Neurophysiology, University Medical Center, Georg-August-University, Robert-Koch-Str. 40, Goettingen 37099, Germany
e-mail: Mnitsch1@gwdg.de

H. Knotkova and D. Rasche (eds.), *Textbook of Neuromodulation*,
DOI 10.1007/978-1-4939-1408-1_9,

[21, 22]. Due to the tenfold higher sensitivity to electrical stimulation of the retina compared to the brain, frontopolar stimulation in particular elicits retina phosphenes perceived at the start and the end of stimulation [23]. These are eliminated by starting and terminating the stimulation gradually (ramping up and down for 8–30 s) [24].

Approximately 50 % of the transcranially applied current enters the brain through the skull both in monkeys [3] and in humans [4]. Modelling studies suggest a nonlinearity of induced current flow dependent on electrode size, configuration, and other factors [25, 26].

The relevant parameters determining the efficacy, direction, and focality of the excitability changes induced by tDCS are *stimulation polarity/electrode position, current density* (i.e., current strength/stimulated area), *stimulation duration, electrode size,* and *configuration*, which are discussed below.

Impact of Stimulation Polarity/Electrode Position on the Effects of tDCS

Stimulation polarity determines the direction of cortical excitability changes elicited by tDCS. In most studies, both in humans and animals, anodal DC stimulation enhances cortical excitability and activity, whereas cathodal stimulation results in reversed effects [12, 13, 27]. However, deviating results have also been reported for subgroups of neurons [27, 28], hippocampal slice preparations [29], specific stimulation durations [30] or return electrode positions [31], and for combination of the stimulation with different types of tasks [32]. One explanation for these heterogeneous effects is the fact that not so much the polarity of the electrode over the stimulated area is the decisive factor for the net effects of tDCS on excitability, but rather the *direction of current flow*: the respective current has to flow along the longitudinal axis of a given neuron to induce relevant effects on membrane polarity [33]. Polarization of the soma and axon might determine the direction of the effects more than dendritic polarization, because of higher receptor and ion channel density at the soma and axon level. Consequently, the position of the return electrode is critical for achieving the intended excitability shifts, because together with the stimulation electrode it determines the electric field orientation in relation to neuronal orientation. In accordance, the position of the return electrode determines direction of the effects, and efficacy of tDCS to induce cortical excitability alterations for motor and visual cortex stimulation [12, 34, 35]. Moreover, for motor cortex stimulation it was demonstrated that positioning of the return electrode at the shoulder or arm resulted in diminished efficacy, as compared to the "classical" bipolar electrode configuration with the return electrode positioned over the contralateral orbit [36].

Impact of Current Density on the Effects of tDCS

A *current density* of about 0.03 mA/cm^2 at the electrode-skin interface is sufficient to induce relevant excitability shifts in the human primary motor cortex (M1) [12]. Similar current densities have also been shown to alter physiological, perceptual, and cognitive processes in prefrontal, parietal, temporal, and occipital cortices [14, 15]. Increasing current density might increase efficacy of stimulation due to a larger membrane polarization shift [12], but might also affect additional neuronal populations because of a greater efficacy of the electrical field in deeper cortical layers and different sensitivities of specific neuronal populations to DC stimulation [27]. Current density for effective stimulation so far has varied between 0.029 and 0.08 mA/cm^2 in most published studies [14]. These limits will probably continue to expand with experience.

Impact of Stimulation Duration on the Effects of tDCS

Stimulation duration determines the occurrence and length of aftereffects of DC stimulation in animals and humans. In humans, the standard protocol to induce acute effects of tDCS on cortical excitability without generating aftereffects is applied with stimulation duration of 4 s [12]. This stimulation protocol induces the respective excitability alterations only during stimulation. tDCS for more than 3 min seems necessary to induce cortical excitability and activity alterations, which outlast the stimulation [12]. Hereby, at least within certain limits extended stimulation protocols induce prolongation of the resulting aftereffects. tDCS from 3 to 7 min results in polarity-specific excitability alterations for some minutes after the end of stimulation, whereas anodal tDCS for 13 min and cathodal tDCS for 9 min results in aftereffects lasting for about 1 h in the human motor cortex ([13, 17], Fig. 9.1). This relationship between stimulation duration, and duration of aftereffects, is however not linear under all conditions: recently it was shown that anodal tDCS for 26 min results in excitability-diminishing, and not enhancing aftereffects, most probably caused by intraneuronal calcium overflow ([30], Fig. 9.2). Thus for the induction of aftereffects lasting relevantly longer than 1 h after tDCS, which are desirable especially to achieve therapeutic effects in clinical studies, simply prolonging stimulation duration seems not to be the optimal strategy. The alternative might be the repetition of stimulation sessions. Indeed, repeating cathodal or anodal tDCS within a time-window of 30 min increases and prolongs the aftereffects of both anodal and cathodal tDCS relevantly, for anodal tDCS for more than 24 h after stimulation [30, 37]. On the other hand, tDCS-intervals of 3 and 24 h diminished the

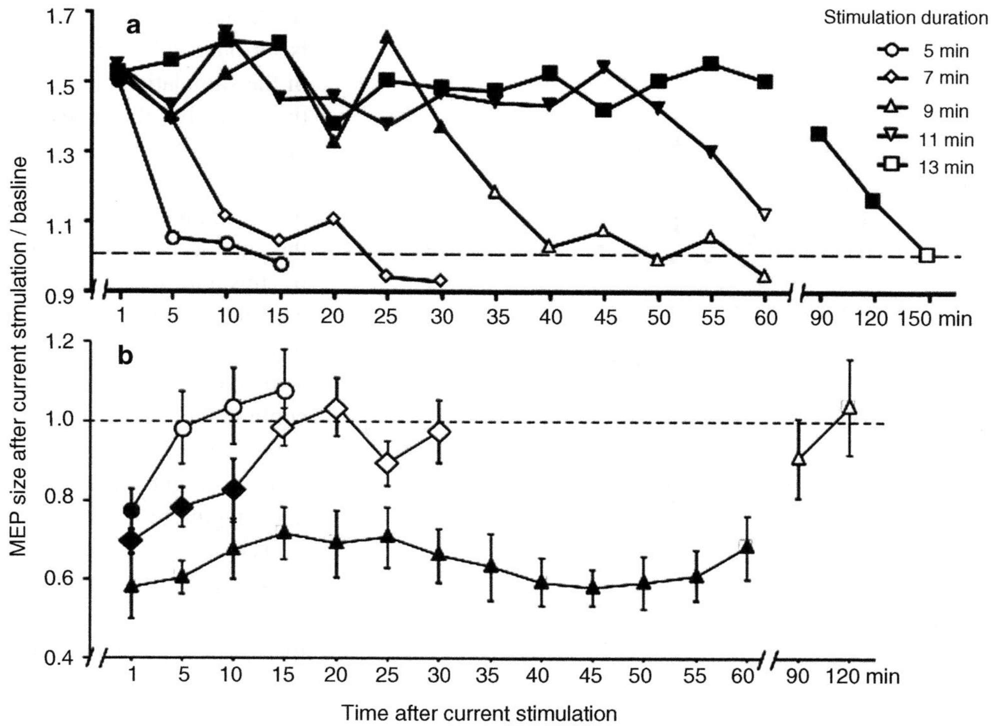

Fig. 9.1 Aftereffects of tDCS. tDCS of the human motor cortex modulates TMS-elicited MEP-amplitudes after stimulation for up to an hour, depending on stimulation duration. Anodal stimulation (**a**) enhances, while cathodal (**b**) diminishes cortical excitability. Note that 5 to 7 min of stimulation result in short-lasting aftereffects, while prolonged tDCS increases the duration of the aftereffects over-proportionally ([13, 17], with permission of Neurology and Clin Neurophysiol)

aftereffects of the second protocol in both studies. Thus specific timing is important for prolongation of tDCS effects on cortical excitability. Moreover, the results of these studies suggest that consecutive tDCS protocols might interact even when the overt impact on cortical excitability has vanished. Therefore, a sufficient interval between experimental sessions is recommended, when it is not intended to induce cumulative aftereffects. It should be kept in mind that the physiological effects might not necessarily translate one-to-one to functional effects of stimulation. In contrast to the physiological effects, it has been shown that repeated tDCS, in most studies conducted once a day for 5 or more consecutive days, induces effects on motor performance, pain, depression, and other functions, or symptoms, which can last for 1 month or more after stimulation [38–40].

Impact of Electrode Configurations on the Focality of tDCS

The "classical" tDCS protocols to induce neuroplastic excitability alterations involve stimulation with two relatively large electrodes (usual size between 25 and 35 cm^2) positioned on the head. These electrodes induce relatively non-focal effects of the underlying cortex, but also at remote areas, as shown experimentally for stimulation of the primary motor cortex [41, 42], and via modelling approaches [43]. Low focality is not necessarily a problem for each application of tDCS. In clinical syndromes, modulation of pathologically altered excitability of larger regions might be preferable, and in some cases, where the intended effects are thought to originate from an interaction of task- and stimulation-generated activity alterations, *functional* focality might result from this interaction. However, focality is crucial for the basic studies aiming to explore the contribution of a specific area to brain function. Thus new tDCS protocols suited to increase focality of stimulation have been developed. At least two factors contribute to the low focality of tDCS, the size of the relative large electrode positioned over the target area, and the physiological effects of the return electrode, if positioned at the scalp. Focality of tDCS over the target area can be enhanced by reducing electrode size, and keeping current density constant. By this modification of the stimulation protocol it has been shown for the motor cortex that a more selective alteration of excitability of specific hand muscle representations is accomplished ([42], Fig. 9.3). Following the same rationale, increasing the size of the return electrode at constant current strength from 35 to 100 cm^2 makes this electrode functionally inefficient, most probably due to reduced current density, and thus results in an at least functionally monopolar stimulation [42]. Alternatively, the return electrode can be positioned at another location than the scalp, e.g., the neck, shoulder, arm, or knee [6, 31, 44]. However, this remote position of the return

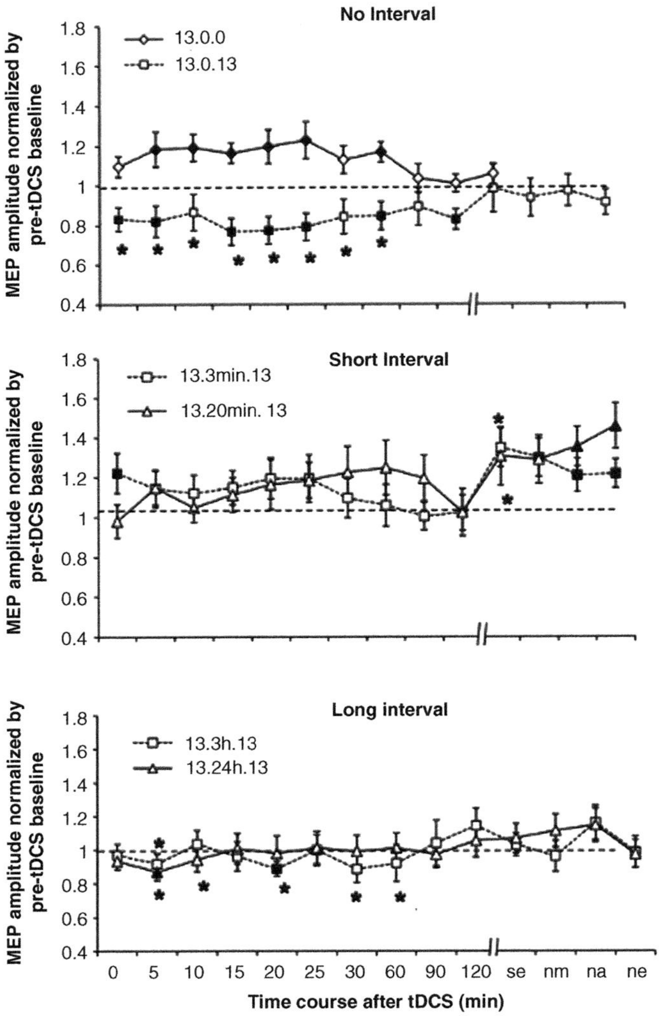

Fig. 9.2 Effects of repetitive tDCS on the impact of tDCS on motor cortex excitability. Interval duration determines the effects of repeated anodal tDCS on motor cortex excitability. A single session of 13 min anodal tDCS (13-0-0) enhances excitability up to 60 min after DC stimulation. Prolonging stimulation duration for 26 min (13-0-13) however converts the aftereffects into excitability diminution (**a**). An inter tDCS-interval of 3 or 20 min (13-3-13, 13-20-13 protocols) primarily diminishes the efficacy of tDCS to enhance excitability, which however is present trendwise up to about 90 min after tDCS. From the evening of the stimulation day on for up to the next evening, however, motor cortex excitability is again enhanced significantly (**b**). Prolonging the inter-tDCS intervals for 3 or 24 h (13-3 h-13, 13-24 h-13 protocols) abolishes the excitability enhancement, and turns it slightly into inhibition (**c**). *se* same evening; *nm* next morning, *na* next afternoon, *ne* next evening (Monte-Siva et al., 2012, with permission of Brain Stimulation)

electrode might diminish the efficacy of stimulation [36], and it is unclear if other sets of neurons would be affected by these approaches due to different electrical field orientation.

Based on modelling of electrical field strength, alternative electrode configurations have been developed to optimize stimulation focality, the so-called high-definition tDCS (HD-tDCS) is one of these approaches. Here relatively small electrodes are used, and a central stimulation electrode is surrounded by four return electrodes placed in the vicinity of the stimulation electrode [43]. Since the distance between the respective electrodes is relatively short, and thus shunting is enhanced relative to the more conventional electrode arrangements, current density has to be relatively high to obtain similar effects as with the large electrodes. Taking this into account, the cortical excitability alterations induced by this protocol seem to be similar to those elicited by conventional tDCS [80]. However, information about the physiological focality of these excitability alterations is not available so far. The functional efficacy of this electrode configuration has been demonstrated in some pilot studies, including pain perception [45]. Another optimizing future strategy might be multi-electrode approaches, which show encouraging results in modelling [46].

Taken together, for tDCS various protocols are available, which differ with regard to stimulation polarity, current density, stimulation duration, as well as electrode size and locations. Dependent on these parameters, stimulation protocols can be customized at least to a certain extent to achieve the desired direction, strength, focality, and duration of effects on cortical activity and excitability. However, systematic studies about optimized physiological and functional effects are rare so far. For functional effects, the development of optimized protocols might have to take into account not only the impact of tDCS on cortical processes, but also the interaction between stimulation, and task-related cortical activity alterations, which might not be trivial in each case. Another future challenge might be the development of individually adapted stimulation protocols, which take interindividual difference of anatomy and physiology into account.

Mechanisms of Action of tDCS

A multitude of studies has been conducted to explore the physiological effects of tDCS in the last years. The motor cortex, especially the primary motor hand area (M1), has been widely used as a model system in order to study modulation of cortical excitability by tDCS. Reasons for this are that M1 lies on the cortical convexity of the precentral gyrus with a minimal distance to the scalp surface and can thus easily be reached with TMS pulses. Furthermore, for motor cortex TMS, specific stimulation protocols have been developed to monitor different types of intracortical neurons as well as cortical output neurons [47]. Therefore, most of our knowledge about basic physiology of tDCS originates from studies in the human motor cortex. However, physiological effects of tDCS on other cortical areas have also been explored, and beyond TMS, evoked potential measures, EEG, and functional imaging have contributed to our understanding of the physiological background of tDCS. Whereas

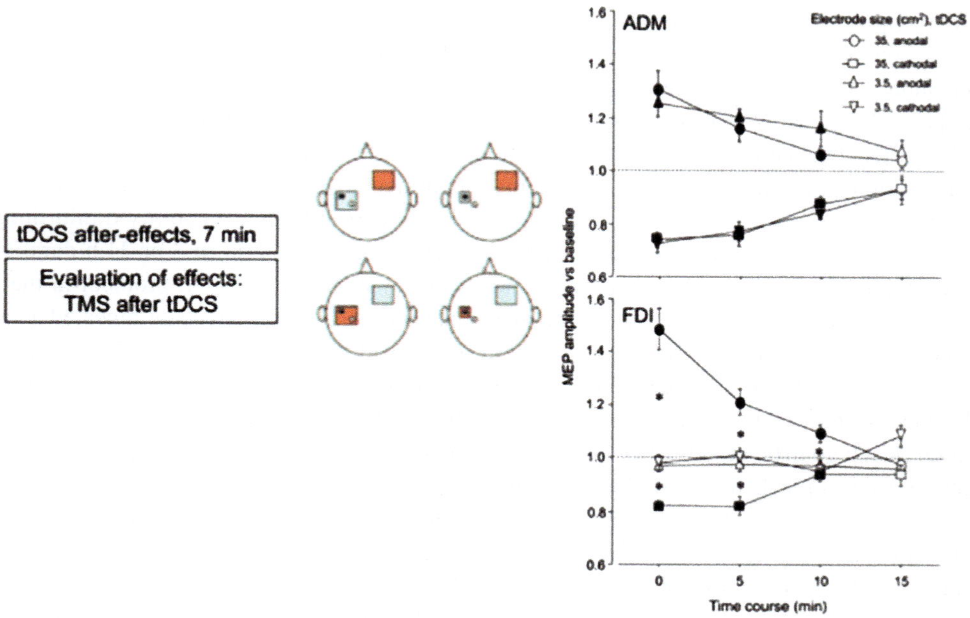

Fig. 9.3 Focusing the effects of tDCS by reducing electrode size. Depicted are baseline-standardized mean motor evoked potential (MEP) amplitude sizes of the abductor digiti minimi (ADM) and first dorsal interosseus (FDI) muscles after 7 min of anodal or cathodal tDCS. In the 35 cm^2 electrode size condition, in which the tDCS electrode covers the motor cortex representation of the ADM and the FDI, anodal tDCS enhances and cathodal tDCS diminishes excitability of both areas for some minutes after the end of stimulation. When tDCS is performed selectively over the motor cortex representation of the ADM (electrode size 3.5 cm^2), the excitability change for the ADM is identical to the former condition, but TMS over the representation of the FDI reveals no excitability changes as compared to baseline. Filled symbols indicate deviations of the post-tDCS MEP amplitudes relative to baseline, the asterisks mark differences between MEP amplitudes of the ADM or FDI obtained with different tDCS electrode sizes. Error bars are standard error of mean ([42], with permission of J Neurophysiol)

regional effects of tDCS were in the focus of investigations during the first years, the impact of tDCS on cortical network activity became a new topic of research recently.

Regional Effects of tDCS on Cortical Excitability

Acute Effects of tDCS on Cortical Activity and Excitability

The primary mechanism of DC stimulation on the cerebral cortex is a subthreshold modulation of neuronal resting membrane potential. In animal experiments anodal stimulation results in a subthreshold depolarisation, while cathodal stimulation hyperpolarises neuronal membranes [27, 28]. However, this polarity-dependent effect, which has been described in most animal studies, has to be qualified. As mentioned above, orientation of electrical field relative to neuronal orientation determines the direction of the effects. Accordingly, antagonistic effects of DC stimulation were described not only for subgroups of neurons, but also for specific preparations, such as hippocampal slice experiments [28, 29]. In humans, similar stimulation polarity-dependent effects have been shown for short stimulation durations of few seconds, which do not induce aftereffects. Anodal tDCS enhances cortical excitability, while cathodal stimulation diminishes it in the human motor cortex, as demonstrated by TMS. These effects are largely restricted to global parameters of corticospinal excitability, which are determined by ion channel conductivity, such as single pulse MEP amplitudes induced by medium TMS intensity and recruitment curves. They do not involve major alterations of intracortical facilitation, and inhibition, as monitored by TMS double-pulse stimulation protocols [12, 48]. Accordingly, blocking voltage-gated sodium and calcium channels abolishes the excitability enhancement accomplished by anodal tDCS, but block of glutamatergic NMDA receptors or enhancement of GABAergic inhibition does not affect the acute effects of tDCS [17, 49]. Thus, taken together, the primary effects of tDCS seem to involve polarity-specific membrane potential alterations, but no synaptic effects.

Aftereffects of tDCS on Cortical Activity, and Excitability

In experiments in anesthetized rats, Bindman and colleagues described prolonged enhancements of cortical activity and excitability lasting for hours after anodal stimulation, while cathodal DC stimulation had antagonistic effects, if stimulation was conducted for 5 min or longer [2]. Identically directed aftereffects of tDCS are accomplished when stimulation duration exceeds 3 min in humans. Here tDCS over the motor cortex for up to 7 min results in aftereffects of about 5–10 min duration, while longer stimulation durations for up to 13 min induce excitability alterations stable for about 60–90 min [12, 13, 17]. However, the duration of the aftereffects might differ between cortical regions, with somewhat shorter lasting effects induced by tDCS over the visual cortex [35, 50].

At the corticospinal level, tDCS elicits similar aftereffects as those accomplished during short stimulation. The slope of the recruitment curve is reduced after cathodal tDCS, but enhanced after anodal stimulation [48]. For intracortical effects, anodal tDCS enhances intracortical facilitation and reduces intracortical inhibition, whereas cathodal tDCS induces antagonistic effects [48]. Most probably, these effects are accomplished by combined modulation of motor cortical afferents and motor cortex output neurons with conventional large electrodes, since selective premotor stimulation induces only the above-mentioned intracortical effects in M1, while focal stimulation over M1 with a small electrode only resulted in the above-mentioned corticospinal effects [51]. Because block of glutamatergic NMDA receptors abolishes the aftereffects of tDCS, and the NMDA receptor agonist d-cycloserine prolonged the aftereffects of anodal stimulation [52, 53], it can be assumed that tDCS induces plasticity of the glutamatergic system. Further indirect evidence for an effect of tDCS on glutamatergic neurons comes from a study showing that block of voltage-gated calcium channels abolishes the aftereffects of anodal tDCS [52], as glutamatergic neuroplasticity is induced by modulation of neuronal calcium influx (Fig. 9.4). These results are in accordance with animal experiments, in which it was shown that anodal tDCS enhances neuronal calcium content [54]. Beyond modulation of the glutamatergic system, it has recently been shown that both—anodal and cathodal tDCS—reduce free gamma-aminobutyric acid (GABA) in the cortical areas under the electrodes [55]. This result fits with an enhancing effect of both anodal and cathodal tDCS on TMS-induced I-wave facilitation, which is controlled by the GABAergic system [48]. GABA-reduction has been shown to enhance glutamatergic plasticity in animal slice experiments, and could have a facilitating effect on tDCS-induced plasticity in humans as well. This might also explain why enhancement of GABAergic receptor activity by lorazepam had no effect on cathodal tDCS-induced plasticity however led to a rebound anodal excitation [49], because benzodiazepines only enhance efficacy of already active GABAergic receptors (Table 9.1).

Beyond the "classic" tDCS protocols, which induce aftereffects of about one hour duration, recently stimulation protocols have been developed to induce excitability enhancements lasting for at least 24 h after the end of anodal tDCS. For such effects, repeated stimulation for 13 min within a time window of 30 min seems to be critical [30]. This fits nicely with the results of animal experiments where it was shown that an intervention within about 30 min after the first plasticity induction procedure results in late-phase long-term potentiation (LTP) effects [56]. Interestingly, continuous anodal tDCS with doubled stimulation protocol duration results in excitability-diminishing plasticity, and increasing the interval to 3 or 24 h duration diminishes the efficacy of the stimulation protocol in the same study. The late-phase LTP-like effects of repeated anodal tDCS depend on the glutamatergic system. The excitability diminution induced by 26 min continuous stimulation might result from intracellular calcium overflow, since calcium channel block abolished this effect [30].

Taken together, it can thus be concluded that the aftereffects of tDCS depend on glutamatergic mechanisms, and that tDCS-induced reduction of GABA might serve as a "gating" mechanism.

Beyond these primary effects, neuromodulators have been shown to have a relevant impact on glutamatergic plasticity in animal models, and humans [57]. In accordance, monoamines have a prominent impact also on tDCS-induced plasticity. The nonselective monoaminergic enhancer amphetamine increases anodal tDCS-induced excitability-enhancing plasticity [58]. This effect might be partially due to its impact on ß-adrenergic receptors, because antagonizing these receptors reduces the duration of the aftereffects of anodal and cathodal tDCS [58]. Moreover, dopamine and serotonin have a prominent impact on tDCS-induced plasticity. For dopamine, physiological receptor activity is critical for the induction of aftereffects, because D2 receptor antagonist abolishes any aftereffects of tDCS [59]. Interestingly, increasing dopamine receptor activation by the nonselective precursor L-dopa has dosage-dependent nonlinear effects on tDCS-generated plasticity. Whereas low- and high-dosage L-dopa abolished excitability-enhancing and -diminishing plasticity, medium dosage prolonged the excitability-diminishing aftereffects, and converted anodal tDCS-induced facilitation into inhibition [60, 61]. Similar effects were accomplished with a D2 receptor agonist with the exception that the medium dose did reestablish the anodal tDCS-induced facilitation, and high dosage medication combined with cathodal tDCS resulted in an excitability enhancement [62]. Additionally, D1 receptor activation under D2 receptor block reestablished tDCS-induced plasticity of both stimulation polarities [63]. Taken together, dopamine has prominent nonlinear effects on tDCS-induced plasticity, which depend on dosage, and subreceptor activity. Interestingly, conversion of the excitability-enhancing effects of anodal tDCS to excitability diminution seems to require activation of both D1- and D2-like receptors. For serotonin, activation by a respective reuptake-inhibitor enhanced and prolonged the aftereffects of anodal tDCS, and converted

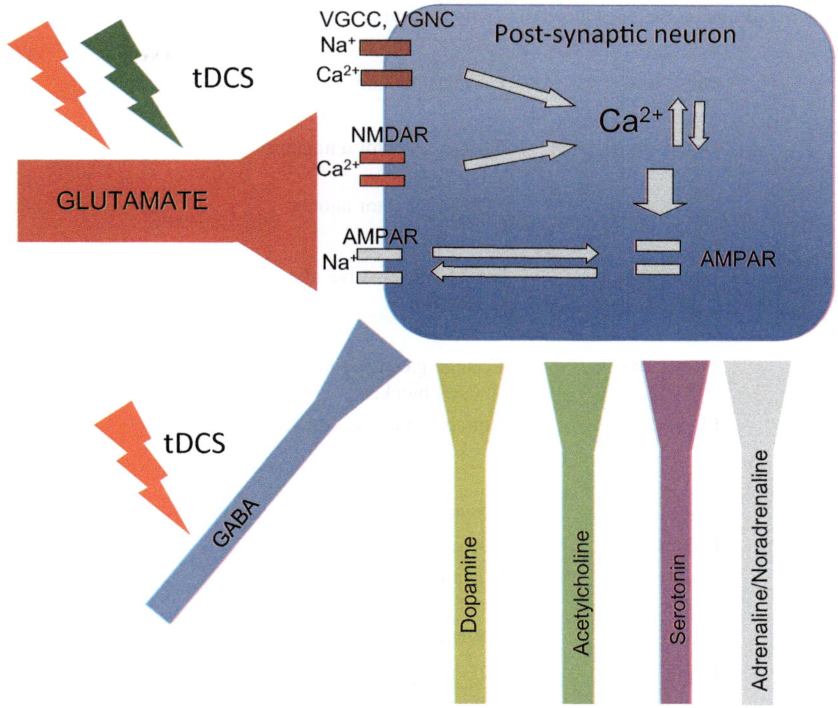

Fig. 9.4 tDCS-generated mechanisms of action of glutamatergic plasticity, including modulatory effects. In this figure, the main plasticity mechanism of glutamatergic synapses, and the modulatory impact of other neurotransmitters and ion channels are displayed. As far as explored, tDCS alters glutamatergic neurons dependent on stimulation polarity, while reducing GABAergic activity independent from stimulation polarity. Glutamate release activates *N*-methyl-D-aspartate receptors (NMDAR), which have calcium (Ca^{2+}) channel properties if it is sufficiently strong. Dependent on the amount of the consecutive intraneuronal calcium increase, enzyme cascades are activated which result in postsynaptic insertion or removal of glutamatergic α-amino-3-hydroxy-5-methyl-4-isoxazolepropionic acid receptors (AMPAR). The amount of postsynaptic AMPA receptors determines if a given activation of a presynaptic neuron leads to supra-threshold postsynaptic activation. Consequently, the modification of AMPA receptor density is the main basis for LTP and LTD. The activity of voltage-dependent calcium channels (VGCC) contributes to intracellular calcium alterations, and the activation of sodium (Na) channels (VGNC) contributes to the resting membrane potential which affects the probability of NMDA receptors activation, and presynaptic activity results in a postsynaptic action potential. Various neurotransmitters such as GABA, dopamine, acetylcholine, serotonin, adrenaline, and noradrenaline affect these principle mechanisms of action in a complex, sometimes nonlinear way, via their specific receptors, and they also have an impact on glutamatergic receptors and ion channels

plasticity induced by cathodal stimulation into facilitation [64]. For the cholinergic system, enhancement of global cholinergic activation resulted in a similar effect as medium-dosage L-dopa on tDCS-generated plasticity, i.e., a slight prolongation of cathodal tDCS-induced excitability diminution, and a conversion of anodal tDCS-induced aftereffects from facilitation into excitability reduction [65]. For anodal tDCS, activation of nicotinic receptors resulted in similar effects, but it abolished the aftereffects of cathodal tDCS [66]. Dosage-dependent effects of serotonin and acetylcholine/nicotine on tDCS-induced plasticity have not been explored so far. While the detailed mechanisms of action of these neuromodulators on tDCS-induced plasticity are waiting to be explored, one relevant potential mechanism might be their impact on intraneuronal calcium concentration.

The above-mentioned studies were performed in the human primary motor cortex, but the effects of tDCS are not restricted to this region. In the last years, numerous studies have been conducted, which show a similar functional or physiological impact of tDCS on a multitude of cortical regions. Neurophysiological effects have been demonstrated for the visual cortex, where anodal and cathodal tDCS have similar effects on cortical excitability as motor cortex stimulation; however, antagonistic effects were also observed if the return electrode is positioned at the neck [31]. tDCS over the visual cortex results in shorter duration of the aftereffects, as compared to the stimulation over M1. For tDCS of the somatosensory cortex, anodal tDCS increased respective SEP amplitudes for at least 60 min after stimulation in one study [67], and cathodal tDCS reduced those in another one [68]. For auditory cortex stimulation, anodal tDCS over the temporal, and cathodal tDCS over the temporoparietal cortex enhanced the respective evoked potentials [69]. Beyond the principle effects on cortical excitability, however, no further studies are available exploring the physiological mechanisms of tDCS in these areas into larger detail.

Table 9.1 Impact of CNS active drugs on tDCS-induced plasticity in human cortex

Study	Substance	Pharmacodynamic effect	Dosage (mg)	LTP-like plasticity	LTD-like plasticity
Glutamate					
Liebetanz et al. [79], Nitsche et al. [52]	Dextromethorphan	NMDA receptor antagonist	150	↓	↓
Nitsche et al. [53]	D-cycloserine	NMDA receptor agonist	100	↑	•
GABA					
Nitsche et al. [49]	Lorazepam	GABAAR: positive allosteric modulator	2	↑, Initial delay	•
Voltage-gated ion channels					
Liebetanz et al. [79], Nitsche et al. [52]	Carbamazepine	Voltage-gated sodium channel blocker	300 + 300	↓	•
Nitsche et al. [52]	Flunarizine	Voltage-gated calcium channel blocker	10	↓	•
Dopamine					
Nitsche et al. [59]	Sulpiride	D2 receptor antagonist	400	↓	↓
Monte-Silva et al. [61]	L-dopa	Dopamine precursor	25	↓	↓
Kuo et al. [60], Monte-Silva et al. [61]	L-dopa	Dopamine precursor	100 mg	↓ Conversion to LTD	↓
Monte-Silva et al. [61]	L-dopa	Dopamine precursor	200 mg	↓	↓
Monte-Silva et al. [62]	Ropinirole	D2/3 receptor agonist	0.125	↓	↓
Monte-Silva et al. [62]	Ropinirole	D2/3 receptor agonist	0.5	•	•
Monte-Silva et al. [62]	Ropinirole	D2/3 receptor agonist	1	↓	↓
Nitsche et al. [63]	L-dopa + sulpiride	Activation of D1 receptor under D2 receptor blockade	100 + 400	•	•
Acetylcholine					
Kuo et al. [65]	Rivastigmine	Cholinesterase inhibitor	3	↓	↓
Thirugnanasambandam et al. [66]	Nicotine	Nicotinic receptor antagonist	15, Patch	↓	↓

n.t. not tested, *tDCS* transcranial direct current stimulation, *LTP* long-term potentiation, *LTD* long-term depression, *GABAAR* gamma-aminobutyric acid type A receptor, • = no plasticity, ↓ = decrease of plasticity, ↑ = increase of plasticity

Interregional Effects of tDCS: Impact on Functional Connectivity

Apart from the regional effects of tDCS under the stimulation electrodes, remote effects on topographically distant cortical and subcortical areas were described relatively early [41]. However, it was unclear whether those effects are caused by physiological spreading of cortical activity or by current spread. Simulation studies, although not physiologically validated so far, are in favor for at least a partial contribution of spread of current flow [43]. In the meantime, clear physiological effects of tDCS on remote areas have been described. Premotor anodal tDCS was shown to enhance intracortical facilitation of M1, most probably due to the activation of premotor–primary motor cortex afferents [51], and combined dorsal premotor and supplementary motor area (SMA) stimulation alters motor and somatosensory evoked potentials [70]. For parietal cortex stimulation, anodal tDCS enhanced, but cathodal tDCS reduced MEP amplitudes in motor imagery conditions [71]. Recently, functional connectivity approaches have been applied to explore cortical network alterations induced by tDCS. For motor cortex stimulation under resting conditions, an fMRI study revealed that nodal minimum path length increased after anodal tDCS over M1, which means that functional connectivity of this area with topographically distant regions of the whole brain significantly decreased. In contrast to this generally reduced whole brain connectivity of M1, functional connectivity was enhanced between the primary motor cortex on the one hand, and premotor and superior parietal areas on the other [72]. In another study, cathodal tDCS of the primary motor cortex increased functional connectivity between the stimulated M1, and the contralateral M1 and premotor cortices [73]. A similar effect of tDCS was described for anodal stimulation combined with motor practice in an EEG study, where functional connectivity was enhanced between primary motor, premotor, and sensorimotor areas in the high gamma band [74]. Moreover, anodal tDCS of the primary motor cortex alters cortico-subcortical connectivity of the motor cortex at rest. Specifically, it was shown to enhance connectivity with the ipsilateral caudate nucleus, and thalamus [75]. Additionally, alterations of intrinsic motor cortex connectivity by tDCS have been demonstrated: cathodal stimulation increased local connectivity, most likely due to cortical noise reduction accomplished by the respective excitability and activity diminution, while anodal tDCS enhanced long-distance connectivity within this area [76]. Therefore it can be concluded by the results of these studies that motor cortex tDCS alters the connectivity of large parts of the motor network.

Beyond tDCS of the motor cortex, stimulation of the dorsolateral prefrontal cortex has also been demonstrated to induce widespread alterations of functional connectivity, including the default mode network, and attention-related networks in healthy subjects [77, 78].

Taken together, in addition to its regional effects under the stimulation electrodes, tDCS has prominent effects on functional networks at both cortical and subcortical levels. The relevance of these network alterations for cognition and behavior needs to be explored in future studies.

Conclusion

tDCS has been reintroduced as a tool to induce acute and neuroplastic alterations of cortical excitability and activity about 12 years ago. Since then, an increasing number of studies has been conducted to develop protocols enhancing the efficacy of stimulation, and to explore the physiological basics of the effects. For the development of new stimulation protocols, determinants of tDCS efficacy, such as stimulation intensity, duration, and repetition intervals have been identified, and protocols which allow a more focal stimulation have been developed. It has been shown that the dependence of tDCS efficacy on these stimulation parameters is not linear in each case. Future work should focus on further optimizing stimulation protocols, which will be important especially for clinical applications, where stable alterations of cortical excitability and activity are needed. Moreover, given the partial nonlinearity of the effects, exploring optimal combinations of stimulation with performance would be an important, but not trivial, topic of future research. Since most of the studies reported in this review were conducted in the primary motor cortex, the transferability of the respective results to other cortical areas has yet to be explored. With regard to the mechanisms of action, pharmacological, TMS, EEG, and functional imaging studies have revealed the main physiological mechanisms of tDCS, i.e., the primary effect of membrane polarization, the dependence of the aftereffects from alterations of glutamatergic synapses, and the complex alteration of tDCS-induced plasticity by neuromodulators. Furthermore, it became increasingly clear recently that the effects of tDCS are not only restricted to the area under the electrodes. The stimulation also induces alterations of connectivity within cortical and cortico-subcortical networks. Although knowledge about the physiological basis of tDCS is far from being complete, these studies provide a basis for understanding its effects, which might also be important for evaluating new fields of application in future.

Acknowledgements M.A.N. receives funding by the German Research Society (DFG) via grants Ni 683/4-2, and Ni 683/6-1.

References

1. Ziemann U, Paulus W, Nitsche MA, Pascual-Leone A, Byblow WD, Berardelli A, et al. Consensus: motor cortex plasticity protocols. Brain Stimul. 2008;1:164–82.
2. Bindman L, Lippold O, Redfearn JWT. The action of brief polarizing currents on the cerebral cortex of the rat (1) during current flow and (2) in the production of long-lasting after-effects. J Physiol Lond. 1964;172:369–82.
3. Rush S, Driscoll DA. Current distribution in the brain from surface electrodes. Anesth Analg. 1968;47:717–23.
4. Dymond AM, Coger RW, Serafetinides EA. Intracerebral current levels in man during electrosleep therapy. Biol Psychiatry. 1975;10: 101–4.
5. Pfurtscheller G. Spectrum analysis of EEG: before, during and after extracranial stimulation in man. Elektromed Biomed Tech. 1970; 15:225–30. Article in German.
6. Costain R, Redfearn JWT, Lippold OCJ. A controlled trial of the therapeutic effects of polarization of the brain in depressive illness. Br J Psychiatry. 1964;110:786–99.
7. Lippold OCJ, Redfearn JWT. Mental changes resulting from the passage of small direct currents through the human brain. Br J Psychiatry. 1964;1964:768–72.
8. Redfearn JWT, Lippold OCJ, Costain R. A preliminary account of the clinnical effects of polarizing the brain in certain psychiatric disorders. Br J Psychiatry. 1964;110:773–85.
9. Lolas F. Brain polarization: behavioral and therapeutic effects. Biol Psychiatry. 1977;12:37–47.
10. Elbert T, Lutzenberger W, Rockstroh B, Birbaumer N. The influence of low-level transcortical DC-currents on response speed in humans. Int J Neurosci. 1981;14:101–14.
11. Jaeger D, Elbert T, Lutzenberger W, Birbaumer N. The effects of externally applied transcephalic weak direct currents on lateralization in choice reaction tasks. J Psychophysiol. 1987;1:127–33.
12. Nitsche M, Paulus W. Excitability changes induced in the human motor cortex by weak transcranial direct current stimulation. J Physiol. 2000;527(Pt 3):633–9.
13. Nitsche M, Paulus W. Sustained excitability elevations induced by transcranial DC motor cortex stimulation in humans. Neurology. 2001;57:1899–901.
14. Nitsche MA, Cohen LG, Wassermann EM, Priori A, Lang N, Antal A, et al. Transcranial direct current stimulation: state of the art 2008. Brain Stimul. 2008;1:206–23.
15. Nitsche MA, Paulus W. Transcranial direct current stimulation: update 2011. Restor Neurol Neurosci. 2011;29:463–92.
16. Dundas JE, Thickbroom GW, Mastaglia FL. Perception of comfort during transcranial DC stimulation: effect of NaCl solution concentration applied to sponge electrodes. Clin Neurophysiol. 2007;118: 1166–70.
17. Nitsche M, Nitsche M, Klein C, Tergau F, Rothwell J, Paulus W. Level of action of cathodal DC polarisation induced inhibition of the human motor cortex. Clin Neurophysiol. 2003;114:600–4.

18. Nitsche M, Niehaus L, Hoffmann K, Hengst S, Liebetanz D, Paulus W, et al. MRI study of human brain exposed to weak direct current stimulation of the frontal cortex. Clin Neurophysiol. 2004; 115:2419–23.
19. Iyer M, Mattu U, Grafman J, Lomarev M, Sato S, Wassermann E. Safety and cognitive effect of frontal DC brain polarization in healthy individuals. Neurology. 2005;64:872–5.
20. Liebetanz D, Koch R, Mayenfels S, Konig F, Paulus W, Nitsche MA. Safety limits of cathodal transcranial direct current stimulation in rats. Clin Neurophysiol. 2009;120:1161–7.
21. Ambrus GG, Antal A, Paulus W. Comparing cutaneous perception induced by electrical stimulation using rectangular and round shaped electrodes. Clin Neurophysiol. 2011;122:803–7.
22. Ambrus GG, Al-Moyed H, Chaieb L, Sarp L, Antal A, Paulus W. The fade-in—short stimulation—fade out approach to sham tDCS—reliable at 1 mA for naive and experienced subjects, but not investigators. Brain Stimul. 2012;5:499–504.
23. Paulus W. On the difficulties of separating retinal from cortical origins of phosphenes when using transcranial alternating current stimulation (tACS). Clin Neurophysiol. 2010;121:987–91.
24. Gandiga PC, Hummel FC, Cohen LG. Transcranial DC stimulation (tDCS): a tool for double-blind sham-controlled clinical studies in brain stimulation. Clin Neurophysiol. 2006;117:845–50.
25. Miranda PC, Faria P, Hallett M. What does the ratio of injected current to electrode area tell us about current density in the brain during tDCS? Clin Neurophysiol. 2009;120:1183–7.
26. Faria P, Hallett M, Miranda PC. A finite element analysis of the effect of electrode area and inter-electrode distance on the spatial distribution of the current density in tDCS. J Neural Eng. 2011;8: 066017.
27. Purpura DP, McMurtry JG. Intracellular activities and evoked potential changes during polarization of motor cortex. J Neurophysiol. 1965;28:166–85.
28. Creutzfeldt OD, Fromm GH, Kapp H. Influence of transcortical d-c currents on cortical neuronal activity. Exp Neurol. 1962;5:436–52.
29. Kabakov AY, Muller PA, Pascual-Leone A, Jensen FE, Rotenberg A. Contribution of axonal orientation to pathway-dependent modulation of excitatory transmission by direct current stimulation in isolated rat hippocampus. J Neurophysiol. 2012;107:1881–9.
30. Monte-Silva K, Kuo MF, Hessenthaler S, Fresnoza S, Liebetanz D, Paulus W, et al. Induction of late LTP-like plasticity in the human motor cortex by repeated non-invasive brain stimulation. Brain Stimul. 2012;6:424–32.
31. Accornero N, Li Voti P, La Riccia M, Gregori B. Visual evoked potentials modulation during direct current cortical polarization. Exp Brain Res. 2007;178:261–6.
32. Antal A, Terney D, Poreisz C, Paulus W. Towards unravelling task-related modulations of neuroplastic changes induced in the human motor cortex. Eur J Neurosci. 2007;26:2687–91.
33. Roth BJ. Mechanisms for electrical stimulation of excitable tissue. Crit Rev Biomed Eng. 1994;22:253–305.
34. Priori A, Berardelli A, Rona S, Accornero N, Manfredi M. Polarization of the human motor cortex through the scalp. Neuroreport. 1998;9:2257–60.
35. Antal A, Kincses TZ, Nitsche MA, Bartfai O, Paulus W. Excitability changes induced in the human primary visual cortex by transcranial direct current stimulation: direct electrophysiological evidence. Invest Ophthalmol Vis Sci. 2004;45:702–7.
36. Moliadze V, Antal A, Paulus W. Electrode-distance dependent after-effects of transcranial direct and random noise stimulation with extracephalic reference electrodes. Clin Neurophysiol. 2010; 121:2165–71.
37. Monte-Silva K, Kuo M-F, Liebetanz D, Paulus W, Nitsche MA. Shaping the optimal repetition interval for cathodal transcranial direct current stimulation (tDCS). J Neurophysiol. 2010;103: 1735–40.
38. Fregni F, Gimenes R, Valle AC, Ferreira MJ, Rocha RR, Natalle L, et al. A randomized, sham-controlled, proof of principle study of transcranial direct current stimulation for the treatment of pain in fibromyalgia. Arthritis Rheum. 2006;54:3988–98.
39. Loo CK, Alonzo A, Martin D, Mitchell PB, Galvez V, Sachdev P. Transcranial direct current stimulation for depression: 3-week, randomised, sham-controlled trial. Br J Psychiatry. 2012;200:52–9.
40. Reis J, Schambra HM, Cohen LG, Buch ER, Fritsch B, Zarahn E, et al. Noninvasive cortical stimulation enhances motor skill acquisition over multiple days through an effect on consolidation. Proc Natl Acad Sci U S A. 2009;106:1590–5.
41. Lang N, Siebner H, Ward N, Lee L, Nitsche M, Paulus W, et al. How does transcranial DC stimulation of the primary motor cortex alter regional neuronal activity in the human brain? Eur J Neurosci. 2005;22:495–504.
42. Nitsche MA, Doemkes S, Karakose T, Antal A, Liebetanz D, Lang N, et al. Shaping the effects of transcranial direct current stimulation of the human motor cortex. J Neurophysiol. 2007;97:3109–17.
43. Datta A, Bansal V, Diaz J, Patel J, Reato D, Bikson M. Gyri-precise head model of transcranial direct current stimulation: improved spatial focality using a ring electrode versus conventional rectangular pad. Brain Stimul. 2009;2:201–7. 207.e201.
44. Cogiamanian F, Marceglia S, Ardolino G, Barbieri S, Priori A. Improved isometric force endurance after transcranial direct current stimulation over the human motor cortical areas. Eur J Neurosci. 2007;26:242–9.
45. Borckardt JJ, Bikson M, Frohman H, Reeves ST, Datta A, Bansal V, et al. A pilot study of the tolerability and effects of high-definition transcranial direct current stimulation (HD-tDCS) on pain perception. J Pain. 2012;13:112–20.
46. Dmochowski JP, Datta A, Bikson M, Su Y, Parra LC. Optimized multi-electrode stimulation increases focality and intensity at target. J Neural Eng. 2011;8:046011.
47. Hallett M. Transcranial magnetic stimulation: a primer. Neuron. 2007;55:187–99.
48. Nitsche M, Seeber A, Frommann K, Klein C, Rochford C, Nitsche M, et al. Modulating parameters of excitability during and after transcranial direct current stimulation of the human motor cortex. J Physiol. 2005;568(Pt 1):291–303.
49. Nitsche M, Liebetanz D, Schlitterlau A, Henschke U, Fricke K, Frommann K, et al. GABAergic modulation of DC stimulation-induced motor cortex excitability shifts in humans. Eur J Neurosci. 2004;19:2720–6.
50. Antal A, Paulus W. Investigating neuroplastic changes in the human brain induced by transcranial direct (tDCS) and alternating current (tACS) stimulation methods. Clin EEG Neurosci. 2012;43: 175.
51. Boros K, Poreisz C, Münchau A, Paulus W, Nitsche MA. Premotor transcranial direct current stimulation (tDCS) affects primary motor excitability in humans. Eur J Neurosci. 2008;27:1292–300.
52. Nitsche M, Fricke K, Henschke U, Schlitterlau A, Liebetanz D, Lang N, et al. Pharmacological modulation of cortical excitability shifts induced by transcranial direct current stimulation in humans. J Physiol. 2003;553:293–301.
53. Nitsche M, Jaussi W, Liebetanz D, Lang N, Tergau F, Paulus W. Consolidation of human motor cortical neuroplasticity by D-cycloserine. Neuropsychopharmacology. 2004;29:1573–8.
54. Islam N, Aftabuddin M, Moriwaki A, Hattori Y, Hori Y. Increase in the calcium level following anodal polarization in the rat brain. Brain Res. 1995;684:206–8.
55. Stagg CJ, Best JG, Stephenson MC, O'Shea J, Wylezinska M, Kincses ZT, et al. Polarity-sensitive modulation of cortical neurotransmitters by transcranial stimulation. J Neurosci. 2009;29: 5202–6.

56. Reymann KG, Frey JU. The late maintenance of hippocampal LTP: requirements, phases, 'synaptic tagging', 'late-associativity' and implications. Neuropharmacology. 2007;52:24–40.
57. Nitsche MA, Müller-Dahlhaus F, Paulus W, Ziemann U. The pharmacology of neuroplasticity induced by non-invasive brain stimulation: building models for the clinical use of CNS active drugs. J Physiol. 2012;590:4641–62.
58. Nitsche M, Grundey J, Liebetanz D, Lang N, Tergau F, Paulus W. Catecholaminergic consolidation of motor cortical neuroplasticity in humans. Cereb Cortex. 2004;14:1240–5.
59. Nitsche M, Lampe C, Antal A, Liebetanz D, Lang N, Tergau F, et al. Dopaminergic modulation of long-lasting direct current-induced cortical excitability changes in the human motor cortex. Eur J Neurosci. 2006;23:1651–7.
60. Kuo M-F, Paulus W, Nitsche MA. Boosting focally-induced brain plasticity by dopamine. Cereb Cortex. 2008;18:648–51.
61. Monte-Silva K, Liebetanz D, Grundey J, Paulus W, Nitsche MA. Dosage-dependent non-linear effect of L-dopa on human motor cortex plasticity. J Physiol Lond. 2010;588:3415–24.
62. Monte-Silva K, Kuo M-F, Thirugnanasambandam N, Liebetanz D, Paulus W, Nitsche MA. Dose-dependent inverted U-shaped effect of dopamine (D2-like) receptor activation on focal and nonfocal plasticity in humans. J Neurosci. 2009;29:6124–31.
63. Nitsche MA, Kuo M-F, Grosch J, Bergner C, Monte-Silva K, Paulus W. D1-receptor impact on neuroplasticity in humans. J Neurosci. 2009;29:2648–53.
64. Nitsche MA, Kuo M-F, Karrasch R, Wächter B, Liebetanz D, Paulus W. Serotonin affects transcranial direct current-induced neuroplasticity in humans. Biol Psychiatry. 2009;66:503–8.
65. Kuo M-F, Grosch J, Fregni F, Paulus W, Nitsche MA. Focusing effect of acetylcholine on neuroplasticity in the human motor cortex. J Neurosci. 2007;27:14442–7.
66. Thirugnanasambandam N, Grundey J, Adam K, Drees A, Skwirba AC, Lang N, et al. Nicotinergic impact on focal and non-focal neuroplasticity induced by non-invasive brain stimulation in non-smoking humans. Neuropsychopharmacology. 2011;36:879–86.
67. Matsunaga K, Nitsche MA, Tsuji S, Rothwell JC. Effect of transcranial DC sensorimotor cortex stimulation on somatosensory evoked potentials in humans. Clin Neurophysiol. 2004;115:456–60.
68. Dieckhofer A, Waberski TD, Nitsche M, Paulus W, Buchner H, Gobbele R. Transcranial direct current stimulation applied over the somatosensory cortex: differential effect on low and high frequency SEPs. Clin Neurophysiol. 2006;117:2221–7.
69. Zaehle T, Beretta M, Jancke L, Herrmann CS, Sandmann P. Excitability changes induced in the human auditory cortex by transcranial direct current stimulation: direct electrophysiological evidence. Exp Brain Res. 2011;215:135–40.
70. Kirimoto H, Ogata K, Onishi H, Oyama M, Goto Y, Tobimatsu S. Transcranial direct current stimulation over the motor association cortex induces plastic changes in ipsilateral primary motor and somatosensory cortices. Clin Neurophysiol. 2011;122:777–83.
71. Feurra M, Bianco G, Polizzotto NR, Innocenti I, Rossi A, Rossi S. Cortico-cortical connectivity between right parietal and bilateral primary motor cortices during imagined and observed actions: a combined TMS/tDCS study. Front Neural Circuits. 2011;5:10.
72. Polania R, Paulus W, Antal A, Nitsche MA. Introducing graph theory to track for neuroplastic alterations in the resting human brain: a transcranial direct current stimulation study. Neuroimage. 2011;54:2287–96.
73. Stagg CJ, O'Shea J, Kincses ZT, Woolrich M, Matthews PM, Johansen-Berg H. Modulation of movement-associated cortical activation by transcranial direct current stimulation. Eur J Neurosci. 2009;30:1412–23.
74. Polania R, Nitsche MA, Paulus W. Modulating functional connectivity patterns and topological functional organization of the human brain with transcranial direct current stimulation. Hum Brain Mapp. 2011;32:1236–49.
75. Polania R, Paulus W, Nitsche MA. Modulating cortico-striatal and thalamo-cortical functional connectivity with transcranial direct current stimulation. Hum Brain Mapp. 2011;32(8):1236–49.
76. Polania R, Paulus W, Nitsche MA. Reorganizing the intrinsic functional architecture of the human primary motor cortex during rest with non-invasive cortical stimulation. PLoS ONE. 2012;7: e30971.
77. Keeser D, Meindl T, Bor J, Palm U, Pogarell O, Mulert C, et al. Prefrontal transcranial direct current stimulation changes connectivity of resting-state networks during fMRI. J Neurosci. 2011;31: 15284–93.
78. Pena-Gomez C, Sala-Lonch R, Junque C, Clemente IC, Vidal D, Bargallo N, et al. Modulation of large-scale brain networks by transcranial direct current stimulation evidenced by resting-state functional MRI. Brain Stimul. 2012;5:252–63.
79. Liebetanz D, Nitsche MA, Tergau F, Paulus W. Pharmacological approach to the mechanisms of transcranial DC-stimulation-induced after-effects of human motor cortex excitability. Brain. 2002;125:2238–47.
80. Kuo HI, Bikson M, Datta A, Minhas P, Paulus W, Kuo MF, et al. Comparing cortical plasticity induced by conventional and high-definition 4x1 ring tDCS: a neurophysiological study. Brain Stimul. 2012;6:644–8.

A Role of Computational Modeling in Customization of Transcranial Direct Current Stimulation for Susceptible Populations

10

Dennis Truong, Preet Minhas, Albert Mokrejs, and Marom Bikson

Introduction to Computational Models of Noninvasive Neuromodulation

Renewed interest in transcranial electrical stimulation has been accompanied by a general modernization of the technique including the use of computational models. This chapter introduces the rationale behind modeling transcranial direct current stimulation (tDCS) as well as the technical development and limitations of models currently in use. This chapter is intended to provide a broad introduction to both clinical researchers and engineers interested in translational work to develop and apply computational models of customized tDCS. Transcranial electrical stimulation is a promising tool in symptom management based on the growing evidence that delivery of current to specific brain regions can promote desirable plastic changes [1, 2]. However, stimulation should be applied using low intensity current in a manner that is safe and well tolerated. In complement to other brain stimulation approaches (Fig. 10.1), tDCS has been gaining considerable interest because it is well tolerated, and can be used as add-on therapy and has low maintenance costs [3].

In contrast to pharmacotherapy, noninvasive electrotherapy offers the potential for both anatomically specific brain activation and complete temporal control. Temporal control is achieved since electricity is delivered at the desired dose instantly and there is no electrical "residue" as the generated brain current disappears when stimulation is turned off. Spatial control is based on from rational selection of electrode number, shape, and position. As explained below, using computational models, tDCS can be customized and individualized to specific brain targets in ways not possible with other interventions in order to optimize a particular therapeutic or rehabilitative outcome. Specifically, the "dose" of electrotherapy (see Peterchev et al. [4] for definition) is readily adjustable by determining the location of electrodes (which determines spatial targeting) and selecting the stimulation waveform (which determines the nature and timing of neuromodulation). Indeed, a single programmable electrotherapy device can be simply configured to provide a diversity of dosages. Though this flexibly underpins the utility of neuromodulation, the myriad of potential dosages (stimulator settings and combinations of electrode placements) makes the optimal choice very difficult to readily ascertain. The essential issue in dose design is to relate each externally controlled dose with the associated brain regions targeted (and spared) by the resulting current flow—and hence the desired clinical outcome. Computational forward models aim to provide precisely these answers to the first part of this question (Fig. 10.2), and thus need to be leveraged in the rational design, interpretation, and optimization of neuromodulation.

The precise pattern of current flow through the brain is determined not only by the stimulation dose (e.g., the positions of the electrodes) but also by the underlying anatomy and tissue properties. In predicting brain current flow using computational models, it is thus important to precisely model both the stimulation itself and the relevant anatomy upon which it is delivered on an individual basis. The latter issue remains an area of ongoing technical development and is critical to establishing the clinical utility of these models. For example, cerebral spinal fluid (CSF) is highly conductive (a preferred "super highway" for current flow) such that details of CSF architecture profoundly shape current flow through adjacent brain regions (see later discussion).

D. Truong (✉) • P. Minhas
Department of Biomedical Engineering, The City College of New York, 160 Convent Avenue, ST-462, New York 10031, NY, USA
e-mail: dtruong01@ccny.cuny.edu

A. Mokrejs
Stuyvesant High School, Class 2016, 345 Chambers Street, New York, NY 10282, USA

M. Bikson
Neural Engineering Laboratory, Department of Biomedical Engineering, The City College of New York of CUNY, New York, NY, USA

H. Knotkova and D. Rasche (eds.), *Textbook of Neuromodulation*,
DOI 10.1007/978-1-4939-1408-1_10, © Springer Science+Business Media, LLC 2015

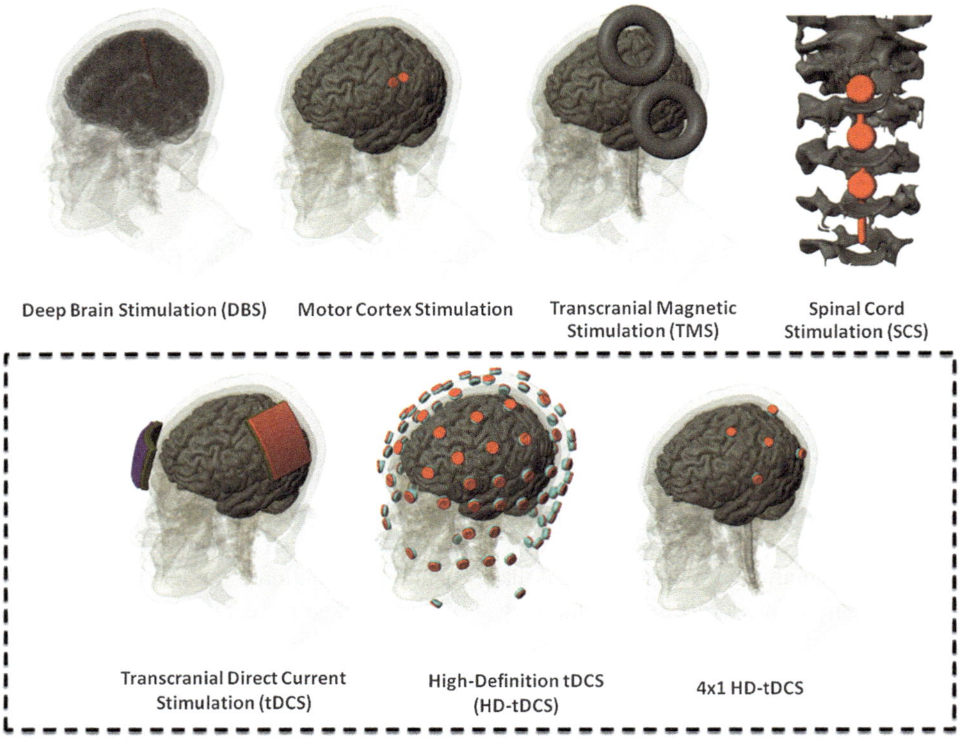

Fig. 10.1 Comparable stimulation techniques: Deep Brain Stimulation, Motor Cortex Stimulation, Transcranial Magnetic Stimulation, and Spinal Cord Stimulation (*top row*); classic transcranial Direct Current Stimulation (tDCS) via sponge pads, optimized High Definition-tDCS (HD-tDCS), and 4 × 1 HD-tDCS (*bottom row*). Transcranial Direct Current Stimulation is an increasingly popular investigational form of brain stimulation, in part, due to its low cost, portability, usability, and safety. However, there are still many of unanswered questions. The number of potential stimulation doses is practically limitless. Stimulation can be varied by simply changing the electric current waveform and electrode shape, size, and position. These variations can thus be analyzed through computational modeling studies that have resulted in montages such as HD-tDCS and 4 × 1 HD-tDCS

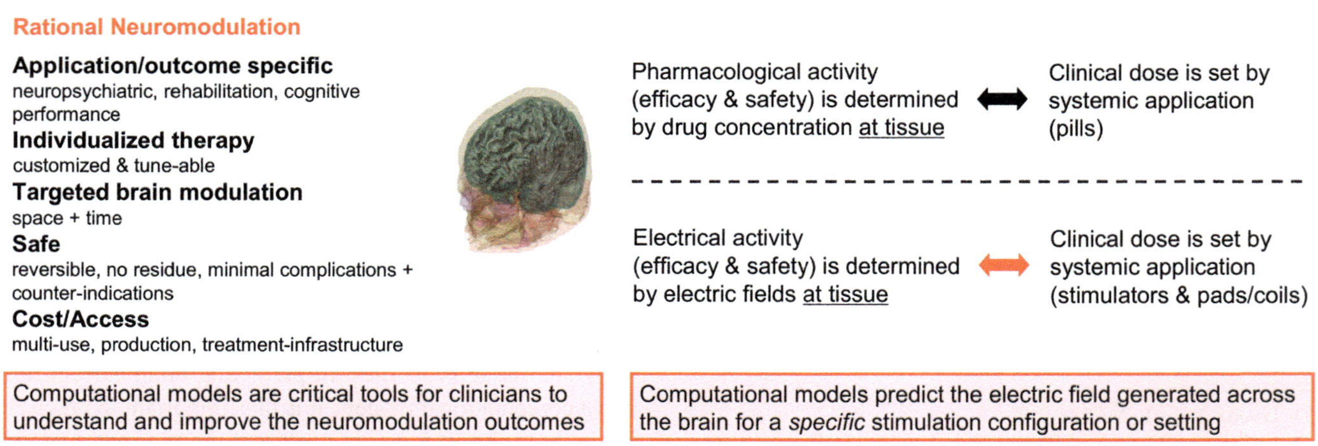

Fig. 10.2 Role of computational models in rational electrotherapy: (*left*) Neuromodulation is a promising therapeutic modality as it affects the brain in a way not possible with other techniques with a high degree of individualized optimization. The goal of computational models is to assist clinicians in leveraging the power and flexibility of neuromodulation (*right*). Computational forward models are used to predict brain current flow during transcranial stimulation to guide clinical practice. As with pharmacotherapy, electrotherapy dose is controlled by the operator and leads a complex pattern of internal current flow that is described by the model. In this way, clinicians can apply computational models to determine which dose will activate (or avoid) brain regions of interest

Especially relevant for rehabilitative applications is the recognition that individual anatomical idiosyncrasies can result in significant distortions in current flow. This is particularly apparent when skull defects and brain lesions occur. The final section of this review highlights the nature and degree of distortions in brain current flow produced by defects and lesions, as well as dose considerations for susceptible populations such as children.

Methods and Protocols in the Generation of Computational Forward Models of tDCS

During tDCS, current is generated in the brain. Because different electrode montages result in distinct brain current flow, researchers and clinicians can adjust the montage to target or avoid specific brain regions in an application specific manner. Though tDCS montage design often follows basic rules-of-thumb (e.g., increased/decreased excitability under the anode/cathode electrode), computational forward models of brain current flow provide more accurate insight into detailed current flow patterns and in some cases, can even challenge simplified electrode-placement assumptions [5–8]. For example, clinical studies are often designed by placing the anode electrode directly over the target region desired to be excited, while the cathode electrode is placed over a far removed region from the target to avoid unwanted reverse effects. This region could be the contralateral hemisphere or in some cases even extra cephalic locations like the neck, shoulder or the arm. Researchers have used smaller stimulation electrode sizes and bigger reference electrode sizes to offset the focality limitations of tDCS. With the increased recognized value of computational forward models in informing tDCS montage design and interpretation of results, there have been recent advances in modeling tools and a greater proliferation of publications [9–22].

Initial models of transcranial current flow assumed simplified geometries such as concentric spheres that could be solved analytically as well as numerically. Miranda et al. [15] was the first numerical modeling effort specifically looking at tDCS montages and intensities. In another spherical head paper, focality of cortical electrical fields was compared across various small electrode configurations and configurations proposed to achieve targeted modulation [10]. Wagner et al. [22] was the first computer-aided design (CAD) rendered head model where current density distributions were analyzed for various montages including healthy versus cortical stroke conditions. The more recent efforts have been mostly MRI derived. Oostendorp et al. [16] was the first to consider anisotropy in the skull and the white matter. Datta et al. [11] built the first high-resolution head model with gyri/sulci specificity. Using diffusion tensor imaging (DTI), Suh et al. [20] concluded that skull anisotropy causes a large shunting effect and may shift the stimulated areas. Fine resolution of gyri/sulci leads to current "hotspots" in the sulci, thereby reinforcing the need for high-resolution modeling [19]. Sadleir et al. [18] compared modeling predictions of frontal tDCS montages to clinical outcomes. Datta et al. [9] studied the effect of tDCS montages on TBI and skull defects. Parazzini et al. [17] was the first to analyze current flow patterns across subcortical structures. Dmochowski et al. [23] showed how a multi-electrode stimulation can be optimized for focality and intensity at the target.

Recent efforts have focused to build patient-specific models and compare modeling predictions to experimental outcomes. In considering new electrode montages, and especially in potentially vulnerable populations (e.g., in patients with skull damage or in children), forward models are the main tool used to relate the externally controllable dose parameters (e.g., electrode number, position, size, shape, current) with resulting brain current flow. While the specific software applications can vary across groups, in general, the approach and workflow for model generation follow a similar pattern (Fig. 10.3).

The steps for generating high-resolution (anatomically specific) forward models of noninvasive neuromodulation are adapted from extensive prior work on computational modeling. These involve: (1) Demarcation of individual tissue types (masks) from high-resolution anatomical data (e.g., magnetic resonance imaging slices obtained at 1 mm slice thickness) using a combination of automated and manual segmentation tools. Specifically, from the perspective of stimulating current flow, it is necessary to distinguish tissues by their resistivity. A majority of effort in the development and implementation of models has involved this step (see also next section) [18]. The number and precision of the individual masks obtained is pivotal for the generation of accurate 3D models in order to capture critical anatomical details that may influence current flow. (2) Modeling of the exact physical properties of the electrodes (e.g., shape and size) and precise placement within the segmented image data (i.e., along the skin mask outer surface). (3) Generation of accurate meshes (with a high-quality factor) from the tissue/electrode masks whilst preserving resolution of subject anatomical data. The generation of meshes is a process where each mask is divided into small contiguous "elements" which allow the current flow to then be numerically computed—hence the term "Finite Element Method" stimulations. (4) Resulting volumetric meshes are then imported into a commercial finite element (FE) solver. (5) At this step, resistivity is assigned to each mask (every element in each mask) and the boundary conditions are imposed including the current applied to the electrodes. (6) The standard Laplacian equation is solved using the appropriate numerical solver and tolerance settings. (7) Data is

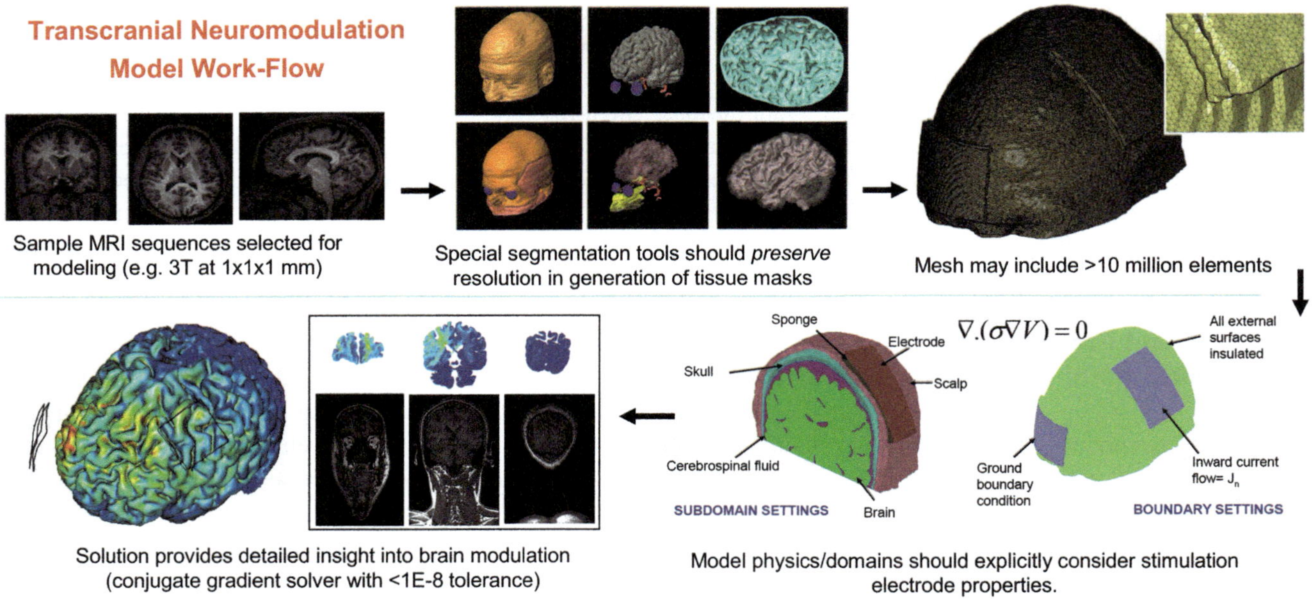

Fig. 10.3 Imaging and computational work-flow for the generation of high-resolution individualized models: Though the specific processes and software packages will vary across technical groups and applications, in each case high-resolution modeling initiated with precise anatomical scans that allow demarcation of key tissues. Tissues with distinct resistivity are used to form "masks." These masks along with the representation of the physical electrodes are "meshed" to allow FEM calculations. The boundary conditions (generally simply reflecting how the electrodes are energized) and the governing equations (related to Ohms law) are well established. The reproduction of the stimulation dose and the underlying anatomy thus allow for the prediction of resulting brain current. These current flow patterns are represented in false-color map and analyzed through various post-processing tools

plotted as induced cortical electric field or current density maps (Fig. 10.3).

Though each of the above steps is required for high-resolution modeling, there remains technical expertise and hence variation in protocols across groups and publications [22]. These variations are relevant to clinical practice only in the sense that they change predictions in current flow that meaningfully effect dose decisions. The sources and impact of these variations is addressed in the next section.

Only a few studies have attempted to more directly link clinical outcomes and model predictions—and thus validate model utility. Clinical evaluation was combined with model predictions to investigate the effects of different montages in clinical conditions such as fibromyalgia [13]. Patient-specific models have been used to retrospectively analyze the therapeutic success of a given experimental stimulation montage [7] and compare model predictions with patterns of activation revealed by functional magnetic resonance imaging (fMRI) [12]. Postmortem "current flow imaging" was also used to validate general model prediction [24]. A focalized form of tDCS called 4 × 1 high-definition tDCS was developed through computational models and then validated in a clinical neurophysiology trial [25]. These example applications open the door for potentially customizing tDCS on a subject to subject basis within the clinical setting [26]. Table 10.1 summarizes the various tDCS montages explored in computational modeling studies.

For clinicians interested in using computational forward models to inform study design or interpretation several options are available. (1) A collaboration with a modeling group [21] or a company can allow for customized exploration of montage options; (2) referencing existing published reports or databases (Table 10.1) for comparable montages (with careful consideration of the role of individual variation and other caveats presented in the next section); (3) using a novel process where a desired brain region can be selected and the optimized electrode montage is proposed within a single step has been developed [23]; (4) a graphical user interface (GUI)-based program to stimulate arbitrary electrode montages in a spherical model is now available (www.neuralengr.com/spheres). This last solution illustrates an important trend: even as increasingly complex and resource expensive modeling tools are developed, parallel efforts to simplify and automate (high-throughput) model workflow are needed to facilitate clinical translation. If tDCS continues to emerge as an effective tool in clinical treatment and cognitive neuroscience, and concurrent modeling studies emphasize the need for rational (and in cases individualized) dose decisions, then it will become incumbent for tDCS researchers to understand the applications (and limitations) of computational forward models [27].

Table 10.1 Synopsis of numerical tDCS computer models[a]

Study	Masks	Electrode montage	Additional methods
Concentric sphere			
Miranda et al. (2006) [15]	4	4 montages	
Datta et al. (2008) [10]	4	6 montages	
Dmochowski et al. (2012) [23] Neuralengr.com/ spheres	4	Arbitrary, user specific, optimized montages	
CAD rendered			
Wagner (2007) [22]	5	Healthy and stroke models with varied montages	
MRI derived			
Oostendorp et al. (2008) [16]	5	C3–SO montage	Anisotropic conductivities for skull and white matter. Model derived from Wolters et al. (2006) [49]
Datta et al. (2009b) [11]	4	C3–SO and HD	High-resolution with gyrisulci topography
Suh et al. (2009) [8]	5	C3–SO montage using point source stimulation electrodes	Anisotropic conductivity for white matter
Datta et al. (2009b) [10]	4	Tissue temperature increases of C3–SO montage and HD montage	
Sadleir [10, 18]	11	F3–SO and F4–SO montage and comparison to reported clinical outcomes in literature	
Datta et al. (2010) [9]	4	Effect of skull defects and skull plates for C3–SO and 01–SO montages	
Bikson et al. (2010) [5]	7	C3–SO and C3-contralateral montages	Effect of "return electrode" position and size
Salvador et al. (2010) [19]	5	C3–SO montage	High-resolution gyrisulci model
Parazzini et al. (2011) [17]	26 unique tissue types	Analysis of current flow through cortical, subcortical, and brain stem regions for C3–SO montage	Model derived from virtual family open source database
Mendonca et al. (2011) [13]	8	C3-extracephalic, SO-extracephalic and C3–SO montages	Correlation of clinical effects in a fibromyalgia study with model predictions
Halko et al. (2011) [12]	7	Oz–Cz montage	Patient-specific visual stroke model of a hemianopia patient undergoing tDCS. Correlation of high-resolution current flow model
Datta et al. (2011) [7]	8	Retrospective analysis comparing experimental outcome with model predictions. LFC-RS, LFC-contralateral mastoid, LFC-SO, RFC-LS	Patient-specific left hemisphere stroke model of a tDCS responder.
DaSilva et al. (2012) [6]	15	C3–SO montage analysis of current flow through subcortical structures	High-resolution individualized model
Turkeltaub et al. (2011) [21]	8	Analysis of left pTC and right pTC montage in dyslexia study	
Bonsai—model solution analyzer	6–8	Healthy and stroke model with varied montages	Online database of solved patient-specific head models. Overlaid views of 2D MRI scans and model solutions
Dmochowski et al. (2011) [23]	6	Healthy Head models with need-specific montages	Two distinct selections, focality based or intensity based
Wagner et al. (2011) [50]	3	Conventional tDCS montages	Inclusion of multicompartment/tissue layer anisotropy
Minhas et al. (2012) [48]	2	Conventional tDCS montages	Pediatric brain modeling

[a]This table summarizes tDCS forward head models using FEM techniques. Head models have progressed from being spherical based to being MRI derived. The most recent ones have employed patient-specific models. The second, third, and fourth columns list number of tissue types, the montage used, and particular model specifics, respectively

C3, C4, F3, F4, O1, Oz, Cz correspond to 10/20 EEG system

LFC left frontal cortex, *LS* left shoulder, *pTC* posterior temporal cortex, *RFC* right frontal cortex, *RS* right shoulder, *SO* contralateral supra-orbital

Pitfalls and Challenges in the Application and Interpretation of Computational Model Predictions

Computational models of tDCS range in complexity from concentric sphere models to high-resolution models based on individuals MRIs (as described above). The appropriate level of modeling detail depends on the clinical question being asked, as well as the available computational resources. Whereas simple geometries (e.g., spheres) may be solved analytically [28], realistic geometries employ numerical solvers, namely, Finite Element Methods (FEM). Regardless of complexity, all forward models share the goal of correctly predicting brain current flow during transcranial stimulation to guide clinical therapeutic delivery. Special effort has been recently directed towards increasing the precision of tDCS models. However, it is important to note that increased model complexity does not necessarily equate with greater accuracy or clinical value.

To meaningfully guide clinical utility, attempts to enhance model precision must rationally balance detail (i.e., complexity) and accuracy. (1) Beginning with high-resolution anatomical scans, the entire model workflow should preserve precision. Any human head model is limited by the precision and accuracy of tissue segmentation (i.e., "masks") and of the assigned conductivity values. One hallmark of precision is that the cortical surface used in the final FEM solver should capture realistic sulci and gyri anatomy. (2) Simultaneously, a priori knowledge of tissue anatomy and factors known to influence current flow should be applied to further refine segmentation. Particularly critical are discontinuities not present in nature that result from limited scan resolution; notably both unnatural perforations in planar tissues (e.g., ventricular architecture, discontinuities in CSF where brain contacts skull, misrepresented skull fissures,) and microstructures (e.g., incomplete or voxelized vessels) can produce significant deviations in predicted current flow. Moreover, because of the sensitivity of current flow to any conductivity boundary, increasingly detailed segmentation (e.g., globe of the eye and related structures, glands, and deeper midbrain structures) without reliable reported human conductivity values in literature (especially at static frequency) may also lead to errors. It is worth noting that the respective contribution of the automated/manual interventions also depends on: (a) sophistication of the particular database or automated algorithm employed since they are usually not optimized for forward transcranial modeling [7] and (b) the need for identification of anomalies in suspect populations like skull defects, lesions, shunts, etc. Thus, addition of complexity without proper parameterization can evidently decrease prediction accuracy. An improper balance between these factors can introduce distortions in predicted brain current flow.

Divergent modeling methods illustrate existing outstanding issues including: (1) detail in physically representing the stimulation electrodes and leads, including shape and material [8], and energy source boundary conditions; (2) differences between conductivity values derived from static resistivity measures and those extrapolated from 10 Hz data; (3) sufficient caudal head volume representation (such that the caudal boundary condition does not affect relevant model prediction), including potential use of synthetic volumes [7, 13]; (4) optimal imaging modalities/sequences to differentiate amongst tissue types; (5) appropriate incorporation of anisotropy (from DTI); (6) suitability of existing image segmentation algorithms (generally developed for other applications) [29]; (7) the degree and nature of manual correction; (8) the adequacy of the numerical solver (especially when making detailed predictions at tissue boundaries); (9) detail in segmenting true lesion borders [7] versus idealized defects; and (10) the need for parametric and interindividual analysis (see below). The optimization of the above issues remains open questions and inevitably reflects available resources (e.g., imaging, computational, anatomical expertise) and the specific clinical question addressed in each modeling effort. Even as computational and engineering groups continue developing more modeling sophistication, clinicians must be aware of the limitations in any modeling approach and the inevitability of technical methodology effecting the predictions made.

Having mentioned the importance of balancing increased complexity with clinical access to modeling, it is also important to emphasize a difference between the "value" of adding precision (complexity) as it is evaluated in engineering papers versus clinical translation. Increasingly detailed computational approaches have been proposed in recent years of varying anatomical and physiological details [16, 30, 17]. At the same time, computational models indicate subject specific variability in susceptibility to the same dose [26, 31, 32], indicating the value of individualized modeling, or at least modeling across a set of archetypes. Real clinical translational utility must therefore balance the value of increased sophistication with the cost associated with clinical scanning, computational time, and human resources/intervention (e.g., manual correction/pre and post-processing etc.). Thus the question is not if "different models will yield different predictions" (as must be posed in an engineering paper) but rather does increased complexity change model predictions in a way that is clinically meaningful—will complexity influence clinical decisions in study design. While this is a complex and application specific question, a first step toward systematizing value, across a myriad of groups and efforts, is to develop a metric of change versus a simpler approach, and then applying a threshold based on perceived clinical value and added cost versus the simpler approach.

A priori, it is assumed that added detail/complexity will enhance model precision and, if done rationally, model accuracy [33]. Though an engineering group can devote extended resources and time to a "case" modeling study, the myriad of potential electrode combinations (dose) and variation across normal head [26] and pathological heads, means that in clinical trial design the particular models will likely now be solved (e.g., 4×1 over FP3 in a female head). Moreover, while "different models will yield different" predictions; practical dose decision is based on clinical study specific criterion "a meaningful clinical difference." Thus, two clinical applications of modeling are considered (1) Deciding across montages—namely, which montage is expected to achieve the optimal clinical outcomes in a given subject or on average across subjects; (2) Deciding on dose variation across subjects—namely, if and how to vary dose based on subject specific anatomy. It is further necessary to consider if the clinician is concerned with optimizing (a) intensity at the target (maximum current at the target regardless of overall brain current flow) or/and (b) focality at the target (intensity at the target relative to other brain regions); consideration of intensity of focality may lead to fundamentally different "best" dose [23]. In the first application, the clinician will compare different montages for their intensity and/or targeting of a brain region. Therefore, additional complexity and detail is only clinical meaningful if it results in a different selection of optimal montage based on either intensity or focality criterion.

Assuming accurate and precise representation of all tissue compartments (anatomy, resistivity, anisotropy) relevant to brain current flow, it is broadly assumed that using modern numerical solvers that the resulting prediction is independent of the numerical technique used. Our own experience across various commercial solvers confirms this implicit assumption when meshes are of sufficient detail—precise description in methods (use of publically available programs) and representation of resulting mesh density and quality (in figures or methods) as well as tests using various solvers provides explicit control for errors generated by the computation itself.

Literature regarding forward modeling—or more broadly the dissemination of modeling analysis to the clinical hands—introduces still further issues in regards to (1) interpretability, reproducibility, and accuracy (tissue masks) and (2) graphical representation of regions of influence (degree of "activation"). As there is no standard protocol for tissue imaging or segmentation, diversity in the nature of resulting tissue masks will invariably influence predicted current flow. As such, it is valuable to illustrate each 3D tissue mask in publication methods and/or classified serial sections. In regards to representation of relative activation, studies employ either maps of current density (unit of A/m^2) or electric field (unit of V/m). Because the two are related linearly by local tissue resistivity, when plotting activation in a region with uniform resistivity (for example the cortical surface), the spatial profile is identical. When plotting activation across tissues (e.g., coronal section), current density may be advantageous to illustrate overall brain current flow. However, the electric field in the brain is directly related to neuronal activation (e.g., for varied resistivity, the electric field, but not current density, provides sufficient information to predict activation). Despite best efforts, figure preparation invariably restricts tissue mask perspectives and comprehensive display of volumetric current flow, which can be supplemented with online data publication (http://www.neuralengr.com/bonsai).

When interpreting simulation predictions, it is important to recognize that the intensity of current flow in any specific brain region does not translate in any simple (linear) manner to the degree of brain activation or modulation (even when considering current direction). Moreover, recent neurophysiological studies indicate changes in "excitability" may not be monotonic with stimulation [34]. For example increasing stimulation amplitude or duration can invert the direction of modulation, as can the level of neuronal background activity [35]. However, to a first approximation, it seems reasonable to predict that regions with more current flow are more likely to be "effected" by stimulation while regions with little or no current flow will be spared the direct effects of stimulation. As the first step to understand mechanism of action of tDCS, a relationship between model predicted regional current flow and changes in functional activation was recently demonstrated [12]. The "quasi-uniform" assumption considers that if the electric field (current density) is uniform on the scale of a region/neuron of interest, then "excitability" may be modulated with local electric field intensity [36] (see discussion in [10] and [37]). Though efforts to develop suitable biophysical detailed models considering myriad of neurons with distinct positions and morphologies or "continuum" approximations [38] of modulation are pending, the current state-of-the-art requires (implicit) application of the "quasi-uniform" assumption.

Much of the theoretical and technical foundations for modeling brain stimulation were established through modeling studies on peripheral nerve stimulation ("Functional Electrical Stimulation," FES) and then Spinal Cord Stimulation (SCS) and Deep Brain Stimulation (DBS) (reviewed in[39–41]). In light of the challenges to tDCS modeling cited above, we note that FES and DBS use electrodes implanted in the body such that relatively small volume of brain is needed to be modeled, and with none of the complication associated with precisely representing gross anatomy (e.g., skull, fat, or CSF). From the perspective of computational burden, the volume, number of masks, and mask complexity results in tDCS models with >5 million elements, compared to <200,000 elements for FES and DBS models. In addition, FES and DBS are suprathreshold allowing modeling studies to represent simply demarcated "regions of influence," inside which action potentials are triggered. tDCS affects large areas of superficial and deep brain structures (many types of cells and processes) and is subthreshold interacting with ongoing activity rather than driving action potentials, making it challenging to simply delineate "black-and-white" regions of influence.

Forward modeling studies and analysis are often published as "case reports" with predictions only on a single head [13, 17, 19, 21]. The suitability of single subject analysis reflects available (limited) resources and the clinical question being addressed. For a given electrode montage and stimulation dose, the sensitivity of global brain current to normal variation in anatomy (including across ages, gender) is unknown; however high-resolution modeling suggest gyri-specific dispersion of current flow, which could potentially account for individual variability. More generally, gross differences in tissue dimensions, notably skull thickness and CSF architecture, are expected to influence current flow. In some cases, modeling efforts specifically address the role of individual anatomical pathology, such as skull defects [9] or brain lesions [7]; it is precisely because these studies have shown the importance of specific defect/lesion details, that findings cannot be arbitrarily generalized. This in turn stresses the importance of individualized modeling as illustrated in the next section.

Though this section focused on the technical features of modeling, there is a broader concern in promoting effective collaboration between engineers and clinicians. For analogy, clinicians are generally aware of the challenges and pitfalls in post-processing and feature selection of fMRI data—and indeed, are thus intimately involved in data analysis rather than blindly relying on a technician. For computational "forward" models of neuromodulation, where results may inform study design and patient treatment, it is evidently as important to consider the uses and technical limitations of modeling approaches—and vigilance and skepticism on the part of clinicians will only enhance model rigor. Critically, for this reason, clinician/investigator experience and "judgment" supersedes all model predictions, even as these models form one important tool in dose design.

Example Results of Computational Analysis in Susceptible Populations

Case 1: Skull Defects

There is interest in the application of tDCS during rehabilitation of patients with brain lesions or skull defects (i.e., with or without skull plates); for example subjects with traumatic brain injury (TBI) or patients undergoing neurosurgery. As some of the neurological sequelae are presumably consequences of disrupted cortical activity following the traumatic event, the use of tDCS to deliver current to both damaged and compensatory regions in such circumstances can be a useful tool to reactivate and restore activity in essential neural networks associated with cognitive or motor processing. In addition, because of the reported antiseizure effects of tDCS [42], this technique might be useful for patients with refractory epilepsy who underwent surgery and have skull plates or decompressive craniectomy for trauma and cerebrovascular disease.

Despite rational incentives for investigation of tDCS in TBI or patients with other major neurological deficits and skull defects, one perceived limitation for the use of tDCS in these patients is the resulting modification of current flow by the skull defects and presence of surgical skull plates. Modeling studies can provide insight into how skull defects and skull plates would affect current flow through the brain and how to modify tDCS dose and/or electrode locations in such cases (Fig. 10.4). For example, a skull defect (craniotomy) that is filled with relatively highly conductive fluid or tissue represents a "shunt" pathway for current entering the brain but in a manner highly dependent on defect position relative to electrode montage. In such cases, the underlying cortex would then be exposed to a higher intensity of focused current flow. This in turn might be either beneficial in targeting the underlying brain region or hazardous if the increased current levels resulted in undesired neurophysiologic or pathological changes. Our modeling results confirm the notion that skull defects and skull plates can change the distribution of the current flow induced in cortical areas by tDCS. However, the details of current modulation depend entirely on the combination of electrode configuration and nature of the defect/plate, thus indicating the importance of individual analysis. Based on model predictions, application of tDCS without accounting for skull defects can lead to suboptimal and undesired brain current.

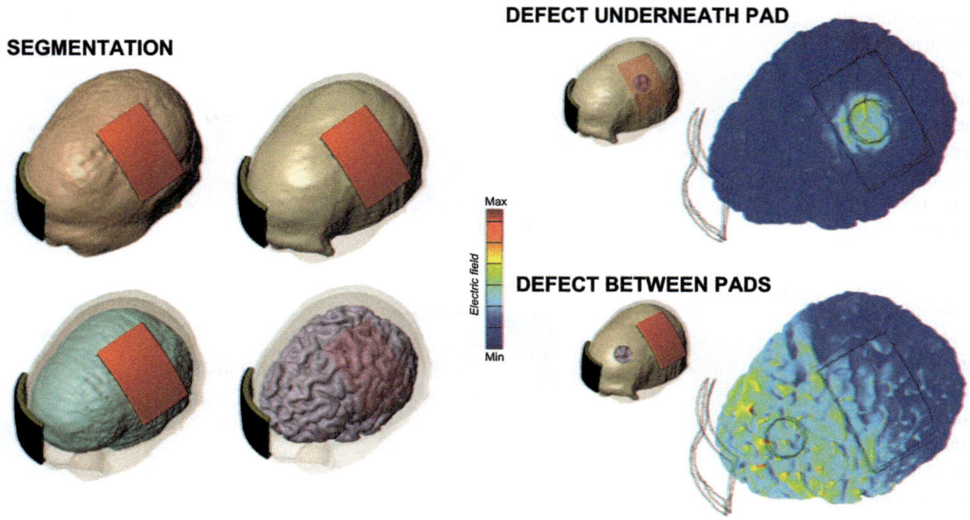

Fig. 10.4 Computational model of current flow in subjects with skull defects/plates. A defect in skull tissue which is the most resistive tissue in the head would hypothetically effect current flow in the underlying brain regions. Furthermore, the exact location of the defect (under/between the stimulation pads) in combination with the "material" filling up the defect with the stimulation montage employed will influence induced current flow. Sample segmentation masks are shown on the *left*. A small defect under the anode pad (*top right*) leads to current flow in the cortex restricted to directly under the defect (avoiding the intermediate regions). A similar sized defect placed between the pads (*bottom right*) does not significantly alter current flow patterns in comparison with a healthy head with no defect. (Adapted from Datta et al. [9])

Case 2: Brain Lesions (Stroke)

tDCS has been shown to modulate cognitive, linguistic, and motor performance in both healthy and neurologically impaired individuals with results supporting the feasibility of leveraging interactions between stimulation-induced neuromodulation and task execution [3]. As emphasized throughout this review, electrode montage (i.e., the position and size of electrodes) determines the resulting brain current flow and, as a result, neurophysiological effects. The ability to customize tDCS treatment through electrode montage provides clinical flexibility and the potential to individualize therapies. However, while numerous reports have been published in recent years demonstrating the effects of tDCS upon task performance, there remain fundamental questions about the optimal design of electrode configuration, especially around lesioned tissue [43]. Several modeling studies have predicted a profound influence of stroke related brain lesions on resulting brain current produced by tDCS [7, 12, 22].

Figure 10.5 illustrates an example of predicted current flow during tDCS from two subjects with a lesion due to stroke located with motor-frontal cortex (a) and occipital cortex (b) (adapted from [7] and [12]). Computational modeling suggests that current flow pattern during tDCS may be significantly altered by the presence of the lesion as compared to intact neurological tissue. Importantly, significant changes in the resulting cortical electric fields were observed not just around peri-lesional regions but also within wider cortical regions beyond the location of the electrodes. In a sense, the lesion itself acts as a "virtual" electrode modulating the overall current flow pattern [7].

Case 3: Pediatric Populations

There is increasing interest in the use of neuromodulation in pediatric populations for a range of indications including rehabilitation, cognitive performance, and epilepsy treatment [44–46]. However, a rational protocol/guideline for the use of tDCS on children has not been formally established. Previous modeling studies have shown that current flow behavior is dependent on *both* the tDCS dose (montage and current intensity) and the underlying brain anatomy. Because of anatomical differences (skull thickness, CSF volume, and gray/white matter volume) between a growing child and an adult it is expected that the resulting brain current intensity in a child would be different as compared to that in an adult. Evidently, it would not be prudent to adjust stimulation dose for children through an arbitrary rule of thumb (e.g., reduce electrode size and current intensity by the ratio of head diameter). Again, computational forward models provide direct insight into the relation between external tDCS dose and resulting brain current and thus can inform dose design in children. Figure 10.6 shows an example of a model of tDCS in a 12-year old compared to that of a standard adult model. Both the peak and spatial distribution of current in the

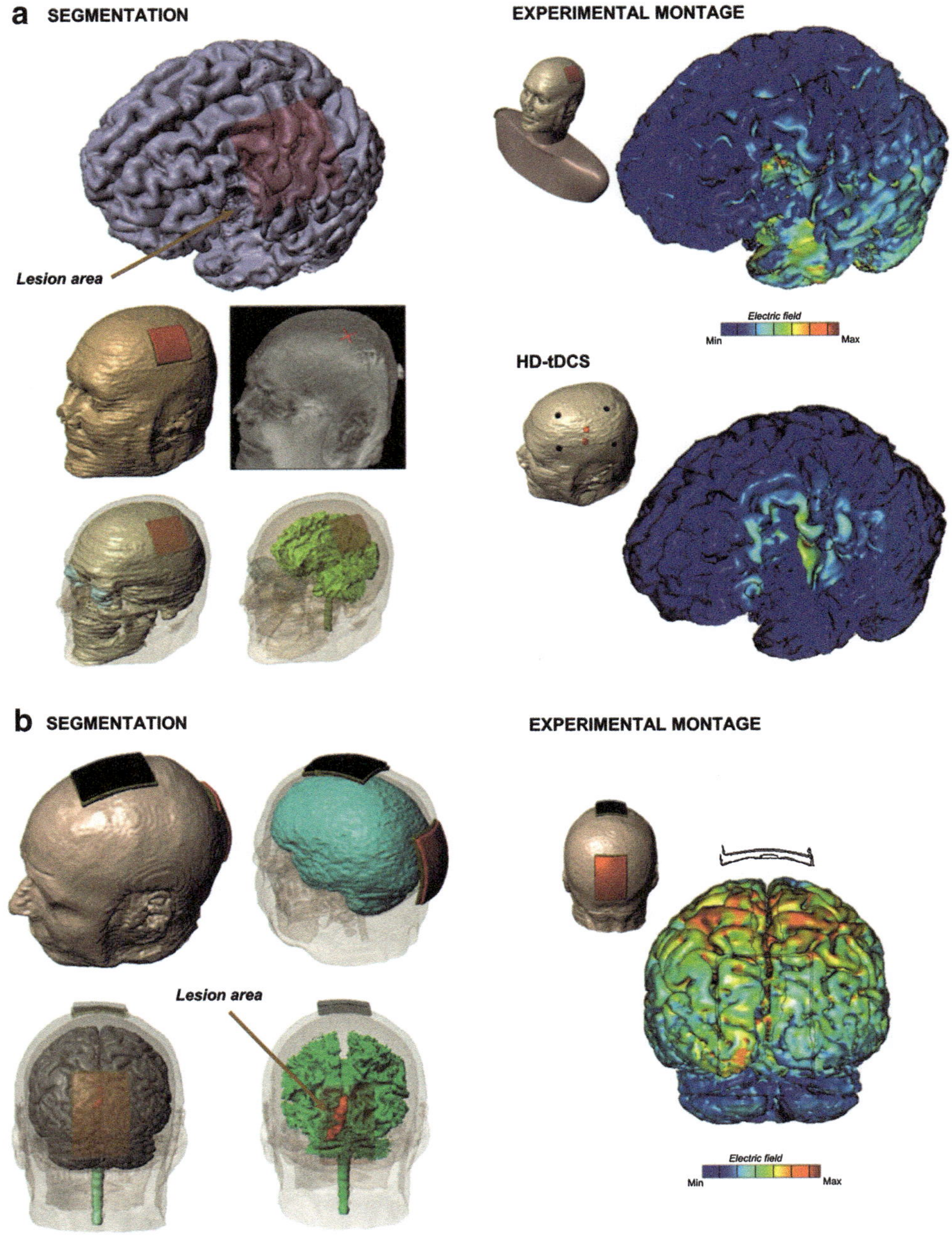

Fig. 10.5 Computational models predict current flow during tDCS in subjects with lesions. Brain lesions, as occur during stroke, are considered to be largely cannibalized and replaced by CSF, which is significantly more conductive than brain. For this reason, brain current flow during tDCS is expected to be altered. (**a**) Patient-specific left hemisphere stroke model. Two stimulation montages are illustrated, a conventional sponge montage (*top right*) and a high-definition montage (*bottom right*). (**b**) Patient-specific visual stroke model. Segmentation masks (*left*) and induced current flow using the experimental montage (*right*). (Adapted from Datta et al. [7] and Halko et al. [12])

brain is altered compared to the typical adult case. In fact, for this particular case, the peak electric fields, at a given intensity, were nearly double in the 12-year-old as compared to the adult. Though questions remain about the impact of gross anatomical differences in altering generated brain current flow during neuromodulation, computational "forward" models provide direct insight into this question, and may ultimately be used to rationally adjust stimulation dose.

Case 4: Obesity

The wide range of uses for tDCS makes it applicable to a diverse population that can include obese subjects. Montages that have been evaluated for pain, depression, or appetite suppression have been modeled in average adults, but unique challenges exist in the obese model (Fig. 10.7). The additional subcutaneous fat present in the obese model warranted an additional layer of complexity beyond the commonly used five tissue model (skin, skull, CSF, gray matter, white matter). Including fat in the model of a super-obese subject led to an increase in cortical electric field magnitude of approximately 60 % compared to the model without fat (Fig. 10.7, a.1–a.3). A shift was also seen in the spatial distribution of the cortical electric field, most noticeable on the orbitofrontal cortex.

To gain an intuition for how subcutaneous fat influences cortical electric field and current density, additional models

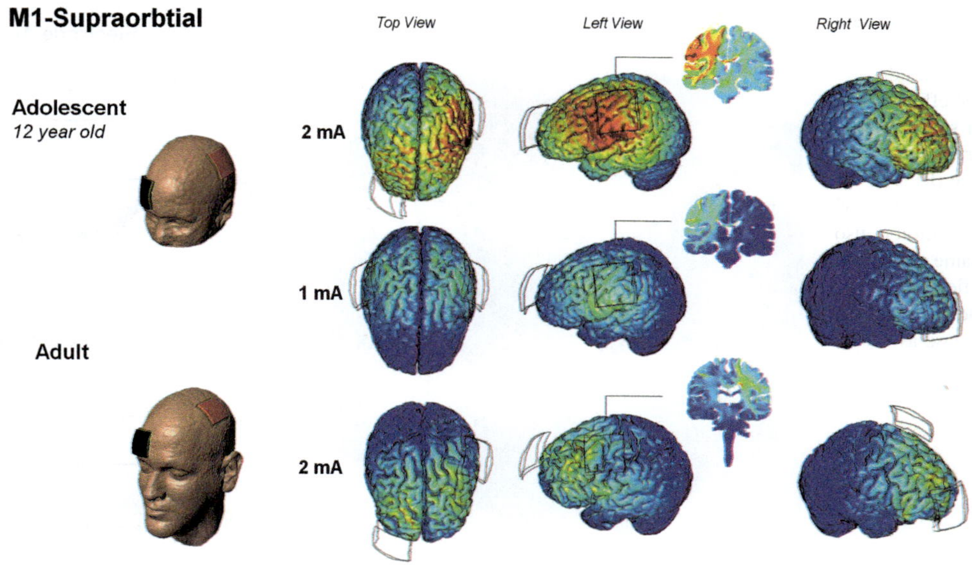

Fig. 10.6 Individualized head model of a two adolescents as compared to an adult: Induced current flow for motor cortex tDCS at different intensities 1 mA of stimulation in the adolescent is comparable to 2 mA of stimulation in an adult

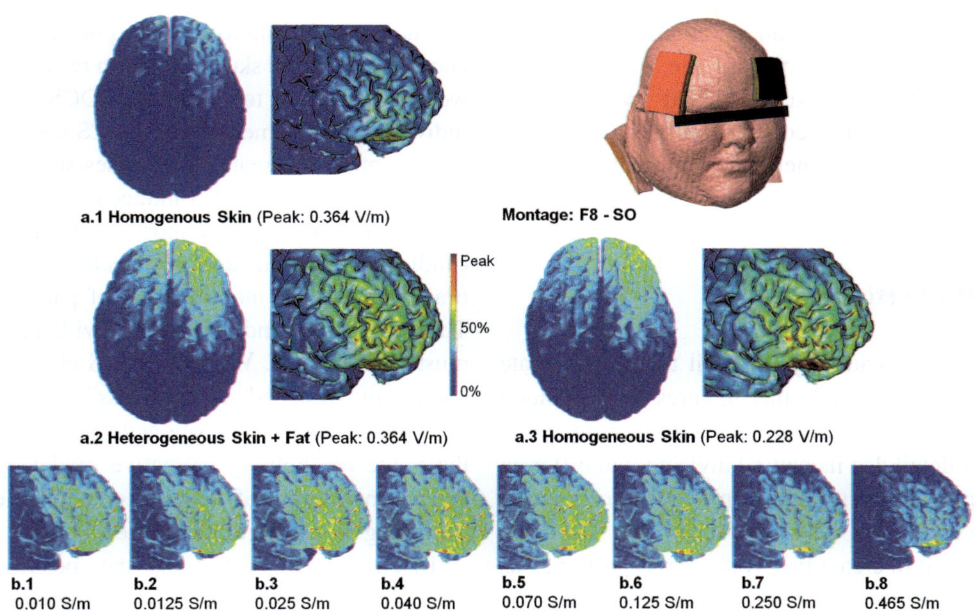

Fig. 10.7 Predicted cortical electric field during inferior prefrontal cortex stimulation via 5″ × 7″ pads. Two conditions, homogenous skin (**a**.1) and heterogeneous skin (**a**.2), are contrasted on the same scale (0.364 V/m/mA peak). The homogeneous skin condition is displayed (**a**.3) at a lowered scale (0.228 V/m/mA peak) to compare the spatial distribution to the heterogeneous condition (**a**.2). The effect due to a range of varying fat conductivities (**b**.1–8) is compared on a fixed scale (0.364 V/m/mA peak). The conductivity of fat (0.025 S/m) is within an "optimum" range of influence that causes an increase in peak cortical electric field when included (Adapted from [47])

examined a range of conductivity values from the conductivity of skull (0.010 S/m, Fig. 10.7 b.1) to the conductivity of skin (0.465 S/m, Fig. 10.7 b.8). Coincidentally, the conductivity commonly used for fat (0.025 S/m, Fig. 10.7 b.4) was in the range that causes a peak increase in cortical electric field magnitude. It was postulated that more current was blocked by subcutaneous fat at an extremely low conductivity (b.1), while more current was redirected at an extremely high conductivity. This, in effect, led to an "optimum" range of influence where the conductivity of fat is believed to reside.

Ultimately, the need to precisely parameterize models rests hand-in-hand with the intended use of the model. From an engineering perspective, the increased complexity

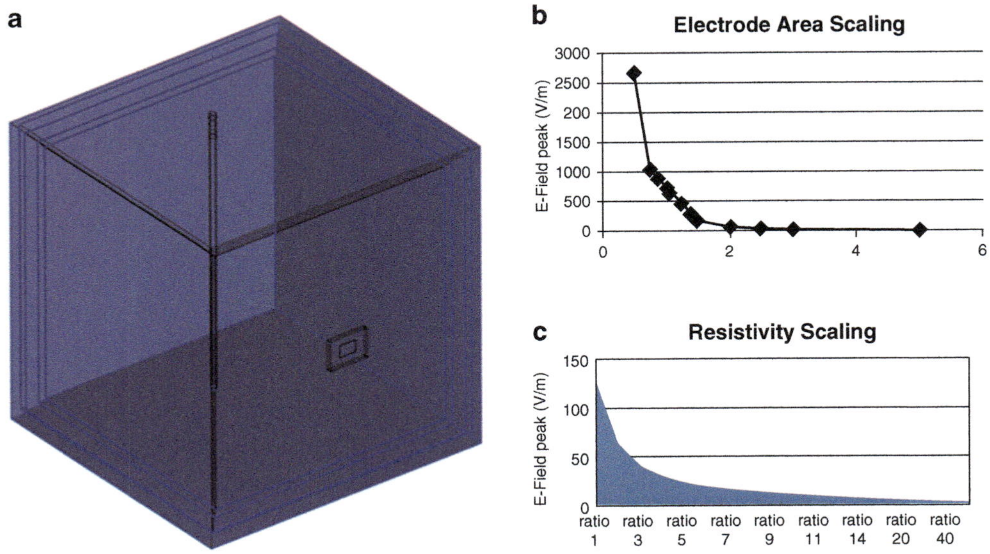

Fig. 10.8 Predicted electric field peak from a model relative to the factor of scaling to electrode sponge size (**a**). The effect is mapped on a linear scale, which shows a visible curve of exponential decrease (**b**). The effect of scaling the resistance of skin layers at a fixed ration is also graphed from the same model and relative to electric field peak. The curve formed by the data points is of exponential decrease as well (**c**)

of this model caused a noteworthy change within the subject modeled, but this change would not be clinically noteworthy if stimulation dose does not change from subject to subject. This clinical analysis requires an additional comparison between subjects and consideration of the wide variation already inherent in "typical" subjects [26]. What can be concluded, however, is that a comparison between models would require consistent parameterization of subcutaneous fat.

Case 5: Skin Properties

Computational models can vary in detail to accommodate various amounts of layers and other features such as blood vessels or sweat pores. Skin in particular can be rendered in varying levels of detail due its natural division into different layers, although even personalized models often simply make it a single layer.

In the model used to create Fig. 10.8, skin is portrayed as two layers one constituting the dermis and the other the epidermis and there are five layers in total. The model was solved for Electric-Field Peak for two separate characteristics, the ratio between tissue resistivity (The ratios between the various tissues being kept fixed, but scaled to see how the scale affected Electric Field), and for the scale of the area of the electrode sponges (The electrodes keeping their dimensional ratios but having their surface area scaled to determine the relationship between surface area and Electric field). Both models showed visible trends which are displayed in the graphs of Fig. 10.8 respectively.

While MRI-derived models are the standard for subject specific modeling, generalized models can be used to deduce trends applicable across populations. This is especially beneficial in cases where personalized cranial models are not necessary or not available. These simplified models allow for the observation and prediction of data in more complex personalized models.

These cases demonstrate the potentially profound influence of lesions and skull defects on resulting current flow, as well as the need to customize tDCS montages to gross individual head dimensions. If tDCS continues to become a viable option for treatment in cases such as chronic stroke, the consideration of tDCS-induced current flow through the brain is of fundamental importance for the identification of candidates, optimization of electrotherapies for specific brain targets, and interpretation of patient-specific results. Thus, the ability and value of individualized tDCS therapy must be leveraged. Whereas, tDCS electrode montages are commonly designed using "gross" intuitive general rules (*eg*, anode electrode positioned "over" the target region), the value of applying predictive modeling as one tool in the rational design of safe and effective electrotherapies is becoming increasingly recognized.

Electrode montage (i.e., the position and size of electrodes) determines the resulting brain current flow and, as a result, neurophysiological effects. The ability to customize tDCS treatment through electrode montage provides clinical flexibility and the potential to individualize therapies [5, 7, 13]. However, while numerous reports have been published in recent years demonstrating the effects of tDCS upon task performance, there remain fundamental questions about the optimal design of electrode configurations with computational "forward" models playing a pivotal role.

Conclusion

While numerous published reports have demonstrated the beneficial effects of tDCS upon task performance, fundamental questions remain regarding the optimal electrode configuration on the scalp. Moreover, it is expected that individual anatomical differences in the extreme case manifest as skull defects and lesioned brain tissue which consequently will influence current flow and should therefore be considered (and perhaps leveraged) in the optimization of neuromodulation therapies. Heterogeneity in clinical responses may result from many sources, but the role of altered bran current flow due to both normal and pathological is tractable using computational "forward" models, which can then be leveraged to individualize therapy. Increasing emphasis on high-resolution (subject specific) modeling, provides motivation for individual analysis leading to optimized and customized therapy.

References

1. Ardolino G, Bossi B, Barbieri S, Priori A. Non-synaptic mechanisms underlie the after-effects of cathodal transcutaneous direct current stimultion of the human brain. J Physiol. 2005;568:653–63.
2. Zentner J. Noninvasive motor evoked potential monitoring during neurosurgical operations on the spinal cord. Neurosurgery. 1989;24:709–12.
3. Brunoni AR, Nitsche MA, Bolognini N, Bikson M, Wagner T, Merabet L, Edwards DJ, et al. Clinical research with transcranial direct current stimulation (tDCS): challenges and future directions. Brain Stimul. 2012;5(3):175–95.
4. Peterchev A, Wagner T, Miranda P, Nitsche M, Paulus W, Lisanby S, et al. Fundamentals of transcranial electric and magnetic stimulation dose: definition, selection, and reporting practices. Brain Stimul. 2012;5:435–53.
5. Bikson M, Datta A, Rahman A, Scaturro J. Electrode montages for tDCS and weak transcranial electrical stimulation: role of "return" electrode's position and size. Clin Neurophysiol. 2010;121:1976–8.
6. DaSilva AF, Mendonca ME, Zaghi S, Lopes M, Dossantos MF, Spierings EL, et al. tDCS-induced analgesia and electrical fields in pain-related neural networks in chronic migraine. Headache. 2012;52:1283–95.
7. Datta A, Baker J, Bikson M, Fridriksson J. Individualized model predicts brain current flow during transcranial direct-current stimulation treatment in responsive stroke patient. Brain Stimul. 2011;4:169–74.
8. Datta A, Bansal V, Diaz J, Patel J, Reato D, Bikson M. Gyri-precise head model of transcranial direct current stimulation: improved spatial focality using a ring electrode versus conventional rectangular pad. Brain Stimul. 2009;2:201–7.
9. Datta A, Bikson M, Fregni F. Transcranial direct current stimulation in patients with skull defects and skull plates: high-resolution computational FEM study of factors altering cortical current flow. Neuroimage. 2010;52:1268–78.
10. Datta A, Elwassif M, Battaglia F, Bikson M. Transcranial current stimulation focality using disc and ring electrode configurations: FEM analysis. J Neural Eng. 2008;5:163–74.
11. Datta A, Elwassif M, Bikson M. Bio-heat transfer model of transcranial DC stimulation: comparison of conventional pad versus ring electrode. Conf Proc IEEE Eng Med Biol Soc. 2009;2009:670–3.
12. Halko MA, Datta A, Plow EB, Scaturro J, Bikson M, Merabet LB. Neuroplastic changes following rehabilitative training correlate with regional electrical field induced with tDCS. Neuroimage. 2011;57:885–91.
13. Mendonca ME, Santana MB, Baptista AF, Datta A, Bikson M, Fregni F, et al. Transcranial DC stimulation in fibromyalgia: optimized cortical target supported by high-resolution computational models. J Pain. 2011;12:610–7.
14. Miranda PC, Faria P, Hallett M. What does the ratio of injected current to electrode area tell us about current density in the brain during tDCS? Clin Neurophysiol. 2009;120:1183–7.
15. Miranda PC, Lomarev M, Hallett M. Modeling the current distribution during transcranial direct current stimulation. Clin Neurophysiol. 2006;117:1623–9.
16. Oostendorp TF, Hengeveld YA, Wolters CH, Stinstra J, van Elswijk G, Stegeman DF. Modeling transcranial DC stimulation. Conf Proc IEEE Eng Med Biol Soc. 2008;2008:4226–9.
17. Parazzini M, Fiocchi S, Rossi E, Paglialonga A, Ravazzani P. Transcranial direct current stimulation: estimation of the electric field and of the current density in an anatomical head model. IEEE Trans Biomed Eng. 2011;58:1773–80.
18. Sadleir RJ, Vannorsdall TD, Schretlen DJ, Gordon B. Transcranial direct current stimulation (tDCS) in a realistic head model. Neuroimage. 2010;51:1310–8.
19. Salvador R, Mekonnen A, Ruffini G, Miranda PC. Modeling the electric field induced in a high resolution head model during transcranial current stimulation. Conf Proc IEEE Eng Med Biol Soc. 2010;2010:2073–6.
20. Suh HS, Kim SH, Lee WH, Kim TS. Realistic simulation of transcranial direct current stimulation via 3-d high resolution finite element analysis: effect of tissue anisotropy. Conf Proc IEEE Eng Med Biol Soc. 2009;2009:638–41.
21. Turkeltaub PE, Benson J, Hamilton RH, Datta A, Bikson M, Coslett HB. Left lateralizing transcranial direct current stimulation improves reading efficiency. Brain Stimul. 2012;5:201–7.
22. Wagner T, Fregni F, Fecteau S, Grodzinsky A, Zahn M, Pascual-Leone A. Transcranial direct current stimulation:a computer-based human model study. Neuroimage. 2007;35:1113–24.
23. Dmochowski JP, Datta A, Bikson M, Su Y, Parra LC. Optimized multi-electrode stimulation increases focality and intensity at target. J Neural Eng. 2011;8:046011.
24. Antal A, Bikson M, Datta A, Lafon B, Dechent P, Parra LC, et al. Imaging artifacts induced by electrical stimulation during conventional fMRI of the brain. NeuroImage. 2014;85:1040–7.
25. Kuo HI, Bikson M, Datta A, Minhas P, Paulus W, Kuo MF, et al. Comparing cortical plasticity induced by conventional and high-definition 4 x 1 ring tDCS: A neurophysiological study. Brain Stimul. 2013;6:644–8.
26. Datta A, Truong D, Minhas P, Parra LC, Bikson M. Inter-individual variation during transcranial direct current stimulation and normalization of dose using MRI-derived computational models. Front Psychiatry. 2012;3:91.
27. Borckardt JJ, Bikson M, Frohman H, Reeves ST, Datta A, Bansal V, et al. A pilot study of the tolerability, safety and effects of high-definition transcranial direct current stimulation (HD-tDCS) on pain perception. J Pain. 2012;13:112–20.
28. Rush S, Driscoll DA. Current distribution in the brain from surface electrodes. Anesth Analg. 1968;47:717–23.
29. Smith SM. Fast robust automated brain extraction. Hum Brain Mapp. 2002;17(3):143–55.
30. Parazzini M, Fiocchi S, Ravazzani P. Electric field and current density distribution in an anatomical head model during transcranial direct current stimulation for tinnitus treatment. Bioelectromagnetics. 2012;33:476–87.
31. Shahid S, Wen P, Ahfock T. Numerical investigation of white matter anisotropic conductivity in defining current distribution under tDCS. Comput Methods Programs Biomed. 2013;109 (1):48–64.

32. Bikson M, Datta A. Guidelines for precise and accurate computational models of tDCS. Brain Stimul. 2012;5(3):430–1. doi:10.1016/j.brs.2011.06.001.
33. Bikson M, Rahman A, Datta A. Computational models of transcranial direct current stimulation. Clin EEG Neurosci. 2012;43(3):176–83.
34. Lindenberg R, Zhu LL, Schlaug G. Combined central and peripheral stimulation to facilitate motor recovery after stroke: the effect of number of sessions on outcome. Neurorehabil Neural Repair. 2012;26(5):479–83.
35. Nitsche MA, Paulus W. Sustained excitability elevations induced by transcranial DC motor cortex stimulation in humans. Neurology. 2001;57:1899–901.
36. Bikson M, Inoue M, Akiyama H, Deans JK, Fox JE, Miyakawa H, et al. Effects of uniform extracellular DC electric fields on excitability in rat hippocampal slices in vitro. J Physiol. 2004;557:175–90.
37. Miranda PC, Correia L, Salvador R, Basser PJ. The role of tissue heterogeneity in neural stimulation by applied electric fields. Conf Proc IEEE Eng Med Biol Soc. 2007;2007:1715–8.
38. Joucla S, Yvert B. The "mirror" estimate: an intuitive predictor of membrane polarization during extracellular stimulation. Biophys J. 2009;96(9):3495–508.
39. McIntyre CC, Miocinovic S, Butson CR. Computational analysis of deep brain stimulation. Expert Rev Med Devices. 2007;4:615–22.
40. Holsheimer J. Computer modelling of spinal cord stimulation and its contribution to therapeutic efficacy. Spinal Cord. 1998;36:531–40.
41. Rattay F. Analysis of models for external stimulation of axons. IEEE Trans Biomed Eng. 1986;33:974–7.
42. Fregni F, Thome-Souza S, Nitsche MA, Freedman SD, Valente KD, Pascual-Leone A. A controlled clinical trial of cathodal DC polarization in patients with refractory epilepsy. Epilepsia. 2006;47:335–42.
43. Fridriksson J. Measuring and inducing brain plasticity in chronic aphasia. J Commun Disord. 2011;44(5):557–63.
44. Mattai A, Miller R, Weisinger B, Greenstein D, Bakalar J, Tossell J, et al. Tolerability of transcranial direct current stimulation in childhood-onset schizophrenia. Brain Stimul. 2011;4:275–80.
45. Schneider HD, Hopp JP. The use of the Bilingual Aphasia Test for assessment and transcranial direct current stimulation to modulate language acquisition in minimally verbal children with autism. Clin Linguist Phon. 2011;25(6–7):640–54.
46. Varga ET, Terney D, Atkins MD, Nikanorova M, Jeppesen DS, Uldall P, et al. Transcranial direct current stimulation in refractory continuous spikes and waves during slow sleep: a controlled study. Epilepsy Res. 2011;97:142–5.
47. Truong DQ, Magerowski G, Pascual-Leone A, Alonso-Alonso M, Bikson M. Finite element study of skin and fat delineation in an obese subject for transcranial direct current stimulation. Conf Proc IEEE Eng Med Biol Soc. 2012;2012:6587–90.
48. Minhas P, Bikson M, Woods AJ, Rosen AR, Kessler SK. Transcranial direct current stimulation in pediatric brain: a computational modeling study. Conf Proc IEEE Eng Med Biol Soc. 2012;2012:859–62.
49. Wolters CH, Anwander A, Tricoche X, Weinstein D, Koch MA, MacLeod RS. Influence of tissue conductivity anisotropy on EEG/MEG field and return current computation in a realistic head model: a simulation and visualization study using high-resolution finite element modeling. Neuroimage. 2006;30(3):813–26.
50. Wagner TA, Eden UT. Systems and methods for stimulating and monitoring biological tissue. U.S. Patent Application 13/162,047, filed June 16, 2011.

Cranial Electrical Stimulation

11

Janet Mindes, Marc J. Dubin, and Margaret Altemus

Introduction

Cranial electrical stimulation (CES) is a noninvasive brain stimulation technology that uses a low intensity (0.1–16 mAmp) alternating current (AC) applied to the head through one or more electrodes. Preset, often patented stimulus frequency patterns vary across different CES devices. Treatment typically is given once or twice per day for 20–60 min, although some newer versions of CES devices designed to stimulate cranial nerves stimulate overnight for 8 h per day. CES frequencies range from 0.5 to 15,000 Hz, often with bursts of high-frequency stimulation separated by low frequency stimulation to produce recurring high-frequency pulse bursts. The higher frequencies are better able to overcome the high impedance of the skull. Some commercial devices offer several intensity settings for individual titration for efficacy and comfort, and for different clinical applications. Many CES devices use two electrodes on opposite sides of the head (e.g., at the temples, on the mastoid processes, on the earlobes using ear clips), and some include a third or fourth electrode as well (e.g., on the forehead). Newer devices designed to stimulate cranial nerves may use one or two electrodes, supraorbitally (centrally on the forehead above the eye sockets). Other devices used clinically or in research may use one electrode over a target area of cortex and a reference electrode on the top of the head (vertex) or on the neck, arm or another location.

Stimulation parameters vary greatly among CES instruments and experimental paradigms. Commercial devices often use special patented patterns of stimulation that combine a range of low to high frequencies, which the original inventors believed produced therapeutically potent stimulation. The alternating current can be sinusoidal or square waves. Alternating current stimulation used in laboratory experiments to probe brain function usually involves a single frequency sinusoidal alternating current applied to the head/scalp, or earlobes and usually is known as transcranial alternating current stimulation (tACS).

Use of diverse forms of low intensity electrical stimulation of the brain—both alternating and direct (galvanic) current—goes back to antiquity [1, 2]. Roman physicians Galen and Scribonius Largus prescribed application of Mediterranean electric fishes to the human head to alleviate melancholia, and to the feet for gout and headaches. More recently in the eighteenth and nineteenth centuries, Volta, Aldini, and others studied medical and physiological effects of direct current (DC). Aldini reported the successful galvanic treatment of patients with melancholia in 1804 [2]. In the twentieth century, various low intensity AC and DC current devices applied to the head have been investigated periodically. Electroconvulsive Therapy (ECT), a high intensity, high frequency AC therapy, introduced in the 1930s by Bini and Cerletti, had been the dominant psychiatric and neurological device until the development of Transcranial Magnetic Stimulation (TMS), Deep Brain Stimulation (DBS) Magnetic Seizure Therapy (MST), and Vagus Nerve Stimulation (VNS), along with revived interest in transcranial Direct Current Stimulation (tDCS), and in diverse forms of Cranial Electrical Stimulation (CES) in recent decades [2].

CES has been studied and used clinically for over 60 years in North America, Europe, Russia and the former Soviet Union, to treat insomnia, anxiety, depression, drug withdrawal, headache, other types of pain, and hypertension. Early Russian interest sprang from the work of Ivan Pavlov, who observed that his dogs frequently fell asleep during experiments using a similar electrical conditioning stimulus,

J. Mindes (✉)
Department of Psychiatry, Center for Bioethics, College of Physicians and Surgeons, Columbia University, 3rd Floor, Suite 3-470, 630 West 168th Street, New York, NY 10032, USA
e-mail: jm653@columbia.edu

M.J. Dubin • M. Altemus
Department of Psychiatry, Weill Medical College, Cornell University, New York, NY, USA

H. Knotkova and D. Rasche (eds.), *Textbook of Neuromodulation*,
DOI 10.1007/978-1-4939-1408-1_11, © Springer Science+Business Media, LLC 2015

hence the earlier term, electrosleep. This was hypothesized to happen because of spreading inhibition over the cortex, from a specific locus to generalized inhibition [3, 4]. Electrical stimulation to treat insomnia in humans was first reported by Robinovitch in 1914, [5]; he used rectangular pulses of 6–8 kHz, of approximately 4.0 mA (35 V) between forehead (−) and hand (+) electrodes.

Interest in electrosleep and other applications of CES in Russia has remained high throughout the twentieth century and continues to the present ([6–10] and many others). However, potentially useful information from a large body of work conducted in the former Soviet Union over many decades mostly has not been translated and therefore is little known in the West. The methodology of many Soviet era studies appears to predate modern clinical research standards. Klawansky et al. [11] considered some of this literature for their meta-analysis, and found that most of the published studies were uncontrolled and were therefore excluded from the meta-analysis. Some more recent Russian studies occasionally have been published in English (e.g., [8, 10, 12]).

From the early twentieth century to the present, many names have been used for low intensity alternating current devices applied to the head, including: cranial electrical stimulation (CES) [13], cranial electrotherapy stimulation (CES); transcranial alternating current stimulation (tACS) [14]; transcranial pulsed current stimulation (tPCS) [15]; transcutaneous cranial electrical stimulation (TCES), [16–18]; transcranial electrostimulation or transcranial electrical stimulation (TES) [8, 9]; cranial or cerebral electrotherapy (CET) [19, 20]; transcerebral electrotherapy (TCET); transcranial electric treatment (TET) [21]; neuroelectric therapy (NET); cranial transcutaneous electrical nerve stimulation (TENS); and descriptives such as electrosleep; brief high intensity pulsed stimulation [17, 22]; and auricular electrical stimulation [20].

In recent years, it has become customary to call this class of devices either CES (for example during the 2012 FDA hearings on possible re-classification of three of these devices; see below), or transcutaneous stimulation for devices intended to stimulate cranial nerves rather than directly stimulate the brain. However, based on stimulation parameters of transcutaneous devices, it is likely that these two categories of devices act through similar mechanisms. At this point, the relative importance of cranial nerve afferent stimulation vs. direct effects of current on brain tissue is unknown.

Compared to the other classes of brain stimulating devices, both FDA-approved for neuropsychiatric indications (Deep Brain Stimulation, Electroconvulsive Therapy, Vagus Nerve Stimulation, Transcranial Magnetic Stimulation) and still in development (Magnetic Seizure Therapy, transcranial Direct Current Stimulation), among commercial CES devices there is less standardization and less transparency regarding stimulation parameters. Among CES devices there is more variability in stimulus intensity (Amperage or Voltage), stimulus frequency (Hz), pattern and duration of stimulus delivery, size, number, and type of electrodes, and cranial placement of electrodes. CES stimulation is delivered at 16 mA or below, because intolerable scalp discomfort and pain are experienced at the electrode site as the intensity rises close to 16 mA. These doses are far below the seizure threshold.

Concerning the potential significance of the pattern of electrical stimulation, Datta et al. [15, 23] draw a distinction between clinical devices that use pulsed, varying frequencies of stimulation, as opposed to very low, constant frequency stimulation used in experimental laboratory studies to probe brain function, which is often called transcranial alternating current stimulation (tACS). They therefore advocate that CES be referred to instead as tPCS (transcranial pulsed current stimulation), a term Alon et al. also employ [24, 25] and the term tACS be used for stable frequencies used in experimental studies. To date, there has been little head-to-head comparison among stimulation parameters to determine differential biophysical or therapeutic effects [13–15, 23, 26, 27]. If differential therapeutic benefits related to the various parameters and methods of current delivery become clearer, this will likely lead to a more standardized device nomenclature.

CES types of devices have been in use for many years for a variety of clinical and subclinical symptoms, and a substantial and diverse body of information has accumulated. As of 2002, a bibliography by Kirsch listed 145 scientific studies of CES involving human subjects, reportedly encompassing over 8,800 people receiving active CES [28]. Nonetheless, poor understanding of CES efficacy and mechanism of action persists [29]. Potential mechanisms and brain areas affected may vary considerably according to all the aforementioned stimulation parameters. Stimulation doses may also vary due to individual skull and brain anatomy [15, 23]. Confusion has persisted concerning the degree to which various devices stimulate brain structures by electrical fields directly reaching brain tissue, or through stimulation of afferent fibers of cranial nerves. Recent research, from modeling [15, 23, 30, 31] and human [24, 25, 32] data indicates that CES devices can modulate cortical and subcortical functions. However, the modeling studies do not account for afferent neural input, and human studies cannot establish whether that modulation is the result of direct cortical stimulation or cranial nerve afferent stimulation.

Despite the long history of CES use in Europe and the USA, there have not been large, well-controlled clinical trials to establish efficacy for neuropsychiatric and other indications. Clinical studies to date have been primarily open trials or randomized trials limited by low subject number, poor subject characterization, inclusion of subjects with mixed diagnoses or subclinical levels of symptoms, inactive sham controls, inadequate blinding, and lack of systematic collection of side effects and adverse events [11, 38]. As devices, stimulation parameters and outcome measures also vary, this makes comparisons and meta-analyses difficult. Even the few well-controlled human studies that do exist often have small numbers of subjects and thus provide constrained evidence of effectiveness for some indications (insomnia, depression, withdrawal from drug addiction) and safety overall.

Earlier in the twentieth century, CES was attempted as a treatment for a variety of of psychosomatic and "psychophysiological" disorders, including encephalitis, preeclampsia, enuresis, acid-peptic disease, essential hypertension, neurodermatitis [33]; and wound healing [9]. In recent decades, the research and clinical focus has been on withdrawal from addictive substances, anxiety, depression, headache, pain, and sleep disorders. More recent studies finally are bringing mainstream clinical trial methodologies to the study of CES, and new indications are under study. However, scientifically unsupported claims continue to be promoted.

There is an extensive literature of animal data using transcranial, auricular and implanted electrodes, supporting efficacy of CES for treatment of pain, drug dependency, and for anesthesia. This literature is not summarized here, except to note that as of 2005, Gilula and Kirsch [34] reported 29 CES animal studies in the literature. Typical examples are the study of Dougherty et al. [35], who found that auricular transcranial electrical stimulation attenuated the severity of naloxone-precipitated morphine withdrawal in rats; and the study of Mantz et al. [36] who found that TCES significantly reduced halothane (a general anesthetic) requirements in a rat model.

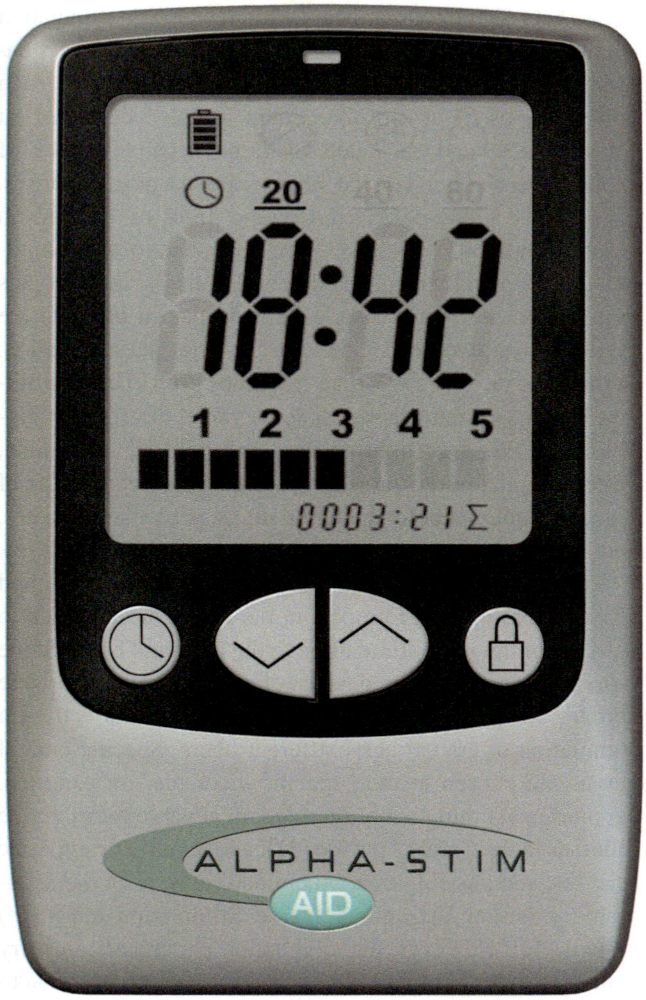

Fig. 11.1 The Alpha-Stim AID cranial stimulator

Contemporary Devices and Clinical Applications

The previous most active period of interest in research on CES was in the 1960s and 1970s, evidenced by the International Symposia for Electrotherapeutic Sleep and Electroanesthesia, held in Graz, Austria, in 1966 and 1969 [11, 37]. In 1975, there were at least seven American-made commercially available CES devices. In 1995, eight commercial CES devices were on the market [11]. The two most widely used CES devices today in the USA are the Alpha-Stim® devices (Electromedical Products Int. Inc.), which deliver stimulation up to 0.6 mA through earclip electrodes with pulsed frequencies which can be set at 0.5, 1.5, or 100 Hz; and the Fisher-Wallace Cranial Stimulator (Fisher-Wallace Laboratories), which delivers pulsed higher frequency stimulation through sponge electrodes placed at both temples. Current range for the Fisher Wallace device is 1.0–4 mA and frequencies are 15, 500, and 15,000 Hz. The Fisher-Wallace device uses the same patented frequencies as the former Liss Cranial Stimulator. CES-Ultra (Neuro-Fitness LLC), also marketed in the USA, delivers an adjustable current amplitude from 0 to 1.5 mA, a current intensity up to 1 A, as a 100 Hz square wave, with 2 ms pulse duration. CES Ultra gives the option to use ear clip electrodes or gel electrodes placed on the mastoid processes. These three devices have 510 K approval status from the FDA to be marketed for treatment of anxiety, depression, and insomnia. They are available in the USA only with a prescription from a licensed health care practitioner (Fig. 11.1).

The "Limoge's current" was reportedly satisfactorily used for several years mostly in France and Russia, to produce anesthesia (electroanesthesia) and pain control [18].

Lefaucheur [17] has described the highly specific stimulation parameters of Limoge's current, primarily used for electroanesthesia. Trains of stimuli are applied at 77–100 Hz, each train composed of positive sharp pulses, delivered at 125–167 kHz and separated by large negative pulses of smaller intensity but with the same area as the positive pulses. This yields a non-polarized stimulus train of 3–4 ms in duration and 30–35 V (200–350 mA) in peak-to-peak amplitude. A specifically engineered device delivers the Limoge's current into the brain, using a cathode placed between the eyebrows and two anodes on each posterior mastoid region. In the years prior to 1990, high frequency (166 kHz) intermittent Limoge-current transcutaneous cranial electrical stimulation (TCES) was used in cardiac, thoracic, abdominal, urological, and micro-surgery, based on observed benefits of reduced requirement for analgesic drugs, particularly opiates, and long-lasting postoperative analgesia [39, 40].

The CES devices commercially available in the USA and CES devices used in Europe and the USSR are intended to deliver non-targeted stimulation to the head and brain. Some more recent CES-like devices, currently only available abroad, are proposed to modulate the brain indirectly via stimulation of cranial nerve afferent fibers. Specific cranial nerves are chosen to treat specific disorders, for example, supraorbital stimulation of the trigeminal nerve for migraine relief, as in the Cefaly® device [41], and to mitigate epileptic seizures, and possibly treat other conditions, as in the Monarch™ external Trigeminal Nerve Stimulation (eTNS™) system [42]. However, the stimulation parameters are very similar to those of older CES devices, raising the question to what degree these devices and CES devices also act at least in part through direct stimulation of brain tissue vs. stimulation of afferent cranial nerves.

The Cefaly® device (STX-Med, Liège, Belgium) uses a single frontal self-adhesive electrode contained within a rigid headband that is placed horizontally over the forehead and over the ears. Cefaly's model indicates the device works by stimulating the bifurcation of the trigeminal nerve centrally just above the orbits (the supratrochlear and supraorbital nerves); this cranial nerve transmits sensation from the face and scalp to the brainstem. The device is thought to stimulate endorphin release, and stimulation of sensory afferents is thought to block headache or migraine pain pathways into the central nervous system. Cefaly® asserts that its technology is very safe. The Cefaly® device generates biphasic rectangular impulses with 250 μs pulse width, 60 Hz frequency, and 16 mA current intensity. Stimulation sessions are recommended to last 20 min, once/day. Case reports and research papers are available on the Cefaly® site, which states that more than 5,000 treatment sessions occurred in the cited 25 laboratory, case, pilot, and blinded studies of Cefaly's clinical effectiveness and safety (http://www.cefaly.ca/site/studies). The Cefaly® device has been submitted for FDA approval in the USA and currently is available in Canada and Europe without a prescription.

The NeuroSigma Monarch™ external Trigeminal Nerve Stimulation (eTNS™) system, also designed to stimulate the trigeminal nerve at both the infraorbital and supraorbital branches. Based on prior research [42–44], FDA has just permitted initiation of a Phase III clinical trial of the Monarch™ system for epilepsy. The manufacturer points out that trigeminal nerve afferents project indirectly to multiple brain areas playing key roles in seizure inhibition and initiation, but also implicated in depression, anxiety, and pain circuits: the nucleus solitarius, locus coeruleus, anterior cingulate, and cerebral cortex. Based on mood improvement in patients treated for epilepsy, this device now also is being investigated for treatment of depression [45]; a Phase II clinical trial is underway in the USA. In addition, a Phase I clinical trial has just been begun of the Monarch ™ device for Post-Traumatic Stress Disorder (PTSD), and for Attention Deficit Hyperactivity Disorder (ADHD) in children. An implantable form of the same technology also is being developed, sTNS™, using subcutaneous electrodes and an implantable pulse generator. The Monarch™ eTNS™ System, not yet available in the USA, is available in Canada and the European Union but only with a physician's prescription (www.neurosigma.com; http://www.monarch-etns.com).

Finally, the Transair device (abbreviated from (*TRAN*scranial electrotherapy *S*timulator for *A*nalgesia, *I*mmunity and *R*eparation), created at the Pavlov Institute of Physiological Sciences of the Russian Academy of Sciences, Center TES (http://neurotes.com) and marketed in Russia and Eastern Europe (see e.g., Onkocet), is reportedly widely used in clinics in those regions. The Transair devices stimulate via four electrodes, two on the mastoids and two on the forehead. Five devices are mentioned on the site. They have multiple-programmed settings to treat a very wide range of illnesses and conditions. Four devices are for clinic use, including one device specialized for audiological use, and one is for home use. Two Transair devices are described with some detail. The types of electric current used are: TRANSAIR-05: pulsed monopolar current and pulsed bipolar current with frequency modulation control, direct current in combination with pulsed monopolar current, and direct current, with intensity up to 5 mA, at a frequency of 50 Hz; TRANSAIR-04: pulsed bipolar current, pulsed monopolar current and combination monopolar and direct currents in 1:1 ratio, with intensity up to 5 mA, at a frequency of 50 Hz (Table 11.1).

Additional novel electrode sites may be used in future forms of cranial and transcranial stimulators. Drawing on earlier research [46, 47], Kraus and colleagues [48] investigated BOLD fMRI effects in response to transcutaneous electrical stimulation of two different zones in the left outer auditory canal. This area is rich in vagal afferents.

Table 11.1 Leading commercially available CES devices, USA and abroad: device type, electrode number, type and placement, clinical applications

Device Name	Device Type	Electrode Number	Electrode Type	Electrode Placement	Clinical applications
Alpha-Stim® AID (does not treat pain) M (treats pain) Electromedical Products Int., Inc	CES	2	Earclip electrodes	Earlobes	Anxiety, depression, insomnia, chronic pain
CES-Ultra Neuro-Fitness, LLC	CES	2	Earclip electrodes Pre-gelled electrodes	Earlobes Mastoid processes	Anxiety, depression, insomnia
Fisher-Wallace Cranial Stimulator® Fisher-Wallace Laboratories	CES	2	Sponge electrodes	Temples, above zygomatic arch	Anxiety, depression, insomnia, chronic pain
Transair DOCTOR TES-03 TRANSAIR-03 TRANSAIR-04 TRANSAIR-05 TRANSAIR-07 Pavlov Institute, Russian Academy of Sciences, Center TES	CES (TES)	4	Electrode pads or Solid gel electrodes (for home use DOCTOR TES-03 model only)	Central forehead/ supraorbital (2) and Mastoid processes (2)	Pain (neuro, other), anxiety, depression, "correction of psychophysiological state," PTSD, addictions, stress, hypertension, tinnitus, many others
Cefaly® STX-Med (Canada, EU only)	Cranial nerve stimulator	1	Self-adhesive electrode patch with connector	Central forehead/ supraorbital	Migraine headache
Monarch™ e-TNS™ NeuroSigma (Canada, EU only)	Cranial nerve stimulator	2	External conductive patch	Central forehead/ supraorbital	Epilepsy, depression, ADHD (ped.), PTSD

Stimulation parameters were pulse width 20 ms, frequency 8 Hz, individually titrated to be well tolerated; and mean stimulation intensity was 32.6 V (min 14 V, max 57 V). They found robust BOLD signal decreases in limbic structures and the brain stem during electrical stimulation of the left anterior auditory canal, including BOLD signal decreases in the area of the nuclei of the vagus nerve, which may indicate an effective stimulation of vagal afferents. Stimulation at the posterior wall of the auditory canal resulted in changes of the BOLD signal within the nucleus solitarius, a key relay station of vagal neurotransmission. Kraus and colleagues concluded that there is promise in this specific novel method of cranial nerve X or vagal stimulation, and that it could be beneficial for treatment of psychiatric conditions. A similar in-ear electrode location was demonstrated by Datta et al. [23] in a modeling study to produce higher induced electrical field magnitudes in the midbrain, pons, hypothalamus, and insula than some conventional CES stimulation sites.

Evidence of CES Efficacy from Open and Randomized Clinical Trials

Clinical conditions for which there is preliminary evidence of CES benefit from human data include, e.g., anxiety [49–51], review; [11], meta-analysis for anxiety indications [52], anxiety in addicts [53] and dental patients [54]; bipolar II disorder [55]; depression [51, 56–58]; hypertension [59, 60]; fibromyalgia [61]; insomnia [62, 63]; migraine headache [41] and tension headache [64]; nightmares, aggression/irritability [62, 65]; pain [66–68]; surgical and post-surgical analgesia [69–71] and anesthesia [18]; Parkinson's disease [25] and pain in PD [72]; substance abuse withdrawal and relapse prevention [21, 53, 73–78, Smith, 1982]; and visual field deficits after optic nerve injury [79, 80].

Some focused [50, 38, 81–83] and fairly comprehensive reviews of CES [11, 13, 18] also have appeared in recent years. According to Klawansky[11], as of 1995, evidence for efficacy, as measured by effect size based on the 14 included pooled studies, was strongest for anxiety disorders (CES > sham, $p < 0.05$).

The more robust clinical trials among the above include studies of CES for fibromyalgia [61, Taylor, 2011]; migraine headache [41]; addictions (e.g., [53, 74]); dental procedure anxiety [54]; surgical analgesia [70, 71]; pain [66] and visual field deficits after optic nerve injury [79, 80].

The Cefaly device reduced migraine frequency during daily treatment for 2 months [41]. Compared to stimulation with a 30 μs pulse width, 1 Hz frequency and 1 mA current intensity. The Cefaly device also was found to promote a sedative effect [84].

The NeuroSigma Monarch™ external Trigeminal Nerve Stimulation (eTNS™) currently is marketed for treatment of epilepsy and depression in Canada and the European Union, but published data supporting efficacy is weak. DeGiorgio [42, 43, 85] conducted a double-blind randomized active-control trial in drug-resistant epilepsy to test the suitability of the NeuroSigma type of CES treatment, and to try to establish control parameters in preparation for a phase III multicenter clinical trial. Fifty subjects with long-term epilepsy (mean age approx. 22 years) and two or more partial onset seizures per month first had a 6-week baseline period, and then were evaluated at 6, 12, and 18 weeks during the acute treatment period. Participants were randomized to treatment (eTNS™ 120 Hz) or control (eTNS™ 2 Hz) parameters, and were matched on key variables; they were highly drug-resistant, having failed on average more than three antiepileptic drugs prior to enrollment. eTNS™ (NeuroSigma) was well-tolerated; side effects included anxiety (4 %), headache (4 %), and skin irritation (14 %). The responder rate (50 % reduction in seizure frequency) was 30 % for the treatment group vs. 21 % for the active control group for the 18-week treatment period (n.s., $p = 0.31$). However, the treatment group experienced a significant within-group improvement in responder rate over the 18-week treatment period (from 18 % at 6 weeks to 41 % at 18 weeks, $p < 0.01$). eTNS™ also was associated with improvements in mood on the Beck Depression Inventory ($p < 0.02$). The authors concluded that this Class II evidence suggests that eTNS™ is safe and may be effective in subjects with drug resistant epilepsy. A larger multicenter phase III clinical trial is being planned.

Using methods and stimulation parameters similar to those in the NeuroSigma epilepsy studies [43, 85]. Schrader et al. [45], examined the effects of the Neuro Sigma device as an adjunct to pharmacotherapy for major depression. Five adults (mean age 47 years), all with persistent depressive symptoms despite adequate pharmacotherapy, participated in an 8-week open-label outpatient trial. Nightly stimulation for a minimum of 8 h over the V1 branch of the trigeminal nerve was well tolerated, although some participants developed skin irritation under the device contact site. The clinician-rated Hamilton Depression Rating Scale ($p = 0.006$) and self-rated Beck Depression Inventory ($p = 0.0004$) detected significant symptomatic improvement over baseline. The authors concluded that eTNS™ may be a useful adjunct to pharmacotherapy in major depressive disorder, and call for larger trials. It should be noted that nightly stimulation for 8–12 h is much more extensive than stimulation periods in most CES studies for mood-related problems, of typically 20–30 min/day.

A number of important treatment parameters remain to be investigated for all CES devices. Some studies suggest that response to CES stimulation can be rapid, occurring after 2–10 sessions [8], but it is not clear how long benefits persist after cessation of treatment. Feighner et al. [33] examined the duration of clinical benefit after terminating use of CES for indications such as depression and anxiety. Their double blind, randomized controlled study tested the efficacy of electrosleep on patients with chronic (>2 years) psychiatric illness refractory to treatment, with symptoms of anxiety, insomnia and depression not caused by medical illness. In a crossover design, patients were randomly assigned to either Group I, ten active electrosleep treatments followed by ten sham treatments over a 4-week period, or Group II, ten sham electrosleep treatments, followed by ten active electrosleep treatments over a 4-week period. Repeated, blinded objective and subjective ratings were acquired to assess clinical improvement, and follow-up ratings were done on a monthly basis for 6 months. Results indicated that active electrosleep treatments significantly improved sleep, anxiety, depression, and psychosocial adjustment. However, only one patient had sustained remission; all other patients who initially responded relapsed during the first month following treatment cessation, and of these, only two responded to a further intensive course of electrosleep therapy, and did well with maintenance treatments.

Further research is needed to identify optimal schedules and duration of treatment—daily use for a specific duration in months, or brief bursts of CES application for a few days, then cessation of use for a specific period of time, then repeated, or simply used *ad libitum* as desired. The effects of tapering of CES treatment either at initiation or termination on efficacy, adverse events, or relapse have not been studied, and should be. A rat model study [27] investigated the effect of varying transcranial AC stimulus frequency, pulse width, charge balance and polarity, electrode placement, and time of day of stimulation on tail flick response to heat. A biphasic, charge balanced waveform with a first phase duration of 2 ms, current 10 mu Amp and repetition rate 10 Hz was found to induce maximum tail flick latency changes from baseline.

There has been almost no systematic examination of whether and how severity of depression or anxiety affects response to CES. In the study of Feighner et al. [33], patients diagnosed as having primary depression (major depressive disorder) did worse with active electrosleep treatment. They concluded that in patients with primary depression, electrosleep therapy should be used with caution, and may be contraindicated. Whether there are sustained or only short term benefits of CES requires much more extensive scientific study.

Lebedev et al. [8] reported that fatigue, stress, and related psycho-physiological disturbances were significantly improved or abolished after 2–5 transcranial electrical stimulation (TES) sessions (TRANSAIR device), in mixed groups of stressed workers, military members, patients with PTSD and other conditions, and others (total $N = 808$), and according to Lebedev et al., more noticeably in cases of more serious disturbance. Better response in patients with more severe illness seems to contradict the report of Feighner et al. of worse response in more severe depression, but not enough detail is provided in either study to compare severity of illness.

Many patients increasingly seek less invasive and less expensive forms of treatment.

Because CES has not been adequately tested in individuals with major depression or specific anxiety disorders [38], there is appropriate concern that more severely ill individuals may avoid proven interventions in favor of CES self-treatment. Schrader et al. [45] are investigating the NeuroSigma eTNS™ trigeminal nerve stimulating device for major depression, but as an adjunct to pharmacotherapy. A more appropriate role for CES might be to help maintain remission after a course of a proven treatment, for example for depression, but little data is available to address the question of efficacy for more severe symptoms.

A new approach which could be particularly productive for clinical use of CES is to target pain, depression, insomnia and fatigue as a group of symptoms, which commonly co-occur in inflammatory disorders, other medical illnesses, and in situations of chronic stress [57, 86]. Anecdotally, CES users often have reported feelings of increased energy, mild euphoria, and a lack of concern about minor problems [87, 88]. Anecdotal documentation of this response to CES is widespread in many studies over the decades of its use, and also can be found on commercial device Web sites that post consumer endorsements and informal tabulations of benefits and side effects. There also is some evidence that a single session of CES can attenuate acute stress responses [8], reduce physiological and psychological arousal in healthy subjects, and reduce vigilance and increase drowsiness in healthy volunteers [84]. Concerning other applications of CES for stress reduction, some human resources professionals have suggested that CES might be used in nonclinical populations to help alleviate workplace stress [89].

Interestingly, relaxation benefits of CES also are reported in animals. It was Pavlov's early observation of the soporific effects on dogs in his experiments that stimulated early Russian interest in electrosleep [3]. Fisher-Wallace Laboratories also offers an equine version of a CES device called the Happy Halter, which is marketed to veterinarians and trainers of high performance horses. It reputedly is useful in calming nervous horses and in pain reduction [90]. The Alpha-Stim device reportedly is also successfully being used to calm horses [91].

Taylor and Lee [92], in a double-blind protocol, administered to ninety healthy volunteers 30 min of constant current sine-wave cranial transcutaneous electrical nerve stimulation (TENS) of 5, 100, or 2,000 Hz frequency (current maintained below 0.5 mA for safety), placebo TENS, or no treatment. The five groups were compared on pretreatment to posttreatment changes in blood pressure, heart rate, peripheral temperature, and anxiety. Analysis showed significant reductions in systolic and diastolic blood pressure and heart rate after 100 Hz cranial TENS as compared to the other groups. No other differences achieved significance.

The military has shown interest in CES, in particular for treatment of PTSD [93–95]. Both the Alpha-Stim and Fisher-Wallace company Web sites indicate military use of the devices and Armed Forces funding of clinical trials.

Clinicaltrials.gov posts the following trials of CES as of July 2013: Cranial Stimulation for Chemotherapy Symptoms in Breast Cancer (Virginia Commonwealth University, National Cancer Institute); Efficacy and Safety of Cranial Electrical Stimulation (CES) for Major Depressive Disorder (MDD) (Massachusetts General Hospital, Fisher Wallace Labs, LLC); Cranial Electrical Stimulation Effects on Symptoms in Persons With Fibromyalgia (University of Virginia); Use of Alpha-Stim Cranial-Electrotherapy Stimulation (CES) in the Treatment of Anxiety (Wyndhurst Counseling Center, Liberty University); A Pilot Study of Cranial Electrotherapy Stimulation [CES] for Generalized Anxiety Disorder (University of California, Los Angeles); Cranial Electrotherapy Stimulation (CES) to treat PTSD (CES-fMRI-PTSD) (McLean Hospital, Mending Minds Foundation).

Contraindications for Use and Safety of CES

There are few contraindications for use of CES on the device manufacturers' Web sites. Interestingly, the Russian company Transair is the only one that lists extensive contraindications (see Table 11.2 below). This makes sense in that Transair seeks to treat much more varied conditions.

Table 11.2 Contraindications for CES device use reported on manufacturer Web sites

CES device name	Contraindications mentioned on Web sites
Alpha-Stim®, Electromedical Products Intl., Inc	Cardiac pacemaker
CES-Ultra, Neuro-Fitness, LLC	None mentioned
Fisher-Wallace Cranial Stimulator®, Fisher-Wallace Laboratories	None mentioned
Transair, Pavlov Institute, Russian Academy of Sciences, Center TES	Seizures, epilepsy; acute brain injuries and tumors, central nervous system infections, stage III hypertension, hypertensive emergency; hydrocephalus; acute psychiatric disorders; thyrotoxicosis; atrial fibrillation; broken or damaged skin on forehead, area of electrode application; implanted electrostimulators; in children under 5 years of age
Cefaly®	Driving, recent brain or facial trauma, skin conditions/rashes/abrasions on face, head, Meniere's disease
STX-Med (Canada, EU only)	
Monarch™ e-TNS™	None mentioned
NeuroSigma (Canada, EU only)	

Transair TES therapy is contraindicated in: seizures, epilepsy; acute brain injuries and tumors, central nervous system infections; stage III hypertension, hypertensive emergency; hydrocephalus; acute psychiatric disorders; thyrotoxicosis; atrial fibrillation; broken or damaged skin on forehead, area of electrode application; implanted electrostimulators; in children under 5 years of age.

No serious adverse events have been reported in the past 50 years of CES use in clinical and research settings. However, few trials to date have systematically and prospectively recorded side effects. In 1974, a review of the research on safety of cranial electrotherapy stimulation (CES) was commissioned by FDA and conducted by the National Research Council, Washington, DC. The NRC reviewers concluded that "significant adverse events or complications attributable" to the application of electric current of approximately 1 mA or less for "therapeutic effect to the head" (cranial electrotherapy stimulation) were "virtually nonexistent" [96].

Electronic Products International (EPI), the manufacturer of the Alpha-Stim device, indicates that consumer reports to EPI in 2007–2011 concerning adverse events were associated with <1 % of a reported 58,030 Alpha-Stim units sold in that same period. Also drawing from 14 published studies using the Alpha-Stim device and involving a total of 2,389 subjects who had active treatment, they further reported that adverse events occurred in less than <1 % of all study treatments. Side effects included pain or itching at the earlobes, vertigo, drowsiness, nausea, headache, tinnitus and others. However, for many of these studies current was set at 0.1 mA, for 60 min, to reduce the chance that subjects could discriminate active treatment from sham. Recently, studies have more systematically collected data on side effects, detecting higher rates of side effects. Even at the low 0.1 mA intensity of stimulation, a recent controlled study with the Alpha-Stim device found that 30 % of subjects reported ear pain or itching at the electrode sites [97]. Of note, at that low stimulation intensity, recent well-controlled trials found no reduction in target symptoms of neuropathic pain [97], insomnia or depression [98].

The NeuroSigma trigeminal nerve stimulation device, intended to be used for 24 h continuously, was associated with mild to moderate skin irritation under the electrodes in eight of 13 subjects [99]. Irritation was relieved by hydrocortisone cream, reduction of length of exposure to stimulation from 24 to 12 h, and alternation of the location from supraorbital to infraorbital.

Studies using higher stimulation frequencies and intensity (4–16 mA) have found that all subjects reported intense paresthesias [41] or flickering lights [24, 100, 101].

Decades ago, electrodes sometimes were applied to the eyes, to bypass skull impedance. but this was associated with blurred vision which persisted for some minutes after treatment.

Other rare, possibly related safety concerns were noted in prior studies. A study of rural law enforcement personnel using CES for depression reported one participant developed increased levels of agitation, and was removed from the study [102]. One participant in a study of CES for chronic mental illness reported an increase in auditory hallucinations but was able to finish the study [103].

Although CES has been suggested as a safer alternative to antidepressant and antianxiety medication during pregnancy, there has been one report of a frequency-dependent reduction in fetal weight and increased fetal death in rats, as a consequence of 1 h of daily CES treatment at 0.125 mA and 0.22 ms pulse width during pregnancy [104].

In 1975, Jordan and Morris investigated safety of a combined AC and DC stimulation paradigm in young male beagle dogs, using an electrosleep (ES) machine manufactured by Hoffman-LaRoche Corporation. This paradigm was based on a human protocol that called for one eye and one occipital electrode at a strength of 1 mA of AC current and 0.33 mA of DC current. The canine protocol involved comparable stimulation sites, with three dogs assigned to each of the three experimental conditions: 1 mA of AC current and 0.33 mA of DC current; 5 mA AC and 1.33 mA DC; and Sham. Frequency was 100 Hz with a pulse width of 5 ms. While the dogs were anesthetized, 13 daily treatments of 1 h duration were applied over a 3-week period, at fixed AM and PM times, with extensive physiologic sampling on days 1, 7, and 13. At the end of the protocol the dogs were sacrificed and both eyes and the brain were examined grossly and microscopically. No clinically significant neurologic signs were observed. Pathological data revealed some suspicious findings (oligodendroglia, areas of calcification) most often in the striate cortex, caudate nucleus and septum, but these were deemed small and of questionable significance, except for one instance. A dose–response relationship was observed, with the high dose condition producing the majority of all lesions (approximately 14/dog), compared to low dose and sham (between approximately 7 and 9/dog), again the majority deemed not likely significant. Other major findings included EEG slowing, depression of B-wave amplitude, and a chronic increase in pulse rate. The authors cited the small number of animals as a reason to replicate the study on a large scale, for valid statistical analysis [105]. Unfortunately this study could not determine whether the AC or DC stimulation was more likely to cause the lesions and other changes observed.

The peak electric field magnitudes generated during CES (<1 V/m) are approximately 100–1,000-fold lower than electric fields induced by transcranial magnetic stimulation (TMS) or electroconvulsive therapy (ECT), which also is AC stimulation [15]. The lack of evidence of brain injury associated with electroconvulsive therapy provides support for the likely safety of CES. ECT uses currents in the range of 2–4 A applied for approximately 30 s per session, designed to induce a seizure. CES uses a 1,000-fold smaller current (0.1–16 mA) for a longer duration (typically, 20–60 min daily) and a greater number of therapeutic sessions (30–60), compared to ECT (6–20). Because CES stimulation is too low intensity to produce seizures, it also does not produce the memory impairment often associated with ECT. There has been no evidence of structural brain injury associated with the far more powerful ECT, as measured by CT or MRI scans [106, 107]. Dwork et al. [108] presented preliminary findings, in what was then the first well-controlled nonhuman primate neuropathological study of ECT to use perfusion fixation, and the first to compare ECT with magnetic seizure therapy (MST); neither modality produced histological lesions in the brain.

There is a literature on transcranial electrical stimulation (TES) used for intraoperative motor evoked potential (MEP) monitoring (although the term TES also has been used by Lebedev for more conventional applications of CES, [7–10]). Journee [22] pointed out that the TES used in intraoperative monitoring differs in several respects from conventional cranial electrical stimulation, for example, it administers brief pulses of several hundreds of volts and currents may exceed 1 A, whereas conventional CES stimulators are limited to <20 mA. Due to the strong scalp pain generated, clinical use of high-intensity TES has been restricted to monitoring of motor pathways under general anesthesia. Transcranial magnetic stimulation, which also causes brief scalp pain in conscious subjects, stimulates a relatively small part of the brain. TES may elicit action potentials in many neural structures in a large volume of the brain, in complex intraoperative stimulation paradigms with increasing numbers of pulses. Therefore, Journee believes that concern about the risk of adverse or irreversible functional changes in the brain is appropriate. High intensity TES would seem to lie on a safety continuum between CES and ECT. MacDonald [109] reviewed the safety of high intensity TES, in comparison with other clinical and experimental brain stimulation methods and in light of clinical experience, in more than 15,000 cases. According to MacDonald, remarkably few adverse events were reported. Journee [22] pointed out that adverse events may have been underreported, but also concluded that with appropriate oversight and stimulation parameters, TES for intraoperative monitoring can be safe and beneficial. The minimal adverse events associated with the more powerful TES device offers some comparative support for the likely safety of the much weaker current of conventional cranial stimulators, although TES is not used chronically.

Research experience with tDCS also provides support for likely safety of CES. The alternating current delivered by CES is of similar amplitude (0.1–16 mA) to the direct current of tDCS. Since the development of tDCS in the 1960s, many hundreds of subjects have participated in studies. tDCS has been very well tolerated, with no significant adverse effects reported after a comprehensive review [110], other than scalp burns. In a more recent review and meta-analysis of studies reporting tDCS-caused adverse events, itching, tingling, burning sensation, headache, and discomfort were reported, more often in older and less healthy subjects and those who got higher current intensities [111]. Of note, scalp burns have never been associated with CES stimulation. Use of alternating current and usually no skin abrasion at the stimulation site are characteristic of CES administration, which may explain why skin burns do not occur with CES, although occasional mild skin reddening does. Additional tDCS safety findings include no elevation of neuron-specific enolase, a sensitive marker of neuronal damage [112]. Bikson et al. [113] discuss animal model data showing brain lesions from use of tDCS at high intensities (higher than would be used therapeutically in humans). The lesions are hypothesized to result from heating of tissue. Further discussion of safety issues for CES and tDCS can be found for example in Bikson et al. [113] and Lefaucheur [16, 17].

Further work will be needed to determine whether there are interactions between CES and neuropsychiatric medications, that could impact efficacy or tolerability of either CES or the concurrent medications. This has not been studied in CES, but has been somewhat examined in tDCS and TMS. Lefaucheur [16] points out that medication is likely to be a major source of changes in cortical function and patients with neuropsychiatric disorders are rarely free of drugs affecting brain excitability. For example, a recent study found that tDCS results improve with concurrent antidepressant administration [114]. The authors' conclusions were that in major depressive disorder, the combination of tDCS and sertraline increases the efficacy of each treatment; and the efficacy and safety of tDCS and sertraline did not differ. Lefaucheur [16] discusses several kinds of interactions of neurotransmitter agonists and antagonists with tDCS stimulation, and additionally mentions that duration of drug administration and drug plasma levels also influence modulatory effects of cortical stimulation on the excitability of a target area [16]. As mentioned above, Schrader et al. [45] are investigating the NeuroSigma trigeminal nerve stimulating device to treat major depression as an adjunct to pharmacotherapy.

Future work also is needed to determine the risk to patients with bipolar disorder of becoming manic. There is one published report of mania being induced in a bipolar II patient being treated with tDCS [115]. Research on CES for bipolar II is in its infancy [55].

CES Regulatory Status (FDA)

Over the past 35 years, several CES devices were granted 510 K clearance in the USA to be marketed for the treatment of depression, anxiety, and insomnia, because the designs are equivalent to devices which were approved prior to 1976, when FDA began to require evidence of efficacy. In 1989, FDA amended its device regulations to require all devices that had not already done so to go through a formal premarket approval process, including submission of evidence of efficacy, and if requested, safety as well. As of 1993, FDA formally requested that CES device manufacturers comply with this requirement; they did not do so at the time [11]. Despite having received 510 K status in 1991 (e.g., the Fisher-Wallace device) to be marketed for the treatment of depression, anxiety, insomnia, and also chronic pain, due to the revised FDA approval process, CES devices remained in the Class III category. They remain in Class III after FDA hearings in February 2012 (Table 11.3).

Given the rise of interest in all forms of electrical and magnetic stimulation, more and better data for CES should gradually become available. However, because existing devices are close to the end of their patents, there is little incentive for conducting high quality, large-scale clinical trials. Device reclassification for CES types of technologies likely will be revisited in the coming years, particularly given an emerging generations of new low intensity, high frequency, alternating current devices, such as the Cefaly® and Monarch™ eTNS™ devices, and others currently in the experimental stage [15].

Proposed Mechanisms of Action of CES

Though the mechanisms by which CES may have impact on the brain and periphery still are minimally characterized, several have been proposed to date. Below we consider factors that influence the nature of the stimulation, that shape its proposed impact on the brain, and therefore the potential mechanisms of action of CES. We summarize evidence for several biological pathways that may be the source of proposed clinically relevant effects, in the hope as well of identifying clearer targets for scientific study. Proposed mechanisms of action include stimulation of cortical and subcortical regions; effects on endogenous brain oscillations and cortical excitability; impact on neurotransmitters, hormones and endorphins; and impact on autonomic nervous system.

A key question regarding mechanism of action is whether CES can penetrate through the skull (high impedance) and cerebrospinal fluid (CSF; low impedance) to stimulate brain tissue directly, whether CES stimulates peripheral nerves that transmit afferent signals to the central nervous system, or whether CES can stimulate via both pathways. For back pain, stimulation with higher current of 60–100 mA at 50–200 Hz (i.e., a TENS device), at the skin surface is thought to relieve pain by stimulation of afferent sensory nerves. Implanted electrodes for stimulation of peripheral nerves in the spine and forehead have been used for relief of visceral pain [116] and headache [117]. Although device makers claim that cranial nerve stimulation sites are chosen for relief of specific symptoms based on anatomical neural relays, there have been no comparative studies with CES demonstrating differential efficacy based on electrode placement. For example, frontal electrodes have been reported to relieve migraine symptoms [41] and to have sedative effects [84]; but bi-temporal electrodes also have relieved migraine pain [118]. If varied electrode placements have similar clinical effects, this would argue for a more diffuse effect of CES on brain tissue, possibly by modulation of endogenous oscillatory rhythms.

Figure 11.2 illustrates the range of stimulation patterns among published studies using different devices that may differentially shape CES effects [15, 23, 26].

Table 11.3 Regulatory status of CES compared to other brain stimulation devices

Device name	FDA status	FDA approved indications for clinical use	Device description
Cranial electrical stimulation (CES)	Class III device	FDA sanctioned: 510(k) clearances (1991), can be marketed to treat anxiety, depression, insomnia, chronic pain	Electrical
			External
			Non-convulsive
Electroconvulsive therapy (ECT)	Class III device	Depression (1979)	Electrical
			External
			Convulsive
Deep brain stimulation (DBS)	Class I device	Essential tremor (1997)	Electrical
		Parkinson's disease (2002)	Implanted/internal
			Non-convulsive
repetitive transcranial magnetic stimulation (rTMS)	Class II device	Depression (2008)	Magnetic
		Migraine prophylaxis (2008)	External
			Non-convulsive
Vagus nerve stimulation (VNS)	Class III device	Epilepsy (1997)	Electrical
		Treatment resistant depression (2005)	External
			Non-convulsive
Magnetic seizure therapy (MST)	None/ investigational use only	No FDA approved indication	Magnetic
			External
			Convulsive
transcranial direct current stimulation (tDCS)	None/ investigational use only	No FDA approved indication	Electrical
			External
			Non-convulsive

Adapted from Novakovic V, Sher L, Lapidus KA, Mindes J, Golier J, Yehuda R (2011). Brain stimulation in posttraumatic stress disorder. Eur J Psychotraumatol. 2: 5609. Review

In order to study the biophysical and clinical significance of varying stimulation parameters on the brain, until now, analytical/spherical-based modeling approaches (see below), animal models, resected skulls, and synthetic phantoms all have been used [23]. However, as Datta and colleagues point out, these are of limited value given the need to study the effects of differing patterns of electrical stimulation in vivo on the human anatomy and its material properties. They cite the 1975 research of Dymond et al. [119] as still the only study that employed direct measurement in humans; the impact of DC electrosleep stimulation-induced intra-cortical current flow was studied in patients undergoing presurgical evaluation for epilepsy [23].

Datta and colleagues characterized scalp voltages caused by administration of CES, to validate subject-specific finite element method (FEM) models of current flow [23]. Each of the four stimulation electrode configurations tested resulted in a distinct distribution of scalp voltages. The authors suggested that monitoring of scalp voltages may be used to optimize electrode placement and current dose to increase transcranial electrical stimulation safety and reproducibility.

Brain Structures Impacted by CES

Computational modeling has been used to estimate intracranial penetration of electrical stimulation [30]. Two studies used finite element modeling (FEM) to estimate the penetration and focality of alternating current compared to a time invariant direct current stimulation [14, 120]. Using 1 mA and 10 or 100 Hz stimulation, Lopes et al. reported that alternating current stimulation generates cerebral fields that are up to ten times larger and 20 % more focused, in part because alternating current minimizes scalp resistance, with less current shunting between electrodes prior to propagating to deeper layers. Ferdjallah et al. [31] created a four-concentric-spheres simulation of CES with all dimensions and electrical properties of the model adapted from clinical data. Results indicated that, with electrode placement on opposite sides of the head to mimic CES application, the penetrating current density was maximized and a small fraction of the modeled CES reached the thalamus.

Datta et al. [15], using an updated, more sophisticated form of modeling, have produced new evidence for the proposed cortical and subcortical impacts of CES. They used a high resolution magnetic resonance imaging (MRI)-derived finite element head model including cortical and subcortical structures. Cortical electric field (current density) peak intensities and distributions were analyzed. They evaluated different electrode configurations of CES, or montages both conventional (ear clip) and novel (in-ear, behind ear (ear hook) and over-ear, all similar to headphone devices; see Fig. 11.3 below). All stimulated at 1 mA intensity (distributed across varying numbers of electrodes).

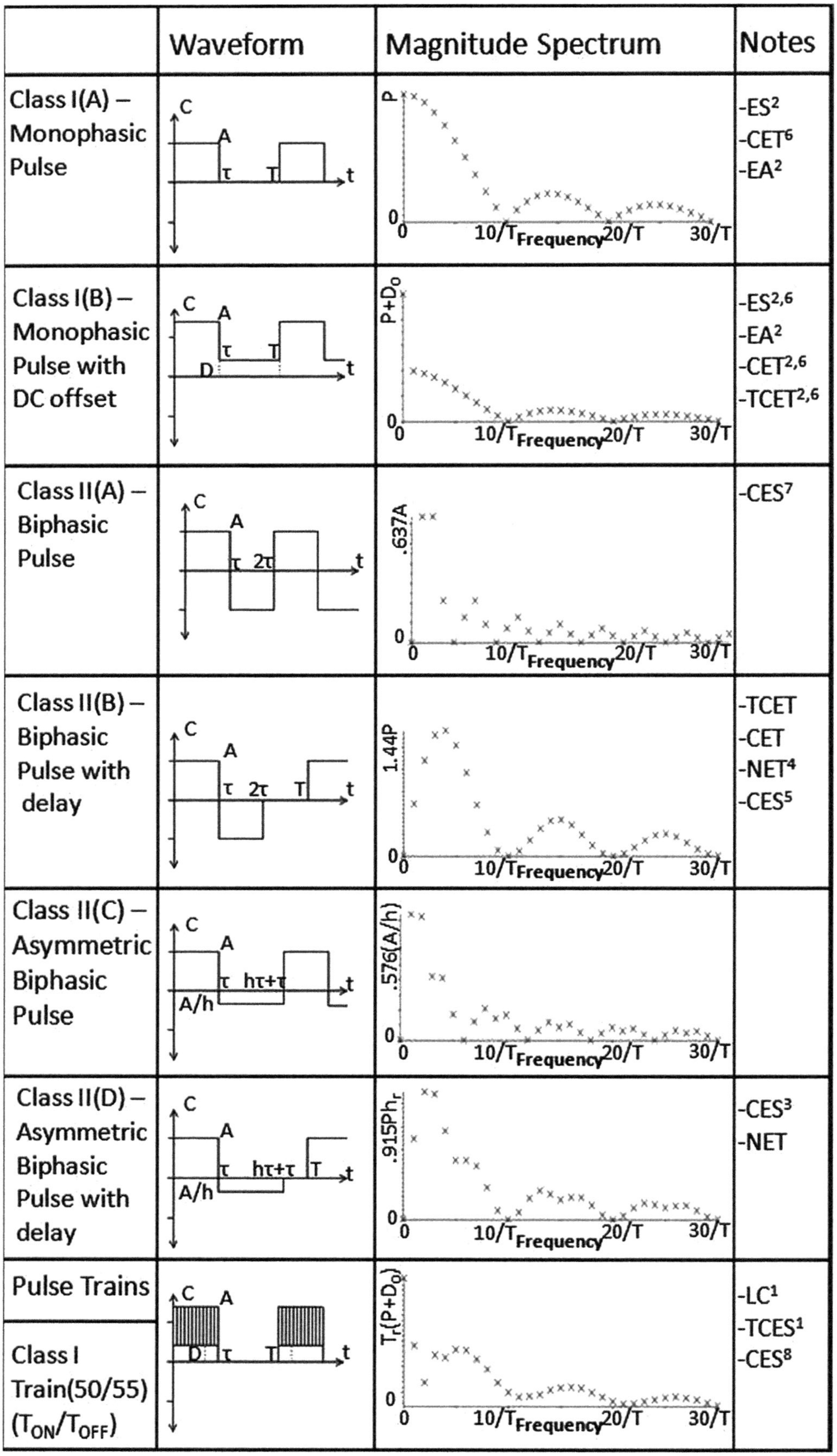

Fig. 11.2 The range of stimulation patterns among published studies using different devices that may differentially shape CES effects (Adapted from [15, 23, 26]). Adapted from: Datta A, Dmochowski JP, Guleyupoglu B, Bikson M, Fregni F (2013a). Cranial electrotherapy stimulation and transcranial pulsed current stimulation: a computer based high-resolution modeling study. Neuroimage. Jan 15;65:280–7

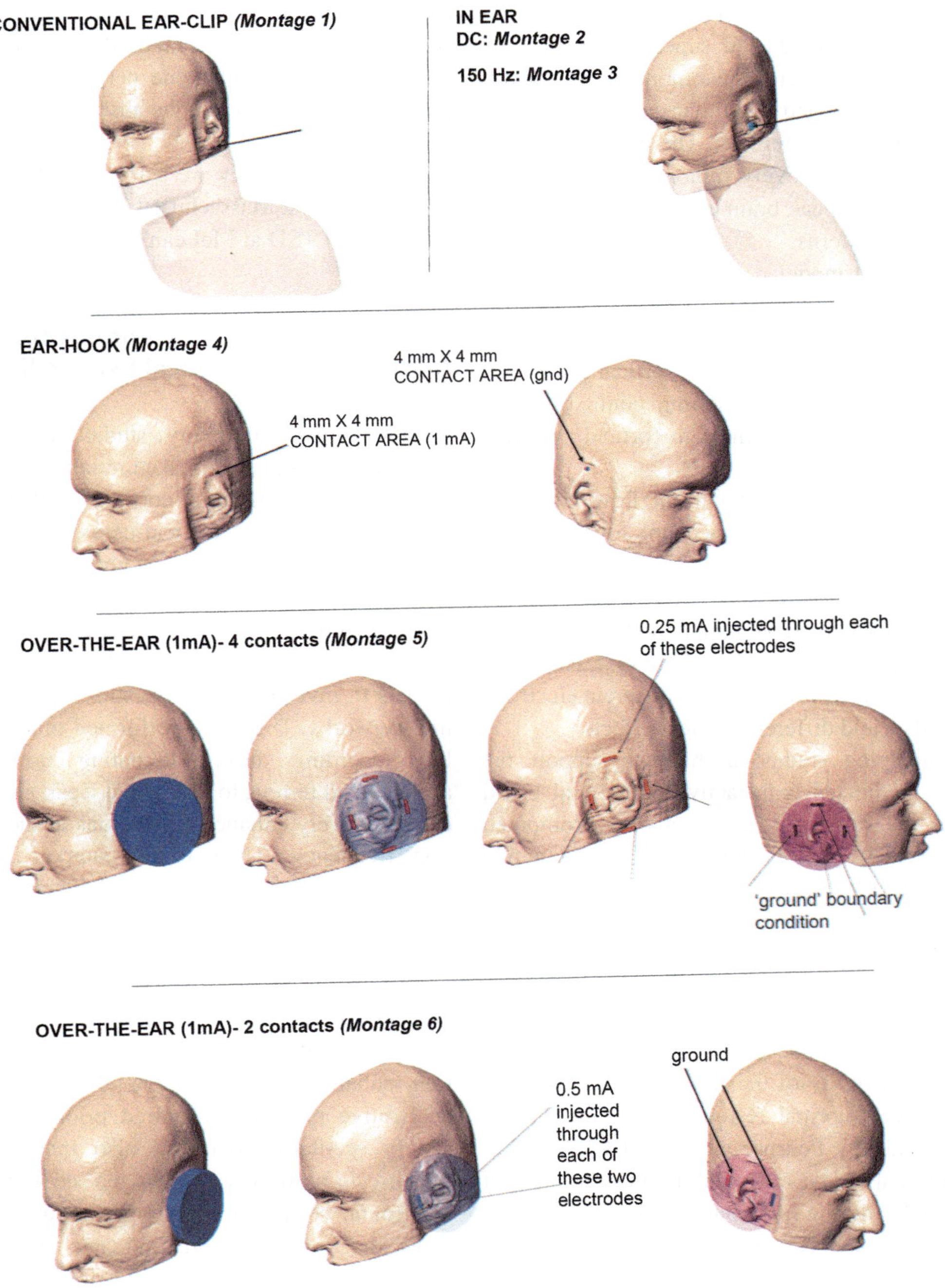

Fig. 11.3 Conventional cranial electrotherapy stimulation (CES) ear clip electrode montage and novel transcranial pulsed current stimulation (tPCS) electrode montages. Adapted from: Datta A, Dmochowski JP, Guleyupoglu B, Bikson M, Fregni F (2013a). Cranial electrotherapy stimulation and transcranial pulsed current stimulation: a computer based high-resolution modeling study. Neuroimage. Jan 15;65:280–7

Their model confirmed that significant amounts of current pass through the skull to reach cortical and subcortical structures. Depending on the electrode placement, induced currents at subcortical areas—midbrain, pons, thalamus, hypothalamus—can be of similar magnitude to those of cortical areas, and occasionally greater.

The conventional ear-clip montage resulted in a 0.10 V/m peak induced cortical electric field. Maximal currents were induced in the temporal cortex and in the medulla oblongata, with diffuse activation in the midbrain, pons, thalamus, insula, and hypothalamus. The in-ear placement resulted in a similar spatial profile of induced currents; however the peak induced electric field in the cortex was higher (0.16 V/m) and in the midbrain, pons, hypothalamus, and insula. The behind ear placement led to the highest peak induced cortical electric fields (0.47 V/m) as well as higher electric field in several deeper brain structures, except the medulla oblongata, possibly due to superior current flow through the mid-brain. The over-the-ear montage placement, either two or four contacts, led to similar current activation in sub-cortical and brainstem regions. The models of Datta et al. suggest that even relatively minor changes in CES electrode placement alter peak brain electric field and overall brain current flow patterns.

In another study that modeled multiple tDCS montages across three normal adult participants, Datta et al. [121] also concluded that current flow profile across all subjects and montages was influenced by details in cortical gyri/sulci, suggesting that subject-specific modeling could optimize effects of tDCS. Individual differences in cortical gyri may also influence CES effects.

Although these models predict current flow based on anatomical structures, they do not account for facilitated flow through afferent nerve pathways. For example, the external ear canal is dense with vagal afferents, and a new, less invasive form of vagus nerve stimulation, transcutaneous VNS (tVNS) also is being developed [46–48]. However, it remains to be determined whether these different electrode placements actually yield different clinical effects.

Recent neuroimaging studies in humans support the notion that CES modulates brain activity. Cerebral blood flow (CBF) was measured by xenon-enhanced computed tomography (XeCT™) before and after 2 h of active ($n = 17$) vs. sham ($n = 19$) TCES. Globally, CBF was unchanged by TCES; however locally, compared to sham stimulation, TCES caused significant CBF decrease in the brainstem (mesencephalon) and thalamus (diencephalon), structures involved in pain and anxiety.

Two MRI studies have shown CES impact on resting state functional connectivity of the Default Mode Network (DMN), which reflects normal resting state brain activity [24, 29]. In the study by Feusner et al. [29] CES at 0.5- and 100 Hz stimulation was applied to the earlobes at subsensory thresholds during functional magnetic resonance imaging in the resting state. Both 0.5 and 100 Hz stimulation yielded significant deactivation in midline frontal and parietal regions. 100 Hz stimulation was associated with both increases and decreases in connectivity within the default mode network (DMN). In the default mode network, nodes oscillate at the frequency of approximately 0.1 Hz [29]. This suggests that direct current or alternating current of frequency different than the DMN can disrupt DMN oscillations. In another study, both tDCS and CES (5, 500, 15,000 Hz) over the primary motor cortex down-modulated the functional connectivity of the associated resting state motor network in a recent study [24]. In major depression, network abnormalities have been reported for both the resting state default mode network (DMN) and the cognitive control network [122, 123]. Both antidepressants [124] and electroconvulsive therapy [125] have been shown to normalize the DMN in depressed individuals. These reports of CES effects on the default mode network represent significant promise for CES, even in the absence of convincing clinical trials data.

MRI data currently are being acquired in a trial of CES for depression at Massachusetts General Hospital, and a trial of CES for PTSD at McLean Hospital, Belmont, Mass.

Evidence for Effects on Endogenous Brain Oscillations and Cortical Excitability

Recent human laboratory studies have suggested that alternating current electrical stimulation is a useful paradigm to modulate endogenous cortical oscillations in order to study the function of cortical networks. However, underlying mechanisms concerning how periodic, weak global perturbations alter spatiotemporal dynamics of large-scale cortical network dynamics are unclear. Ali and colleagues [126] simulated large-scale networks of spiking neuron models to investigate this question in endogenously rhythmic networks. They also performed multichannel extracellular recordings during alternating current stimulation in anesthetized ferrets, to verify that weak global perturbations can selectively enhance oscillations at the applied stimulation frequency. Their results support future design of alternating current paradigms that dynamically tailor stimulation frequency to the spectral peak of ongoing brain activity.

Marshall et al. [127] studied transcranial application of very low frequency (0.75 Hz) AC during early non-REM sleep (a period of emerging slow wave sleep). This stimulation enhanced the retention of hippocampal-dependent declarative memories acquired prior to sleep onset. The slowly oscillating potential also induced an immediate increase in slow wave sleep, and slow spindle activity in the frontal cortex. Brain stimulation at 5 Hz, a frequency band that normally predominates during REM sleep, reduced slow wave sleep and left declarative memory unchanged.

Using constant low frequency AC stimulation, Kanai et al. [101] demonstrated modulation of phosphene thresholds to single-pulse TMS, in a frequency-dependent manner. Of four frequencies tested (5, 10, 20, and 40 Hz) only stimulation at 20 Hz modulated cortical excitability. However, it is possible that referred CES stimulation of the retina rather than occipital cortex produces phosphenes in this [128] and other studies [129].

Schroeder et al. [130] examined CES-induced EEG changes in 12 healthy right handed males receiving 0.5, 100 Hz, or sham in a randomized, double-blind crossover design, using ear clip electrodes, with CES administered for 20 min., adjusting the current level until the subject could feel sensation at the electrode site. The current was then reduced to a subthreshold level. The current settings for all subjects had a mean of 48 mA and a range of 10–100 mA. Relative to sham, 0.5 and 100 Hz caused the alpha band mean frequency to shift downward, and 100 Hz CES also caused a decrease of the alpha band median frequency and beta band power fraction. Other studies have found changes in resting EEG after a single session [20, 130, 131] and also 2 weeks after completing 14 daily 20 min sessions [132]. Directionality of effects have been conflicting, likely due to wide variation in stimulation parameters among studies.

Zaghi and colleagues [13] conducted an experiment that revealed how important specific stimulation parameters—including electrode size, which influences current density—are to producing neurophysiological effects using CES (here, tACS). They cited a previous study [133] in which tACS was applied for 2 and 5 min with current density of 0.16–0.25 A/m2 (0.4 mA, 10 Hz, 16 cm^2 electrodes) that was unable to show robust effects on cortical excitability. Zaghi et al. applied tACS at the significantly higher current density of 0.80 A/m2 (1 mA, 15 Hz, 12.56 cm^2 electrodes), for the considerably longer duration of 20 min, and were able to demonstrate measurable changes to cortical excitability. Their results revealed that active 15 Hz tACS of the motor cortex significantly diminished the amplitude of motor evoked potentials and decreased intracortical facilitation (ICF), as compared to baseline and sham stimulation, supporting the notion that AC stimulation with weak currents can induce significant changes in brain excitability. In this study, 15 Hz tACS led to a pattern of inhibition of cortical excitability. They proposed that tACS may have a dampening effect on cortical networks, and perhaps interfere with the temporal and spatial summation of weak subthreshold electric potentials.

In contrast to tDCS which is thought to hyperpolarize or depolarize neurons by electric-field induced changes in the conformation of membrane proteins and thereby change the resting firing rate [134], CES is thought to not hyperpolarize or depolarize neurons, but to modulate endogenous neurophysiologic activity or oscillations [13, 126, 127, 130, 135]. However, recent experimental laboratory studies using targeted electrode placements shown that lower frequency CES can alter visceral and somatosensory perception [136], motor control [137, 138], and memory [127], matched to the synchronized oscillatory activity of cortical areas engaged in specific cognitive and motor processes recorded through EEG [139]. To date, CES laboratory studies of behavioral effects have not examined head-to-head possible differential CES device efficacy based on electrode placement, or any other specific configurations of stimulation parameters. However, in one recent study, at the theta frequency of 6.5 Hz, CES effects were hemisphere-specific for a risk-assessment task [140].

Radman et al. [141] pointed out that it is remarkable that a weak electric field such as that delivered by CES-like devices has the ability to entrain an oscillating brain network.

Abnormalities in oscillatory function have begun to be recognized in depression, schizophrenia, and other neuropsychiatric disorders. CES theoretically has the potential to reactivate hypoactive neuronal circuits or inhibit overactive circuits. In addition, CES may play a therapeutic role by counteracting deleterious, disease-related synchronization between subcortical structures interconnected with the cortex [16].

Evidence for Impact on Neurotransmitters, Hormones, and Endorphins

PET scanning could reveal brain-based changes in particular neurotransmitters' release and receptor availability as a function of CES stimulation. Although it is frequently suggested that CES raises brain endorphin levels, evidence supporting this assertion still is relatively weak, and primarily based on animal studies.

Two small uncontrolled human studies found increases in cerebrospinal fluid (CSF) beta endorphin and serotonin following CES stimulation [58, 142, 143]. Additional reports of CES-associated changes in urinary or blood plasma level of hormones, neuropeptides, and neurotransmitters, including serotonin, catecholamines, GABA, DHEA, human growth hormone (HGH), cortisol, beta-endorphin, and thyroxine [144–146] are likely to reflect pituitary or peripheral production of these neuromodulators rather than spillover from brain production. However increases in hormones which readily cross the blood brain barrier, such as thyroxine, could impact brain function [144] and peripheral release of neuropeptides could activate the brain through vagal afferents.

A number of animal studies implicate the endogenous opioid system in the analgesic effects of CES [36, 39, 40].

Further animal studies report CES effects on hormones and neurotransmitters [147, 148]. Warner and colleagues [147] found that serotonin (5-HT) was involved in analgesia induced by low current transcranial electrostimulation (TE), 10 mu-Amp, 10 Hz, pulsed current via electrodes in the rat ear, in a tail pressure paradigm. This involves putting progressively increasing pressure on the rat tail 1/4 in. from the tip with a pneumatically driven, right angle wedge. The amount of pressure at which the rat moved its tail was measured both before and after TE, or sham TE, and recorded as the difference in tolerated peak pressure (DTPP). TE produced analgesia as manifested by a 613 %

increase in DTPP compared with sham TE treatment values. Among TE-treated rats, pretreatment with pCPA (para-chlorophenylalanine, a synthetic amino acid which is a selective, irreversible inhibitor of tryptophan hydroxylase, a rate-limiting enzyme in biosynthesis of serotonin) decreased DTPP 91.5 % compared with saline control values, indicating 5HT involvement. 5HTP restored TE-induced analgesia in pCPA-treated rats to the level of saline treated control animals, confirming 5HT involvement. Warner et al. also reported [148] on anesthetized rats exposed either to a 10 Hz, 10 muAmp transcranial electrostimulation treatment (TCET) current for 30 min, via electrodes placed in the ears, or to 0 muAmp sham stimulation. Post-sacrifice, brain levels of several neurotransmitters and their metabolites were measured in selected homogenized brain areas by high performance liquid chromatography. Levels of norepinephrine (NE) and dopamine (DA) were significantly higher in the hypothalamic region of stimulated rats compared to control rats; midbrains of TCET rats contained significantly elevated levels of DA, MHPG (3-Methoxy-4-hydroxyphenylglycol, a metabolite of norepinephrine), and 5HT and 5HIAA (5-Hydroxyindoleacetic acid, the primary metabolite of serotonin); in the hindbrain no significant differences were observed. They did not find any change in serum endorphin levels which they suggest indicated that TCET-induced opioid activity may be confined to the central nervous system.

A small randomized trial of low-frequency (0.5 Hz) CES to try to improve the rest/activity pattern of patients with Alzheimer's disease did not find an effect of CES on salivary cortisol [149].

Evidence for Impact on Autonomic Nervous System

An open trial of CES for hypertensive subjects found an increase in heart rate variability during treatment with CES, suggesting changes in sympathetic and parasympathetic tone [60]. Many studies and consumer anecdotes report relaxation and meditation-like experiences, post-CES, which are in keeping with reduced sympathetic tone and increased parasympathetic tone [20, 88, 145, 146]. An increase in parasympathetic tone, or a decrease in sympathetic tone, could play a role in many of the proposed clinical benefits of CES, including improvements in insomnia, anxiety, and pain.

Whether or not CES methodologies can be developed to target specific brain areas, non-focal modulation of endogenous brain activity also may be an effective approach to depression treatment. ECT is non-focal, and investigators in Denmark have been conducting human clinical studies with a technology called T-PEMF [150, 151], a device using multichannel low voltage transcranial pulsed electromagnetic fields generated by seven coils (R/L anterior temporal, R/L posterior temporal, R/L parietal, and midline occipital) which has shown efficacy in treatment resistant depression [151]. Wires in a housing create a magnetic field orders of magnitude weaker than that generated by TMS; the neural impact of this stimulation is non-focal, similar to CES. Results show a statistically significant benefit for patients with treatment resistant depression treated with T-PEMF plus antidepressant medication [150, 151].

CES and Alternative Medicine

Since the beginnings of the alternative medicine movement in the USA in the 1960s, up to the present, some practices have been mainstreamed, such as acupuncture, meditation, and healthful dietary patterns, while others, including CES, have remained marginalized. The reasons for the failure of CES to enter the mainstream along with acupuncture, yoga, and meditation are not entirely clear but the relatively lower number of individuals, and physicians, aware of and using CES may be a factor. In addition, although we live in an era of ever-proliferating electronic gadgetry, both medical and nonmedical, which now extends to new brain stimulating devices, the decades-old negative reputation of ECT may have biased many against even much more gentle electrical devices to directly stimulate the head and brain. This bias against electrical devices may be receding as new knowledge reaches the alternative medicine community [152] and the wider public.

Of note, sometimes CES is linked to alternative and complementary medicine, and sometimes it is not. The National Center for Complementary and Alternative Medicine (NCCAM) of the National Institutes of Health (NIH) does not list CES as a therapy on its Web site. Perhaps this is because it is an FDA sanctioned device, because it does not fall into existing categories such as interventions derived from World traditional medicine systems, or is not seen as a "natural" treatment. The Wikipedia page for CES (http://en.wikipedia.org/wiki/Cranial_Electrotherapy_Stimulation), a primary source for many people researching the topic, lists it under the heading "Alternative medicine /fringe therapies."

The association of CES with alternative medicine also may have contributed to the relative lack of academic neuropsychiatric research interest over the past 50 years. CES has had longstanding acceptance within the alternative medicine community due to interest in therapies perceived to be gentler, less invasive, and more likely to support the body's endogenous systems and properties [153, 154], including Chi (Xi), the body's endogenous life force as understood in Chinese and other Eastern medical traditions [155].

Another factor contributing to the popularity of CES in the alternative medicine community is that it can be prescribed by non-M.D. practitioners, including nurses, acupuncturists, chiropractors, and psychologists, in contrast to pharmaceuticals and more invasive devices and procedures which require prescription by a physician. For medical professionals, even if CES might be helpful, this understandably raises the concern that non-physician practitioners will use CES for more severely ill individuals who would be better served by pharmaceuticals or more powerful electric or magnetic interventions.

A related issue is that CES, because of its minimal side effects, and availability to nonmedical practitioners, often has been applied to subclinical conditions, which have not been well characterized, and often fall outside diagnostic categories of conventional medicine. While this use is mostly not scientifically documented, patient testimonials and other information on company and alternative medicine Web sites and online communities offer evidence of benefit. In addition, many who are coping with hard-to-diagnose or treat conditions, such as withdrawal from addictive substances and fibromyalgia, have turned to CES and other alternative medicine approaches for symptom relief, for a sense of personal control, and to avoid side effects of mainstream treatments [151].

Rehabilitation medicine has long employed both mainstream and alternative low intensity, high frequency, alternating current devices for peripheral nerve stimulation, typically for pain relief, although their efficacy and optimal stimulation sites and parameters continue to be debated: e.g., transcutaneous electrical nerve stimulation at noncranial sites (TENS); implantation of subcutaneous electrodes or percutaneous electrical nerve stimulation (PENS); and electroacupuncture, a form of acupuncture in which a weak alternating electric current is passed between pairs of acupuncture needles [156]. Both PENS and electroacupuncture have been applied to sites on the head, which could be considered a form of CES stimulation as well.. Several trials of electroacupuncture for conditions such as depression are listed on the Web site Clinicaltrials.gov. Stimulated acupuncture points, via traditional needling and electroacupuncture, have been shown to activate diverse brain regions and physiological pathways detectable by brain imaging [156].

Ultimately, major reasons why CES has failed to garner mainstream interest comparable to that in tDCS, despite a century of evidence of therapeutic potential, are circular: the absence of large scale wellcontrolled clinical trials, systematic safety studies, and standardization of parameters of stimulation [155]; proprietary devices with patented frequencies that are not embraced by scientists; the mostly non-targeted nature of CES treatment and therefore non-focal brain effects, if any; and unclear mechanism(s) of action. In addition, because the existing CES devices are coming to the end of existing patents, there is limited motivation to invest in large-scale randomized clinical trials.

Interest in CES devices now may be increasing, as the effects of differing electrode configurations and stimulation parameters are investigated for their varied cranial nerve and brain stimulating effects, and as a new interest in therapeutic cranial nerve stimulation develops. Renewed interest in CES also is being swept along by greatly increased academic research interest in tDCS, and rTMS, which are subject to the current more stringent FDA efficacy and safety criteria for approval, and restricted to use by physicians.

Barriers and Future Directions

It is remarkable that CES has not gained traction in the world of modern brain stimulation research. This has continued to puzzle many, given considerable evidence that it may be therapeutically useful. Another major reason why CES never gained traction—companies were understandably concerned to market their "special patented" waveform, but this then greatly limits the interest of neural scientists. Commercial CES over many decades has been characterized by changing waveforms, as different devices were engineered and patented, therefore any safety and efficacy data applies only to the characteristics of that device, and to the specific dose used in a given study using a specific CES device [26, 158]. By comparison, tACS, where the waveforms are simple, i.e., constant sinusoidal alternating current and no special patented waveforms, allows for replication of studies using any tACS device or paradigm. Laboratory-designed tPCS stimulation similarly could be controlled and studied just as any other scientifically investigated protocol or device. Put another way—we cannot establish what CES does or does not do, until we can control what CES is.

While regulators (FDA) allow any similar low intensity AC device to call itself CES, to scientists these various devices are not the same and will have different neural and clinical impacts [26]. That said, increasingly there are valid scientific and clinical motivations to systematically study a range of low intensity electrical devices, and vary a range of stimulation parameters, using both constant (i.e., tACS) and pulsed (i.e., tPCS) alternating current stimulation, as well as DC stimulation (tDCS), and low intensity magnetic devices such as T-PEMF (Table 11.4).

It remains to be seen whether CES will attain the degree of scientific and commercial interest which has been focused on tDCS, which is undergoing continued

Table 11.4 Comparison of low-intensity electrical and magnetic brain stimulating devices: CES (tPCS; tACS), eTNS, tDCS, tPEMF

Stimulation device	Number of electrodes Stimulation sites	Stimulation type Current source Current type	Safety profile	Current intensity Duration of stimulation	Frequency	Proposed mechanisms of action	Clinical applications	Research applications
CES (Cranial Electrical Stimulation) tPCS; tACS (transcranial Pulsed Current Stimulation; transcranial Alternating Current Stimulation)	2, 3, or 4 Earlobes, mastoid processes, temples, other	*Electrical* AC Pulsed square wave or sinusoidal	Minimal side effects, adverse events (headache, itching, flickering lights)	0.5–16 mA *Home use* (various patented devices): 1–2×/day, 20–60"/day	0.5–15,000 Hz	Transcranial stimulation, cranial nerve stimulation Stimulate thalamus, subcortical areas, entrain endogenous brain rhythms: synchronize (single resonance frequency), desynchronize (several frequencies) Upregulate parasympathetic nervous system	*FDA sanctioned*: anxiety, depression, insomnia, pain fibromyalgia ? PTSD ?	CES—clinical studies (device-specific outcomes) tACS—modulate endogenous brain oscillations; modulate ANS
eTNS (external Trigeminal Nerve Stimulation)	1 or 2 Forehead supraorbitally	*Electrical* AC Pulsed	Minimal side effects, adverse events (headache, itching, irritation under electrode)	16 mA (*Cefaly*) *Home use* (*Cefaly*): 1×/day, 20"/day *Home use* (*Monarch eTNS*): 8, 12, 24 h/day	60 Hz (Cefaly) 120 Hz (NeuroSigma Monarch eTNS)	eTNS for epilepsy: mechanism not well understood; cranial (trigeminal) nerve stimulation: extensive connections w. *locus coeruleus* (LC), *nucleus tractus solitarius* (NTS), both involved in seizure initiation eTNS for migraine: relaxing effect of repeated stimulation of trigeminal nerve, diverse subcortical afferent pathways eTNS may share common pathways, mechanisms with vagus nerve stimulation (VNS)	*EU, Canada*: epileptic seizures, migraine headache depression ? other? [Cefaly may be available in US in 2014]	Clinical studies investigate trigeminal nerve pathways, mechanisms of action in depression, epilepsy
tDCS (experimental) (transcranial Direct Current Stimulation)	2 Anode, cathode at region of interest [and	*Electrical* DC	Occasional scalp burns, headache, itching; nausea	<1 mA–max 2 mA *Study*: 20" Wait 48 h before	N/A	Transcranial stimulation Anode—neural hyperpolarization Cathode—neural	? anxiety, depression, schizophrenia, cognitive enhancement (focus),	Clinical studies Investigate cortical function via TMS-like targeted

	multi-electrode HD-tDCS; MtCS]		(mastoid electrodes)	repeating stimulation		depolarization LTP, LTD	fibromyalgia, Parkinson's, post-stroke motor deficits, tinnitus	stimulation Investigate LTP, LTD, synaptic transmission; modifications of intracellular cAMP, calcium; protein synthesis
tPEMF (experimental) (transcranial Pulsed Electromagnetic Fields) [peripheral PEMF commercially available]	Plastic stimulation cap 7 coils connected in parallel w. pulse generator	*Magnetic* 220 V pulse generator; alternating magnetic field (+50 to −50 V) Induces electrical fields in tissue	Well tolerated, treatment-emergent side effects few and mild	*Study*: 30" daily	55 Hz	Stimulation below level of intensity that could cause depolarization; increase cortical excitability Increase receptor tyrosine kinase, effects on signal pathways controlling cell growth, metabolism, survival	depression ? [Peripherally: pain, bone and tissue healing, osteoarthritis, angiogenesis, increase microcirculation, enhance *in vitro* neurite growth]	Clinical studies investigate intracellular signaling, cortical excitability

technical development with an aim to target specific brain areas more effectively [134]. The ability to localize tDCS stimulation has made it more attractive to researchers. The degree to which transcranial CES/external and cranial nerve stimulation can have well-documented localized and therapeutically focal effects within the brain remains to be determined, as does the potential usefulness of deliberately using more generalized stimulation for therapeutic ends.

As of October 2013, searching Pubmed.org for "direct and current and stimulation and treatment and human and brain" yields 637 references, one quarter of them published in 2012–2013. Substituting "alternating" for "direct" yields only 40 references, 11 of them published in 2012–2013, although this particular search does not capture all CES papers in part due to the highly variable nomenclature for AC devices. Among the numerous publications for tDCS are several reporting positive results of double-blind randomized sham-controlled trials for depression [159], Parkinson's disease [160], epilepsy [161], memory function [162], and addiction [163]. Additional open label evidence exists for pain and fibromyalgia [164].

Although bioengineering modeling studies indicate that electrode placement can affect how CES impacts the brain with respect to which cortical and subcortical areas are stimulated, with what intensity and magnitude [15, 23, 165], it remains to be determined whether different electrode placements actually yield different clinical effects. In Fig. 11.3 above, schematic images depict one conventional CES electrode placement and several novel ones. Placement of CES electrodes bilaterally in the ear canal yielded, as one might expect, enhanced transcranial stimulation [15]. Even if CES stimulation has less potential for localization compared to tDCS, synchronization of brain oscillatory currents by CES may have unique therapeutic effects, such as ability to beneficially modulate aberrant CNS activity patterns, and enhanced anti-inflammatory and autonomic action. Much work needs to be done to identify any such generalizing neural and physiological effects of CES.

Despite remaining barriers, the future of minimally invasive, low intensity electric therapeutics looks bright. Bioelectronics is a rapidly developing collaboration among engineers, computer scientists, and biomedical scientists. Proponents envision more rapid development of new and potentially more effective electrical and magnetic therapeutics [86]. Medical treatment of the future increasingly may include what some now are calling electroceuticals, disease-specific low intensity electrical therapeutics designed as an alternative to pharmaceuticals ([86, 166]. The proliferation of neuromodulating devices may increase, not decrease, as some classes of devices become sub-specialized for specific therapeutic tasks and targets. CES devices recently developed (Cefaly®, Neuro Sigma Monarch eTNS™) to stimulate cranial afferents for relief of specific ills (migraine; epilepsy and depression, respectively) are an example. Modulating cranial nerves for narrow therapeutic purposes has been called the "low-hanging fruit" of the next generation of brain stimulation [86]).

Conclusion

In summary, CES variants and other low intensity brain stimulation technologies such as tDCS, tVNS and T-PEMF, may hold significant promise for the treatment of neuropsychiatric disorders. Given the proliferation of these devices, and unclear mechanisms of action, much work lies ahead to establish possible therapeutic rationales and roles for each of them in mainstream psychiatry, neurology, and rehabilitation medicine. Experimental and modeling studies are providing new insights into putative mechanism(s) of action of CES, which should shed light on pathophysiology of target conditions and at the same time help to refine CES device designs and treatment protocols. Rapidly growing interest, industry funding [167] and academic scientific involvement in investigating the so-called electroceuticals [86, 152] should hasten the emergence of better science and new understanding of the multiple ways therapeutic electricity can be used to modulate brain function [15, 23, 26].

If efficacy is established, CES could be an attractive primary or augmentation treatment for psychiatric and neurological conditions, with potentially fewer side effects than medications, and potentially lower cost than medications and more invasive forms of brain stimulation (ECT, TMS, VNS) , and psychotherapy. CES devices are inexpensive and can be used in the home, making this treatment approach relatively affordable and convenient. Because of low side effect burden and expense, CES may be very useful when it would be preferable to avoid use of medications, such as in the elderly, in individuals with substance abuse disorders, and for pregnant and nursing women. In addition to a possible role in treating diagnosed neuropsychiatric conditions, CES also may be useful for less disabling degrees of anxiety, depression, and insomnia, to help prevent clinical levels of illness from developing in the first place, and to help maintain remission. These potential therapeutic uses have not yet been studied.

In conclusion, a great deal more research on CES—mechanistic studies, well-powered, rigorously designed clinical trials, and studying updated technologies – is very much needed. All accumulated evidence to date would suggest it is very warranted.

References

1. Stillings D. A survey of the history of electrical stimulation for pain to 1900. Med Instrum. 1975;9:255–9.
2. Zaghi S, Acar M, Hultgren B, Boggio PS, Fregni F. Noninvasive brain stimulation with low-intensity electrical currents: putative mechanisms of action for direct current and alternating current stimulation. Neuroscientist. 2009;16(3):285–307.
3. Pavlov IP. Experimental psychology and other essays. New York: Philosophical Library; 1957.
4. Sergeev GV. The use of electrosleep in clinical medicine. Proceedings of the 1st International Symposium on Electrosleep and Electroanesthesia. 1967;1:115-120.
5. Robinovitch LG. Electrical analgesia, sleep, and resuscitation. In: Gwathmey JT, editor. Anesthesia. New York, NY: Appleton; 1914.
6. Anan'ev MG, Golubeva IV, Gurova EV, Kaschevskaia LA, Levitskaia LA, Khudyi YB. Preliminary data on experimental electronarcosis induced with apparatus of the Scientific Research Institute of Experimental Surgical Apparatus and Instruments. Anesthesiology. 1960;21:215–9.
7. Lebedev VP. [Transcranial electrostimulation: a new approach (experimental and clinical bases and equipment)]. Med Tekh. 1997;2:7–13. Article in Russian.
8. Lebedev VP, Malygin AV, Kovalevski AV, Rychkova SV, Sisoev VN, Kropotov SP, Krupitski EM, Gerasimova LI, Glukhov DV, Kozlowski GP. Devices for noninvasive transcranial electrostimulation of the brain endorphinergic system: application for improvement of human psycho-physiological status. Artif Organs. 2002;26(3):248–51.
9. Lebedev VP, Il'inskiĭ OB, Savchenko AB, Kolosova LI, Kovalevskiĭ AV, Tsirul'nikov EM, Rychkova SV, Malikhova MV, Aleksandrov VA, Gerasimova LI, Pavlov VA. [Noninvasive transcranial electrostimulation of endorphin structures of the brain as a reparation activator: experimental and clinical parallels]. Med Tekh. 2002;6:32–5. Article in Russian.
10. Lebedev VP, Bilichenko SV, Ordyan NE, Pivina SG, Nechiporenko SP, Puzyrev AA, Mikheeva EA, Kubacheva KK. Transcranial electrostimulation activates reparative regeneration and the insulin-producing function of pancreatic B-cells in alloxan diabetes in rats. Neurosci Behav Physiol. 2007;37(4):341–7.
11. Klawansky S, Yeung A, Berkey C, Shah N, Phan H, Chalmers TC. Meta-analysis of randomized controlled trials of cranial electrostimulation: efficacy in treating selected psychological and physiological conditions. J Nerv Ment Dis. 1995;183(7):478–84. Comment in, J Nerv Ment Dis. 1997 Dec;185(12):766–7.
12. Joy ML, Lebedev VP, Gati JS. Imaging of current density and current pathways in rabbit brain during transcranial electrostimulation. IEEE Trans Biomed Eng. 1999;46(9):1139–49.
13. Zaghi S, de Freitas RL, Machado de Oliveira L, El-Nazera R, Menning S, Tadini A, Fregni B. Inhibition of motor cortex excitability with 15 Hz transcranial alternating current stimulation (tACS). Neurosci Lett. 2010;479:211–4.
14. Lopes S, Davies N, Toumazou C, Grossman N. Theoretical investigation of transcranial alternating current stimulation using laminar model. Conf Proc IEEE Eng Med Biol Soc. 2012;4152–5.
15. Datta A, Dmochowski JP, Guleyupoglu B, Bikson M, Fregni F. Cranial electrotherapy stimulation and transcranial pulsed current stimulation: a computer based high-resolution modeling study. Neuroimage. 2013;65:280–7.
16. Lefaucheur JP. Principles of therapeutic use of transcranial and epidural cortical stimulation. Clin Neurophysiol. 2008;119 (10):2179–84.
17. Lefaucheur JP. Methods of therapeutic cortical stimulation. Neurophysiol Clin. 2009;39(1):1–14.
18. Limoge A, Robert C, Stanley TH. Transcutaneous cranial electrical stimulation (TCES): a review 1998. Neurosci Biobehav Rev. 1999;23:529–38.
19. Flemenbaum A. Cerebral electrotherapy (electrosleep): a review. Curr Psychiatr Ther. 1975;15:195–202.

20. Kennerly R. QEEG analysis of cranial electrotherapy: a pilot study. J Neurother. 2004;112–113.
21. Krupitsky EM, Burakov AM, Karandashova GF, Katsnelson JS, Lebedev VP, Grinenko AJ, Borodkin JS. The administration of transcranial electric treatment for affective disturbances therapy in alcoholic patients. Drug Alcohol Depend. 1991;27(1):1–6.
22. Journée HL. Electrical safety in intraoperative monitoring. Proceedings, Intraoperative Neurophysiology 2003, Symposium on Intraoperative Neurophysiology, with the 19th Dr. Janez Faganel Memorial Lecture, Oct 17–18, Ljubljana, Slovenia.
23. Datta A, Zhou X, Su Y, Parra LC, Bikson M. Validation of finite element model of transcranial electrical stimulation using scalp potentials: implications for clinical dose. J Neural Eng. 2013;10 (3):036018.
24. Alon G, Roys SR, Gullapalli RP, Greenspan JD. Non-invasive electrical stimulation of the brain (ESB) modifies the resting-state network connectivity of the primary motor cortex: a proof of concept fMRI study. Brain Res. 2011;1403:37–44.
25. Alon G, Yungher DA, Shulman LM, Rogers MW. Safety and immediate effect of noninvasive transcranial pulsed current stimulation on gait and balance in Parkinson disease. Neurorehabil Neural Repair. 2012;26(9):1089–95. Epub 2012 May 10.
26. Guleyupoglu B, Schestatsky P, Edwards D, Fregni F, Bikson M. Classification of methods in transcranial Electrical Stimulation (tES) and evolving strategy from historical approaches to contemporary innovations. J Neurosci Methods. 2013;219(2):297–311.
27. Wilson OB, Hamilton RF, Warner RL, Johnston CM, deFriece R, Harter L, Schweitzer C, Talaverra J, Hymel CM, Skolnick MH. The influence of electrical variables on analgesia produced by low current transcranial electrostimulation of rats. Anesth Analg. 1989;68(5):673–81.
28. Kirsch DL. The science behind cranial electrotherapy stimulation. 2nd ed. Edmonton, AL: Medical Scope; 2002.
29. Feusner JD, Madsen S, Moody TD, Bohon C, Hembacher E, Bookheimer SY, Bystritsky A. Effects of cranial electrotherapy stimulation on resting state brain activity. Brain Behav 2012;1–10.
30. Bai S, Loo C, Dokos S. A review of computational models of transcranial electrical stimulation. Crit Rev Biomed Eng. 2013;41:21–35.
31. Ferdjallah M, Bostick Jr FX, Barr RE. Potential and current density distributions of cranial electrotherapy stimulation (CES) in a four-concentric-spheres model. IEEE Trans Biomed Eng. 1996;43(9):939–43.
32. Gense de Beaufort D, Sesay M, Stinus L, Thiebaut R, Auriacombe M, Dousset V. Cerebral blood flow modulation by transcutaneous cranial electrical stimulation with Limoge's current. J Neuroradiol. 2011;39(3):167–75.
33. Feighner JP, Brown SL, Olivier JE. Electrosleep therapy. A controlled double blind study. J Nerv Ment Dis. 1973;157(2):121–8.
34. Gilula MF, Daniel L. Kirsch DL. Cranial electrotherapy stimulation review: a safer alternative to psychopharmaceuticals in the treatment of depression. J Neurotherapy. 2005;9(2).
35. Dougherty PM, Dafny N. Trans-cranial electrical stimulation attenuates the severity of naloxone-precipitated morphine withdrawal in rats. Life Sci. 1989;44(26):2051–6.
36. Mantz J, Azerad J, Limoge A, Desmonts JM. Transcranial electrical stimulation with Limoge's currents decreases halothane requirements in rats. Evidence for the involvement of endogenous opioids. Anesthesiology. 1992;76:253–60.
37. Wageneder FM, Iwanovsky A, Dodge CH. Electrosleep (cerebral electrotherapy) and electroanesthesia: the international effort at evaluation. Foreign Sci Bull. 1969;5:1–104.
38. Kavirajan HC, Lueck K, Chuang K. Alternating current cranial electrotherapy stimulation (CES) for depression. Cochrane Database Syst Rev. 2014;7, CD010521.
39. Auriacombe M, Tignol J, Le Moal M, Stinus L. Transcutaneous electrical stimulation with Limoge current potentiates morphine analgesia and attenuates opiate abstinence syndrome. Biol Psychiatry. 1990;28(8):650–6.
40. Stinus L, Auriacombe M, Tignol J, Limoge A, Le Moal M. Transcranial electrical stimulation with high frequency intermittent current (Limoge's) potentiates opiate-induced analgesia: blind studies. Pain. 1990;42(3):351–63.
41. Schoenen J, Vandersmissen B, Jeangette S, Herroelen L, Vandenheede M, Gérard P, Magis D. Migraine prevention with a supraorbital transcutaneous stimulator: a randomized controlled trial. Neurology. 2013;80(8):697–704.
42. DeGiorgio CM, Soss J, Cook IA, Markovic D, Gornbein J, Murray D, Oviedo S, Gordon S, Corralle-Leyva G, Kealey CP, Heck CN. Randomized controlled trial of trigeminal nerve stimulation for drug-resistant epilepsy. Neurology. 2013;80(9): 786–91.
43. DeGiorgio CM, Murray D, Markovic D, Whitehurst T. Trigeminal nerve stimulation for epilepsy: long-term feasibility and efficacy. Neurology. 2009;72(10):936–8.
44. Editors. Medgadget Sep 7, 2012 • 2:38 pm. http://www.medgadget.com/2012/09/neurosigmas-monarch-etns-system-for-epilepsy-depression-cleared-in-europe.html (2012). Accessed 5 Oct 2013.
45. Schrader LM, Cook IA, Miller PR, Maremont ER, DeGiorgio CM. Trigeminal nerve stimulation in major depressive disorder: first proof of concept in an open pilot trial. Epilepsy Behav. 2011;22 (3):475–8.
46. Fallgatter AJ, Neuhauser B, Herrmann MJ, Ehlis AC, Wagener A, Scheuerpflug P, Reiners K, Riederer P. Far field potentials from the brain stem after transcutaneous vagus nerve stimulation. J Neural Transm. 2003;110(12):1437–43. Epub 2003.
47. Kraus T, Hösl K, Kiess O, Schanze A, Kornhuber J, Forster C. BOLD fMRI deactivation of limbic and temporal brain structures and mood enhancing effect by transcutaneous vagus nerve stimulation. J Neural Transm. 2007;114(11):1485–93.
48. Kraus T, Kiess O, Hösl K, Terekhin P, Kornhuber J, Forster C. CNS BOLD fMRI effects of sham-controlled transcutaneous electrical nerve stimulation in the left outer auditory canal – a pilot study. Brain Stimul. 2013;6(5):798–804.
49. Bystritsky A, Kerwin L, Feusner J. A pilot study of cranial electrotherapy stimulation for generalized anxiety disorder. J Clin Psychiatry. 2008;69:412–7.
50. DeFelice EA. Cranial electrotherapy stimulation (CES) in the treatment of anxiety and other stress-related disorders: a review of controlled clinical trials. Stress Med. 1997;13(1): 31–42.
51. Barclay TH, Barclay RD. A clinical trial of cranial electrotherapy stimulation for anxiety and comorbid depression. J Affect Disord. 2014;164:171–7.
52. Overcash SJ. Cranial electrotherapy stimulation in patients suffering from acute anxiety disorders. Am J Electromed. 1999;16(1):49–51.
53. Schmitt R, Capo T, Boyd E. Cranial electrotherapy stimulation as a treatment for anxiety in chemically dependent persons. Alcohol Clin Exp Res. 1986;10(2):158–60.
54. Winick RL. Cranial electrotherapy stimulation (CES): a safe and effective low cost means of anxiety control in a dental practice. Gen Dent. 1999;47(1):50–5.
55. Koppolu SS, Kazariants G, Varvara M, McClure D, Yaseen Z, Lee AMR, Galynker I. A single blind, randomized, sham controlled study of Cranial Electrical Stimulation in Bipolar II disorder. Poster presented at the Annual Meeting of the American Psychiatric Association, May 10, 2013.

56. Hearst ED, Cloninger CR, Crews EL, Cadoret RJ. Electrosleep therapy: a double-blind trial. Arch Gen Psychiatry. 1974;30 (4):463–6.
57. Lyon DE, Schubert C, Taylor AG. Pilot study of cranial stimulation for symptom management in breast cancer. Oncol Nurs Forum. 2010;37(4):476–83.
58. Shealy CN, Cady RK, Wilkie RG, Cox R, Liss S, Clossen W. Depression: a diagnostic, neurochemical profile and therapy with cranial electrical stimulation (CES). J Neurolo Orthop Med Surg. 1989;10(4):319–21.
59. Danilova I, Orekhova E.[The use of sinusoidal modulated currents as a method of electrosleep] Russian. Vopr Kurortol Fizioter Lech Fiz Kult 6;1989.
60. Podzolkov VI, Mel'nikova TS, Suvorova IA, Churganova LI, Starovoĭtova SP. [Cranial electrostimulation–a new nondrug method of treating the initial stage of hypertension]. Ter Arkh. 1992;64(1):24–7. Article in Russian.
61. Lichtbroun AS, Raicer MC, Smith RB. The treatment of fibromyalgia with cranial electrotherapy stimulation. J Clin Rheumatol. 2001;7(2):72–8.
62. Koegler RR, Hicks SM, Barger JH. Medical and psychiatric use of electrosleep: transcerebral electrotherapy. Dis Nerv Syst. 1971;32:100–4.
63. Lande RG, Gragnani C. Efficacy of cranial electric stimulation for the treatment of insomnia: a randomized pilot study. Complement Ther Med. 2013;21(1):8–13.
64. Mousavi SA, Mirbod SM, Khorvash F. Comparison between efficacy of imipramine and transcutaneous electrical nerve stimulation in the prophylaxis of chronic tension-type headache: a randomized controlled clinical trial. J Res Med Sci. 2011;16:923–7.
65. Childs A, Price L. Cranial electrotherapy stimulation reduces aggression in violent neuropsychiatric patients. Prim Psychiatr. 2007;14:50–6.
66. Capel ID, Dorrell HM, Spencer EP, Davis MW. The amelioration of the suffering associated with spinal cord injury with subperception transcranial electrical stimulation. Spinal Cord. 2003;41:109–17.
67. Gabis L, Shklar B, Baruch YK, Raz R, Gabis E, Geva D. Pain reduction using transcranial electrostimulation: a double-blind "active placebo" controlled trial. J Rehabil Med. 2009;41:256–61.
68. Holubec JT. Cumulative response from Cranial Electrotherapy Stimulation (CES) for chronic pain. Prac Pain Manag. 2009;9 (9):80–3.
69. Mignon A, Laudenbach V, Guischard F, Limoge A, Desmonts JM, Mantz J. Transcutaneous cranial electrical stimulation (Limoge's currents) decreases early buprenorphine analgesic requirements after abdominal surgery. Anesth Analg. 1996;83:771–5.
70. Stanley TH, Cazalaa JA, Atinault A, Coeytaux R, Limoge A, Louville Y. Transcutaneous cranial electrical stimulation decreases narcotic requirements during neurolept anesthesia and operation in man. Anesth Analg. 1982;61(10):863–6.
71. Stanley TH, Cazalaa JA, Limoge A, Louville Y. Transcutaneous cranial electrical stimulation increases the potency of nitrous oxide in humans. Anesthesiology. 1982;57(4):293–7.
72. Rintala DH, Tan G, Willson P, Bryant MS, Lai ECH. Feasibility of using Cranial Electrotherapy Stimulation for pain in persons with Parkinson's Disease. Parkinsons Dis. 2010;2010:569154.
73. Eidelman WS. Control of cigarette cravings with cranial electrotherapy stimulation. The Townsend Letter for Doctors. 2009;311:81–5.
74. Gomez E, Mikhail AR. Treatment of methadone withdrawal with cerebral electrotherapy (electrosleep). Br J Psychiatr. 1978;134:111–3.
75. Overcash SJ, Siebenthall A. The effects of cranial electrotherapy stimulation and multisensory cognitive therapy on the personality and anxiety levels of substance abuse patients. Am J Electromed. 1989;105–111.
76. Patterson MA, Firth J, Gardiner R. Treatment of drug, alcohol and nicotine addiction by neuroelectric therapy: analysis of results over 7 years. J Bioelectr. 1984;3(1&2):193–221.
77. Patterson MA, Patterson L, Patterson SI. Electrostimulation: addiction treatment for the coming millennium. J Altern Complement Med. 1996;2(4):485–91.
78. Schmitt R, Capo T, Frazier H, Boren D. Cranial electrotherapy stimulation treatment of cognitive brain dysfunction in chemical dependence. J Clin Psychiatry. 1984;45:60–063.
79. Gall C, Sgorzaly S, Schmidt S, Brandt S, Fedorov A, Sabel BA. Noninvasive transorbital alternating current stimulation improves subjective visual functioning and vision-related quality of life in optic neuropathy. Brain Stimul. 2011;4:175–88.
80. Schmidt S, Mante A, Rönnefarth M, Fleischmann R, Gall C, Brandt SA. Progressive enhancement of alpha activity and visual function in patients with optic neuropathy: a two-week repeated session alternating current stimulation study. Brain Stimul. 2013;6 (1):87–93.
81. Gilula MF. Cranial electrotherapy stimulation and fibromyalgia. Expet Rev Med Dev. 2007;4(4):489–95.
82. Kirsch DL. Cranial electrotherapy stimulation: a safe and effective treatment for anxiety. Med Scope Mon. 1996;3:1–26.
83. O'Connell NE, Wand BM, Marston L, Spencer S, Desouza LH. Non-invasive brain stimulation techniques for chronic pain. Cochrane Database Syst Rev. 2010;9, CD008208. Review.
84. Piquet M, Balestra C, Sava SL, Schoenen JE. Supraorbital transcutaneous neurostimulation has sedative effects in healthy subjects. BMC Neurol. 2011;11:135.
85. DeGiorgio CM, Shewmon DA, Whitehurst T. Trigeminal nerve stimulation for epilepsy. Neurology. 2003;61(3):421–2.
86. Solon O. Electroceuticals. WIRED Magazine. 28 May http://www.wired.co.uk/news/archive/2013-05/28/electroceuticals (2013). Accessed Jul 22 2013.
87. Rosenthal SH, Wulfsohn NL. Electrosleep: a preliminary communication. J Nerv Mental Dis. 1970;151(2):146–51.
88. Schappi J. Aging and Parkinson's and me. http://parkinsonsand5htp.blogspot.com/2012/06/cranial-electrotherapy-stimulation.html(2012). Accessed Jul 24 2013.
89. Matteson MT, Ivancevich JM. An exploratory investigation of CES as an employee stress management procedure. J Health Hum Resour Admin. 1986;9(1):93–109.
90. Fisher-Wallace Labs. http://www.happyhalter.com/uploads/Brochure.pdf (undated).
91. Clarke N, Mills D, Marchant J. Evaluation of the potential efficacy of the Alpha-Stim SCS in the horse. Caythorpe, UK: De Montfort University Lincoln; 2000.
92. Taylor DN, Lee CT. Frequency-dependent effects of sine-wave cranial transcutaneous electrical nerve stimulation in human subjects. Acupunct Electrother Res. 1992;17(3):221–7.
93. Kirsch DL, Price LR, Nichols F, Marksberry JA, Platoni KT. Efficacy of Cranial Electrotherapy Stimulation for anxiety, PTSD, insomnia and depression: US Military service members and veterans self-reports. Poster presented at the Annual Meeting of the Chinese Society of Psychiatry; co-sponsored by the Chinese Medical Association, Psychiatry Branch of the Chinese Medical Association and the Nanjing Brain Hospital. October 18–21, Nanjing, Jiangsu Province, China; 2012.
94. Kirsch DL, Price LR, Nichols F, Marksberry JA, Platoni KT. Efficacy of cranial electrotherapy stimulation for anxiety, PTSD,

insomnia and depression: US M3litary service members and veterans self-reports. The Army Medical Dept Journal. 2014;(In Press).
95. Xenakis SN. It's time to move beyond the cliches. October 16 Huffington Post. http://www.huffingtonpost.com/brigadier-general-stephen-n-xenakis-md/veterans-ptsd_b_4099070.html (2013). Accessed Oct 17 2013
96. National Research Council (December 14, 1974, p. 42). Petitioner presentation to Neurological Devices Panel for reclassification of Alpha-Stim® CES devices from Class III to Class II. In: Alpha-Stim. http://www.alpha-stim.com/wp-content/uploads/EPIs-fda-presentation.pdf(2012). Accessed Aug 1 2013.
97. Tan G, Rintala D, Jensen MP, Richards JS, Holmes SA, Parachuri R, Lashgari-Saegh S, Price LR. Efficacy of cranial electrotherapy stimulation for neuropathic pain following spinal cord injury: a multi-site randomized controlled trial with a secondary 6-month open-label phase. J Spinal Cord Med. 2011;34(3):285–96.
98. Rose K, Taylor AG, Bourguignon C. Effects of cranial electrical stimulation on sleep disturbances, depressive symptoms, and caregiving appraisal in spousal caregivers of persons with Alzheimer's disease. Appl Nurs Res. 2009;2:119–25.
99. Pop J, Murray D, Markovic D, DeGiorgio CM. Acute and long-term safety of external trigeminal nerve stimulation for drug-resistant epilepsy. Epilepsy Behav. 2011;22(3):574–6.
100. Kanai R, Chaieb L, Antal A, Walsh V, Paulus W. Frequency-dependent electrical stimulation of the visual cortex. Curr Biol. 2008;18:1839–43.
101. Kanai R, Paulus W, Walsh V. Transcranial alternating current stimulation (tACS) modulates cortical excitability as assessed by TMS-induced phosphene thresholds. Clin Neurophysiol. 2010;121 (9):1551–4. Epub 2010 Apr 9.
102. Mellen RR, Mackey W. Reducing sheriff's officers' symptoms of depression using cranial electrotherapy stimulation (CES): a control experimental study. The Correctional Psychologist. 2009;41 (1):9–15.
103. Strentzsch JA. An examination of cranial electrotherapy stimulation (CES) on alpha-amylase levels, cortisol levels and state-trait anxiety scores in the chronically mentally ill. Doctoral dissertation. Saint Mary's University, San Antonio, Texas; 2008.
104. Little B, Patterson MA. Embryofetal effects of neuroelectric therapy (NET). Electro Magnetobiol. 1996;15(1):1–8.
105. Jordan JE, Morris D. Evaluation of the electrosleep machine. Dis Nerv Syst. 1975;36(12):661–5, 14.
106. Devanand DP, Dwork AJ, Hutchinson ER, Bolwig TG, Sackeim HA. Does ECT alter brain structure? Am J Psychiatry. 1994;151:957–70.
107. Weiner R, Lisanby SH, Husain MM, Morales OG, Maixner DF, Hall SE, Beeghly J, Greden JF, National Network of Depression Centers. Electroconvulsive therapy device classification: response to FDA advisory panel hearing and recommendations. J Clin Psychiatry. 2013;74:38–42.
108. Dwork AJ, Arango V, Underwood M, Ilievski B, Rosoklija G, Sackeim HA, Lisanby SH. Absence of histological lesions in primate models of ECT and magnetic seizure therapy. Am J Psychiatry. 2004;161:576–8.
109. MacDonald DB. Safety of intraoperative transcranial electrical stimulation motor evoked potential monitoring. J Clin Neurophysiol. 2002;19(5):416–29.
110. Iyer MB, Mattu MA, Grafman J, Lomarev M, Sato M, Wasserman E. Safety and cognitive effects of frontal DC brain polarization in healthy individuals. Neurology. 2005;64:872–5.
111. Brunoni AR, Amadera J, Berbel B, Volz MS, Rizzerio BG, Fregni F. A systematic review on reporting and assessment of adverse effects associated with transcranial direct current stimulation. Int J Neuropsychopharmacol. 2011;14(8):1133–45.
112. Nitsche MA, Liebetanz D, Lang N, Antal A, Tergau F, Paulus W. Safety criteria for transcranial direct current stimulation (tDCS) in humans. Clin Neurophysiol. 2003;114(11):2220–2.
113. Bikson M, Datta A, Elwassif M. Establishing safety limits for transcranial direct current stimulation. Clin Neurophysiol. 2009;120(6):1033–4.
114. Brunoni AR, Valiengo L, Baccaro A, Zanão TA, de Oliveira JF, Goulart A, Boggio PS, Lotufo PA, Benseñor IM, Fregni F. The sertraline vs electrical current therapy for treating depression clinical study: results from a factorial, randomized, controlled trial. JAMA Psychiatr. 2013;70:383–91.
115. Galvez V, Alonzo A, Martin D, Mitchell PB, Sachdev P, Loo CK. Hypomania induction in a patient with bipolar II disorder by transcranial direct current stimulation (tDCS). J ECT. 2011;27:256–8.
116. Kapural L, Narouze SN, Janicki TI, Mekhail N. Spinal cord stimulation is an effective treatment for the chronic intractable visceral pelvic pain. Pain Med. 2006;7(5):440–3.
117. Bartsch T, Paemeleire K, Goadsby PJ. Neurostimulation approaches to primary headache disorders. Curr Opin Neurol. 2009;22:262–8.
118. Brotman P. Low-intensity transcranial electrostimulation improves the efficacy of thermal biofeedback and quieting reflex training in the treatment of classical migraine headache. Am J Electromed. 1989;6:120–3.
119. Dymond AM, Coger RW, Serafetinides EA. Intracerebral current levels in man during electrosleep therapy. Biol Psychiatry. 1975;10:101–4.
120. Neuling T, Wagner S, Wolters CH, Zaehle T, Herrmann CS. Finite-element model predicts current density distribution for clinical applications of tDCS and tACS. Front Psychiatr. 2012;3:83.
121. Datta A, Truong D, Minhas P, Parra LC, Bikson M. Inter-individual variation during transcranial Direct current stimulation and normalization of dose using MRI-derived computational models. Front Psychiatry. 2012;3(91).
122. Greicius MD, Flores BH, Menon V, Glover GH, Solvason HB, Kenna H, Reiss AL, Schatzberg AF. Resting-state functional connectivity in major depression: abnormally increased contributions from subgenual cingulate cortex and thalamus. Biol Psychiatry. 2007;62:429–37.
123. Zhu X, Wang X, Xiao J, Liao J, Zhong M, Wang W, Yao S. Evidence of a dissociation pattern in resting-state default mode network connectivity in first-episode, treatment-naive major depression patients. Biol Psychiatry. 2012;71:611–7.
124. Posner J, Hellerstein DJ, Gat I, Mechling A, Klahr K, Wang Z, McGrath PJ, Stewart JW, Peterson BS. Antidepressants normalize the default mode network in patients with dysthymia. JAMA Psychiatr. 2013;70:373–82.
125. Perrin JS, Merz S, Bennett DM, Currie J, Steele DJ, Reid IC, Schwarzbauer C. Electroconvulsive therapy reduces frontal cortical connectivity in severe depressive disorder. Proc Natl Acad Sci U S A. 2012;3:5464–8.
126. Ali MM, Sellers KK, Fröhlich F. Transcranial alternating current stimulation modulates large-scale cortical network activity by network resonance. J Neurosci. 2013;33(27):11262–75.
127. Marshall L, Helgadóttir H, Mölle M, Born J. Boosting slow oscillations during sleep potentiates memory. Nature. 2006;444:610–3.
128. Schwiedrzik CM. Retina or visual cortex? The site of phosphene induction by transcranial alternating current stimulation. Front Integr Neurosci. 2009;3:6.
129. Schutter DJ, Hortensius R. Retinal origin of phosphenes to transcranial alternating current stimulation. Clin Neurophysiol. 2010;121(7):1080–4.

130. Schroeder MJ, Barr RE. Quantitative analysis of the electroencephalogram during cranial electrotherapy stimulation. Clin Neurophysiol. 2001;112(11):2075–83.
131. Zaehle T. Transcranial alternating current stimulation enhances individual alpha activity in human EEG. PLoS One. 2010;5: e13766.
132. Yanmin L, Guiqing Z. qEEG study on the treatment of ADHD with CES. Chinese Journal of Clinicians. 2011;5:2462–3. Electronic Edition.
133. Antal A, Boros K, Poreisz C, Chaieb L, Terney D, Paulus W. Comparatively weak after-effects of transcranial alternating current stimulation (tACS) on cortical excitability in humans. Brain Stimul. 2008;1(2):97–105.
134. Kuo H-I, Bikson M, Datta A, Minhas P, Paulus W, Kuo MF, Nitsche MA. Comparing cortical plasticity induced by conventional and high-definition 4 × 1 ring tDCS: a neurophysiological study. Brain Stimul. 2012;6(4):644–8.
135. Reato D, Gasca F, Datta A, Bikson M, Marshall L, Parra LC. Transcranial electrical stimulation accelerates human sleep homeostasis. PLoS One. 2013;9:e1002898.
136. Feurra M, Paulus W, Walsh V, Kanai R. Frequency specific modulation of human somatosensory cortex. Front Psychol. 2011;2:13.
137. Feurra M, Bianco G, Santarnecchi E, Del Testa M, Rossi A, Rossi S. Frequency-dependent tuning of the human motor system induced by transcranial oscillatory potentials. J Neurosci. 2011;31:12165–70.
138. Pogosyan A, Gaynor LD, Eusebio A, Brown P. Boosting cortical activity at Beta-band frequencies slows movement in humans. Curr Biol. 2009;19:1637–41.
139. Varela F, Lachaux JP, Rodriguez E, Martinerie J. The brainweb: phase synchronization and large-scale integration. Nat Rev Neurosci. 2001;2:229–39.
140. Sela T, Kilim A, Lavidor M. Transcranial alternating current stimulation increases risk-taking behavior in the balloon analog risk task. Front Neurosci. 2012;6:22.
141. Radman T, Datta A, Peterchev AV. In vitro modulation of endogenous rhythms by AC electric fields: syncing with clinical brain stimulation. J Physiol. 2007;584(Pt 2):369–70.
142. Kuzin MI, Avrutskiĭ MI, Shliuznikov BM, Lakhter MA, Panchenko LF. [Effect of transcutaneous transcerebral electrostimulation as electroanesthesia on the beta-endorphin content of the cerebrospinal fluid and blood plasma]. Biull Eksp Biol Med. 1984;97:515–6. Russian.
143. Shealy CN, Cady RK, Culver-Veehoff et al. Cerebrospinal fluid and plasma neurochemicals: response to cranial electrical stimulation. J Neurol Orthop Med Surg. 1988;18:94-97
144. Rosenthal SH. Alterations in serum thyroxine with cerebral electrotherapy (electrosleep). Arch Gen Psychiatry. 1973;28:28–9.
145. Liss S, Liss B. Physiological and therapeutic effects of high frequency electrical pulses. Integr Physiol Behav Sci. 1996;31 (2):88–95.
146. Liss S, Liss B. Modulated electric energy stimulators. Report presented at the American Academy of Pain Management Conference, Las Vegas, NV, Sep; 1999.
147. Warner R, Hudson-Howard L, Johnston C, Skolnick M. Serotonin involvement in analgesia induced by transcranial electrostimulation. Life Sci. 1990;46(16):1131–8.
148. Warner RL, Johnston C, Hamilton R, Skolnick MH, Wilson OB. Transcranial electrostimulation effects on rat opioid and neurotransmitter levels. Life Sci. 1994;54(7):481–90.
149. Scherder E, Knol D, van Someren E, Deijen JB, Binnekade R, Tilders F, Sergeant J. Effects of low-frequency cranial electrostimulation on the rest-activity rhythm and salivary cortisol in Alzheimer's disease. Neurorehabil Neural Repair. 2003;17 (2):101–8.
150. Bech P, Gefke M, Lunde M, Lauritzen L, Martiny K. The pharmacopsychometric triangle to illustrate the effectiveness of T-PEMF concomitant with antidepressants in treatment resistant patients: a double-blind, randomised, sham-controlled trial revisited with focus on the patient-reported outcomes. Depress Res Treat. 2011;806298.
151. Martiny K, Lunde M, Bech P. Transcranial low voltage pulsed electromagnetic fields in patients with treatment-resistant depression. Biol Psychiatry. 2010;68:163–9.
152. HMDI Editors. Heart MD Institute 08 April. http://www.heartmdinstitute.com/health-topics/alternative-medicine/99-electroceuticals (2010). Accessed 5 Oct 2013.
153. Ruggie M. Marginal to mainstream: alternative medicine in America. New York: Cambridge University Press; 2004.
154. Schneirov M, Geczik J. A diagnosis for our times: alternative health, from lifeworld to politics. New York, NY: State University Press of New York; 2003.
155. McCusker C. Cranial Electrotherapy Stimulation (CES), Chi, homeostasis, and the bioelectrical system. http://charlesmccusker.com (2005). Accessed Apr 22 2013.
156. Zhang Z-J, Wang X-M, McAlonan GM. Neural acupuncture unit: a new concept for interpreting effects and mechanisms of acupuncture. Evidence-based complementary and alternative medicine. 2012;2012(429412): 23 pages. Review.
157. Edelmuth RC, Nitsche MA, Battistella L, Fregni F. Why do some promising brain-stimulation devices fail the next steps of clinical development? Expet Rev Med Dev. 2010;7(1):67–97.
158. Peterchev AV, Wagner TA, Miranda PC, Nitsche MA, Paulus W, Lisanby SH, Pascual-Leone A, Bikson M. Fundamentals of transcranial electric and magnetic stimulation dose: definition, selection, and reporting practices. Brain Stimul. 2012;5(4):435–53. Review.
159. Martin DM, Alonzo A, Mitchell PB, Sachdev P, Gálvez V, Loo CK. Fronto-extracephalic transcranial direct current stimulation as a treatment for major depression: an open-label pilot study. J Affect Disord. 2011;134(1–3):459–63.
160. Fregni F, Boggio PS, Santos MC, Lima M, Vieira AL, Rigonatti SP, Silva MT, Barbosa ER, Nitsche MA, Pascual-Leone A. Noninvasive cortical stimulation with transcranial direct current stimulation in Parkinson's disease. Mov Disord. 2006;21:1693–702.
161. Fregni F, Otachi PT, Do Valle A, Boggio PS, Thut G, Rigonatti SP, Pascual-Leone A, Valente KD. A randomized clinical trial of repetitive transcranial magnetic stimulation in patients with refractory epilepsy. Ann Neurol. 2006;60:447–55.
162. Nitsche MA, Nitsche MS, Klein CC, Tergau F, Rothwell JC, Paulus W. Level of action of cathodal DC polarization induced inhibition of the human motor cortex. Clin Neurophys. 2003;114:600–4.
163. Boggio PS, Sultani N, Fecteau S, Merabet L, Mecca T, Pascual-Leone A, Basaglia A, Fregni F. Prefrontal cortex modulation using transcranial DC stimulation reduces alcohol craving: a double-blind, sham-controlled study. Drug Alcohol Depend. 2008;92:55–60.
164. Fregni F, Gimenes R, Valle AC, Ferreira MJ, Rocha RR, Natalle L, Bravo R, Rigonatti SP, Freedman SD, Nitsche MA, Pascual-Leone A, Boggio PS. A randomized, sham-controlled, proof of principle study of transcranial direct current stimulation for the treatment of pain in fibromyalgia. Arthritis Rheum. 2006;54:3988–98.
165. Dmochowski JP, Datta A, Bikson M, Su Y, Parra LC. Optimized multi-electrode stimulation increases focality and intensity at target. J Neural Eng. 2011;8(4):046011.
166. Famm K, Litt B, Tracey KJ, Boyden ES, Slaoui M. Comment: a jump-start for electroceuticals. Nature. 2013;496(7444):159–61.
167. Staff, medcitynews.com. GSK plans $1 M prize to jump-start "electroceuticals." Medcitynews, April 10, 2013 1:00 pm. http://medcitynews.com/2013/04/gsk-plans-1m-prize-to-jump-start-electroceuticals/(2013). Accessed Jul 22 2013.

The Mechanisms and Actions of Motor Imagery Within the Clinical Setting

12

Nicola E. Walsh, Louise Jones, and Candida S. McCabe

What Is Motor Imagery?

Motor imagery (MI) refers to the process of imagining a movement in the absence of either actual movement or execution of the mentally rehearsed task. It is a dynamic simulation of the performed action incorporating temporal, sequential, and biomechanical planning, which changes in content as the action is imagined over time [1, 2]. The mechanisms for imagining movements are diverse and described in terms of the modality and perspective of techniques employed. Modality refers to whether the emphasis is on visualisation of the action (seeing the movement happen), whereas kinaesthetic imagery focusses on the sensation of the movement, including balance mechanisms, force production and the effort of execution (feeling the movement happen) [3]. Visualisation can be further categorised according to perspective and whether the individual sees the movement in the first person, as if they were performing the action, or in the third person, where they are a spectator to the movement being performed either by themselves or somebody else [4]. Furthermore, MI may be "implicit", such as when judging the laterality of a photographed hand (see "Clinical application of MI" below), or "explicit", as when mentally evoking the action of a movement.

Neuroimaging work by Guillot et al. [5] has demonstrated that visual imagery activates the visual cortical pathways whilst kinaesthetic imagery predominantly involves the motor-associated regions and inferior parietal lobe. Previous research suggests that visualisation imagery is easier to perform, but kinaesthetic imagery may be more closely allied to actual movement processes [6]. From a clinical perspective a combination of these two processes may be appropriate.

MI was originally developed as a strategy to improve performance outcomes in sport [7, 8], and today is an accepted part of athletic training used to enhance specific motor skills and improve psychological factors such as confidence, focus, motivation and arousal [9]. Given the requirement of these physical and psychological traits in performance of "normal movement", MI is gaining recognition as a rehabilitation technique to assist motor recovery for movement dysfunction and as a pain management technique.

Neurophysiology of Movement Initiation

The ability to initiate and control motor function involves high-level neural processing and infinite sensorimotor interaction. The cerebral cortex acts as a "central processing unit" integrating information from our environment, previous experiences, sensorimotor feedback and action readiness, the consolidation of which forms the basis for movement initiation. Anatomically the cortex has subdivisions according to functionality, but it is the motor cortices of the frontal lobes, consisting of the primary motor cortex, premotor cortex and supplementary motor areas, that are directly responsible for voluntary movement tasks [10]. Figure 12.1 outlines the cortical areas primarily involved.

Primary Motor Cortex

Controls voluntary contractions, each muscular area is mapped out and represented according to the dexterity required within those muscles: The representative area of the hand for example, which performs fine finger movements, is significantly larger than that devoted to the large muscle

N.E. Walsh (✉) • L. Jones • C.S. McCabe
Faculty of Health and Applied Sciences, University of the West of England, Glenside Campus, Blackberry Hill, Bristol BS16 1DD, UK
e-mail: nicola.walsh@uwe.ac.uk

H. Knotkova and D. Rasche (eds.), *Textbook of Neuromodulation*,
DOI 10.1007/978-1-4939-1408-1_12, © Springer Science+Business Media, LLC 2015

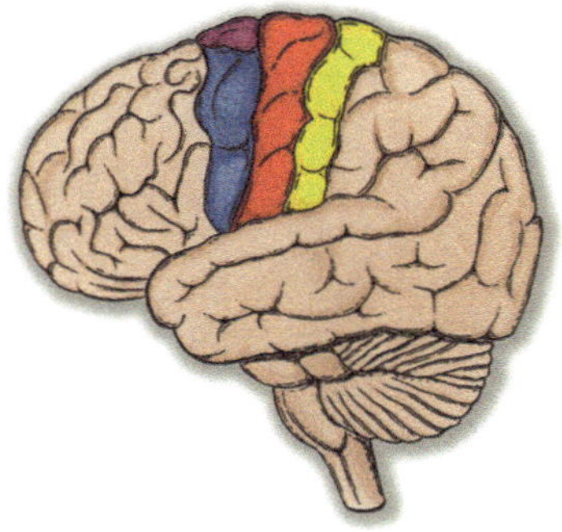

Fig. 12.1 Cortical representation of motor areas

groups of the thigh that have a gross rather than specific movement function. This area funnels considerable amounts of information to the spinal cord which initiates movement via descending tracts.

Premotor Cortex

A motor association area, involved in planning or programming of voluntary movements: The medial region is involved in tasks from memory (neurones here discharge in advance of the onset of self-initiated movement); the lateral area is involved in movement selection, particularly in conditional motor tasks involving visual cueing. Both are generally involved in selecting a movement or pattern of movements.

Supplementary Motor Areas

Involved in planning complex movements, and co-ordinating movements involving both hands: Movements are frequently not associated with the trigger of an external cue.

Other areas that also provide information for motor performance include the basal ganglia, limbic system, cerebellum and thalamus. Figure 12.2 outlines the interactions that occur between the systems to facilitate normal movement.

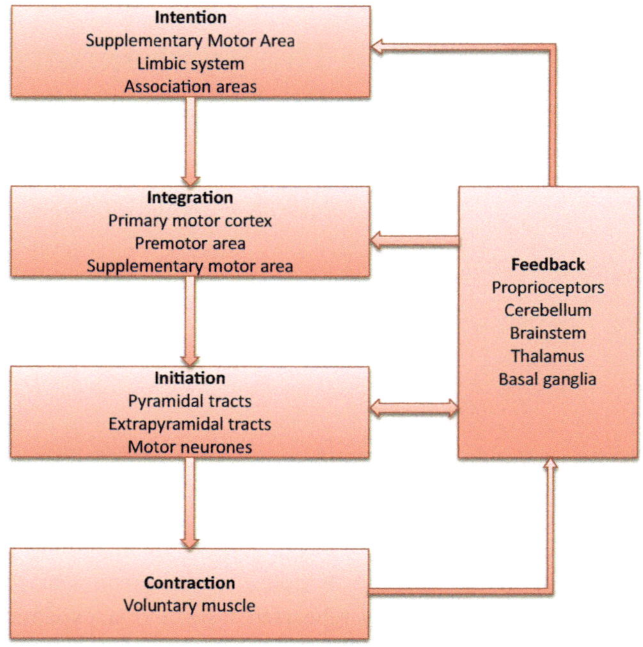

Fig. 12.2 Neurophysiological process of normal movement

Motor Imagery and Movement

Exactly how much of the above movement pathway is actually activated during MI remains unclear. Electroencephalography (EEG) and functional MRI (fMRI) studies have demonstrated that actual movement and MI share similar autonomic, temporal organisation and neural substrates. For example, those with a motor disorder, such as the bradykinesia exhibited in Parkinson's disease, demonstrate a mirroring of these motor problems when conducting MI, so their imagined movements are similarly slow [11]. Neuroimaging studies reveal significant cortical activity in the motor-related areas of the brain (e.g. the supplementary motor area and premotor cortex) when MI is performed, and in those areas required for motor execution (see [1] for review). Isochronicity between actual and imagined movements, even for complex tasks, is well known and in some studies used as a marker of motor imagery ability [12, 13]. Furthermore motor imagery tasks obey Fitts' law (the duration of a task requiring accuracy increases with the degree of accuracy) and share similar autonomic responses to execution [14, 15]. Neuroimaging techniques confirm these psychophysical findings, showing that comparable brain areas are activated during actual performance and mental rehearsal of the same tasks and support the notion of functional equivalence between movement execution and imagination [16].

However, MI involves the inhibition of movement and this inevitably leads to variation in neural patterns between movement performance and MI. Quite at what level this inhibition occurs is unclear but Guillot and colleagues [1] have proposed three possible routes: (1) as an integral part of mental representation; (2) suppression by cortical regions once the motor command has been constructed and (3) within the cerebellar and spinal networks. Electromyography (EMG) data has demonstrated peripheral muscle activation during MI, and although this activity is reduced compared to actual movement data, it provides evidence that inhibition is not complete [17–19].

Clinical Application of Motor Imagery (See Table 12.1 for Summary of Studies)

The potential therapeutic benefits of MI are thought to be associated with the activation of neural networks that are, as described above, remarkably comparable to those activated during physical execution. Recent reviews provide guidance on the elements most observed in successful interventions [20, 21]. Precisely how MI has a positive rehabilitative effect is unclear as there is no objective evidence to date of an association between activation of muscles during MI and improvement of motor performance [1]. However, recent research suggests that cortical disorganisation in the primary and premotor cortices, secondary to neuropathic and musculoskeletal pain, may be ameliorated through visualisation of motor patterns resulting in cell plasticity, neural reorganisation and subsequent enhanced sensorimotor function [22–24]. Rehearsal of movement in patients with movement dysfunction may help to reverse cortical changes resulting from inactivity via the recruitment of intact neurones, thus allowing earlier commencement of rehabilitation when little or no actual movement is possible [25, 26]. However, it should be noted that MI is not an innocuous intervention and has been shown to increase pain and oedema in some patients with chronic pain [27].

Clinical use of MI for functional rehabilitation post-stroke suggests that it improves motor processing and perhaps function, even in those with chronic symptoms (see [28] for review). Improvements have been found in acute, subacute and chronic stroke [29–33]. Similar improvements in motor performance with MI have been reported in those with Parkinson's disease [34, 35].

In addition to improvements in function, there is also evidence of MI improving chronic pain and aberrant cortical reorganisation [36–38]. MacIver and colleagues [36] demonstrated a reversal of cortical reorganisation, and a significant reduction in pain interference and intensity in 13 patients with amputee phantom limb pain after a 6-week motor imagery training intervention. In addition, all participants found MI to be a relaxing technique to undertake. MI has also been shown to reduce pain in complex regional pain syndrome (CRPS), a chronic pain condition of unknown aetiology with associated movement disorders that commonly affects a single limb [39]. MI is most commonly used for CRPS within a three-stage graded motor imagery programme (see below) designed to correct the individual's disrupted body schema, thereby reducing pain and disability [24, 40]. The positive results of motor imagery interventions may help to benefit other chronic pain conditions such as osteoarthritis where emerging evidence suggests that altered cortical activity is similar in nature to CRPS and phantom limb pain [41].

Graded Motor Imagery

Graded motor imagery (GMI) comprises three progressive stages. Devised by Moseley (2004), it is designed to improve cortical organisation [24, 40] and ultimately function. Research studies suggest improvements in pain and function in patients with CRPS and amputee phantom limb pain [24, 43]. However, further research regarding the application of GMI techniques within a routine clinical setting is required as a prospective clinical audit has demonstrated limited benefit using GMI for pain management in CRPS patients [42].

In the first stage of the GMI, the patient performs Parsons' left-right judgement tasks where they identify pictures of left or right hands or feet in a variety of orientations [44]. The left-right orientation of a hand is determined via the assimilation of the visual representation of the pictured hand and a proprioceptive representation of the observer's own hand. The calibration of this data evokes the perception of ownership, or movement if observing a moving imaging, by the observer and recognition of the laterality of that hand. This task is considered an example of implicit MI, though recent research by Viswanathan and colleagues [45] has challenged this, demonstrating an ability to evoke ownership and perceived movement in the "wrong" hand when the subject's attention is experimentally manipulated. The underlying principle is that an intact body image is required to undertake laterality tasks [40], and that rehearsal of such tasks will assist in facilitating an accurate cortical representation of their own body. Progress on to stage two is determined by accurate and pain-free recognition [46].

The progressive second stage requires the patient to visualise matching specific hand postures; they actively imagine moving the affected hand to match the orientation of a hand on a picture [24]. The goal is for the imagined movement to be pain free.

The third stage integrates mirror therapy into the programme. The affected hand is placed behind the mirror (or inside a "mirror box") and the unaffected hand positioned in front of the mirror. The patient is asked to move the unaffected hand and observe it in the mirror—the mirror provides the illusion that the affected hand is moving. Once the patient is able to perform movements with the unaffected hand pain free, the exercise can be progressed to perform the same movements with the affected hand whilst still observing the reflected contralateral hand in the mirror. This protocol differs somewhat from the original trial of mirror visual feedback for CRPS [47]. In this study, the participants performed bilateral synchronised movements at each time point. Subsequent research has demonstrated increased/new pain and reduced function in some participants when asynchronous movements are

Table 12.1 Studies addressing the clinical application of motor imagery

Patient group	Study	Participant numbers	Methodology	Outcome measures	Main findings
CRPS	Johnson et al. [43]	$n = 41$	Prospective audit Graded motor imagery (GMI) treatment in two clinical practices	Brief pain inventory Accuracy and response time of left-right hand judgements Function Hospital anxiety and depression scale	No improvement in pain with GMI Significant functional improvement with GMI at one practice
CRPS	Moseley [40]	$n = 20$	Randomised trial Graded motor imagery in different orders	Neuropathic pain scale (NPS) Function numerical rating scale	Significant improvement in pain and disability in hand laterality, imagined movements, mirror movement group compared to other groups
CRPS	Moseley [48]	$n = 13$	RCT 6-week GMI versus therapy	NPS	Significant improvement in NPS with GMI
CRPS or phantom limb pain	Moseley [24]	Control ($n = 26$) Intervention ($n = 25$)	Graded motor imagery versus physiotherapy	Function numerical rating scale. McGill pain questionnaire	Significant improvement in pain and function with GMI compared to control
Parkinson's disease	Braun et al. [65]	Control ($n = 22$) Intervention ($n = 25$)	RCT 6-week physiotherapy with relaxation versus 6-week physiotherapy with mental practice	Walking performance (VAS) Timed "up and go" 10 m walk	No significant difference
Parkinson's disease	Subramanian et al. [34]	Control ($n = 5$) Intervention ($n = 5$)	RCT Motor imagery with ×2 neurofeedback session versus motor imagery without neurofeedback	Unified Parkinson's disease rating scale (UPDRS) Finger tapping test Functional magnetic resonance imaging (fMRI)	Significantly increased movement speed during motor imagery with feedback compared to no feedback Significantly increased activity in the supplementary feedback area of the brain during motor imagery with neurofeedback
Parkinson's disease	Tamir et al. [35]	Control ($n = 11$) Intervention ($n = 12$)	RCT 1 h, ×2/week for 12-week physiotherapy versus physiotherapy with motor imagery	Timed sequence of movements Balance test UPDRS Cognitive tests	Significantly reduced bradykinesia with motor imagery group compared to control
Phantom limb pain	MacIver et al. [36]	Control ($n = 6$) Intervention ($n = 13$)	×6 1-h mental imagery sessions once a week or fortnight	fMRI Phantom limb pain questionnaire Vividness of imagery scale Pain	Significant reduction in pain and reversed neuroplasticity following MI training
Spinal cord injury	Cramer et al. [66]	Control ($n = 10$) Intervention ($n = 10$)	×2 60-min sessions per day for 7-day motor imagery training tongue and foot	fMRI Tapping test Transcranial magnetic stimulation	Significantly improved speed of movement in non-paralysed muscles Increased left putamen activation in SCI and control group
Stroke	Lee et al. [67]	Control ($n = 11$) Intervention ($n = 13$)	3 × 30-min treadmill training plus motor imagery versus treadmill training alone	Gait ability	Motor imagery significantly improved gait ability

(*continued*)

Table 12.1 (continued)

Patient group	Study	Participant numbers	Methodology	Outcome measures	Main findings
Stroke	Page et al. [29]	Control ($n = 8$) 20 min ($n = 8$) 40 min ($n = 6$) 60 min ($n = 7$)	RCT Comparison of 20-, 40- or 60-min taped mental practice sessions or no mental practice	Fugl-Meyer motor assessment (FMA) Action research arm test (ARA)	Significantly increased FMA score with increased treatment duration No significant effect of increased duration on ARA score Larger score changes on the FMA and ARA with mental practice
Stroke	Page et al. [30]	Control ($n = 5$) Intervention ($n = 6$)	RCT 30-min therapy ×2/week plus 30 mental practice delivered by tape versus 30-min relaxation delivered by tape for 6 weeks	Motor activity log ARA	Increased use of affected upper limb following mental practice Significantly greater change in ARA score in mental practice group
Stroke	Dijkerman et al. [31]	Control 1 ($n = 5$) Control 2 ($n = 5$) Intervention ($n = 10$)	4-week upper limb mental practice ×3/daily versus control group 1; imagery using pictures and control group 2; no imagery	Motor function Locus of control Attention ADL independence	All groups improved motor function Greater improvement in training task in motor imagery group
Stroke	Liu et al. [32]	Control ($n = 22$) Intervention ($n = 27$)	RCT ×5 1-h MI sessions/week for 3 weeks versus conventional functional training	Performance of 15 trained and five untrained tasks FMA Color trails test	Improved relearning of trained and untrained tasks in MI group compared with the control group
Stroke	Page et al. [33]	Control ($n = 5$) Intervention ($n = 8$)	RCT Mental imagery of ADLs delivered by tape; ×3/week at home, ×2/week in clinic versus taped stroke information	FMA ARA	Significant improvement in FMA and ARA in mental practice group compared to control

performed whilst viewing a mirror image [41, 49, 50]. Although mirror visual feedback is not a direct representation of motor imagery it does signify an important component of GMI.

Outcome Measures in Motor Imagery

The ability of an individual to use MI determines the effectiveness of its use in practice [51], as a subject who is unable or finds it difficult to engage in MI practice may not benefit from this form of therapy. The assessment of ability is particularly important in presentations such as stroke where subjects with parietal lobe lesions have been found to have MI impairment [52]. Various ways of assessing the ability to perform MI have been developed, each of which evaluates a different dimension of MI tasks.

Questionnaires

Questionnaires aim to establish the vividness of motor imagery [53] and are either self-administered or assessor led (Table 12.2). One of the earliest questionnaires was the Vividness of Movement Imagery Questionnaire (VMIQ) [54]. This 24-item questionnaire is commonly used in sport and involves the participant imagining movements such as jumping off a high wall or running downhill. Firstly the participant imagines that they are watching someone perform the movement, after which they imagine that they are performing the movement themselves. The vividness of the image is reported on a five-point scale (1 = clear and vivid as normal vision; 5 = no vision at all). The VMIQ originally intended to measure visual and kinaesthetic imagery; however a structured factor analysis suggested that it only measures the vividness of visual imagery [55]. Given the nature of the tasks included in this questionnaire its clinical utility is questionable.

The Revised Movement Imagery Questionnaire (MIQ-R), used in healthy adult populations to measure motor imagery vividness in the visual and kinaesthetic dimensions [56], was created as a revision of the earlier Movement Imagery Questionnaire (MIQ) [57]. In this self-administered questionnaire, the subject assumes a starting position and performs a movement after reading a description of the movement. After resuming the starting position,

Table 12.2 Outcome measures to determine the ability to undertake motor imagery tasks

Outcome	Population	Administration	Type of imagery measured	Type of measure
KVIQ	Stroke or physical disabilities	5-point scale	Visual and kinaesthetic	20-item assessor-administered questionnaire
KVIQ-10	Stroke or physical disabilities	5-point scale	Visual and kinaesthetic	10-item assessor-administered questionnaire
MIQ-R	Able bodied	7-point scale	Visual and kinaesthetic	8-item self-administered questionnaire
MIQ-RS	Stroke or physical disabilities	7-point scale	Visual and kinaesthetic	14-item self-administered questionnaire
VMIQ	Able bodied	5-point scale	Visual	24-item self-administered questionnaire
Laterality test	All	Orientation and reaction time	Accuracy	Mental rotation test
Temporal congruence	All (task dependent)	Timed	Timing	Mental chronometry
TDMI	All (task dependent)	Timed	Timing	Mental chronometry

the subject has to imagine the movement and report the ease or difficulty at which he or she could imagine the movement on a 7-point scale (7 = very easy to see/feel; 1 = very hard to see/feel). Due to the complexity of some of the tasks the questionnaire is unlikely to be suitable for affected populations.

More recently the Movement Imagery Questionnaire-Revised, Second Edition (MIQ-RS), has been developed to assess movement imagery in the stroke population [58]. The action of jumping was removed from the MIQ-R and eight functional items were added to the questionnaire. The questionnaire has been found to be both valid when compared to the KVIQ-10 and reliable with test–retest analysis ranging from 0.83 to 0.99 [59].

The Kinaesthetic and Visual Imagery questionnaire (KVIQ) has been specifically developed for people with physical disabilities [60]. As with the MIQ-R and MIQ-RS it measures visual and kinaesthetic dimensions in the first person perspective. The questionnaire consists of 20 different movements, split into 10 visual and 10 kinaesthetic subscales, which are performed in sitting. The subject is shown a movement and then asked to repeat. They are invited to answer questions regarding the clarity and intensity of the sensation of the movement on a five-point ordinal scale. Unlike the MIQ-R and the VMIQ, the questionnaire is not self-administered and can take up to 45 min to complete. A shorter KVIQ-10 was developed by the authors to reduce the completion time. Test–retest reliability in both the KVIQ and KVIQ-10 has been measured in healthy subjects and those who have sustained a stroke. A high level of internal consistency has been found. Bifactorial structure analysis indicates that the questionnaires do assess the two dimensions (visual and kinaesthetic) of motor imagery [60].

Mental Chronometry

Mental chronometry investigates temporal coupling between real and imagined movements [53]. Differences in timing between the two test conditions may indicate an inability to perform MI [61]. The Time Dependent Motor Imagery screening test (TDMI) records the number of a predefined movements performed over three different time periods (e.g., 15, 25, and 45 s). The TDMI indicates that subjects who are able to imagine an increase in the number of movements over an increase in time are able to understand instructions and perform motor imagery. Malouin et al. [62] confirmed reliability in a TDMI involving stepping in a seated position in both stroke and able-bodied subjects.

Temporal congruence tests record the duration of a number of real and imagined movements. This method of testing has been found to be reliable (ICC 0.77–0.97) in a test timing real and imagined five stepping movements whilst seated in both stroke and able-bodied subjects [62]. It is important to note that subjects who pass chronometric tests may have difficulty generating vivid imagined movements; therefore it is important to measure several aspects of motor imagery to gain an understanding of a person's ability [53].

Mental Rotation

Mental rotation tasks are thought to assess the accuracy of motor imagery performance [62]. One of the most common assessments is the laterality tasks where subjects are shown images of hands or feet in different orientations [44] and asked to determine whether it is a left or right hand or foot. The time taken to make a decision and the orientation is recorded. This method of assessment is also used as part of the GMI programmes as described above [24, 40].

In summary, there are many ways to assess the domains of MI. In a clinical setting it is best to consider several different aspects of motor imagery to gain a better understanding of an individual's ability to perform it prior to commencing with therapy [53].

Conclusion

Research to date suggests that MI is an important addition to the therapeutic "toolbox" of rehabilitation techniques. It can provide functional and analgesic benefits in selected populations and may yet prove to have benefit in other chronic pain groups where central mechanisms are thought to play a role, such as osteoarthritis. Furthermore, MI is "easy to learn and apply and is neither physically exhausting nor harmful" [63]. The therapeutic benefit of MI is thought to occur by training the neural correlates of movement without actual muscle contraction and therefore enhancing motor output without the deleterious effects of pain and fatigue [5, 64].

Further research is required to understand precisely which peripheral and central networks are engaged when MI is performed so as to better understand which conditions may be best helped by this technique. Furthermore, the relative novelty of MI training in rehabilitation means that training parameters have yet to be optimised, even in the conditions it has proven beneficial for. These successful trials of MI also demonstrate that MI is not beneficial or even practically possible for all, and may in some cases worsen pain and other symptoms. Therefore future research should focus on identifying the clinical phenotypes that gain most from MI and at what time point in a condition MI is optimal.

From a clinical perspective, MI is a potentially exciting new therapy which can deliver functional and analgesic gains in some chronic diseases that have proven intractable to more traditional interventions.

Acknowledgements N. Walsh is funded by an Arthritis Research UK Career Development Fellowship, L. Jones is funded by the Chartered Society of Physiotherapy Charitable Trust, and C. McCabe is funded by an NIHR Career Development Fellowship. Stephen Tate provided the original line drawing.

References

1. Guillot A, Di Rienzo F, MacIntyre T, Moran A, Collet C. Imagining is not doing but involves specific motor commands: a review of experimental data related to motor inhibition. Front Hum Neurosci. 2012. doi:10.3389/fnhum.2012.00247.
2. Jeannerod M. Motor cognition. What actions tell the self. Oxford: Oxford University Press; 2006. p. 21–44.
3. Callow N, Waters A. The effects of kinesthetic imagery on the sports confidence of flat-race horse jockeys. Psychol Sport Exerc. 2005;6:443–59.
4. Voisin JIA, Mercier C, Jackson P, Richards CL, Malouin F. Is somatosensory excitability more affected by the perspective or modality content of the motor imagery? Neurosci Lett. 2011;493:33–7.
5. Guillot A, Colles C, Nguyen VA, Malouin F, Richards C, Doyon J. Brain activity during visual versus kinaesthetic imagery: an fMRI study. Hum Brain Mapp. 2009;30:2157–72.
6. Stinear CM, Byblow WD, Steyvers M, Levin O, Swinnen SP. Kinesthetic, but not visual, motor imagery modulates corticomotor excitability. Exp Brain Res. 2011;168:157–64.
7. Richardson A. Mental practice: a review and discussion. Part I Research Quarterly. 1967;38:95–107.
8. Richardson A. Mental practice: a review and discussion. Part II Research Quarterly. 1967;38:264–73.
9. Weinberg R. Does imagery work? Effects on performance and mental skills. J Imagery Res Sport Phys Activ. 2008;3(1):1–21.
10. Rothwell JC. Overview of neurophysiology of movement control. Clin Neurol Neurosurg. 2012;114:432–5.
11. Dominey P, Decety J, Broussolle E, Chazot G, Jeannerod M. Motor imagery of a lateralized sequential task is asymmetrically slowed in hemi-Parkinson's patients. Neuropsychologia. 1995;33:727–41.
12. Schott N, Munzert J. Mental chronometry in the elderly. J Exerc Sport Psychol. 2002;24:109.
13. Malouin F, Richards CL, Desrosiers J, Doyon J. Bilateral slowing of mentally simulated actions after stroke. Neuroreport. 2004;15:1349–53.
14. Decety J, Jeannerod M. Fitts law in mentally simulated movements. Behav Brain Res. 1996;72:127–34.
15. Decety J, Jeannerod M, Durozard D, Baverel G. Central activation of autonomic effectors during mental simulation of motor actions in man. J Physiol. 1993;461:549–63.
16. Mulder T, de Vries S, Zijlstra S. Observation, imagination and execution of an effortful movement: more evidence for a central explanation of motor imagery. Exp Brain Res. 2005;344–351.
17. Lebon F, Rouffet D, Collet C, Guillot A. Modulation of EMG power spectrum frequency during motor imagery. Neurosci Lett. 2008;25:181–5.
18. Guillot A, Lebon F, Rouffet D, et al. Muscular responses during motor imagery as a function of muscle contraction types. Int J Psychophysiol. 2007;66:18–27.
19. Jowdy DP, Harris DV. Muscular responses during mental imagery as a function of motor skill level. J Sport Exerc Psychol. 1990;12:191–201.
20. Schuster C, Hilfiker R, Amft O, et al. Best practice for motor imagery: a systematic literature review on motor imagery training elements in five different disciplines. BMC Med. 2011;9(1):75.
21. Malouin F, Richards C. Mental practice for relearning locomotor skills. Phys Ther. 2010;90(2):240–51.
22. Beaumont G, Mercier C, Michon PE, Malouin F, Jackson PL. Decreasing phantom limb pain through observation of action and imagery: a case series. Pain Med. 2011;12(2):289–99.
23. De Vries S, Mulder T. Motor imagery and stroke rehabilitation: a critical discussion. J Rehabil Med. 2007;39(1):5–13.
24. Moseley GL. Graded motor imagery for pathologic pain: a randomized controlled trial. Neurology. 2006;67:2129–34.
25. Munzert J, Lorey B, Zentgraf K. Cognitive motor processes: the role of motor imagery in the study of motor representations. Brain Res Rev. 2009;60:306–26.
26. Mulder T. Motor imagery and action observation: cognitive tools for rehabilitation. J Neural Transm. 2007;114:1265–78.
27. Moseley GL. Imagined movements cause pain and swelling in a patient with complex regional pain syndrome. Neurology. 2004;62(1):1644.
28. Sharma N, Pomeroy VM, Baron JC. Motor imagery: a backdoor to the motor system after stroke? Stroke. 2006;37:1941–52.
29. Page SJ, Dunning K, Hermann V, Leonard A, Levine P. Longer versus shorter mental practice sessions for affected upper extremity movement after stroke: a randomized controlled trial. Clin Rehabil. 2011;25(7):627–37.
30. Page SJ, Levine P, Sisto S, Johnston MV. A randomized efficacy and feasibility study of imagery in acute stroke. Clin Rehabil. 2005;86:399–402.
31. Dijkerman HC, Letswaart M, Johnston M, MacWalter RS. Does motor imagery training improve hand function in chronic stroke patients? A pilot study. Clin Rehabil. 2004;18:538–49.
32. Liu KP, Chan CC, Lee TM, Hui-Chan CW. Mental imagery for promoting relearning for people after stroke a randomized controlled trial. Arch Phys Med Rehabil. 2004;85:1403–8.

33. Page SJ, Levine P, Sisto S, Johnston MV. A randomized efficacy and feasibility study of imagery in acute stroke. Clin Rehabil. 2001;15:233–40.
34. Subramanian L, Hindle JV, Johnston S, et al. Real-time functional magnetic resonance imaging neurofeedback for treatment of Parkinson's disease. J Neurosci. 2011;31:16309–17.
35. Tamir R, Dickstein R, Huberman M. Integration of motor imagery and physical practice in group treatment applied to subjects with Parkinson's disease. Neurorehabil Neural Repair. 2007;21:68–75.
36. MacIver K, Lloyd DM, Kelly S, Roberts N, Nurmikko T. Phantom limb pain, cortical reorganization and the therapeutic effect of mental imagery. Brain. 2008;131(8):2181–91.
37. Lacourse MG, Orr EL, Cramer SC, Cohen MJ. Brain activation during execution and motor imagery of novel and skilled sequential hand movements. Neuroimage. 2005;27(3):505–19.
38. Jackson PL, Lafleur MF, Malouin F, Richards CL, Doyon J. Functional cerebral reorganization following motor sequence learning through mental practice with motor imagery. Neuroimage. 2003;20(2):1171–80.
39. Harden RN, Bruelh S, Perez RS, et al. Validation of proposed diagnostic criteria (the Budapest Criteria) for Complex Regional Pain Syndrome. Pain. 2010;150:268–74.
40. Moseley GL. Is successful rehabilitation of complex regional pain syndrome due to sustained attention to the affected limb? A randomised clinical trial. Pain. 2005;1–4:54–61.
41. Cohen H, Harris N, McCabe CS. Distorting proprioception in patients with rheumatic diseases exacerbates sensory disturbances: further evidence for central pain mechanisms. Rheumatology. 2010;49(S1):i62.
42. Swart K, Stins JF, Beek PJ. Cortical changes in complex regional pain syndrome (CRPS). Eur J Pain. 2009;13:902–7.
43. Johnson S, Hall J, Barnett S, et al. Using graded motor imagery for complex regional pain syndrome in clinical practice: failure to improve pain. Eur J Pain. 2012;16(4):550–61.
44. Parsons LM, Fox PT, Downs JH, et al. Use of implicit motor imagery for visual shape discrimination as revealed by PET. Nature. 1995;375:54–8.
45. Viswanathan S, Fritz C, Grafton ST. Telling the right hand from the left hand: multisensory integration, not motor imagery, solves the problem. Psychol Sci. 2012;23(6):598–607.
46. Priganc VW, Stralka SW. Graded motor imagery. J Hand Therapy. 2011;24(2):164–9.
47. McCabe CS, Haigh RC, Ring EFR, Halligan PW, Wall PD, Blake DR. A controlled pilot study of the utility of mirror visual feedback in the treatment of Complex Regional Pain Syndrome (Type 1). Rheumatology. 2003;42:97–101.
48. Moseley GL. Graded motor imagery is effective for long-standing complex regional pain syndrome: a randomised controlled trial. Pain. 2004;108(1–2):192–8.
49. McCabe CS, Haigh RC, Halligan PW, Blake DR. Simulating sensory-motor incongruence in healthy volunteers: implications for a cortical model of rheumatology pain. Rheumatology. 2005;44:509–16.
50. McCabe C, Bodamyali T, Cohen H, Blake DR. Somaesthetic disturbances in fibromyalgia are exaggerated by sensory-motor conflict: implications for chronicity of the disease? Rheumatology. 2007;46:1587–92.
51. Hall CR. Imagery in sport and exercise. In: Singer RN, Hausenblas HA, Janelle CM, editors. Handbook of sport psychology. 2nd ed. New York, NY: Wiley; 2001. p. 529–49.
52. Sirigu A, Duhamel JR, Cohen L, Pillon B, Dubois B, Agid Y. The mental representation of hand movements after parietal cortex damage. Science. 1996;273:1564–8.
53. Malouin F, Richards CL, Durand A, Doyon J. Clinical assessment of motor imagery after stroke. Neurorehabil Neural Repair. 2008;22:330–40.
54. Isaac A, Marks DF, Russell DG. An Instrument for assessing imagery of movement; the Vividness of Movement Imagery Questionnaire (VMIQ). J Ment Imag. 1986;10(4):23–30.
55. Campos A, Perez MJ. A factor analysis study of two measures of mental imagery. Percept Mot Skills. 1990;71:995–1001.
56. Hall CR, Martin KA. Movement imagery abilities: a revision of the Movement Imagery Questionnaire. J Ment Imag. 1997;21:143–54.
57. Hall CR, Pongrac J. Movement imagery questionnaire. Faculty of Physical Education. London, ON: The University of Western Ontario; 1983.
58. Gregg M, Hall C, Butler A. The MIQ-RS, A suitable option for examining movement imagery ability. Evid Base Compl Alternative Med. 2010;7(2):249–57.
59. Butler A, Cazeaux J, Fidler A, et al. The movement imagery questionnaire-revised, second edition (MIQ-RS) is a reliable and valid tool for evaluating motor imagery in stroke populations. Evid Base Compl Alternative Med. 2012;2012:1–11.
60. Malouin F, Richards CL, Jackson P, Lafleur M, Durand A, Doyon J. The Kinesthetic and Visual Imagery Questionnaire (KVIQ) for Assessing Motor Imagery in Persons with Physical Disabilities: A Reliability and Construct Validity Study. Journal of Neurologic Physical Therapy. 2007;31(1):20–9.
61. McAvinue LP, Robertson IH. Measuring motor imagery ability: a review. Eur J Cogn Psychol. 2008;20(2):232–51.
62. Malouin F, Richards CL, Durand A, Doyon J. Reliability of Mental Chronometry for Assessing Motor Imagery Ability After Stroke. Arch Phys Med Rehabil. 2008;89:311–9.
63. Zimmermann-Schlatter A, Schuster C, Puhan MA, Siekierka E, Steurer J. Efficacy of motor imagery in post-stroke rehabilitation: a systematic review. J Neuroeng Rehabil. 2008;5:8.
64. Roosink M, Zijdewind I. Corticospinal excitability during observation and imagery of simple and complex hand tasks: implications for motor rehabilitation. Behav Brain Res. 2010;213:35–41.
65. Braun S, Beurskens A, Kleynen M, Schols J, Wade D. Rehabilitation with mental practice has similar effects on mobility as rehabilitation with relaxation in people with Parkinson's disease: a multicentre randomised trial. J Physiother. 2011;57:27–34.
66. Cramer SC, Orr EL, Cohen MJ, Lacourse MG. Effector of motor imagery training after chronic complete spinal cord injury. Exp Brain Res. 2006;177:233–42.
67. Lee G, Song C, Lee Y, Cho H, Lee S. Effects of motor imagery training on gait ability of patients with chronic stroke. J Phys Ther Sci. 2011;23(2):197–200.

Recommended Reading

68. Halpern SD, Ubel PA, Caplan AL. Solid-organ transplantation in HIV-infected patients. N Engl J Med. 2002;347(4):284–7.
69. Lorant J, Nicolas A. Validation of the French translation of the Movement Imagery Questionnaire-Revised (MIQ-R). Science Motricité. 2004;53:57–68.

Neuroprosthesis and Sensorimotor Training 13

Martin Diers

Introduction

An injury- or stimulation-related increase or decrease of sensory input into the brain leads to changes in the respective primary sensory and usually also the motor areas and these alterations can be associated with unpleasant sensations such as pain. In these disorders sensory or motor training seems to be useful and is increasingly employed. In this review we will focus on sensorimotor training in states of chronic pain such as phantom limb pain, complex regional pain syndrome, chronic back pain, or fibromyalgia. First, we will briefly describe cortical changes that are characteristic for these disorders and will then discuss sensorimotor training including stimulation methods and will focus on their effects, potential mechanisms, and future developments.

Brain Changes in Chronic Pain

Injury-Related Brain Changes in Neuropathic Pain Disorders

In persons with amputations it has been shown that the region of the somatosensory cortex that formerly received input from the now amputated limb reorganizes and receives input from neighboring regions [1–3]. These changes are mirrored in the motor cortex [4–7]. Interestingly, reorganizational changes were only found in amputees with phantom limb pain after amputation, but not in amputees without pain. This suggests that pain may contribute to the changes observed and that the persisting pain might also be a consequence of the plastic changes that occur. In several studies carried out on human upper-extremity amputee patients, displacement of the lip representation in the primary motor and somatosensory cortex was positively correlated with the intensity of phantom limb pain and was not present in pain-free amputee patients or healthy control subjects. In addition, in the patients with phantom limb pain, but not in the pain-free amputee patients, imagined movement of the phantom hand was shown to activate the neighboring face area [7]. This co-activation probably occurs due to the high overlap of the hand, arm, and mouth representations.

Similar observations have been made in patients with complex regional pain syndrome (CRPS). In these patients, the representation of the affected hand tended to be smaller compared with that of the unaffected hand, and the individual digit representations had moved closer together [8–12]. The extent of the pathological changes in the cortical representations correlated with the intensity of pain or motor dysfunction [10, 13, 14] but was additionally related to a degradation of sensibility in the affected hand. It was, however, unrelated to a loss of motor function [14]. It is so far not known how an expansion of adjacent representations and a shrinking of adjacent representations as observed in phantom limb pain and CRPS, respectively, can both be associated with pain. However, it is possible that a degradation of the representations resembles a reduction of representational areas, whereas an expansion and overlap is visible as enlargement.

Brain Changes in Musculoskeletal Pain Disorders

Not only decreased input related to deafferentation but also increased behaviorally relevant input related to non-neuropathic pain leads to changes in the cortical map or different processing of pain in chronic musculoskeletal pain syndromes such as chronic back pain (CBP) or fibromyalgia (FM) [15–21]. For example, Flor et al. [16] reported a close association between the chronicity of back pain and

M. Diers (✉)
Department of Cognitive and Clinical Neuroscience, Central Institute of Mental Health/Medical Faculty Mannheim, Heidelberg University, Mannheim, Germany
e-mail: martin.diers@zi-mannheim.de

H. Knotkova and D. Rasche (eds.), *Textbook of Neuromodulation*,
DOI 10.1007/978-1-4939-1408-1_13, © Springer Science+Business Media, LLC 2015

enhanced excitability and map expansion of the back representation in the primary somatosensory cortex in patients with non-neuropathic back pain. The back representation had expanded and shifted toward the leg representation the longer the pain had persisted. This was site specific since the hand representation was unaffected. Similar changes were reported by Giesecke et al. [17] using functional magnetic resonance imaging. Recently, Tsao et al. [19] observed a close interaction between changes in the motor cortex and postural control in patients with CBP suggesting an intricate interaction between peripheral and central traces of plastic changes related to chronic pain.

In patients with fibromyalgia greatly enhanced representations of painful stimulation were found. Gracely et al. [18] reported that comparable levels of subjectively reported painful pressure stimulation resulted in cerebral activation patterns that were similar in FM patients and healthy controls. However, similar stimulation intensities resulted in stronger activation in regions specific for pain processing in FM patients, supporting the hypothesis of augmented pain processing in FM patients. Cook et al. [22] examined painful heat stimuli (47 °C) to the nondominant thenar in patients with FM and healthy controls and observed activations in the primary and secondary somatosensory cortices, the anterior cingulate cortex, the supplementary motor area, and the insular cortex. Contrasts between both groups revealed significantly more activation for the FM group in the contralateral insular cortex. A repetitive injection of protons (low pH) and prostaglandin E_2 (PGE_2) in isotonic solution into the left extensor carpi radialis brevis muscle of FM patients revealed significantly stronger activation for FM patients in the left anterior insula and a more prolonged perception of pain compared to controls [23]. For perceptually equivalent pain ratings, FM patients failed to respond to pain provocation in the descending pain regulating system (the rostral anterior cingulate cortex) [24].

These changes were present in cortical activation maps as well as in areas involved in the affective and cognitive processing of pain [15]. Catastrophizing was found to be significantly associated with increased activity in brain areas related to anticipation of pain (medial frontal cortex, cerebellum), attention to pain (dorsal anterior cingulate cortex, dorsolateral prefrontal cortex), emotional aspects of pain (claustrum, closely connected to amygdala), and motor control when depressive symptomatology was controlled for [25]. Symptoms of depression and the presence of major depressive disorder were associated with the magnitude of pain-evoked neuronal activations in brain regions associated with affective pain processing (the amygdalae and contralateral anterior insula) [26]. Patients with major depressive disorder show hyperalgesia, but the hyperalgesia is more pronounced in FM and a deficit in pain inhibition is specific to FM [27, 28]. A recent study with 83 subjects showed that depressive symptoms, anxiety, and catastrophizing scores were correlated, but did not correlate with ratings of clinical pain or with sensitivity to pressure pain [29]. Brain activity during experimental pain was not modulated by depressive symptoms, anxiety, or catastrophizing [29]. The general and widespread nature of pain in FM suggests the involvement of central mechanisms via spinal and/or supraspinal modulation of experimental peripheral input. The exact interplay of pain, anxiety, depression, and catastrophizing needs to be further investigated and can be different in different subgroups of patients [30].

Interventions

Sensory and Motor Training

In amputees with phantom pain, several stimulation-related procedures were found to be effective. Intense input into the cortical amputation zone by the use of a myoelectric prosthesis or other prosthetic devices like a Sauerbruch prosthesis, for example, was found to reduce both cortical reorganization and phantom limb pain [31, 32]. By wearing a Sauerbruch prosthesis, the use of the amputation stump is increased and could produce a countervailing use-dependent, afferent increase [31]. A myoelectric prosthesis directly controls the prosthesis trough electromyography signals of the stump, increasing the efferent input into the stump [32]. The negative correlation between prosthesis use and phantom limb pain became nonsignificant when the effect of cortical reorganization was removed by partial correlation. This is interpreted that the phantom limb pain reduction is mediated by cortical reorganization [32]. In a longitudinal study Dietrich et al. [33] showed that a sensory feedback prosthesis effectively reduces phantom limb pain, modulated by visual and sensory feedback to the brain via the prosthesis, combining efferent input into the stump with afferent increase into the brain. The results of these studies suggest that muscular training and stimulation of the stump combined with visual feedback from the prosthesis might have a beneficial effect on maladaptive cortical reorganization and phantom limb pain. This is also in accordance with animal experiments which showed that the cortical representation of the stimulated body region expands through input from behaviorally relevant tactile stimulation [34, 35].

In patients in whom the use of prosthesis is not possible, sensory discrimination training might be beneficial. In one study, electrodes were closely spaced over the amputation stump in a region where stimulation excites the nerve that supplies the amputated portion of the arm (see Fig. 13.1). Patients then had to discriminate the frequency and location of the stimulation in an extended training period that lasted 90 min/day over a 2-week period. Substantial improvements

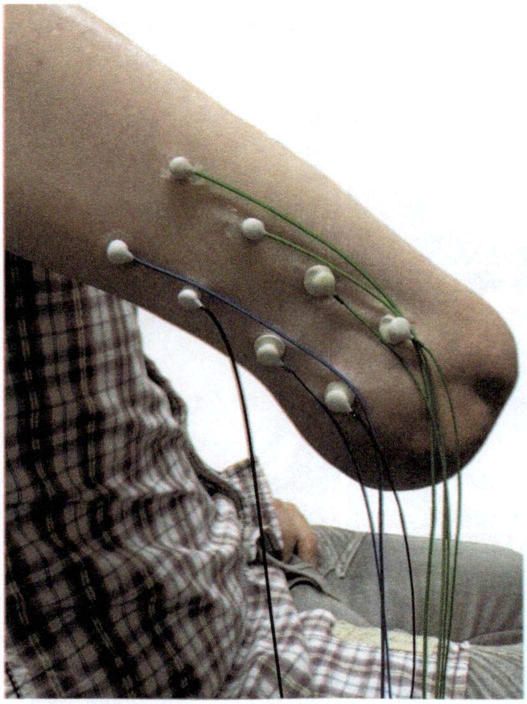

Fig. 13.1 Sensory discrimination training: four pairs of electrodes were closely spaced over the amputation stump in a region where stimulation excites the nerve that supplies the amputated portion of the arm. Patients then had to discriminate the frequency and location of the stimulation in an extended training period that lasted 90 min/day over a 2-week period [36]

to both two-point discrimination and phantom limb pain were demonstrated in the trained patients. These improvements were accompanied by changes in cortical reorganization, indicating a normalization of the shifted mouth representation [36]. An asynchronous stimulation of the stump and lip area also yielded a significant reduction in phantom limb pain suggesting that the separation of overlapping cortical networks involved in pain may be important [37].

Similar results were found in CRPS patients where active discrimination between tactile stimuli led to an improvement in pain intensity and two-point discrimination compared to passive stimulation alone [38]. When patients watch the reflected image of their unaffected limb during training, the effect of tactile discrimination training is enhanced [39]. Tactile spatial acuity also improved when a Hebbian stimulation protocol of tactile coactivation [40] was used. The question arises whether active stimulation is necessary or if passive stimulation is sufficient. In rats it could be shown that associative (Hebbian) pairing of passive tactile stimulation leads to a selective enlargement of the areas of cortical neurons representing the stimulated skin fields and of the corresponding receptive fields [41]. In humans paired tactile stimulation goes along with an improved spatial discrimination performance [41, 42] matched by alterations of the primary somatosensory cortex [43] indicating that fast

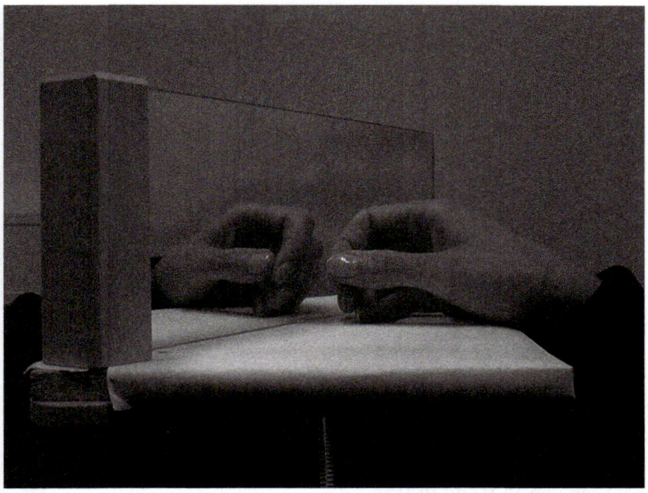

Fig. 13.2 Mirror box: viewing movements of one's intact hand in a mirror provides the impression of viewing the amputated or affected hand

plastic processes based on coactivation patterns act on a cortical and perceptual level. It is possible that in healthy controls passive stimulation without a task is sufficient for changes on the perceptual and cortical level, whereas patients, who are less able to discriminate stimuli [38, 40], may need active stimulation for an improvement in discrimination ability (and pain intensity). These training effects can be enhanced by the use of pharmacological agents. For example, two-point discrimination after a coactivation protocol was doubled by amphetamine and was blocked by a *N*-methyl-D-aspartate-receptor blocker [44], or lorazepam, a GABAA receptor agonist [45]. However, these pharmacological modulation effects are not easily translated into clinical practice. In stroke patients amphetamine showed mixed results [46].

Mirror and Motor Imagery Training

Ramachandran et al. [47] suggested that the use of a mirror might reverse the reorganizational changes observed in patients with phantom limb pain, and they provided anecdotal evidence that viewing movements of one's intact hand in a mirror, which provides the impression of viewing the amputated hand, led to better movement of and less pain in the phantom limb (see Fig. 13.2). In lower limb amputees Brodie [48] reported a significantly greater number of movements in the phantom when a mirror box was used. Hunter et al. [49] showed that a single trial mirror box intervention led to a more vivid awareness of the phantom and a new or enhanced ability to move the phantom. Contrasting a mirror box with executed movement, Brodie et al. [50] reported that movements in front of a mirror as well as movements without a mirror attenuated phantom

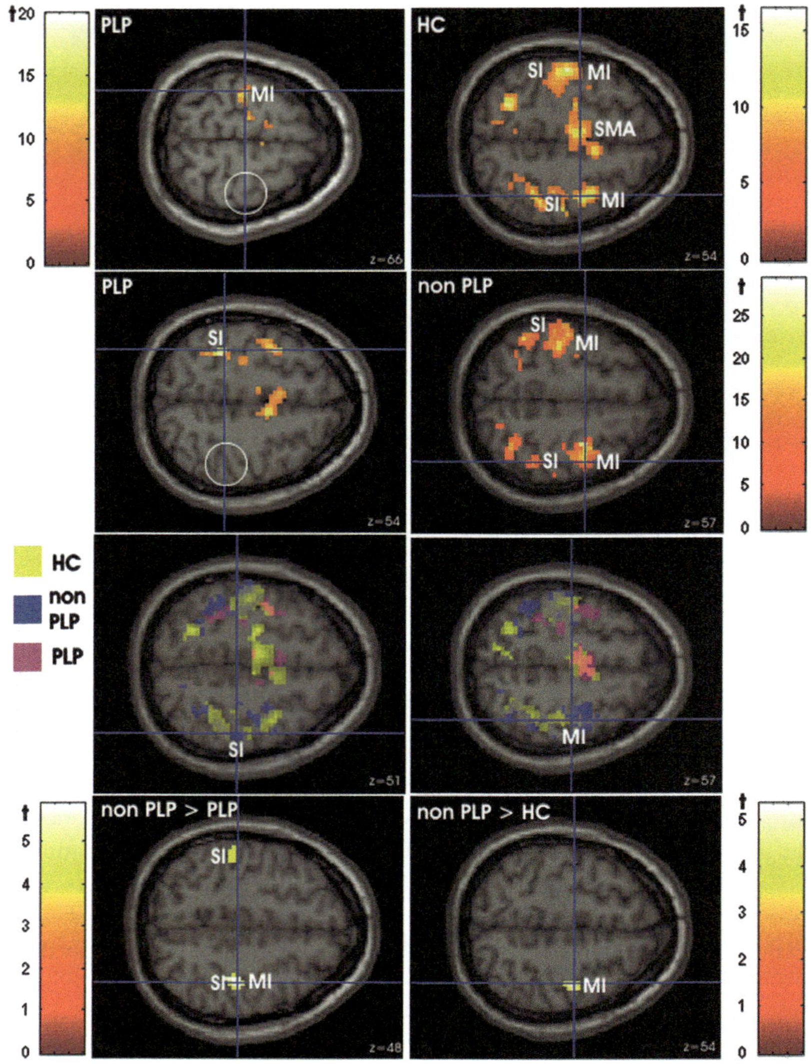

Fig. 13.3 Subjects executed movements with the right/intact hand. The reflection in the mirror showed a left hand. First and second rows show brain activations for amputees' with phantom limb pain (PLP) without PLP (non-PLP) and healthy controls (HC). The circles show the missing activation in the primary sensorimotor cortex in the PLP group. The third row shows overlays of these three groups. PLP failed to activate the primary somatosensory (SI) and primary motor (MI) cortices contralateral to the mirror image. The fourth row shows contrast between non-PLP and PLP as well as non-PLP and HC with differences in SI and MI contralateral to the mirror image. Montreal Neurological Institute (MNI) coordinates [54]

limb pain and phantom sensation. Contrary to these findings, which were based on a single trial, 4 weeks of mirror training led to significantly more decrease in phantom limb pain than training with a covered mirror or using mental visualization in lower limb amputees [51] suggesting that phantom pain can be altered by visual feedback. The visual system has a perceptual dominance in intersensory conflicts. The reason is the better spatial solution provided by vision compared to other senses (including touch) [38, 52, 53]. We recently observed in an fMRI session that amputees with phantom limb pain were unable to activate the sensorimotor cortex opposite to the amputated limb when the intact hand was moved in front of a mirror (appearing as movement of the phantom, see Fig. 13.3). A similar lack of activation was, however, also present with executed movements of the intact hand and with imagery of the phantom hand [54]. Moreover, phantom limb pain was inversely correlated with activation on the hemisphere contralateral to the amputation suggesting that mirror training may not be special [55].

Other reports on imagined phantom movements in amputees [7, 56–59] showed activation in the primary sensorimotor cortex representing the amputated limb in the pain-free amputees and the healthy controls but not in the patients with phantom limb pain [54] and were supported by results from transcranial magnetic stimulation (TMS), which showed that perceived phantom hand movement could be triggered by stimulation over the motor cortex in an area that represented the now amputated limb [60]. Both Giraux and Sirigu [61] and MacIver and colleagues [62] showed that imagery alone also affects the cortical map representing the amputated limb and relieves phantom limb pain in contrast to Chan and colleagues [51] who did not find changes in phantom pain related to imagery but did not assess cortical changes. These studies suggest that several types of modification of input into the affected brain region may alter pain sensation. For a review on the effects of mirrored and imagined movements, see [63].

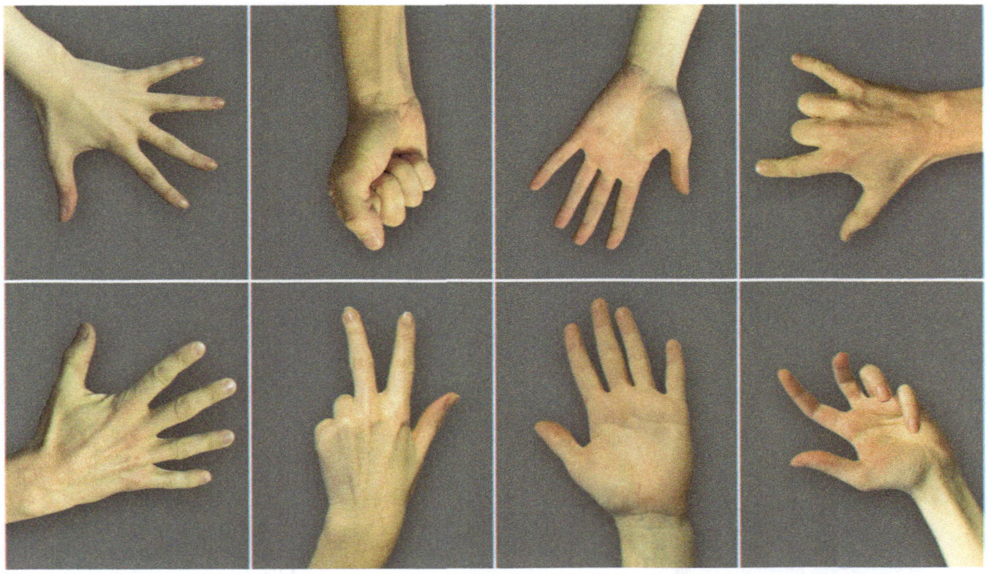

Fig. 13.4 The graded motor imagery consisted of a hand laterality recognition task, imagined hand movements, and mirror therapy. Displayed are examples of hand postures used in the hand lateralization task. Patients have to decide if the presented hand is a left or right hand [64]

Moseley used a tripartite program to treat patients with CRPS [64, 65]. This program consisted of a hand laterality recognition task (a pictured hand was to be recognized as left or right, see Fig. 13.4), imagined movements of the affected hand, and mirror therapy (patients were asked to adopt the hand posture of both hands shown on a picture in a mirror box while watching the reflection of the unaffected hand). After a 2-week treatment, pain scores were found to be significantly reduced. They replicated this result in CRPS and phantom limb pain patients [66]. In addition, McCabe and colleagues [67] found a reduction in pain ratings during and after mirrored visual feedback of movement of the unaffected limb in CRPS patients. Gieteling and colleagues [68] asked CRPS patients with dystonic postures of the right upper extremity to execute or imagine movements during a functional magnetic resonance (fMRI) measurement. Compared with controls, imaginary movement of the affected hand in patients showed reduced activation in the ipsilateral premotor and adjacent prefrontal cortex and, in a cluster comprising the frontal operculum, the anterior part of the insular cortex and the superior temporal gyrus. On the contralateral side, reduced activation was seen in the inferior parietal and adjacent primary sensory cortices. There were no differences between patients and controls when they executed movements, nor when they imagined moving their unaffected hand. Watching an enlarged view of the limb during movement significantly increased the pain and swelling evoked by movements while shrinking the view of the limb decreased pain and swelling [69]. These observations were interpreted as being due to a top-down effect of body image on the integration of incoming sensory information [69]. Transcranial motor cortex stimulation (TMS) contralateral to the CRPS-affected side has also been found to reduce pain intensities in CRPS [70].

Until now only little research has focused on mirror training, distorted body image, and cortical representations in chronic musculoskeletal pain. A recent study suggested the use of mirror training to treat fibromyalgia and found anecdotal evidence for reduced pain ratings [71]. In chronic back pain a disrupted body image and decreased tactile acuity, measured by two-point discrimination, in the area of usual pain was found [72]. Patients in this study reported that they could not find the outline of their trunk in the region of chronic pain. The larger two-point discrimination threshold in patients with chronic back pain could be positively related to worse performance on voluntary lumbopelvic movements, suggesting that a tactile acuity training might support recovery of normal motor performance [73]. In another study patients with chronic back pain participated on a left/right trunk rotation judgment task and a left/right hand judgment [74]. The patients made more mistakes and were less accurate in the trunk rotation task. No differences were found for the hand judgment task. This gives further evidence of a disrupted working body schema of the trunk in patient with chronic musculoskeletal pain. By visualizing the back in chronic back pain patients, it could be shown that seeing the back during repeated lumbar spine movements reduces movement-evoked pain [75]. This approach works not only for movements but also for visualizing one's own back on experimental pain perception at this site (see Fig. 13.5). Therefore, online video feedback of the back during painful stimulation of the trapezius muscle was implemented. Visual feedback of the back reduced perceived pain intensity compared to feedback of the hand in both chronic back pain patients and controls [76]. These findings suggest that multisensory modulation could enhance pain treatments as previously suggested [77–79] and may lead to novel intervention modes for chronic back

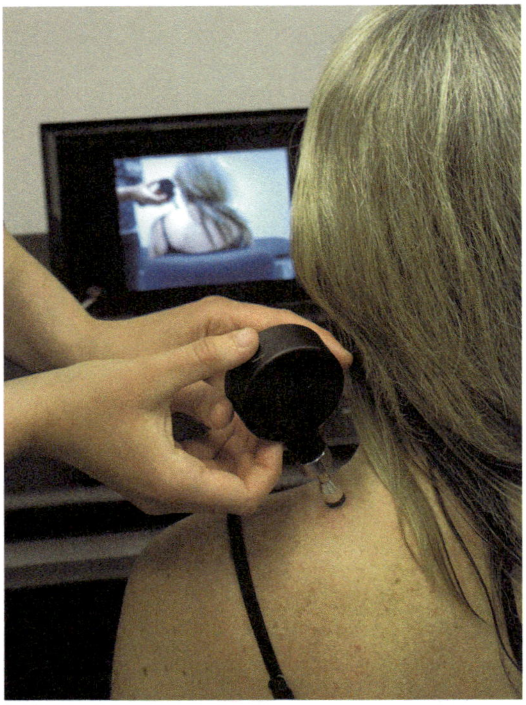

Fig. 13.5 Experimental setup of site-specific visual feedback: stimuli were applied to the upper back, while subjects watched the online image taken by a video camera placed behind them. Seeing the back reduces pain perception compared to seeing the hand [76]

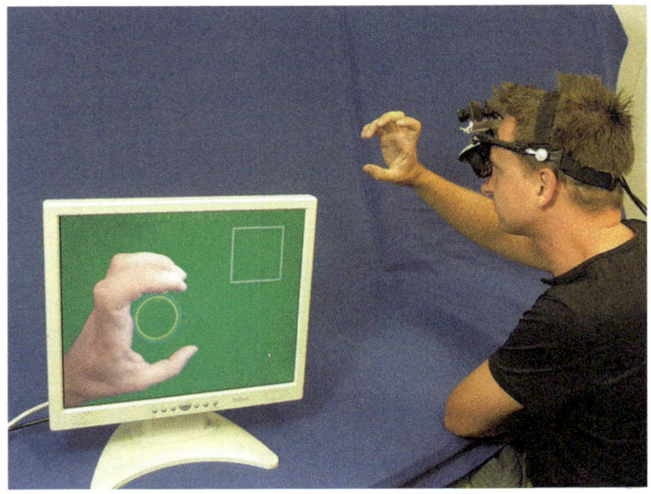

Fig. 13.6 Augmented reality mirror box: ball grasping task. The image shows a participant performing the tasks and an external screen, which is not part of the standard setup, showing the view presented to the head-mounted display [89, 90]. The subjects have to grasp a ball by forming a "C" with thumb and index finger and carry it to a quadratic target area

pain based on visualization of body parts by augmented reality applications.

In these disorders also another kind of visual feedback is used in behavioral treatments that focus on the extinction of pain behaviors and the acquisition of healthy behaviors. There video feedback of patients' pain behaviors and activity trainings as well as spouse trainings are used to extinguish pain and to increase healthy behaviors [80, 81] with concomitant positive brain changes [82]. Of particular interest was the activation in the insula which shifted bilaterally from a more anterior site before treatment to a more posterior location after treatment. The pre- to posttreatment reduction in both interference related to pain and pain severity were significantly associated with bilateral activation in pain-evoked activity in the posterior insula, the ipsilateral caudate nucleus/striatum, the contralateral lenticular nucleus, the left thalamus, and the primary somatosensory cortex contralateral to the stimulated side [82].

Virtual Reality Approaches to Mirror Training and Robotic Applications

Using a mirror box has some technical limitations. The intact limb has to move symmetrically with the mirrored limb. This is especially highly unnatural for the leg. This led to the invention of virtual reality (VR) and augmented reality (AR) mirror boxes (for a review see [83]). In a first approach the perceived phantom arm was presented on a flat screen in 3D and controlled via a wireless data glove on the intact arm [84]. The advantage of the VR mirror box was the possibility of incongruent movements between the intact hand with the data glove and the virtual phantom hand. For example, some of the virtual/phantom fingers were frozen and movements of the complete phantom led to more pain. The number of moved phantom fingers was thus gradually increased, and it came to a relaxation and less pain sensation in two of the three cases. A different approach used immersive virtual reality (IVR) to transpose the movements made by an amputee's remaining anatomical limb into movements of a virtual limb [85]. These authors found a reduction of phantom pain intensity in two of three cases [86, 87]. The advantage of this system is that the entire body is implemented in the IVR, and thus, complex hand-eye coordination is possible. A novel variation on this method is using motion capture to collect data directly from a patient's stump and then transform it into goal-directed, virtual action in the VR environment [88]. In a first experimental study with 14 patients, 72 % reported the ability to move the phantom and a reduction in phantom limb pain. Another possibility is an augmented reality home training systems. Here several training tasks could be implemented to make the training more exciting and increase the commitment of the patients (for an example of a task, see Fig. 13.6). Therefore, a head-mounted display equipped with cameras captures one hand held in front of the body, mirrors it, and displays it in real time [89–91]. These VR applications are promising and could be extended in the future. With the rubber hand illusion, it could be shown that the transfer of tactile sensations from the stump to a prosthetic limb by tricking the brain is possible [92]. This is an important contribution to the field of neuroprosthetics where a major goal is to develop artificial limbs that feel like a real part of the body. Another possibility is a flexible multielectrode implantation for multi-movement prosthesis control and sensory feedback. The multielectrodes were implanted in the median and ulnar nerves of an amputee and led to real-time control of motor output [93].

Conclusions

Based on neuroscientific evidence on alterations in the primary sensory and motor areas in sensory and motor disorders such as chronic pain, sensory and motor training methods have been developed. They include training of perceptual abilities, motor function, direct cortical stimulation, as well as behavioral approaches and have been shown to reorganize altered sensory and motor maps. The cellular mechanisms underlying these changes still need to be determined, but they involve changes in inhibitory circuits and long-term synaptic changes. In addition, treatments that combine several modalities such as imagery or mirror treatment as well as use of prostheses seem to have beneficial effects. Direct brain stimulation methods such as TMS or tDCS have also been employed successfully in these disorders. Further, much work still needs to be done to demonstrate the efficacy of these plasticity-related treatment approaches, which were usually tested in small heterogeneous samples without adequate controls and without adequate follow-ups. However, they may point out new approaches to treatment of chronic disorders and rehabilitation for the future. Future research should explore additional benefits which might arise from using brain stimulation methods in conjunction with behavioral trainings, virtual reality applications, or plasticity-modifying pharmacological interventions.

Acknowledgments The completion of this chapter was facilitated by a grant from the Deutsche Forschungsgemeinschaft DI 1553/3 and an Early Career Research Grant offered by the International Association for the Study of Pain as well as by the PHANTOM MIND project, which receives research funding from the European Community's Seventh Framework Programme (FP7/2007-2013)/ERC grant agreement no. 230249. This chapter reflects only the author's views, and the Community is not liable for any use that may be made of the information contained therein.

References

1. Elbert TR, Flor H, Birbaumer N, Knecht S, Hampson S, Larbig W, et al. Extensive reorganization of the somatosensory cortex in adult humans after nervous system injury. Neuroreport. 1994;5:2593–7.
2. Yang TT, Gallen C, Schwartz B, Bloom FE, Ramachandran VS, Cobb S. Sensory maps in the human brain. Nature. 1994;368 (6472):592–3.
3. Flor H, Elbert T, Knecht S, Wienbruch C, Pantev C, Birbaumer N, et al. Phantom-limb pain as a perceptual correlate of cortical reorganization following arm amputation. Nature. 1995;375 (6531):482–4.
4. Cohen LG, Bandinelli S, Findley TW, Hallett M. Motor reorganization after upper limb amputation in man. Brain. 1991;114:615–27.
5. Kew JJ, Ridding MC, Rothwell JC, Passingham RE, Leigh PN, Sooriakumaran S, et al. Reorganization of cortical blood flow and transcranial magnetic stimulation maps in human subjects after upper limb amputation. J Neurophysiol. 1994;72(5):2517–24.
6. Karl A, Birbaumer N, Lutzenberger W, Cohen LG, Flor H. Reorganization of motor and somatosensory cortex in upper extremity amputees with phantom limb pain. J Neurosci. 2001;21 (10):3609–18.
7. Lotze M, Flor H, Grodd W, Larbig W, Birbaumer N. Phantom movements and pain. An fMRI study in upper limb amputees. Brain. 2001;124:2268–77.
8. Juottonen K, Gockel M, Silen T, Hurri H, Hari R, Forss N. Altered central sensorimotor processing in patients with complex regional pain syndrome. Pain. 2002;98(3):315–23.
9. Schwenkreis P, Janssen F, Rommel O, Pleger B, Volker B, Hosbach I, et al. Bilateral motor cortex disinhibition in complex regional pain syndrome (CRPS) type I of the hand. Neurology. 2003;61 (4):515–9.
10. Pleger B, Tegenthoff M, Ragert P, Forster AF, Dinse HR, Schwenkreis P, et al. Sensorimotor retuning [corrected] in complex regional pain syndrome parallels pain reduction. Ann Neurol. 2005;57(3):425–9.
11. Maihöfner C, Handwerker HO, Neundorfer B, Birklein F. Patterns of cortical reorganization in complex regional pain syndrome. Neurology. 2003;61(12):1707–15.
12. Maihöfner C, Handwerker HO, Birklein F. Functional imaging of allodynia in complex regional pain syndrome. Neurology. 2006;66 (5):711–7.
13. Maihöfner C, Handwerker HO, Neundorfer B, Birklein F. Cortical reorganization during recovery from complex regional pain syndrome. Neurology. 2004;63(4):693–701.
14. Maihöfner C, Baron R, DeCol R, Binder A, Birklein F, Deuschl G, et al. The motor system shows adaptive changes in complex regional pain syndrome. Brain. 2007;130(Pt 10):2671–87.
15. Burgmer M, Pogatzki-Zahn E, Gaubitz M, Wessoleck E, Heuft G, Pfleiderer B. Altered brain activity during pain processing in fibromyalgia. Neuroimage. 2009;44(2):502–8.
16. Flor H, Braun C, Elbert T, Birbaumer N. Extensive reorganization of primary somatosensory cortex in chronic back pain patients. Neurosci Lett. 1997;224(1):5–8.
17. Giesecke T, Gracely RH, Grant MA, Nachemson A, Petzke F, Williams DA, et al. Evidence of augmented central pain processing in idiopathic chronic low back pain. Arthritis Rheum. 2004;50 (2):613–23.
18. Gracely RH, Petzke F, Wolf JM, Clauw DJ. Functional magnetic resonance imaging evidence of augmented pain processing in fibromyalgia. Arthritis Rheum. 2002;46(5):1333–43.

19. Tsao H, Galea MP, Hodges PW. Reorganization of the motor cortex is associated with postural control deficits in recurrent low back pain. Brain. 2008;131(Pt 8):2161–71.
20. Diers M, Koeppe C, Diesch E, Stolle AM, Hölzl R, Schiltenwolf M, et al. Central processing of acute muscle pain in chronic low back pain patients: an EEG mapping study. J Clin Neurophysiol. 2007;24 (1):76–83.
21. Diers M, Koeppe C, Yilmaz P, Thieme K, Markela-Lerenc J, Schiltenwolf M, et al. Pain ratings and somatosensory evoked responses to repetitive intramuscular and intracutaneous stimulation in fibromyalgia syndrome. J Clin Neurophysiol. 2008;25 (3):153–60.
22. Cook DB, Lange G, Ciccone DS, Liu WC, Steffener J, Natelson BH. Functional imaging of pain in patients with primary fibromyalgia. J Rheumatol. 2004;31(2):364–78.
23. Diers M, Schley MT, Rance M, Yilmaz P, Lauer L, Rukwied R, et al. Differential central pain processing following repetitive intramuscular proton/prostaglandin E(2) injections in female fibromyalgia patients and healthy controls. Eur J Pain. 2011;15(7):716–23.
24. Jensen KB, Kosek E, Petzke F, Carville S, Fransson P, Marcus H, et al. Evidence of dysfunctional pain inhibition in Fibromyalgia reflected in rACC during provoked pain. Pain. 2009;144 (1–2):95–100.
25. Gracely RH, Geisser ME, Giesecke T, Grant MA, Petzke F, Williams DA, et al. Pain catastrophizing and neural responses to pain among persons with fibromyalgia. Brain. 2004;127(Pt 4):835–43.
26. Giesecke T, Gracely RH, Williams DA, Geisser ME, Petzke FW, Clauw DJ. The relationship between depression, clinical pain, and experimental pain in a chronic pain cohort. Arthritis Rheum. 2005;52(5):1577–84.
27. de Souza JB, Potvin S, Goffaux P, Charest J, Marchand S. The deficit of pain inhibition in fibromyalgia is more pronounced in patients with comorbid depressive symptoms. Clin J Pain. 2009;25 (2):123–7.
28. Normand E, Potvin S, Gaumond I, Cloutier G, Corbin JF, Marchand S. Pain inhibition is deficient in chronic widespread pain but normal in major depressive disorder. J Clin Psychiatry. 2010;72:219–24.
29. Jensen KB, Petzke F, Carville S, Fransson P, Marcus H, Williams SC, et al. Anxiety and depressive symptoms in Fibromyalgia are related to low health esteem but not to pain sensitivity or cerebral processing of pain. Arthritis Rheum. 2010;62:3488–95.
30. Flor H, Turk DC. Chronic pain. An integrated biobehavioral approach. Seattle: IASP Press; 2011.
31. Weiss T, Miltner WH, Adler T, Bruckner L, Taub E. Decrease in phantom limb pain associated with prosthesis-induced increased use of an amputation stump in humans. Neurosci Lett. 1999;272 (2):131–4.
32. Lotze M, Grodd W, Birbaumer N, Erb M, Huse E, Flor H. Does use of a myoelectric prostesis prevent cortical reorganisation and phantom limb pain? Nat Neurosci. 1999;2(6):501–2.
33. Dietrich C, Walter-Walsh K, Preissler S, Hofmann GO, Witte OW, Miltner WH, et al. Sensory feedback prosthesis reduces phantom limb pain: proof of a principle. Neurosci Lett. 2012;507(2):97–100.
34. Jenkins WM, Merzenich MM, Ochs MT, Allard T, Guic-Robles E. Functional reorganization of primary somatosensory cortex in adult owl monkeys after behaviorally controlled tactile stimulation. J Neurophysiol. 1990;63(1):82–104.
35. Recanzone GH, Merzenich MM, Jenkins WM, Grajski KA, Dinse HR. Topographic reorganization of the hand representation in cortical area 3b owl monkeys trained in a frequency-discrimination task. J Neurophysiol. 1992;67(5):1031–56.
36. Flor H, Denke C, Schaefer M, Grüsser S. Effect of sensory discrimination training on cortical reorganisation and phantom limb pain. Lancet. 2001;375:1763–4.
37. Huse E, Preissl H, Larbig W, Birbaumer N. Phantom limb pain. Lancet. 2001;358(9286):1015.
38. Moseley GL, Zalucki NM, Wiech K. Tactile discrimination, but not tactile stimulation alone, reduces chronic limb pain. Pain. 2008;137 (3):600–8.
39. Moseley GL, Wiech K. The effect of tactile discrimination training is enhanced when patients watch the reflected image of their unaffected limb during training. Pain. 2009;144(3):314–9.
40. Maihöfner C, DeCol R. Decreased perceptual learning ability in complex regional pain syndrome. Eur J Pain. 2007;11(8):903–9.
41. Godde B, Spengler F, Dinse HR. Associative pairing of tactile stimulation induces somatosensory cortical reorganization in rats and humans. Neuroreport. 1996;8(1):281–5.
42. Godde B, Stauffenberg B, Spengler F, Dinse HR. Tactile coactivation-induced changes in spatial discrimination performance. J Neurosci. 2000;20(4):1597–604.
43. Godde B, Ehrhardt J, Braun C. Behavioral significance of input-dependent plasticity of human somatosensory cortex. Neuroreport. 2003;14(4):543–6.
44. Dinse HR, Ragert P, Pleger B, Schwenkreis P, Tegenthoff M. Pharmacological modulation of perceptual learning and associated cortical reorganization. Science. 2003;301(5629):91–4.
45. Dinse HR, Ragert P, Pleger B, Schwenkreis P, Tegenthoff M. GABAergic mechanisms gate tactile discrimination learning. Neuroreport. 2003;14(13):1747–51.
46. Carter AR, Connor LT, Dromerick AW. Rehabilitation after stroke: current state of the science. Curr Neurol Neurosci Rep. 2010;10 (3):158–66.
47. Ramachandran VS, Rogers Ramachandran D, Cobb S. Touching the phantom limb. Nature. 1995;377(6549):489–90.
48. Brodie EE, Whyte A, Waller B. Increased motor control of a phantom leg in humans results from the visual feedback of a virtual leg. Neurosci Lett. 2003;341(2):167–9.
49. Hunter JP, Katz J, Davis KD. The effect of tactile and visual sensory inputs on phantom limb awareness. Brain. 2003;126(Pt 3):579–89.
50. Brodie EE, Whyte A, Niven CA. Analgesia through the looking-glass? A randomized controlled trial investigating the effect of viewing a "virtual" limb upon phantom limb pain, sensation and movement. Eur J Pain. 2007;11(4):428–36.
51. Chan BL, Witt R, Charrow AP, Magee A, Howard R, Pasquina PF, et al. Mirror therapy for phantom limb pain. N Engl J Med. 2007;357(21):2206–7.
52. Rock I, Victor J. Vision and touch: an experimentally created conflict between the two senses. Science. 1964;143:594–6.
53. Halligan PW, Hunt M, Marshall JC, Wade DT. When seeing is feeling; acquired synaesthesia or phantom touch? Neurocase. 1996;2:21–9.
54. Diers M, Christmann C, Koeppe C, Ruf M, Flor H. Mirrored, imagined and executed movements differentially activate sensorimotor cortex in amputees with and without phantom limb pain. Pain. 2010;149(2):296–304.
55. Moseley GL, Gallace A, Spence C. Is mirror therapy all it is cracked up to be? Current evidence and future directions. Pain. 2008;138(1):7–10.
56. Lotze M, Montoya P, Erb M, Hülsemann E, Flor H, Klose U, et al. Activation of cortical and cerebellar motor areas during executed and imagined hand movements: an fMRI study. J Cogn Neurosci. 1999;11(5):491–501.
57. Ersland L, Rosén G, Lundervold A, Smievoll AI, Tillung T, Hugdahl S, et al. Phantom limb imaginary fingertapping causes primary motor cortex activation: an fMRI study. Neuro Report. 1996;8(1):207–10.
58. Roux FE, Lotterie JA, Cassol E, Lazorthes Y, Sol JC, Berry I. Cortical areas involved in virtual movement of phantom limbs:

comparison with normal subjects. Neurosurgery. 2003;53 (6):1342–53.
59. Roux FE, Ibarrola D, Lazorthes Y, Berry I. Virtual movements activate primary sensorimotor areas in amputees: report of three cases. Neurosurgery. 2001;49(3):736–42.
60. Mercier C, Reilly KT, Vargas CD, Aballea A, Sirigu A. Mapping phantom movement representations in the motor cortex of amputees. Brain. 2006;129(Pt 8):2202–10.
61. Giraux P, Sirigu A. Illusory movements of the paralyzed limb restore motor cortex activity. Neuroimage. 2003;20 Suppl 1: S107–11.
62. MacIver K, Lloyd DM, Kelly S, Roberts N, Nurmikko T. Phantom limb pain, cortical reorganization and the therapeutic effect of mental imagery. Brain. 2008;131(Pt 8):2181–91.
63. Moura VL, Faurot KR, Gaylord SA, Mann JD, Sill M, Lynch C, et al. Mind-body interventions for treatment of phantom limb pain in persons with amputation. Am J Phys Med Rehabil. 2012;91 (8):701–14.
64. Moseley GL. Graded motor imagery is effective for long-standing complex regional pain syndrome: a randomised controlled trial. Pain. 2004;108(1–2):192–8.
65. Moseley GL. Is successful rehabilitation of complex regional pain syndrome due to sustained attention to the affected limb? A randomised clinical trial. Pain. 2005;114(1–2):54–61.
66. Moseley GL. Graded motor imagery for pathologic pain: a randomized controlled trial. Neurology. 2006;67(12):2129–34.
67. McCabe CS, Haigh RC, Ring EF, Halligan PW, Wall PD, Blake DR. A controlled pilot study of the utility of mirror visual feedback in the treatment of complex regional pain syndrome (type 1). Rheumatology (Oxford). 2003;42(1):97–101.
68. Gieteling EW, van Rijn MA, de Jong BM, Hoogduin JM, Renken R, van Hilten JJ, et al. Cerebral activation during motor imagery in complex regional pain syndrome type 1 with dystonia. Pain. 2008;134(3):302–9.
69. Moseley GL, Parsons TJ, Spence C. Visual distortion of a limb modulates the pain and swelling evoked by movement. Curr Biol. 2008;18(22):R1047–8.
70. Pleger B, Janssen F, Schwenkreis P, Volker B, Maier C, Tegenthoff M. Repetitive transcranial magnetic stimulation of the motor cortex attenuates pain perception in complex regional pain syndrome type I. Neurosci Lett. 2004;356(2):87–90.
71. Ramachandran VS, Seckel EL. Using mirror visual feedback and virtual reality to treat fibromyalgia. Med Hypotheses. 2010;75:495–6.
72. Moseley GL. I can't find it! Distorted body image and tactile dysfunction in patients with chronic back pain. Pain. 2008;140 (1):239–43.
73. Luomajoki H, Moseley GL. Tactile acuity and lumbopelvic motor control in patients with back pain and healthy controls. Br J Sports Med. 2011;45(5):437–40.
74. Bray H, Moseley GL. Disrupted working body schema of the trunk in people with back pain. Br J Sports Med. 2010;45(3):168–73.
75. Wand BM, Tulloch VM, George PJ, Smith AJ, Goucke R, O'Connell NE, et al. Seeing it helps: movement-related back pain is reduced by visualization of the back during movement. Clin J Pain. 2012;28(7):602–8.
76. Diers M, Zieglgänsberger W, Trojan J, Drevensek AM, Erhardt-Raum G. Flor H Site-specific visual feedback reduces pain perception. Pain. 2013;154:890–6.
77. Flor H, Nikolajsen L, Staehelin Jensen T. Phantom limb pain: a case of maladaptive CNS plasticity? Nat Rev Neurosci. 2006;7 (11):873–81.
78. Wand BM, Parkitny L, O'Connell NE, Luomajoki H, McAuley JH, Thacker M, et al. Cortical changes in chronic low back pain: current state of the art and implications for clinical practice. Man Ther. 2011;16(1):15–20.
79. Moseley GL, Flor H. Targeting cortical representations in the treatment of chronic pain: a review. Neurorehabil Neural Repair. 2012;26(6):646–52.
80. Thieme K, Flor H, Turk DC. Psychological pain treatment in fibromyalgia syndrome: efficacy of operant behavioural and cognitive behavioural treatments. Arthritis Res Ther. 2006;8(4):R121.
81. Thieme K, Gromnica-Ihle E, Flor H. Operant behavioral treatment of fibromyalgia: a controlled study. Arthritis Rheum. 2003;49 (3):314–20.
82. Diers M, Yilmaz P, Rance M, Thieme K, Gracely RH, Rolko C, et al. Treatment-related changes in brain activation in patients with fibromyalgia syndrome. Exp Brain Res. 2012;218(4):619–28.
83. Cole J. Virtual & augmented reality, phantom experience and prosthetics. In: Gallagher P, Desmond DM, MacLachlan M, editors. Neuroprostheses. London: Springer; 2007. p. 141–53.
84. Desmond DM, O'Neill K, De Paor A, McDarby G, MacLachlan M. Augmenting the reality of phantom limbs: three case studies using an augmented mirror box procedure. J Prosthet Orthot. 2006;18 (3):74–9.
85. Murray CD, Patchick E, Pettifer S, Caillette F, Howard T. Immersive virtual reality as a rehabilitative technology for phantom limb experience: a protocol. Cyberpsychol Behav. 2006;9 (2):167–70.
86. Murray CD, Patchick EL, Caillette F, Howard T, Pettifer S. Can immersive virtual reality reduce phantom limb pain? Stud Health Technol Inform. 2006;119:407–12.
87. Murray CD, Pettifer S, Howard T, Patchick EL, Caillette F, Kulkarni J, et al. The treatment of phantom limb pain using immersive virtual reality: three case studies. Disabil Rehabil. 2007;29(18):1465–9.
88. Cole J, Crowle S, Austwick G, Slater DH. Exploratory findings with virtual reality for phantom limb pain; from stump motion to agency and analgesia. Disabil Rehabil. 2009;31(10):846–54.
89. Bach F, Buschmann J, Schmitz B, Maaß H, Çakmak H, Diers M et al. Using interactive immersive VR/AR for the therapy of phantom limb pain. 13th International conference on humans and computers; 08.12.2010–10.12.2010; University of Aizu: University of Aizu Press; 2010. p. 183–7.
90. Bach F, Cakmak H, Maass H. Vision-based hand representation and intuitive virtual object manipulation in mixed reality. Biomed Tech. 2012;57,(SI-1 Track-B):462–465.
91. Trojan J, Diers M, Fuchs X, Bach F, Bekrater-Bodmann R, Foell J, Kamping S, Rance M, Maaß H. Flor H (2014) An augmented reality home-training system based on the mirror training and imagery approach. Behav Res Methods. 2014;46(3):634–40. doi:10.3758/s13428-013-0412-4.
92. Ehrsson HH, Rosen B, Stockselius A, Ragno C, Kohler P, Lundborg G. Upper limb amputees can be induced to experience a rubber hand as their own. Brain. 2008;131(Pt 12):3443–52.
93. Rossini PM, Micera S, Benvenuto A, Carpaneto J, Cavallo G, Citi L, et al. Double nerve intraneural interface implant on a human amputee for robotic hand control. Clin Neurophysiol. 2010;121(5):777–83.

Part III

Clinical Potential and Applications

Clinical Applications of Neuromodulation in Psychiatry

14

Pedro Shiozawa, Rosamaria Raza, Quirino Cordeiro Jr., and André Russowsky Brunoni

Major Depressive Disorder

Major depressive disorder (MDD) is an incapacitating disorder associated with significant personal, social and economic impairment. Patients with MDD present a "double burden," characterized by a lower quality of life associated with a higher prevalence of medical comorbidities [1]. The main symptoms of MDD include persistent low mood, anhedonia (i.e., diminished pleasure in previous significant activities), impairment in sleep, psychomotor retardation, weight changes, and negative thoughts that range from pessimism to guilt and suicidal ideation (Table 14.1). Moreover, although only the most severe spectrum of depression is associated with suicide, its chronic, incapacitating symptoms make depression one of the most incapacitating conditions worldwide. Thus, MDD has been projected to be the second most disabling condition by 2020 [2]. Since MDD is known to be a recurrent and relapsing psychiatric condition, approximately 50 % of the patients who present a depressive episode shall undergo a new episode further in life [3]. Finally, nearly 30 % of patients present themselves in a refractory state, i.e., when depressive symptoms are observed despite the appropriate psychological and pharmacological treatment [4]. For these reasons, continuous research on MDD in terms of newer treatment techniques presents itself as a mandatory need.

P. Shiozawa (✉)
Laboratory of Clinical Neuromodulation, Santa Casa Medical School, 1 Rua Major Magliano 241, Sao Paulo, Brazil
e-mail: pedroshiozawa@gmail.com

R. Raza • Q. Cordeiro Jr.
Department of Psychiatry, Santa Casa Medical School, São Paulo, Brazil
e-mail: rosamaria.raza@yahoo.com.br; qcordeiro@yahoo.com

A.R. Brunoni
Department and Institute of Psychiatry, University of São Paulo, São Paulo, Brazil
e-mail: brunowsky@gmail.com; Brunoni@usp.br

Pharmacotherapy

Antidepressant drugs are considered the pillar stone when analyzing treatment approaches for depression. The pharmacological arsenal includes first-generation antidepressants (tricyclic antidepressants and monoamine oxidase inhibitors), SSRIs (serotonin selective reuptake inhibitors, such as sertraline and fluoxetine), serotonin–norepinephrine reuptake inhibitors (SNRIs) ("dual-inhibitors," such as venlafaxine and duloxetine), and others (e.g., bupropion and mirtazapine). A recent meta-analysis suggested that escitalopram and sertraline are the antidepressants that best combine effectiveness with tolerability and therefore should be the first choice for treatment [5]. Given the multiple pharmacological treatments available, the STAR*-D (Sequenced Treatment Alternatives to Relieve Depression), a NIMH-sponsored trial, enrolled almost 3,000 patients to evaluate the efficacy of several antidepressant treatments [4]. STAR*-D highlighted the importance of refractoriness in pharmacotherapy, i.e., remission rates decay as more antidepressant treatments fail—in fact, after four consecutive antidepressant interventions, 30 % of patients still present depression symptoms. Also, different meta-analyses [6–8] observed that dropout rates are relatively high (20–30 %) irrespective of the drug class assessed—the causes of dropouts are multiple and include side-effects, time gap observed from the initial treatment and consequent improvement of depressive symptoms and patient–physician relationship [9] all of each can increase relapse rates in the long-term. These issues reinforce the need for newer interventions in the treatment of MDD.

Neuromodulation Strategies

Noninvasive brain stimulation (NIBS) stands as a general term used to describe techniques that might aid to overcome some of the current challenges that both pharmacological and psychotherapy undergo. Ideally, NIBS techniques

H. Knotkova and D. Rasche (eds.), *Textbook of Neuromodulation*,
DOI 10.1007/978-1-4939-1408-1_14,

Table 14.1 Diagnostic criteria for MDD and main clinical symptoms of depressive episode according to DSM-IV [122]

Diagnosis criteria for MDD
A. Presence of two or more Major Depressive Episodes.
B. The Major Depressive Episodes are not better accounted for other psychiatric disorder
C. There has never been a Manic Episode, a Mixed Episode, or a Hypomanic Episode.
Main clinical symptoms of Depressive Episode
Depressed mood most of the day, nearly every day, as indicated by either subjective report (e.g., feels sad or empty) or observation made by others
Markedly diminished interest or pleasure in all, or almost all, activities most of the day
Significant weight loss when not dieting or weight gain
Insomnia or hypersomnia
Psychomotor agitation or retardation
Fatigue or loss of energy
Feelings of worthlessness or excessive or inappropriate guilt
Diminished ability to think or concentrate, or indecisiveness
Recurrent thoughts of death (not just fear of dying), recurrent suicidal ideation without a specific plan, or a suicide attempt or a specific plan for committing suicide

MDD major depressive disorder

should not only be as effective as pharmacotherapy but should also present a lower rate of adverse effects, thereby increasing treatment adherence.

Neuromodulation techniques include old techniques such as electroconvulsive therapy (ECT) to novel clinical and preclinical techniques, such as transcranial magnetic stimulation (TMS), vagus nerve stimulation (VNS), transcranial direct current stimulation (tDCS), and trigeminal nerve stimulation (TNS). Since these techniques are still considered to be unfamiliar to both most of the medical community and to the general public, a cited description of its physiological mechanism is necessary.

Electroconvulsive Therapy

ECT is one of the most effective treatments for acute depression, especially when psychotic features and/or severe acute suicidal ideation are present. ECT was the first neuromodulatory therapy, initially described by Cerletti and Bini (1940), who were in fact investigating safer alternative therapies for therapeutic seizures against the most used strategies at the time (e.g., intramuscular injection of camphor oil, malaric fever, and so forth). In 1938, these two psychiatrists successfully treated one psychotic patient with 11 cycles of ECT [10]. This technique, however, would only become widespread by the end of World War II.

The energy provided by the ECT is approximately 100 J with a peak pulse in the order of 8 A, which lasts from 0.5 to 2 ms. In fact, the induced seizure—and not the electric charge itself—is considered responsible for the observed antidepressant effects [11].

The UK ECT review group [12], in a systematic review and meta-analysis of different ECT protocols, found that active ECT was more effective than (a) sham ECT (difference in Hamilton scores of 9.7; Confidence Interval [CI], 95 % between 5.7 and 13.5), (b) antidepressant drugs (difference 5.2 points, 95 % CI 1.4–8.9); and that bilateral ECT was more effective that the unilateral protocol (reduction of 3.6 points, 95 % CI 2.2–5.2). Currently, ECT is considered the most effective treatment for the acute depressive episode and is particularly suitable for severely ill patients with suicidal ideation and/or psychotic depression [13]. ECT devices, in spite of a vast range of clinical protocols, use preestablished and independent (within certain limits) amplitudes of pulse determined by the impedance found in each electrical circuit. Some devices allow the physician to specify the stimulation parameters (frequency, width, current, and duration) towards a more individual approach. Shorter pulse durations appear to be more effective in inducing seizures, and increases in stimulus duration may be more effective than increases in frequency. The main clinical indications for ECT are summarized in Table 14.2.

Nevertheless, ECT has some important limitations. It requires anesthesia and, therefore, specialized personnel and adequate medical apparatus for advanced life support. When considering cognitive effects, although anterograde amnesia is relatively common and self-limiting, Sackeim and colleagues [14], in an observational study with 751 patients with MDD who underwent ECT, showed significant impairment in several neuropsychological tests, with an emphasis on attention and memory performance worsening. In terms of safety, some possible adaptations have been suggested in different studies: right unilateral stimulation (vs. bilateral), short pulse (vs. sinusoidal), ultrashort pulse, use of smaller doses, and limiting the total number of sessions [15–17]. Other frequent ECT collateral effects include headache and myalgia [18].

Therefore, ECT is a biological alternative in the treatment of MDD, particularly suitable for the most severe cases [19]. Moreover, difficulties inherent in the application of the technique (sedation, number of sessions) associated with the side

Table 14.2 Main clinical indications for ECT

Catatonia or other psychotic symptoms
Severe risk of suicide
History of prior good response to ECT
Need for rapid, definitive treatment response on either medical or psychiatric grounds
Risks of other treatments outweigh the risks of ECT (i.e., comorbid medical conditions make ECT the safest treatment alternative)
History of poor response to multiple antidepressants
Intolerable side effects to all classes of antidepressant medications (e.g., seizures, hyponatremia, severe anxiety)
Patient preference

ECT electroconvulsive therapy

Table 14.3 Summary of rTMS parameters for depression protocols

Parameter	Summary
Stimulation site	Regarding left vs. right stimulation, the accumulated evidence favors the former as more studies were performed stimulating the left DLPFC
Frequency of trains	Most low-frequency protocols use 1 Hz or less; while high-frequency stimulation ranges from 5 to 20 Hz with more recent studies favoring the 10 Hz-frequency
Intensity of stimulus	Vary from 80 to 120 % MT; issue of safety needs to be addressed
Frequency of sessions	Usually delivered daily in weekdays (5 sessions per week) although some studies used different protocols such as three times a week or two times per day
Duration of treatment	Vary from 10 to 30 sessions

DLPFC dorsolateral prefrontal cortex, *MT* motor threshold

effects cited previously and the risk of cognitive impairment in the long-term exposure represent a limitation of the technique [20], which is intended to be overruled with newer neuromodulatory therapies.

Repetitive Transcranial Magnetic Stimulation (rTMS)

Transcranial magnetic stimulation (TMS) was first introduced as a neurophysiological technique in 1985, when Anthony Barker and his team developed a compact machine that allowed noninvasive stimulation of the cerebral cortex [21]. TMS is based on the physical property that an electric current can generate a varying magnetic field which in turn induces a new electric current over a conductive material. In humans, the TMS coil is placed over the scalp above the targeted stimulation area. The resulting magnetic field is perpendicular to the electric field. In the case of a circular coil, the magnetic field is stronger near the outer circumference of the coil and weaker near the center. The magnetic field can activate neurons at a depth of 20–30 mm over an area of 30 mm long by 20 mm wide reaching mainly cortical areas.

RTMS for MDD typically involves 10–30 treatment sessions of 15–45 min. duration, administered once a day, 5 days a week on an outpatient basis. For MDD, the dorsolateral prefrontal cortex (DLPFC) is the targeted area; typical protocols apply either high-frequency, excitatory stimulation to the left DLPFC or low-frequency, inhibitory stimulation to the right DLPFC. There are two types of rTMS of interest in MDD: (1) low-frequency rTMS (<1 Hz) that is applied over the right DLPFC to induce a decrease in cortical excitability, and (2) high-frequency (>5 Hz, typically 10–20 Hz) rTMS that is applied on the left DLPC to increase cortical excitability. Both approaches induce neuroplasticity changes in the targeted areas [18] (Tables 14.3 and 14.4).

Table 14.4 Adverse effects related to rTMS

Adverse effects
Seizure and syncope
Cognitive impairment
Headache
Nausea
Pain
Manic episodes
Motor effects
Sleep/tiredness

rTMS repetitive transcranial magnetic stimulation

The rationale for rTMS in the depression treatment is based on the hypothesis that the DLPFC is hypoactive in patients with depression—therefore high-frequency rTMS on this area could restore its activity to physiological levels. The use of low-frequency rTMS over the right DLPFC is based on the prefrontal cortical asymmetry theory that states that the left DLPFC is relatively hypoactive whereas the right DLPFC is relatively hyperactive in MDD [22, 23].

An important phase III study using rTMS for MDD was performed by O'Reardon et al. [24]. In this trial, 301 patients with depressive disorder without concurrent antidepressant therapy were enrolled. RTMS was performed at a 10 Hz frequency (120 % of the motor evoked potential, MEP), 3,000 pulses per session for 4–6 weeks. Active rTMS was statistically superior to sham intervention in terms of improvement in depressive symptoms, which was assessed through the Hamilton Rating Scale for Depression. Despite the positive results obtained, there was only a trend for superior active rTMS efficacy considering the primary outcome that employed the Montgomery–Åsberg Depression Rating Scale (MADRS), which resulted in conflicted doubt regarding rTMS's efficacy. This issue was finally resolved in another multicentric randomized controlled trial [25], which evaluated rTMS effects in 199 depressed patients using a 10 Hz frequency stimulation (120 % MEP), with 3,000 pulses per session for 3–6 weeks. The authors found that patients who underwent active rTMS stimulation had 4.2 times greater chance of meeting remission rates scores than patients receiving sham stimulation (95 % confidence interval, 1.32–13.24), with remission rates of 14.1 % and 5.1 % for active and sham rTMS, respectively. Recent meta-analyses confirmed the efficacy of two rTMS modalities: both high-frequency rTMS over the left and low-frequency rTMS over the right DLPFC are effective for MDD [26, 27].

Long-lasting effects are unclear in medical literature as follow-up studies are still incipient [28]. Cohen and colleagues [29] followed 204 patients performing rTMS every other week. The mean time remission period was of 120 days. Demirtas-Tatlidede et al. [30] followed 16 patients for 4 years performing rTMS protocols when the patients relapsed. The mean period free of depressive symptoms were 5 months. Fitzgerald et al. [31] showed that the time of relapse was 10 months in a sample of 19 patients, who also had clinical response for repetitive rTMS protocols. To some that, O'Reardon and colleagues [32] followed ten patients for a period varying from 6 months to 6 years, with weekly or twice a week maintenance of rTMS sessions. At the end of follow-up, only two patients presented remission of symptoms with exclusive rTMS maintenance therapy. Further studies are necessary to establish the optimal rTMS protocols on the maintenance phase of MDD treatment.

The adverse effects of rTMS procedures are generally well tolerated. Although discomfort and facial pain are common symptoms, only a small percentage of patients discontinued treatment due to these symptoms [33]. Another concern is the risk of seizures, which is, in fact, very low for healthy subjects [33]. There are other potential adverse effects, represented by a more rare incidence, which includes: syncope due to a vasodepressor related mechanism, headache, and acute psychiatric changes such as induced mania for bipolar patients (0.84 % mania for active rTMS vs. 0.73 % for sham rTMS) [34].

Currently, rTMS can be considered an interesting therapeutic tool due to its mild side effects and potentially satisfactory clinical outcomes [28]. However, the relatively high-cost for rTMS application remains as an important limitation. In a study carried by Simpson and colleagues, the cost-effectiveness of the technique in question, was analyzed. They concluded that therapy through rTMS had a satisfactory cost-effectiveness when compared to standard antidepressant regimens [35].

In conclusion, rTMS is a safe, well-tolerated strategy, which has been recently approved in several countries as a treatment for Major Depressive Disorder. Given the high-costs, the need of specialized staff for delivering rTMS and the uncertainty regarding its long-term effects, these current limitations still reinforce the need for further research.

Transcranial Direct Current Stimulation

The rationale behind the use of tDCS for depression is based on its properties for increasing (anode) and decreasing (cathode) cortical excitability [36]. Some initial clinical trials showed significant depression improvement. Fregni et al. in a sham-controlled, randomized clinical trial, found a significant decrease in the Hamilton Depression Rating Scale and Beck Depression Inventory after 5 days of active stimulation with 1 mA for 20 min once a day [37]. The mean reduction in the depression scores were between 60 and 70 % for active tDCS group when compared to the baseline values. Similar results were demonstrated in a posterior study with antidepressant-free patients [38].

Rigonatti et al. [39] compared the clinical effects of active prefrontal tDCS vs. a 6-week treatment protocol with 20 mg/day fluoxetine finding that the effects of both therapies were similar.

Another study investigated the long-lasting antidepressant effects of tDCS. The authors evaluated a protocol of ten tDCS sessions with 2 mA [40]. A total of 40 patients with moderate to severe major depression without current use of antidepressants were included and randomly assigned to prefrontal (21 patients), occipital (9 patients), or sham stimulation (10 patients). Depressive symptoms were assessed before, immediately after, 15 and 30 days after stimulation. Only prefrontal tDCS reduced depressive symptoms significantly—reaching approximately 40 % of baseline ratings, and these effects were stable 30 days after the last stimulation session. Loo et al. [41] did not find significant differences between active tDCS and sham stimulation in a double-blind randomized study including 40 outpatients with depression. Treatment was provided for five treatment sessions, 3 days per week, with anodal stimulation over the left DLPFC at 1 mA for 20 min. In a more recent trial, this same group enrolled 64 participants with current depression to receive active or sham anodal tDCS to the left prefrontal cortex (2 mA, 15 sessions over 3 weeks), followed by a 3-week open-label active treatment phase. There was a significant improvement in mood after active compared to sham treatment ($p < 0.05$).

Ferrucci and colleagues [42] used tDCS in patients with severe depression applying 2 mA per day, twice a day for five consecutive days demonstrating an improvement that reached near 20 % on diminishing depressive symptoms. Brunoni et al., in a study with 31 patients, found that the same protocol was effective in patients with bipolar depression [43], with a mean reduction of 18 % in clinical symptoms. Another recent open study [44], demonstrated the efficacy of the same protocol in a group of 23 patients with refractory depression reducing symptoms in 25 %. Finally, Martin et al. [45] performed tDCS sessions consecutively for 20 days, with 2 mA for 20 min, in 11 patients with depression. In this open study, which placed the cathode on the right deltoid muscle, the reduction of symptoms was around 44 %.

Recently, a systematic review and meta-analysis [46] reviewed the efficacy of tDCS for MDD treatment, showing that active vs. sham tDCS is an effective treatment for MDD. However, there is still a need for further studies investigated tDCS efficacy in depression, as there was significant between-study heterogeneity in the reviewed trials.

Deep Brain Stimulation (DBS)

DBS consists on the implantation of an electrode in subcortical areas, with further application of an electrical current of 130–180 Hz. This preferred region is the subgenual cingulate area, since this area is hyperactive in depression, with partial normalization of its activity after antidepressant treatment [47]. The literature concerning DBS for depression is scarce, since there are few studies on the matter. One recent open label trial enrolled 17 patients with severe depression who were followed for 2 years, with significant improvement of mood symptoms [48]. Another study [49] enrolled six patients with treatment resistant depressive disorder to receive DBS. The authors found a sustained remission of depression among four out of six patients and hypothesized by neuroimaging assessment that disrupting focal activity in limbic-cortical circuits may be a key target of novel neuromodulation approaches.

Further follow-up data was obtained from an extended cohort of 20 patients with treatment resistant depression who underwent DBS for 3–6 years (mean 3.5 years) showing an average response rate of 64.3 % and an average remission rate of 42.9 % in depressive symptoms. Patients showed considerable improvement in social functioning and in the degree of involvement in work-related activity [50].

Cranial Nerve Stimulation

Vagus nerve stimulation (VNS) procedure stands for the disposal of a bipolar electrode around vagus nerve and further dissemination of low frequency electric pulse from the nerve towards central nervous system. The stimulation can be performed in several ways as with surgical implantation of electrodes around vagus nerve or transcutaneously. Electric stimulation of the nerve provides direct modulatory effect in subcortical sites. The specific network activated during the procedure varies according to certain parameters, suggesting that with more extensive knowledge, one could "direct" the VNS signal within groups of patients or even individually.

Recently, Mohr et al. found, in review of four clinical trials ($n = 355$) using VNS for resistant depression, a steadily increasing improvement of depressive symptoms after 6–12 months, which sustained up to 2 years follow-up. Bajbouj and colleagues [51], in an open label study analyzed 74 patients diagnosed with treatment-resistant depression, showing clinical response and benign adverse effects over a 2-year follow-up.

Safety-wise, Gerson et al. [52] described a case in which VNS treatment in a patient with epilepsy and unipolar depression was associated with the rapid development of manic symptoms. Another study described, in a sample of nine patients, transitional changes of time perception with vagus nerve stimulation (VNS), which was considered a minor, but relevant collateral effect [53]. When analyzing the cardiovascular risk, the same research group pointed VNS as a safe therapeutic strategy for treating depressive disorder [54]. Further collateral effects presented in literature include cough and vocal disturbances.

Another site of stimulation is the trigeminal nerve (TNS), which is performed in a 120 Hz frequency with pulse wave duration of 250 μs and cycle of 30 s. Electric stimuli determine an asymmetrical biphasic pulse wave adjustable from 0 to 100 mA. The trigeminal nerve conveys information to important structures in the brain including the nucleus solitarius, the locus coeruleus, the vagus nerve and the cerebral cortex. It also specifically sends signals to the anterior cingulate cortex, which is involved in mood, attention and decision-making. Shraeder et al. treated five patients (60 % female; man age: 49.6 years) with treatment-resistant depression who received TNS for 8 weeks. The authors verified depressive-symptoms remission rates up to 70 % among patients in a 2-month follow-up [55].

Table 14.5 Summary of rTMS studies with bipolar depression

Study	Sample	Age (years)	Stimulation site	Stimulation frequency	Design	MEP (%)	Control	Use of medication
Tamas 2007 [64]	4	44.5	Right DLPFC	1	Double blind, randomized	95	1 Sham, 3 active	Yes
Dell'Osso 2009 [65]	11	54.4	Right DLPFC	1	Open label	110	110	Yes
Nahas 2003 [63]	23	43	Left DLPFC	5	Blind, randomized	110	No	Yes
Huang 2008 [123]	46	44	Left DLPFC	5	Open label	100	No	Yes
Dolberg 2002 [62]	20	54	–	–	Double blind, randomized	–	10 Sham, 10 active	–

DLPFC dorsolateral prefrontal cortex, *MEP* motor evoked potential

Bipolar Disorder

Bipolar disorder (BD) is a recurrent, chronic and severe disease. It causes significant impact in the quality of life and also considerable distress in the relatives of the patients and in the society in general. The prevalence of the BD in the USA varies around 0.4–3.7 %. The functional incapacity of the disease is comparable to most of chronic diseases such as cardiac conditions, since its comorbid both physical and psychiatric are due to low adherence in the prescribed treatment.

Pharmacotherapy

The treatment of bipolar disorder is divided in the acute and maintenance phases. In the acute phase the objective is to treat manic/depression symptoms whereas the maintenance phase aims to decrease relapse with concomitant improvement of general psychological functions. Mainstream treatment is based on the use of mood stabilizers and antipsychotic agents [56]. These pharmacological groups have been clinically used as the first-line treatment for bipolar depression, largely because longer-term preventative therapies with these agents are useful. Depressive episodes that do not respond to lithium, divalproate, or another mood stabilizer, or episodes that "breakthrough" despite preventive treatment, often warrant treatment with further strategies such as antidepressant agents and ECT. Clinical trials suggest that lithium is superior to placebo in treating bipolar depression, but the efficacy of lithium in comparison to antidepressants remains uncertain [57–60].

Electroconvulsive Therapy

Different clinical trials have reported the efficacy of ECT in bipolar depression. Response rates are quite variable among studies with a general tendency of satisfactory clinical outcome. The possibility of shifting from depression to hypomania or mania in patients treated with ECT appears equivalent to that associated with conventional antidepressant treatment [61]. For the manic episode, ECT is an adjuvant treatment in manic/mixed acute states. It can also be used in treatment-resistant patients.

Repetitive Transcranial Magnetic Stimulation (rTMS)

The physiological rationale concerning the use of rTMS for treating BD is the same as for MDD: high-frequency stimulation on the left DLPFC and/or low-frequency stimulation on the right DLFPC. Dolberg et al. [62] randomized 20 patients to receive either active or sham rTMS, finding superiority for active rTMS [62]. Nahas and colleagues, in a study with similar design, did not demonstrate efficacy of the technique in 23 patients with BD [63]. Tamas and colleagues conducted a study with five patients diagnosed with bipolar depression in current use of mood stabilizers. Positive clinical outcomes were observed after 6 weeks of follow-up [64]. A recent open-label study with 11 subjects focused on treatment-resistant bipolar depression. The authors showed improvement in depressive symptoms with low frequency rTMS over the right DLPFC [65] (Table 14.5).

A few studies also investigated rTMS for the treatment of manic episodes. An initial study with 18 patients in mania demonstrated the clinical efficacy of high-frequency rTMS in improving manic symptoms [66]. Other two open-label studies showed significant improvement in manic symptoms [67] and/or mixed episodes [68] in BP patients. Both studies applied rTMS in the right DLPFC. In addition, a sham-controlled study also found significant improvement in manic symptoms also using high-frequency rTMS in the right DLPFC [69]. Another study used rTMS for over 2 weeks, finding improvement of manic symptoms [67].

Table 14.6 Diagnosis criteria for schizophrenia based on DSM-IV [122]

A. Characteristic Symptoms: delusions, hallucinations, disorganized Speech, grossly disorganized or catatonic behavior, negative symptoms of time during a 1-month period
B. Social/Occupational dysfunction
C. Duration: Continuous signs of the disturbance persist for at least 6 months
D. Schizoaffective and Mood Disorder exclusion
E. Substance/General Medical Condition exclusion
F. Relationship to a Pervasive Developmental Disorder exclusion

Transcranial Direct Current Stimulation

Currently, there are no trials that investigated tDCS as a treatment for the manic episode. For the depressive episode, Brunoni et al. [43] used anodal tDCS over the left DLPFC in 31 patients (14 with BD, 17 with MDD). Depressive symptoms in both study groups improved immediately after the fifth session. The beneficial effect persisted after 1 week and 1 month [43].

Schizophrenia

Schizophrenia is a common psychiatric disorder with an overall prevalence of 1–1.5 % and a chronic course through life. The disease onset is in early adulthood although preclinical symptoms might be present in childhood and adolescence [70, 71]. Its symptoms can be grouped into three relatively distinct phenomenological presentations: (a) positive symptoms, (b) impairment or "negative" symptoms, and (c) cognitive dysfunction. Positive symptoms are characterized by hallucinations and delusions; negative symptoms by impairments in sociability, expression of affect and motivation; and cognitive dysfunction by deficits in executive functioning (attention and/or memory) [72, 73].

Diagnostic criteria according to the DSM-IV are based on the presence of at least two of five symptoms (hallucinations, delirium, disorganized speech, disorganized or catatonic behavior and negative symptoms) (Table 14.6) [74]. Traditionally, positive symptoms occur within the first 10–15 years of the disease, while negative and cognitive symptoms exhibit a more chronic, persistent, and sometimes progressive presentation [75].

Patients with schizophrenia have, in general, low-functionality in performing daily life activities, lower quality of life and greater incidence of comorbidities such as depressive symptoms, substance related disorders, suicidal behavior, and cardiovascular risk [76, 77].

Pharmacological Treatment for Schizophrenia

Approximately 25 % of patients with schizophrenia do not respond to conventional drug treatment [78]. Several antipsychotics among "typical" (first generation, developed between 1950 and 1970) and "atypical" (second generation, developed since the 1990s) are available for the pharmacological treatment of schizophrenia. However, recent clinical studies using some of these drugs have failed to show efficacy of any particular medication. The CATIE study (Clinical Antipsychotic Trials of Intervention Effectiveness), sponsored by the National Institute of Mental Health (NIMH) recruited almost 1,500 patients with schizophrenia to receive olanzapine, quetiapine, risperidone, or ziprasidone in a double blind, randomized study. The authors observed high rates of dropouts (74 %), similar effectiveness among different drugs and relevant collateral effects such as metabolic and extrapyramidal symptoms [79]. Another study (the Cost Utility of the Latest Antipsychotic Drugs in Schizophrenia Study [CUtLASS]), sponsored by the National Health System (NHS), randomized 227 people with schizophrenia to receive either first or second generation antipsychotics, which found no differences in quality of life, symptom improvement, or financial costs in 1 year of follow-up [80].

One antipsychotic drug, however, needs to be analyzed separately: clozapine, which is two times more effective than other antipsychotics, according to a meta-analysis [81]. Clozapine also seems to be one of the few, if not the only, antipsychotic that may show some improvement over negative symptoms [82]. Although effective, clozapine use is limited by potentially severe collateral effects such as neutropenia and agranulocytosis. This requires constant monitoring for leukopenia for patients on clozapine [83]. Other side effects include sedation, drowsiness; drooling and weight gain [84]. Nonetheless, approximately 40 % of refractory patients do not respond adequately to clozapine—a condition known as super-refractory [82].

The treatment of schizophrenia usually starts with either a typical or atypical antipsychotic with expected clinical response within 4–6 weeks. Further adjustments may be required and whether symptoms persist, a second antipsychotic is associated. For these cases, lack of clinical response will characterize refractoriness and clozapine should be, therefore, recommended over the following 6 months. If still no response is observed, there are several strategies available, however, with discrete level of evidence such as ECT, rTMS, and tDCS.

Electroconvulsive Therapy

Electroconvulsive therapy alone is less effective than antipsychotics according to trials comparing directly these two therapeutic modalities [85]. It also has better clinical response for patients with positive symptoms or catatonic presentation [11, 86]. In a systematic review performed by Chanpattana et al. [87], the authors suggested that ECT might be effective in acute episodes of certain types of schizophrenia and for the reduction in relapse occurrence.

Repetitive Transcranial Magnetic Stimulation

Several trials evaluated the efficacy of rTMS for auditory hallucinations (AH) and negative symptoms in schizophrenia. For AH, low-frequency rTMS is applied on the left temporoparietal site. Studies addressing the use of rTMS for AH mostly target the temporoparietal cortex region [88], since this area is related to primary auditory processing. Hoffman et al. [89] conducted a double blind, cross-over trial with three schizophrenic patients with persistent AH. They used low frequency rTMS (1 Hz) on the left temporoparietal area (80 % of motor threshold, total of 2,880 pulses). All three patients showed improvement in the intensity of hallucinations, and two had nearly complete remission of hallucinations for 2 weeks. Similar results were found by d'Alfonso et al. [90]. Recently, Hoffman et al. [91] randomized 20 patients with schizophrenia or schizoaffective disorder who had refractory AH to receive either rTMS or sham intervention. The stimulation was performed at 1 Hz for 9 days with 90 % motor threshold. These authors found a response (reduction of at least 50 % in symptoms) in 9 of 12 patients treated with rTMS.

It seems that negative symptoms are related to decreased activity of the left prefrontal lobe. Cohen et al. [92] performed the first study showing improvement of negative symptoms with rTMS. The authors studied six patients with chronic schizophrenia on standard antipsychotic regimen. They received high-frequency rTMS for 2 weeks at 80 % of motor threshold. There was a statistically significant decline in negative symptoms of Positive and Negative Syndrome Scale (PANSS) [92]. Nahas et al. [63] conducted a crossover double-blind study with seven patients with schizophrenia with predominantly negative symptoms. Patients were randomized to receive either active vs. sham rTMS (20 Hz, 100 % motor threshold, 40 pulses at two second intervals over 20 min, total stimuli: 1,600) over the left DLPFC. Results showed that active rTMS improved negative symptoms. A recent meta-analysis was conducted to assess the efficacy of prefrontal rTMS for treating negative symptoms of schizophrenia. The authors evaluated nine trials ($n = 213$) and found that overall mean weighted effect size for rTMS vs. sham was statistically significant ($d = 0.43$; 95 % CI, 0.05–0.80). Studies with a longer duration of treatment (>3 weeks) had a larger mean effect size when compared to studies with shorter treatment duration [93].

Transcranial Direct Current Stimulation

Hitherto, only one trial investigated tDCS for the treatment of AH in schizophrenia. Thirty patients with persistent AH were randomized to receive either active or sham tDCS. The cathode was placed on the left temporoparietal region and the anode on the left DLPFC. The rationale was to simultaneously perform an inhibitory stimulation over the area related to positive symptoms (AH) and an excitatory stimulation over the area correlated with negative symptoms. TDCS was applied twice daily for 5 days. The authors showed an improvement of AH (primary endpoint) after the end of stimulation, with sustained clinical response after 1 and 3 months of treatment [94].

Eating Disorders

Eating disorders present two main diagnostic categories: anorexia nervosa (AN) and bulimia nervosa (BN). There are other categories of Eating Disorders (ED) that are not diagnosis "per se," but rather include partial characteristics of AN and BN, referred as Eating Disorders Not Otherwise Specified.

The DSM-IV criteria for anorexia nervosa consist of intense fear for gaining weight or becoming fat, distortion of one's body shape, intense food restriction, and amenorrhea. Bulimia nervosa is characterized by periods of binge eating when large amounts of food are consumed and a sense of control is absent. Both can be indulged with different types of purging behavior to prevent weight gain.

The physical complications of a long-term eating disorder are important issues, and because of that, anorexia nervosa and bulimia nervosa are illnesses that should involve a more careful approach when considering the course of therapy applied. With limited resources endorsed by the medical community in terms of efficient treatment for eating disorders, neuromodulation techniques may play a role in unveiling the mechanisms behind cerebral functions and as a possible strategic therapeutic treatment tool. In this context, non-pharmacological brain stimulation might aid to overcome current challenges in treating eating disorders. The techniques further discussed aim to increase response and remission rates and also to decrease adverse effects, thereby increasing treatment adherence.

Pharmacotherapy

When analyzing separately the pharmacotherapy used for each type of eating disorder, the literature on medications is sparse and inconclusive [95]. For AN, few trials found positive results in weight outcome and relapse events, even though diverse classes of medications were evaluated. AN might be associated with serotonin dysregulation and often presents comorbid anxiety, depression, and obsessive-compulsive disorders. Thus, several studies have examined the efficacy of SSRIs. It should be noted that SSRIs are preferable over tricyclics given the more common adverse effects of the latter [96–98]. Further, there is limited evidence as to whether antidepressants improve the comorbid disorders as a secondary outcome or if they primarily induce to weight gain and improvement of dysfunctional cognition related to eating [99]. In fact, psychotherapy is the mainstream treatment for AN. Cognitive behavioral therapy (CBT) is the form of psychotherapy best supported by the available evidence [100]. There are limitations when considering psychotherapy, given the cognitive rigidity of patients with AN, this might reflect its limited progress with the cognitive component of treatment [101].

In BN, antidepressants show more positive results than AN [102]. Early studies have analyzed the use of tricyclic medication, which shows efficacy in decreasing binge episodes compared to placebo. However, currently the psychopharmacological research focuses on the SSRIs, since tricyclic have considerable side effects [103–105]. There are several studies showing that the use of fluoxetine at 60 mg/day is also successful in reducing binge/purge frequency as well as concerns with food, drive for thinness and it has been well tolerated by the patients. CBT is also used in BN. Currently, fluoxetine and CBT combined are considered the optimal treatment for BN, although the remission rates are still below the expected, which maintains the need for continued new approaches.

Neuromodulation Strategies

In order to summarize the current neuromodulation techniques, a systematic review of all available studies was carried through (Table 14.7).

In the reviewed studies, only 6.7 % of patients were males. Comorbidity with depression occurred in all studies, except for one, in which no scale was used for assessment. Anxiety was observed in one study concomitantly with depression. These data reinforce the general concept that eating disorders have a significant relationship with mood disorders.

Craving and purging were the primary outcomes assessed in studies with BN, and decrease in symptoms was observed for both. AN was contemplated only in case reports/pilot studies and outcome assessment varied considerably, but all articles observed improvement either in one of the criteria: "feeling full," concern with shape/body, increase of body mass index (BMI). Urge to restrict or urge to exercise was less clear.

The techniques applied appear to be safe and with minimal side effects. Brain modulation might possibly have an effect in the core symptoms of eating disorders. In the majority of the studies, samples were small and larger studies are needed to validate these techniques as adjuvant therapeutic tools. From these preliminary results, it can be speculated that neuromodulation techniques shed a promising filed of treatment in a psychiatric disorders that lacks still nowadays a current effective pharmacological treatment.

Obsessive Compulsive Disorder (OCD)

Obsessive-compulsive disorder (OCD) has a prevalence of approximately 2–3 % in the general population [106, 107]. This makes OCD the fourth most prevalent psychiatric disorder. Among adults the prevalence is equivalent in men and women, differing only in adolescents and children with higher rates for men. The mean age is 20 years. This syndrome is characterized by the presence of obsessions and compulsions sufficiently severe to cause disruption in the patient's life, resulting in considerable suffering. Symptoms are perceived by the patient as intrusive and often cause significant distress [108] Obsessions are described as thoughts, images and impulses undesired and repetitive. Compulsions are behaviors or mental attitudes that the patient feel compelled to execute. This pattern has the objective of reducing the anxiety caused by the obsessions (Table 14.8).

Table 14.7 Studies of noninvasive brain stimulation and eating disorders

Author	Sample	Female (%)	Study	Age real rTMS	Age sham	BMI real rTMS	BMI sham	Comorbid	Eating disorder	Primary outcome
Walpoth [124]	14	1	Between subjects	27.4 ± 4.8	22.6 ± 2.6	19.6 ± 2.4	19.7 ± 1.7	Depression	BN	No difference in both groups in purge behavior and in scales
Van den Eynde [125]	37	86	Between subjects	30.5 ± 11.2	29.5 ± 8.4	25.8 ± 11.5	25.0 ± 8.5	Depression	BN, EDNOS-BN	Reduced cue-induced food craving
Van den Eynde [126]	7	1	Between subjects	22.9 ± 2.9	–	22.2 ± 2.7	–	Depression and anxiety	BN, EDNOSBED	Comparison with right-handed trial group in Van den Eynde, 2010. Mood worsened in left-handed × improved in right handed. Improvement observed in craving with the FCSs measure but not with the VAS. Sham-rTMS with right-handed reduced craving
Claudino [127]	22	1	Between subjects	28.2 ± 9.2	28.9 ± 8.5	26.8 ± 13.2	22.2 ± 3.1	–	BN, EDNOS-BN	Real rTMS showed lower cortisol levels compared with sham, thus real rTMS reduces craving but not superior effect on tension, mood, hunger, urge to binge eat. Real rTMS showed less binge in the 24 h following

HS healthy subjects, *BN* bulimia nervosa, *EDNOS-BN* eating disorder not otherwise specified-bulimia nervosa, *BED* binge eating disorder

Table 14.8 Diagnosis criteria for OCD [122]

Either obsessions or compulsions.
At some point during the course of the disorder, the person has recognized that the obsessions or compulsions are excessive unreasonable.
The obsessions or compulsions cause marked distress, are time-consuming.
If another Axis I disorder is present, the content of the obsessions or compulsions is not restricted to it.
The disturbance is not due to the direct physiological effects of a substance.

Pharmacotherapy

Common treatments include the antidepressant clomipramine, followed by the selective serotonin reuptake inhibitors (SSRIs) such as paroxetine, sertraline, fluoxetine, citalopram, and fluvoxamine. The protocol used for medical intervention consists of starting with SSRIs, followed by the use of three different SSRIs and, after that, by a trial with clomipramine. The addition of an atypical antipsychotic such as risperidone can be used [109].

Cognitive-Behavioral Therapy

It is generally agreed that cognitive-behavioral therapy (CBT) such as exposure and response prevention, should be the first approach to treatment, along with family counseling for children and adolescents [110, 111]. For adults, CBT can be initially combined in association with pharmacotherapy [111].

Transcranial Magnetic Stimulation

Recent studies have reported mixed findings regarding the efficacy of rTMS for OCD treatment. For instance, Sachdev et al. [112] found negative results using high-frequency rTMS over the DLPFC. Conversely, Nauczyciel et al. [113] found positive findings when stimulating the orbitofrontal cortex, in a sham-controlled study. Recently, Volpato et al. [114] investigated the effects of rTMS and tDCS in a case report. They suggested tDCS to be more effective than rTMS in reducing depression and anxiety, although both therapies had no effect on obsessive-compulsive symptoms.

To conclude, given the heterogeneity of the protocols used, it is difficult to directly compare the results. This could indicate that disparate protocols lead to different outcomes (given that the higher frequency used could increase the potential of excitability) and, therefore, more rTMS studies to address the efficacy of the technique are necessary.

Attention Deficit Hyperactivity Disorder (ADHD)

ADHD is a syndrome defined by a persistent pattern of lack of attention and/or hyperactive behavior and impulsiveness, which tends to be more severe than what should be expected in children of the same age and in the same level of cognitive development [115]. Attention Deficit Hyperactivity Disorder (ADHD) is one of the most frequently diagnosis made in neuropsychiatric childhood disorders. A core symptom is a motor hyperactivity. It accounts for approximately 3–8 % of the diagnosis made in childhood. Over the past decade the use of medication for treating ADHD increased considerably.

Pharmacotherapy

The treatment of ADHD involves a multidimensional approach combining psychosocial and psychopharmacological interventions. When considering the psychosocial treatment, efforts should be directed towards information regarding the clinical aspects of the disorder to family members. A special training program for parents in order to learn how to manage their children's symptoms can be endorsed. The school environment also has to be specialized for these children, and teachers should have a special training so that external stimuli can be minimal. Physical activities are an important therapeutic tool in terms of enhancing concentration in other school activities. Also, it can be necessary in some cases psychomotor reeducation for motor control. In terms of psychosocial interventions, clinical psychotherapy can be introduced to cope with comorbidities such as depressive and anxiety symptoms, self-esteem issues, lack of control of hyperactivity, and impulse symptoms [116].

The psychostimulants are the first line of pharmacological treatment for ADHD. Effectiveness is similar for adolescents and children. Methylphenidate is used between 20 and 60 mg/day (0.3 to 1 mg/kg/day); it acts through increasing dopaminergic and noradrenergic synaptic efflux throughout the brain and presents a rapid onset of action [117].

Neuromodulation Strategies

In a preliminary study, 13 adults, who had ADHD diagnosed on DSM IV criteria, participated in a double blind randomized crossover study that compared sham and active rTMS [118]. There was a specific beneficial effect on attention 10 min after a real rTMS course with no effect evident in the sham rTMS. Another study applied rTMS over the right DLPFC at 10 Hz, with 100 % of the observed motor threshold, for 2,000 pulses per session, in a 10-session course over 2 weeks in a sham-controlled crossover design. The patients showed no significant difference in symptoms comparing sham and active stimulation [119]. Niederhofer et al. [120] applied low frequency at 1 Hz, 1,200 pulses per session for 5 days of rTMS and it was observed improvement in attention and hyperactivity symptoms that lasted for 4 weeks. Finally, Bloch et al. [121] found substantial improvement on attention 10 min after active rTMS. This study applied a single session of high-frequency of rTMS in the right DLPFC in a double-blind randomized, sham controlled design. The sham stimulation had no effect in the analyzed patients [121].

Conclusion

Mental disorders are estimated to be the leading cause of disability worldwide. Presently there are still important challenges to optimize psychiatric treatment, which faces high refractoriness and recurrence rates with well-known burden for patients, their families, and society. Neuromodulation strategies have been systematically addressed as valuable tolls to face these challenges as shown by clinical and basic scientific investigations. The development of research in neuromodulation techniques can impact outcome of different neuropsychiatric disorders as major depression. Lower costs, a decreased rate of adverse effects and satisfactory clinical outcomes have been reassuring tDCS as a relevant issue in current neuroscience. Further translational research is also crucial to guide a more practical use of neuromodulation research findings in clinical psychiatric with a broad understanding of advantages and limitations inherent to each treatment strategy. Further research in neuromodulation is a current challenge in psychiatric scenario.

References

1. Wittchen HU, Knauper B, Kessler RC. Lifetime risk of depression. Br J Psychiatry Suppl. 1994:16–22.
2. Murray CJ, Lopez AD. Alternative projections of mortality and disability by cause 1990–2020: Global Burden of Disease Study. Lancet. 1997;349:1498–504.
3. Eaton WW, Anthony JC, Gallo J, et al. Natural history of diagnostic interview schedule/DSM-IV major depression. The Baltimore Epidemiologic Catchment Area follow-up. Arch Gen Psychiatry. 1997;54:993–9.
4. Rush AJ, Trivedi MH, Wisniewski SR, et al. Acute and longer-term outcomes in depressed outpatients requiring one or several treatment steps: a STAR*D report. Am J Psychiatry. 2006;163:1905–17.
5. Cipriani A, La Ferla T, Furukawa TA, et al. Sertraline versus other antidepressive agents for depression. Cochrane Database Syst Rev. 2010;4, CD006117.
6. Mendlewicz J, Massat I, Linotte S, et al. Identification of clinical factors associated with resistance to antidepressants in bipolar depression: results from an European Multicentre Study. Int Clin Psychopharmacol. 2010;25:297–301.
7. Steffens D, Krishnan K, Helms M. Are SSRIs better than TCAs? Comparison of SSRIs and TCAs: a meta-analysis. Depress Anxiety. 1997;6:10–8.
8. Anderson I. SSRIs versus tricyclic antidepressants in depressed inpatients: a meta-analysis of efficacy and tolerability. Depress Anxiety. 1998;7:11–7.
9. Demyttenaere K. Compliance during treatment with antidepressants. J Affect Disord. 1997;43:27–39.
10. Passione R. Italian psychiatry in an international context: Ugo Cerletti and the case of electroshock. Hist Psychiatry. 2004;15:83–104.
11. Mankad M, Beyer J, Krystal A. Clinical manual of electroconvulsive therapy. Washington, DC: American Psychiatric Publishing; 2010.
12. National Institute for Health and Clinical Excellence (NICE) (2003). The clinical effectiveness and cost effectiveness of electroconvulsive Therapy (ECT) for depressive illness, schizophrenia, catatonia and mania. London: National Institute for Health and Clinical Excellence (NICE). Available online: http://www.nice.org.uk/TA059.
13. Fleck MP, Berlim MT, Lafer B, et al. [Review of the guidelines of the Brazilian Medical Association for the treatment of depression (Complete version)]. Rev Bras Psiquiatr. 2009;31 Suppl 1:S7–17.
14. Sackeim HA, Prudic J, Fuller R, Keilp J, Lavori PW, Olfson M. The cognitive effects of electroconvulsive therapy in community settings. Neuropsychopharmacology. 2007;32:244–54.
15. Loo CK, Sainsbury K, Sheehan P, Lyndon B. A comparison of RUL ultrabrief pulse (0.3 ms) ECT and standard RUL ECT. Int J Neuropsychopharmacol. 2008;11:883–90.
16. Loo CK, Schweitzer I, Pratt C. Recent advances in optimizing electroconvulsive therapy. Aust N Z J Psychiatry. 2006;40:632–8.
17. Prudic J. Strategies to minimize cognitive side effects with ECT: aspects of ECT technique. J ECT. 2008;24:46–51.
18. Brunoni AR, Teng CT, Correa C, et al. Neuromodulation approaches for the treatment of major depression: challenges and recommendations from a working group meeting. Arq Neuropsiquiatr. 2010;68:433–51.
19. Pagnin D, de Queiroz V, Pini S, Cassano GB. Efficacy of ECT in depression: a meta-analytic review. J ECT. 2004;20:13–20.
20. Kennedy SH, Milev R, Giacobbe P, et al. Canadian Network for Mood and Anxiety Treatments (CANMAT) clinical guidelines for the management of major depressive disorder in adults. IV. Neurostimulation therapies. J Affect Disord. 2009;117 Suppl 1: S44–53.
21. Barker AT, Jalinous R, Freeston IL. Non-invasive magnetic stimulation of human motor cortex. Lancet. 1985;1:1106–7.
22. Barrett J, Della-Maggiore V, Chouinard P, Paus T. Mechanisms of action underlying the effect of repetitive transcranial magnetic stimulation on mood: behavioral and brain imaging studies. Neuropsychopharmacology. 2004;29:1172–9.
23. Videbech P. PET measurements of brain glucose metabolism and blood flow in major depressive disorder: a critical review. Acta Psychiatr Scand. 2000;101:11–20.
24. O'Reardon JP, Cristancho P, Pilania P, Bapatla KB, Chuai S, Peshek AD. Patients with a major depressive episode responding to treatment with repetitive transcranial magnetic stimulation (rTMS) are resistant to the effects of rapid tryptophan depletion. Depress Anxiety. 2007;24:537–44.
25. George MS, Aston-Jones G. Noninvasive techniques for probing neurocircuitry and treating illness: vagus nerve stimulation (VNS), transcranial magnetic stimulation (TMS) and transcranial

direct current stimulation (tDCS). Neuropsychopharmacology. 2010;35:301–16.
26. Schutter DJ. Antidepressant efficacy of high-frequency transcranial magnetic stimulation over the left dorsolateral prefrontal cortex in double-blind sham-controlled designs: a meta-analysis. Psychol Med. 2009;39:65–75.
27. Schutter DJ. Quantitative review of the efficacy of slow-frequency magnetic brain stimulation in major depressive disorder. Psychol Med. 2010;40:1789–95.
28. Slotema CW, Blom JD, Hoek HW, Sommer IE. Should we expand the toolbox of psychiatric treatment methods to include repetitive transcranial magnetic stimulation (rTMS)? A meta-analysis of the efficacy of rTMS in psychiatric disorders. J Clin Psychiatry. 2010;71:873–84.
29. Cohen RB, Boggio PS, Fregni F. Risk factors for relapse after remission with repetitive transcranial magnetic stimulation for the treatment of depression. Depress Anxiety. 2009;26:682–8.
30. Demirtas-Tatlidede A, Mechanic-Hamilton D, Press DZ, et al. An open-label, prospective study of repetitive transcranial magnetic stimulation (rTMS) in the long-term treatment of refractory depression: reproducibility and duration of the antidepressant effect in medication-free patients. J Clin Psychiatry. 2008;69:930–4.
31. Fitzgerald PB, Benitez J, de Castella AR, Brown TL, Daskalakis ZJ, Kulkarni J. Naturalistic study of the use of transcranial magnetic stimulation in the treatment of depressive relapse. Aust N Z J Psychiatry. 2006;40:764–8.
32. O'Reardon J, Peshek A, Romero R. Neuromodulation and transcranial magnetic stimulation (TMS): a 21st century paradigm for therapeutics in psychiatry. Psychiatry. 2005;3:30–40.
33. Rossi S. The safety of TMS consensus group. Clin Neurophysiol. 2009;120:2008–39.
34. Xia G, Gajwani P, Muzina DJ, et al. Treatment-emergent mania in unipolar and bipolar depression: focus on repetitive transcranial magnetic stimulation. Int J Neuropsychopharmacol. 2008;11:119–30.
35. Simpson KN, Welch MJ, Kozel FA, Demitrack MA, Nahas Z. Cost-effectiveness of transcranial magnetic stimulation in the treatment of major depression: a health economics analysis. Adv Ther. 2009;26:737.
36. Brunoni AR, Nitsche MA, Bolognini N, et al. Clinical research with transcranial direct current stimulation (tDCS): challenges and future directions. Brain Stimul. 2012;5(3):175–95.
37. Fregni F, Boggio PS, Nitsche MA, Marcolin MA, Rigonatti SP, Pascual-Leone A. Treatment of major depression with transcranial direct current stimulation. Bipolar Disord. 2006;8:203–4.
38. Fregni F, Boggio PS, Nitsche MA, Rigonatti SP, Pascual-Leone A. Cognitive effects of repeated sessions of transcranial direct current stimulation in patients with depression. Depress Anxiety. 2006;23:482–4.
39. Rigonatti SP, Boggio PS, Myczkowski ML, et al. Transcranial direct stimulation and fluoxetine for the treatment of depression. Eur Psychiatry. 2008;23:74–6.
40. Boggio PS, Rigonatti SP, Ribeiro RB, et al. A randomized, double-blind clinical trial on the efficacy of cortical direct current stimulation for the treatment of major depression. Int J Neuropsychopharmacol. 2008;11:249–54.
41. Loo CK, Sachdev P, Martin D, et al. A double-blind, sham-controlled trial of transcranial direct current stimulation for the treatment of depression. Int J Neuropsychopharmacol. 2010;13:61–9.
42. Ferrucci R, Bortolomasi M, Brunoni AR, et al. Comparative benefits of transcranial direct current stimulation (tDCS) treatment in patients with mild/moderate vs. severe depression. Clin Neuropsychiatry. 2009;6:246–51.
43. Brunoni AR, Ferrucci R, Bortolomasi M, et al. Transcranial direct current stimulation (tDCS) in unipolar vs. bipolar depressive disorder. Prog Neuropsychopharmacol Biol Psychiatry. 2011;35:96–101.
44. Dell'osso B, Zanoni S, Ferrucci R, et al. Transcranial direct current stimulation for the outpatient treatment of poor-responder depressed patients. Eur Psychiatry. 2011;27(7):513–7.
45. Martin D, Alonzo A, Mitchell P, Sachdev P, Galvez V, Loo C. Fronto-extracephalic transcranial direct current stimulation as a treatment for major depression: an open-label pilot study. J Affect Disord. 2011;134:459–63.
46. Kalu UG, Sexton CE, Loo CK, Ebmeier KP. Transcranial direct current stimulation in the treatment of major depression: a meta-analysis. Psychol Med. 2012;42:1791–800.
47. Mohr P, Rodriguez M, Slavickova A, Hanka J. The application of vagus nerve stimulation and deep brain stimulation in depression. Neuropsychobiology. 2011;64:170–81.
48. Holtzheimer PE, Kelley ME, Gross RE, et al. Subcallosal cingulate deep brain stimulation for treatment-resistant unipolar and bipolar depression. Arch Gen Psychiatry. 2012;69:150–8.
49. Mayberg HS, Lozano AM, Voon V, et al. Deep brain stimulation for treatment-resistant depression. Neuron. 2005;45:651–60.
50. Kennedy SH, Giacobbe P, Rizvi SJ, Placenza FM, Nishikawa Y, Mayberg HS, Lozano AM. Deep brain stimulation for treatment-resistant depression: follow-up after 3 to 6 years. Am J Psychiatry. 2011;168:502–10.
51. Bajbouj M, Merkl A, Schlaepfer TE, et al. Two-year outcome of vagus nerve stimulation in treatment-resistant depression. J Clin Psychopharmacol. 2010;30:273–81.
52. Gerson R, Murray E, Price B, Frankel M, Douglass L, Cunningham M. Mania following vagus nerve stimulation: a case report and review of the literature. Epilepsy Behav. 2011;20:138–40.
53. Biermann T, Kreil S, Groemer T, et al. Time perception in patients with major depressive disorder during vagus nerve stimulation. Pharmacopsychiatry. 2011;44:179–82.
54. Sperling W, Biermann T, Spannenberger R, et al. Changes in gustatory perceptions of patients with major depression treated with vagus nerve stimulation (VNS). Pharmacopsychiatry. 2011;44:67–71.
55. Schrader L, Cook I, Miller P, Maremont E, DeGiorgi OC. Trigeminal nerve stimulation in major depressive disorder: first proof of concept in an open pilot trial. Epilepsy Behav. 2011;22:475–8.
56. Yatham LN, Kennedy SH, Schaffer A, et al. Canadian Network for Mood and Anxiety Treatments (CANMAT) and International Society for Bipolar Disorders (ISBD) collaborative update of CANMAT guidelines for the management of patients with bipolar disorder: update 2009. Bipolar Disord. 2009;11:225–55.
57. Mendels J, Frazer A. Intracellular lithium concentration and clinical response: towards a membrane theory of depression. J Psychiatr Res. 1973;10:9–18.
58. Goodwin FK, Murphy DL, Bunney WE. Lithium-carbonate treatment in depression and mania—a longitudinal double-blind study. Arch Gen Psychiatry. 1969;21:486–96.
59. Greenspan K, Schildkraut J, Gordon E, Baer L, Aronoff M, Durell J. Catecholamine metabolism in affective disorder—III: MHPG and other catecholamine metabolites in patients treated with lithium carbonate. J Psychiatr Res. 1970;7:171–83.
60. Baron M, Gershon E, Rudy V, Jonas W, Buchsbaum M. Lithium carbonate response in depression. Arch Gen Psychiatry. 1975;32:1107–11.
61. Srisurapanont M, Yatham L, Zis A. Treatment of acute bipolar depression: a review of the literature. Can J Psychiatry. 1995;40:533–44.

62. Dolberg OT, Dannon PN, Schreiber S, Grunhaus L. Transcranial magnetic stimulation in patients with bipolar depression: a double blind, controlled study. Bipolar Disord. 2002;4 Suppl 1:94–5.
63. Nahas Z, Kozel FA, Li X, Anderson B, George MS. Left prefrontal transcranial magnetic stimulation (TMS) treatment of depression in bipolar affective disorder: a pilot study of acute safety and efficacy. Bipolar Disord. 2003;5:40–7.
64. Tamas RL, Menkes D, El-Mallakh RS. Stimulating research: a prospective, randomized, double-blind, sham-controlled study of slow transcranial magnetic stimulation in depressed bipolar patients. J Neuropsychiatry Clin Neurosci. 2007;19:198–9.
65. Dell'Osso B, Mundo E, D'Urso N, et al. Augmentative repetitive navigated transcranial magnetic stimulation (rTMS) in drug-resistant bipolar depression. Bipolar Disord. 2009;11:76–81.
66. Grisaru N, Chudakov B, Yaroslavsky Y, Belmaker RH. Transcranial magnetic stimulation in mania: a controlled study. Am J Psychiatry. 1998;155:1608–10.
67. Michael N, Erfurth A. Treatment of bipolar mania with right prefrontal rapid transcranial magnetic stimulation. J Affect Disord. 2004;78:253–7.
68. Saba G, Rocamora JF, Kalalou K, et al. Repetitive transcranial magnetic stimulation as an add-on therapy in the treatment of mania: a case series of eight patients. Psychiatry Res. 2004;128:199–202.
69. Praharaj S, Ram D, Arora M. Efficacy of high frequency (rapid) suprathreshold repetitive transcranial magnetic stimulation of right prefrontal cortex in bipolar mania: a randomized sham controlled study. J Affect Disord. 2009;117:146–50.
70. Loranger A. Sex difference in age at onset of schizophrenia. Arch Gen Psychiatry. 1984;41:157–61.
71. McGlashan T, Johannessen J. Early detection and intervention with schizophrenia: rationale. Schizophr Bull. 1996;22:201–22.
72. Andreasen N. Symptoms, signs, and diagnosis of schizophrenia. Lancet. 1995;346:477–81.
73. Wong A, Van Tol H. Schizophrenia: from phenomenology to neurobiology. Neurosci Biobehav Rev. 2003;27:269–306.
74. APA. Diagnostic and statistic manual of mental disorders, IV-TR ed. Washington, DC: American Psychiatric Association; 2000.
75. Weickert T, Goldberg T, Gold J, Bigelow L, Egan M. Cognitive impairments in patients with schizophrenia displaying preserved and compromised intellect. Arch Gen Psychiatry. 2000;57:907–13.
76. Conley R. The burden of depressive symptoms in people with schizophrenia. Psychiatr Clin North Am. 2009;32:853–61.
77. Bensenor I, Brunoni A, Pilan L, Goulart A, Busatto G. Cardiovascular risk factors in patients with first-episode psychosis in Sao Paulo, Brazil. Gen Hosp Psychiatry. 2012;34:268–75.
78. Bressan R, Chaves A, Pilowsky L, Shirakawa I, Mari J. Depressive episodes in stable schizophrenia: critical evaluation of the DSM-IV and ICD-10 diagnostic criteria. Psychiatry Res. 2003;117:47–56.
79. Lieberman J, Stroup T, McEvoy J, Swartz M, Rosenheck R. Effectiveness of antipsychotic drugs in patients with chronic schizophrenia. N Engl J Med. 2005;353:1209–23.
80. Jones P, Barnes T, Davies L, Dunn G, Lloyd H. Randomized controlled trial of the effect on quality of life of second- vs. first-generation antipsychotic drugs in schizophrenia: Cost Utility of the Latest Antipsychotic Drugs in Schizophrenia Study (CUtLASS 1). Arch Gen Psychiatry. 2006;63:1079–87.
81. Davis J, Chen N, Glick I. A meta-analysis of the efficacy of second-generation antipsychotics. Arch Gen Psychiatry. 2003;60:553–64.
82. Elkis H, Louza M. Psiquiatria Básica. 2nd ed. São Paulo: Atheneu; 2007.
83. Chong S, Remington G. Clozapine augmentation: safety and efficacy. Schizophr Bull. 2000;26:421–40.
84. Taylor D, Paton C, Kapur S. The South London and Maudsley NHS Foundation Trust and Oxleas NHS Foundation Trust: prescribing guidelines. 10th ed. London: Informa Healthcare; 2009.
85. Tharyan P, Adams CE. Electroconvulsive therapy for schizophrenia. Cochrane Database Syst Rev. 2005 Apr 18;(2):CD000076. Review.
86. Kho K, Blansjaar B, de Vries S, Babuskova D, Zwinderman AH, et al. Electroconvulsive therapy for the treatment of clozapine nonresponders suffering from schizophrenia—an open label study. Eur Arch Psychiatry Clin Neurosci. 2004;254:372–9.
87. Chanpattana W. (2007). A questionnaire survey of ECT practice in Australia. *Journal of ECT 23*(2):89-92.
88. Burt T, Lisanby SH, Sackeim HA. Neuropsychiatric applications of transcranial magnetic stimulation: a meta analysis. Int J Neuropsychopharmacol. 2002;5:73–103.
89. Hoffman RE, Boutros NN, Berman RM, et al. Transcranial magnetic stimulation of left temporoparietal cortex in three patients reporting hallucinated "voices". Biol Psychiatry. 1999;46:130–2.
90. d'Alfonso AA, Aleman A, Kessels RP, et al. Transcranial magnetic stimulation of left auditory cortex in patients with schizophrenia: effects on hallucinations and neurocognition. J Neuropsychiatry Clin Neurosci. 2002;14:77–9.
91. Hoffman RE, Hawkins KA, Gueorguieva R, et al. Transcranial magnetic stimulation of left temporoparietal cortex and medication-resistant auditory hallucinations. Arch Gen Psychiatry. 2003;60:49–56.
92. Cohen E, Bernardo M, Masana J, et al. Repetitive transcranial magnetic stimulation in the treatment of chronic negative schizophrenia: a pilot study. J Neurol Neurosurg Psychiatry. 1999;67:129–30.
93. Dlabac-de-Lange J, Knegtering R, Aleman A. Repetitive transcranial magnetic stimulation for negative symptoms of schizophrenia: review and meta-analysis. J Clin Psychiatry. 2010;71:411–8.
94. Brunelin J, Mondino M, Gassab L, et al. Examining transcranial direct-current stimulation (tDCS) as a treatment for hallucinations in schizophrenia. Am J Psychiatry. 2012;169(7):719–24.
95. Berkman N, Bulik C, Brownley K. Management of eating disorders. Evid Rep Technol Assess. 2006;135:1–166.
96. Attia E, Haiman C, Walsh B, Flater S. Does fluoxetine augment the inpatient treatment of anorexia nervosa? Am J Psychiatry. 1998;155:548–51.
97. Kaye W, Nagata T, Weltzin T. Double-blind placebo-controlled administration of fluoxetine in restricting- and restricting-purging-type anorexia nervosa. Biol Psychiatry. 2001;49:644–52.
98. Fassino S, Leombruni P, Daga G. Efficacy of citalopram in anorexia nervosa: a pilot study. Eur Neuropsychopharm. 2002;12:453–9.
99. Brown T, Keel P. Current and emerging directions in the treatment of eating disorders. Subst Abuse. 2012;6:33–61.
100. Herpertz S, Hagenah U, Vocks S, von Wietersheim J, Cuntz U, Zeeck A. The diagnosis and treatment of eating disorders. Dtsch Arztebl Int. 2011;108:678–85.
101. Treasure J, Tchanturia K, Schmidt U. Developing a model of the treatment for eating disorder: using neuroscience research to examine the how rather than the what of change. Couns Psychother Res. 2005;5:191–202.
102. Hudson J, Pope HJ, Jonas J, Yurgelun-Todd D. Family history study of anorexia nervosa and bulimia. Br J Psychiatry. 1983;142:428–9.
103. Milano W, Siano C, Putrella C, Capasso A. Treatment of bulimia nervosa with fluvoxamine: a randomized controlled trial. Adv Ther. 2005;22:278–83.
104. Fichter M, Kruger R, Rief W, Holland R, Dohne J. Fluvoxamine in prevention of relapse in bulimia nervosa: effects on eating-specific psychopathology. J Clin Psychopharmacol. 1996;16:9–18.
105. Milano W, Petrella C, Sabatino C, Capasso A. Treatment of bulimia nervosa with sertraline: a randomized controlled trial. Adv Ther. 2004;21:232–7.

106. Karno M, Golding J, Sorenson S, Burnam M. The epidemiology of obsessive compulsive disorder in five US communities. Arch Gen Psychiatry. 1988;45:1094–9.
107. Weissman M, Bland R, Canino G, Greenwald S, Hwu H, Lee C. The cross national epidemiology of obsessive compulsive disorder. J Clin Psychiatry. 1994;55:5–10.
108. Iancu I, Dannon P, Zohar J. Obsessive–compulsive disorder. Oxford: Oxford University Press; 2003.
109. Shin M, Choi H, Kim H, Hwang J, Kim B, Cho S. A study of neuropsychological deficit in children with obsessive-compulsive disorder. Eur Psychiatry. 2008;23:512–20.
110. March J, Mulle K. OCD in children and adolescents: a Cognitive behavioral treatment manual. New York: The Guilford Press; 1998.
111. Watson H, Rees C. Meta-analysis of randomized, controlled treatment trials for pediatric obsessive-compulsive disorder. J Child Psychol Psychiatry. 2008;49:489–98.
112. Sachdev P, Loo C, Mitchell P, McFarquhar T, Malhi G. Repetitive transcranial magnetic stimulation for the treatment of obsessive compulsive disorder: a double blind controlled investigation. Psychol Med. 2007;37:1645–9.
113. Nauczyciel C, Drapier D. Repetitive transcranial magnetic stimulation in the treatment of obsessive-compulsive disorder. Rev Neurol (Paris). 2012;168:655–61.
114. Volpato C, Piccione F, Cavinato M, et al. Modulation of affective symptoms and resting state activity by brain stimulation in a treatment-resistant case of obsessive-compulsive disorder. Neurocase. 2013;19(4):360–70.
115. Barkley R. Behavioral inhibition, sustained attention, and executive functions: constructing a unifying theory of ADHD. Psychol Bull. 1997;121:65–94.
116. Swanson M, Kraemer C, Hinshaw P, Arnold E, Conners K, Abikoff B. Clinical relevance of the primary findings of the MTA: success rates based on severity of ADHD and ODD symptoms at the end of treatment. J Am Acad Child Psychiatry. 2001;40:168–79.
117. Kujirai T, Caramia M, Rothwell J, et al. Corticocortical inhibition in human motor cortex. J Physiol. 1993;471:501–19.
118. Moll G, Heinrich H, Rothenberger A. Transcranial magnetic stimulation in child and adolescent psychiatry: excitability of the motor system in tic disorders and/or attention deficit hyperactivity disorders. Z Kinder Jugendpsychiatr Psychother. 2001;29:312–23.
119. Weaver L, Rostain A, Mace W, Akhtar U, Moss E, O'Reardon J. Transcranial magnetic stimulation (TMS) in the treatment of attention-deficit/hyperactivity disorder in adolescents and young adults: a pilot study. J ECT. 2012;28:98–103.
120. Niederhofer H. Effectiveness of the repetitive transcranical magnetic stimulation (rTMS) of 1 Hz for attention- deficit hyperactivity disorder (ADHD). Psychiatr Danub. 2008;20:91–2.
121. Bloch Y, Harel E, Aviram S. Positive effects of repetitive transcranial magnetic stimulation on attention in ADHD subjects: a randomized controlled pilot study. World J Biol Psychiatry. 2010;11:755–8.
122. APA. Diagnostic and statistical manual of mental disorders DSM-IV-TR. 4th ed. Washington, DC: American Psychiatric Publishing; 2000.
123. Huang C, Wei I, Chou Y, Su T. Effect of age, gender, menopausal status, and ovarian hormonal level on rTMS in treatment-resistant depression. Psychoneuroendocrinology. 2008;33:821–31.
124. Walpoth M, Hoertnagl C, Mangweth-Matzek B, et al. Repetitive transcranial magnetic stimulation in bulimia nervosa: preliminary results of a single-centre, randomised, double-blind, sham-controlled trial in female outpatients. Psychother Psychosom. 2008;77:57–60.
125. Van den Eynde F, Claudino A, Mogg A, et al. Repetitive transcranial magnetic stimulation reduces cue-induced food craving in bulimic disorders. Biol Psychiatry. 2010;67:793–5.
126. Van den Eynde F, Claudino A, Campbell I, Schmidt U. Immediate cognitive effects of repetitive transcranial magnetic stimulation in eating disorders: a pilot study. Eat Weight Disord. 2011;16:45–8.
127. Claudino AM, Van den Eynde F, Stahl D, et al. Repetitive transcranial magnetic stimulation reduces cortisol concentrations in bulimic disorders. Psychol Med. 2011;41:1329–36.

Applications of Neuromodulation in Pain Management

15

Helena Knotkova, Aaron Greenberg, Eliezer Soto, and Ricardo A. Cruciani

Complex Regional Pain Syndrome (CRPS)

Complex regional pain syndrome (CRPS) is a debilitating pain syndrome that includes CRPS I (formerly known as Reflex Sympathetic Dystrophy), that typically follows trauma without a known nerve-lesion, and CRPS II (formerly called Causalgia), in which the same signs and symptoms are observed together with an identifiable major nerve lesion.

The diagnostic criteria for CRPS were developed by the International Association for the Study of Pain in 1994 [1], and clinical signs of CRPS include pain, allodynia, edema, abnormal regulation of blood flow of the affected area, movement disorders, and changes in the skin trophism, typically affecting a part of a limb. It is estimated that CRPS is twice as common in the upper limb as in the lower limb, and occurs more frequently in adult females [2, 3]. There are approximately 17,000 new cases reported each year, which may actually represent only a fraction of total cases [4, 5].

Numerous trigger mechanisms for CRPS have been identified, including trauma [6, 7], limb immobilization [8, 9], ischemia/reperfusion [10, 11] and genetic factors [12, 13]. The neurophysiological mechanisms underlying CRPS symptoms, including CRPS-related pain, are not well understood but are thought to be multifactorial and may or may not include involvement of the sympathetic symptom. There is evidence indicating that functional and structural properties of pain-processing neurons and neuronal networks undergo pathological changes at peripheral, spinal, and cortical levels [14–23], that may contribute to the development and maintenance of CRPS-related pain. For a comprehensive review see Pappagallo et al. [24].

Recent findings suggest that CRPS patients present with cortical reorganization involving pathological changes of somatotopic maps within the somatosensory and motor cortices. It has been shown that there is a close relationship between the degree of cortical reorganization and the magnitude of pain [14, 25–28], and normalization (or a trend toward normalization) was paralleled by pain relief [14, 16, 27, 29]. This evidence facilitated exploration of neuromodulatory treatments to relieve CRPS-related pain.

Treatment Strategies in CRPS

The usual treatment of CRPS often relies on a multimodality approach, which includes a combination of pharmacological, interventional, and physiotherapeutic strategies, and in selected cases also psychological interventions.

There is no FDA-approved medication specifically for CRPS, and pharmacological pain management in CRPS therefore relies at large on the use of conventional agents for neuropathic and inflammatory pain, such as the gabapentinoid anticonvulsants (gabapentin, pregabalin) [30–32], non-gabapentinoid anticonvulsants such as carbamazepine, lamotrigine [33], topiramate [34], levetiracetam, zonisamide, oxcarbazepine, and tiagabine [35], tricyclic antidepressants (amitriptyline, nortriptyline, and desipramine) [36], $\alpha 2$-adrenergic agonists (e.g., clonidine, tizanidine) [37–40], γ-aminobutyric acid (GABA) agonists (e.g. intrathecal baclofen) [13], local anesthetics (transdermal lidocaine) [41], or opioids (methadone, morphine, fentanyl, and oxycodone) [42–47].

H. Knotkova (✉)
MJHS Institute for Innovation in Palliative Care, 39 Broadway, Suite 1230, New York, NY 10006, USA
e-mail: hknotkov@mjhs.org

A. Greenberg
Department of Pain Medicine and Palliative Care, Beth Israel Medical Center, New York, NY, USA

E. Soto
Anesthesia Pain Care Consultants, 7171 N. University Dr. 3rd Floor, Tamarac, FL 33321, USA

R.A. Cruciani
Center for Comprehensive Pain Management and Palliative Care, Capital Health Medical Center, Pennington, NJ, USA

H. Knotkova and D. Rasche (eds.), *Textbook of Neuromodulation*,
DOI 10.1007/978-1-4939-1408-1_15,

Other medications for CRPS-related pain include nonsteroidal anti-inflammatory drugs (NSAIDs), steroids (methylprednisolone) [48, 49], bisphosphonates [50–55], bone metabolism modulators (calcitonin) [56, 57], neuro-immunomodulatory and anticytokine therapies (thalidomide) [58, 59], *N*-Methyl-D-Aspartate (NMDA) receptor antagonists (dextromethorphan, memantine, ketamine) [60–62], antioxidants (dimethylsulfoxide; *N*-acetylcysteine) [63, 64], or topical capsaicin. Further, selected interventional strategies, such as sympatholytic procedures [65] and nonpharmacological treatments, such as rehabilitation and physiotherapy, have been used in CRPS [66].

Neuromodulation

Repetitive Transcranial Magnetic Stimulation (rTMS)

Up to date, only few studies explored the use of rTMS to relieve CRPS-related pain. Pleger and colleagues [29] applied a high-frequency (10 Hz) rTMS in ten right-handed patients with CRPS in one upper limb (Fig. 15.1). The subjects received one session of real rTMS and one session of sham in the cross-over design on 2 consecutive days. The visual analog scale (VAS) was used for the patients' self-reports of pain intensity. Out of the ten patients, seven responded to verum rTMS and showed significant decreased in pain level starting 30 s after stimulation and reaching maximum analgesic effect 15 min later, but it re-intensified 45 min later. Sham rTMS caused no changes in individual pain intensity.

In the study by Picarelli and colleagues [67], 23 patients with CRPS I-related unilateral pain in upper limb ten sessions or either real rTMS or sham rTMS over the motor cortex were added to the medical treatment regimen consisting of analgesics, adjuvant medications, and physical therapy. Pain intensity was assessed daily during the round of the 10-session rTMS, and 1 week and 3 months after the last rTMS session. The mean reduction of pain during the real rTMS treatment was 50.9 % as compared to 24.7 % in the sham group. The pain relief was most prominent at the last treatment session and correlated with the improvement of the affective and emotional scores measured with the McGill Pain Questionnaire and the Health Survey-36. The findings from the rTMS studies justify further research and explorations of the clinical potential of this neuromodulatory technique in the treatment of CRPS-related pain.

Transcranial Direct Current Stimulation (tDCS)

There is some empirical evidence indicating that tDCS can relieve CRPS-related pain that does not respond to conventional pharmacological treatment [68]. For example, there is a case report [69] of CRPS patient with intractable CRPS-

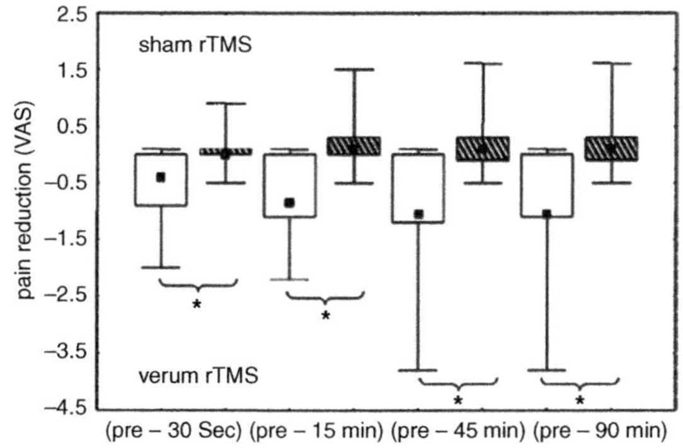

Fig. 15.1 The box-whisker-plot shows the benefit of verum rTMS when compared to sham rTMS. Pain levels (VAS) differences between pre-rTMS and the four successive evaluations over 90 min post-rTMS (the black point within the box gives the median of data. The top and bottom of the box gives the 25 and 75 percentiles, respectively. The top and bottom of the whisker gives the maximum and the minimum, respectively). To elucidate the difference between the two conditions a Student's paired *t*-test was utilized ($p < 0.005$). (From Pleger et al., 2004, with permission [66])

related pain in lower limb who received a total of five blocks of anodal tDCS (2 mA for 20 min, saline-soaked sponge electrodes 25 cm^2) applied over the primary motor cortex over the course of 42 weeks in "as needed" regime. Each block of tDCS resulted in pain relief, which substantially over-lasted the stimulation, by up to 11 weeks. The patient also gained secondary benefits from tDCS (for example improvement in sleep, mood, and activity) that over-lasted the stimulation by weeks. The repeated stimulation (five blocks, each block consisting of tDCS session on 5 consecutive days) did not cause any serious adverse effects, and did not show the effect of "desensitization" to the tDCS treatment.

Further, there is a case report [70] suggesting that not only anodal tDCS over the motor cortex, but also cathodal tDCS over the somatosensory cortex may alleviate CRPS-related chronic pain (Fig. 15.2).

Motor Imagery

Findings on the use of motor imagery for the treatment of CRPS-related pain are mixed. For example, Lagueux and colleagues [71] noted pain relief after the graded motor imagery in series of seven patients with CRPS of upper limb, as did Walz and colleagues [72] in a patient with unilateral CRPS. On contrary, findings by Johnson and colleagues [73] from a prospective evaluation of 32 CRPS patients who received the graded motor imagery treatment at two UK medical centers, reported failure of the motor imagery treatment to improve CRPS-related pain in clinical settings. The failure of the real-world implementation of graded motor imagery suggests that better understanding of both the graded motor imagery methodology and its interaction with other treatment methods is needed in order to

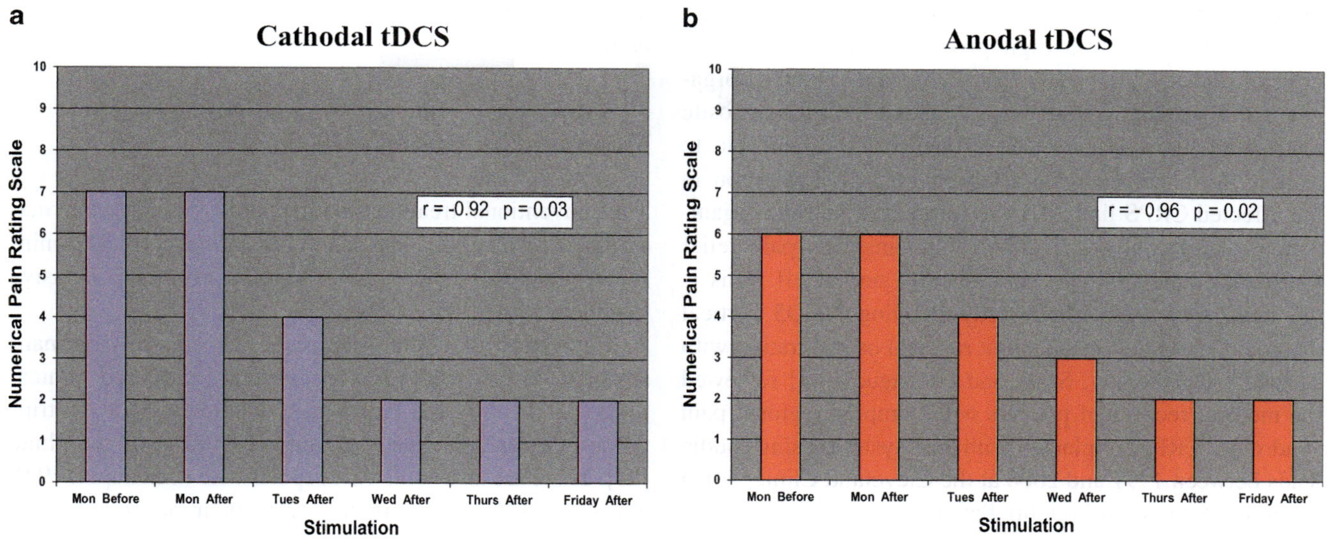

Fig. 15.2 Pain relief was induced by a block (five tDCS sessions on 5 consecutive days) of either cathodal tDCS over the somatosensory cortex (**a**), or anodal tDCS over the motor cortex (**b**) at intensity of 2 mA for 20 min, using saline-soaked sponge electrodes, size 25 cm^2. The interval between the two blocks of stimulation was 6 weeks. Both modalities cathodal tDCS over the somatosensory cortex and anodal tDCS over the motor cortex resulted in significant pain relief. (From Knotkova el al., 2010, with permission [70])

translate the research results of motor imagery into clinical practice.

Motor Cortex Stimulation (MCS)

Fonoff and colleague [74] report on two patients with pain related to CRPS and severe functional deficits treated with motor cortex stimulation (MCS) who not only had significant analgesic effects, but also improvements in sensory and motor symptoms. In the long term (27 and 36 months after surgery), visual analog scale pain scores were improved by 60–70 % as compared to baseline. There was also a significant increase in the range of motion in the joints of the affected limbs and an improvement in allodynia, hyperpathia, and hypoesthesia. Positron emission tomography scan in both subjects revealed that MCS influenced regions involved in the circuitry of pain. Study by Velasco and colleagues [75] analyzed the MCS efficacy in patients with CRPS. Five patients with CRPS of different etiologies underwent a small craniotomy for unilateral 20-grid-contact implantation on MC, guided by craniometric landmarks. Preoperative and postoperative monthly evaluations were performed during 1 year. A double-blind maneuver was introduced assigning two groups. One had stimulators turned OFF from day 30 to 60 and the other from day 60 to 90. Four patients showed important decrease in pain, sensory and sympathetic changes during the therapeutic trial, while one patient did not have any improvement and was rejected for implantation. VAS and McGill pain scales diminished significantly ($p < 0.01$) throughout the follow-up, accompanied by disappearance of the sensory (allodynea and hyperalgesia) and sympathetic signs. MCS is effective not only to treat pain, but also improve the sympathetic changes in CPRS. Son and colleagues [76] report the efficacy of motor cortex stimulation (MCS) in a patient with complex regional pain syndrome (CRPS) Type II, formerly known as causalgia, with hemibody allodynia. Pain and allodynia in the areas associated with this sensation were alleviated significantly. The analgesic effect of stimulation proved to be long lasting and was still present at the 12-month follow-up.

Spinal Cord Stimulation (SCS)

Implantable devices, such as spinal cord stimulators (SCS), have been used successfully to produce symptomatic relief [77]. Systematic review of the literature and meta-analysis support the usefulness of SCS in the management of CRPS [78]. Although spinal cord stimulation can produce inhibition of sympathetic outflow, its mechanism is likely related to neurochemical changes at both spinal and supraspinal targets, and not to sympatholysis [79]. Indeed, it was shown that spinal cord stimulation produced sufficient analgesia even in patients who had undergone previous sympathectomy, suggesting that spinal-cord-stimulation related analgesia might not be mediated by inhibition of the sympathetic function. Spinal cord stimulation may cause inhibition of the A-beta fiber-mediated dorsal horn neuron excitability through a GABA mechanism.

For example, Pahapill and Zhang [80] have shown a reversal of cortical reorganization in CRPS after SCS. Two patients treated with either thoracic or cervical SCS with leg or arm CRPS were studied with MEG. Baseline and tactile-evoked responses were recorded with and without effective

SCS therapy. In the patient with arm CRPS, with the stimulator off, first and fifth digit primary somatosensory (SI) cortical representations (D1/D5) were significantly disorganized and spatially inverted as compared with the opposite unaffected limb. Effective SCS therapy was then able to acutely normalize or restore hand cortical organization in the affected CRPS limb. This restoration of cortical organization was partially maintained with lingering pain relief when the stimulator was subsequently turned off. This is the first report of a MEG study showing D1/D5 cortical disorganization and its apparent reversal or restoration with cervical SCS therapy. Sears and colleagues [81] reviewed the medical records of patients with complex regional pain syndrome (CRPS) implanted with SCS systems using paddle leads between 1997 and 2008 at the Cleveland Clinic with a minimum 6-month follow-up. Patients were contacted to fill out a questionnaire evaluating outcomes with the NRS-11 as well as overall satisfaction. More than 50 % of the CRPS patients with CRPS reported greater than 50 % pain relief at a mean follow-up of 4.4 years, and 77.8 % of patients with CRPS indicated that they would undergo SCS surgery again for the same outcome.

Phantom-Limb Pain

Phantom limb pain (PLP), is commonly defined as pain that is localized to the missing limb [82], and has to be distinguished from other amputation-related pains and abnormal sensations, such as stump-pain or telescoping. While stump pain encompasses pain sensation in the remaining part of the limb [83], telescoping is sensation where the distal part of the phantom is gradually felt to approaching the residual limb and may even perceived to be within the stump [84].

PLP develops in about 80 % of patients with partial or total loss of a limb, affects more women than men, and more often after upper extremity amputation [85]. PLP belongs among neuropathic pain syndromes and the pain sensation in PLP is often described as tingling, itching burning, or aching. Mechanisms underlying PLP are not fully understood, but the recent findings suggest that both peripheral- as well as central mechanisms, including neuroplastic changes in CNS, can contribute to PLP [25, 26, 86]. Notably, a pathological change of the afferent input after amputation represents a significant source of neural plasticity, i.e. dynamic changes in function of neurons and neural networks in CNS, including both spinal and cerebral parts of pain processing network [87, 88]. Indeed, it has been shown that amputees with PLP often present with changes in organization of somatotopic maps in the somatosensory and motor cortices (so called cortical reorganization), and that normalization of the changes was paralleled by pain relief [26]. Therefore it is not surprising that exploration of neuromodulation for management of phantom limb pain is on the rise.

Treatment Strategies in PLP

The conventional treatment options in PLP include pharmacological treatment, supportive nonpharmacological noninvasive strategies, such as physiotherapy, and invasive treatments.

Medications that show significant benefits in pain management of PLP and were assessed in controlled clinical trials specifically in PLP patient-population include amitriptyline [89], gabapentine [84], tramadol [90]; and morphine [91]. There are also some case reports with mitrazapine [92], duloxetine [91], milnacipran [93], memantine [94, 95], and baclofen [96], and buprenorphine [97]. Further, other analgesics that have not been assessed specifically for PLP but show efficacy in other types of neuropathic pain can also be considered in the treatment of PLP. For a review, see Knotkova and colleagues [98]. Some pharmacological treatment strategies in PLP suggest preemptive analgesia, i.e. the administration of analgesic and anesthetics prior to a surgical intervention [99, 100], in order to prevent the development of central sensitization due to impulses generated at the level of the amputation. However, supporting evidence for that varies. Epidural analgesia, ropivacine, and patient-controlled analgesia (PCA), during the perioperative period have shown to decrease PLP, but ketamine and ketamine plus bupivacaine showed conflicting results [101–103].

In selected, pharmacotherapy-resistant cases, nondestructive interventions such as nerve blocks, interscalene blocks, or stellate ganglion blocks for upper extremity phantom limb pain, or lumbar sympathetic blocks for lower extremity phantom limb pain can be considered [104]. Destructive procedures like thermal nerve root destruction, rhizotomy, spinal ganglionectomy, or dorsal root entry zone lesion (DREZ) [105] are reserved only for selected patients with severe refractory PLP, and the overall volume of the invasive destructive procedures is continuously decreasing.

Supportive nonpharmacological therapies include physical therapy, reflexology, hypnosis [106, 107] or various psychotherapeutic approaches [108].

Neuromodulation

rTMS

Although several studies have shown that a single session of rTMS can transiently relieve pain in some patients with chronic neuropathic pain [109–114], and a multiple application on several consecutive days lead to prolongation of the effects [115, 116], evidence on the analgesic effects of rTMS

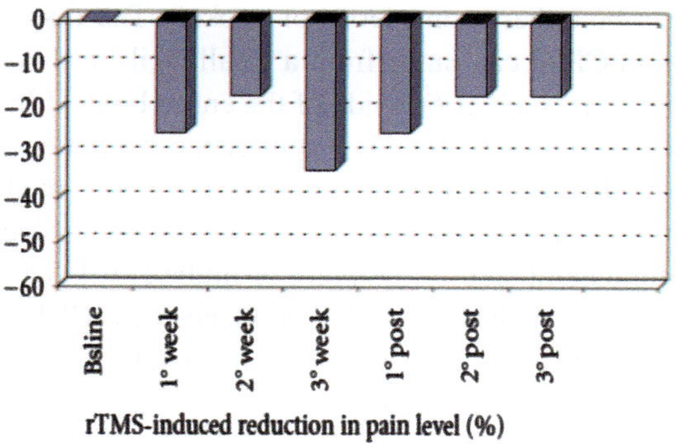

Fig. 15.3 Pain relief induced by low-frequency (1 Hz) rTMS stimulation in a patient with phantom limb pain. The stimulation was delivered over the motor cortex of the unaffected hemisphere (that was not involved in the phantom limb pain). The graph shows a reduction in percentage of pain in time. The percentage of pain level modification was calculated from the VAS score by the following equation (post. rTMS—pre.rTMS pain scores) × 100/(pre.rTMS pain scores). (From Di Rollo et al., 2011, free access article [115])

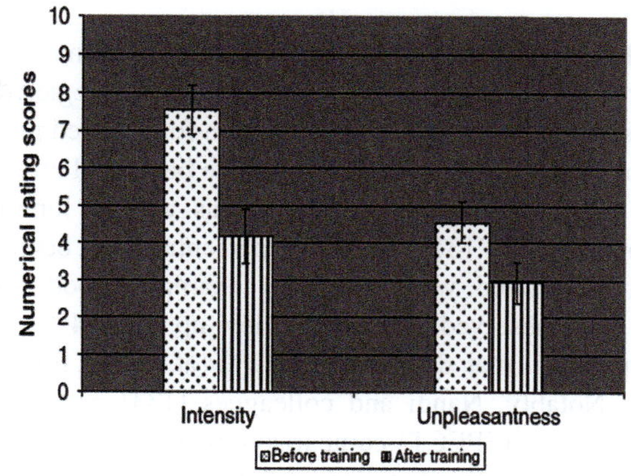

Fig. 15.4 Scores of constant pain intensity and unpleasantness before and after training, measured by daily pain diaries using numerical rating scores. Reduction in pain intensity was significant ($p < 0.0005$), as was reduction in pain unpleasantness ($p < 0.01$). (From McIver et al., 2008; free access article [119])

specifically in patients with PLP are mostly based on case/series reports, such as that reported by DiRollo and Pallanti [117] (Fig. 15.3), and others [115, 116].

However, Ahmed and colleagues [118] report findings from a randomized sham-controlled trial to assess analgesic effects of high-frequency (20 Hz) rTMS of motor cortex in 27 unilateral amputees with PLP, delivered in five daily sessions. The real rTMS lead to more profound decrease of pain scores and to a significant increase of serum beta-endorfine as compared to sham, through different time-points of follow-up for 2 months. The findings indicate that the rTMS 5-day treatment protocol over the motor cortex can produce longer-lasting analgesic effects and be beneficial in PLP.

Visual Feedback Therapy and Motor Imagery

Visual feedback (also called Mirror-box therapy) is based on illusions of movement and touch in a phantom limb by inducing somatosensory and motor pathway coupling between the phantom and real limb [119]. Motor imagery is a dynamic state during which an individual mentally simulates a given action and the subject feels herself/himself performing the action [120]. A rationale of this approach arises from the existence of maladaptive neuroplastic changes underlying PLP, specifically cortical reorganization in the somatosensory and motor cortices, a relation between the cortical reorganization and the occurrence of PLP, and beneficial effects of cortical normalization on PLP. Both the visual feedback therapy (mirror-box therapy) and motor imagery in PLP are based on behaviorally relevant sensory-motor stimulation of the stump [121–125], and can be very beneficial for PLP patients. MacIver and colleagues [121] observed a therapeutic effect of 6-week training in mental imagery in 13 amputees with phantom limb pain. Following training, patients reported a significant reduction in intensity of constant pain (Fig. 15.4), and in exacerbations, with a corresponding elimination of cortical reorganization.

Further, a controlled neuroimaging study of motor imagery in PLP by Brodie and colleagues [123] showed evidence of cortical reorganization of motor and somatosensory cortices and its correlation with patients' pain scores prior the motor imagery training. The training resulted in a significant decrease of intensity and unpleasantness of pain which correlated with reduction (improvement) of cortical reorganization. Overall, the mirror-box therapy and motor imagery are safe and nonexpensive add-on therapies for PLP.

MCS and DBS

On contrary to surgical destructive procedures, invasive neuromodulatory techniques are PLP-mechanisms-driven, specifically addressing maladaptive central neuroplastic changes in pain-processing networks. Nevertheless, invasive neuromodulation is considered the last-resort treatment for patients who failed various trials of noninvasive treatments.

A review of evidence [126] suggests that MCS yields favorable results in about 53 % of PLP patients. MCS for PLP of the upper limb seems to be favorable due to the large representation on the convex part of the precentral gyrus, but interhemispheral lead implantation for the lower limb has also been reported, and PLP is an accepted indication for MCS in many treatment centers [109, 126–129]. As for DBS, evidence up to date is controversial. Nevertheless, some PLP patients clearly benefit from DBS, experiencing long-term pain relief and improved quality of life [130].

SCS

As PLP is difficult-to-treat pain syndrome and many PLP patients do not respond to other treatment strategies, SCS represents a promising treatment option for selected population of patients. Clinical results indicate beneficial effects of SCS in PLP patients on immediate as well as long-term outcomes [129, 131], although percentage of benefiting patients declined with time. For example, good results have been observed at 2-year follow-up in 52.4 % of 64 PLP patients, that decreased to 39 % at 5-year follow-up [132]. Notably, Nandi and colleagues [133] performed a neuroimaging (SPECT) comparison of two PLP cases that have been satisfactorily treated with CNS stimulation; motor cortex stimulation followed by periventricular gray stimulation was used in one case, while SCS in the other. SPECT images were compared before the stimulation, and then during the stimulation with noted pain relief. Interestingly, regardless of the type/site of stimulation in the CNS, pain relief was in both cases associated with blood-flow changes in similar areas of brain, mainly in the parietal and cingulated cortex and also in the thalamic nuclei and the central gray matter. Although further controlled studies are warranted, the findings indicate that different invasive neuromodulatory treatments may at least to some degree trigger a cascade of similar neurohumoral changes that are associated with pain relief.

Central Post-stroke Pain (CPSP)

Central post-stroke pain (CPSP) is a neuropathic pain syndrome following a cerebrovascular accident. CPSP is characterized by pain and sensory abnormalities in the body part that corresponds to the brain territory injured by the cerebrovascular lesion, and where other causes of obvious nociceptive, psychogenic, or peripheral neuropathic origin have been ruled out [134, 135]. CPSP belongs to a class of chronic pain disorders named central neuropathic pain because the pain is due to lesion or dysfunction of the CNS. Besides PSPC, this class includes for example trigeminal neuropathic facial pain, multiple sclerosis related pain, or pain due to spinal cord injuries.

The prevalence of CPSP in patients with stroke is estimated to be between 1 and 12 % [136]. The few epidemiological studies of CPSP indicate that the development of CPSP is associated with the presence of sensory impairment and the location of the lesion. In specific, the occurrence of CPSP is high after the lateral medullary infarction or lesions in the ventroposterior thalamus.

Clinical features of CPSP substantially vary among patients and there are no uniform signs with regard to onset, intensity, presentation, or characteristics, and the pain can be either spontaneous or evoked. The distribution of pain in CPSP can range from a small well-localized area to large areas, such as one side of the entire body [136]. The hemibody pain is frequently experienced by patients with thalamic lesions, while patients with lateral medullary infarction may develop pain involving one side of face and the contralateral side of the body or limbs [136]. The diagnosis of CPSP is based on clear evidence of a CNS injury, pain and sensory alterations, and the exclusion of other possible mechanisms of pain.

Treatment Strategies in CPSP

Central post-stroke pain is among the most intractable types of pain, and is often resistant to conventional pharmacologic strategies which are limited in number and efficacy. Several drug categories have been reported to have an analgesic effect in this patient population including: anticonvulsants, tricyclic antidepressants, NMDA antagonists, GABA agonists, cannabinoid receptor agonists and systemic opioids. However, evidence based on controlled trials for pharmacologic therapies of CPSP is limited.

Results of randomized trials of amitriptyline for the treatment of CPSP were mixed [137, 138]. The efficacy of anticonvulsants such as lamotrigine, phenytoin, and gabapentin, as a treatment options for this syndrome, have been investigated in several small studies [139]. In a randomized, placebo-controlled study, lamotrigine showed a pain reduction of 30 % in 44 % of the patients at doses of 200 mg per day [139], but further clinical trials are needed to evaluate this therapy in the treatment of CPSP.

Several small trials have studied the use of local anesthetic agents as possible therapy for CPSP [140–143]. In a small double-blind, placebo-controlled study in CPSP patients, IV lidocaine resulted in significant short term relief of spontaneous pain, mechanical allodynia and mechanical hyperalgesia; however, the transition to oral mexiletine had no effects on the pain [140]. The injection of the putative GABA agonist propofol has also been shown to reduce spontaneous and evoked pain and allodynia in CPSP using subhypnotic dosages without hemodynamic side effects [144].

Trials of other medications, such as noncompetitive NMDA blockers, (e.g. dextromethorphan and ketamine) and systemic opioids [145–149] provided mixed results.

Therefore pharmacological options for CPSP often follow the consensus guidelines regarding pharmacologic approaches for the treatment of neuropathic pain of all types, that recommend tricyclics and calcium channel ligands (e.g. gabapentin) as the first line of treatment and anticonvulsants drugs and opioids as the second line [150, 151].

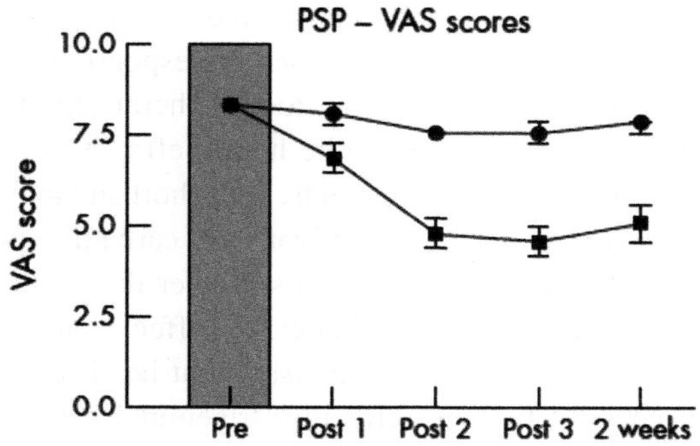

Fig. 15.5 Changes in mean pain rating scores (visual analog scale VAS) at the five assessment points in the post-stroke patients. The first assessment was done immediately prior to commencing rTMS treatment (Pre), the second (Post 1) was immediately after the first session of rTMS, and then the fourth (Post 2) and fifth (Post 3) rTMS sessions, and 15 days after the last session. The mean scores of the patients who received real rTMS decreased more over the course of the treatment than those who received sham rTMS. (From Khedr et al., 2005, with permission [114])

Neuromodulation

rTMS

Although CPSP was mostly treated by invasive neuromodulatory interventions, there are some very limited research findings from applications of noninvasive neuromodulation as well. For example, Khedr and colleagues [116] delivered high-frequency rTMS (20 Hz) or sham over the motor cortex on 5 consecutive days in 48 patients, of which 24 were CPSP patients. Real rTMS resulted in significantly greater pain relief than sham stimulation and the effects were present at a 2-week follow-up (Fig. 15.5).

Saitoh and colleagues [152] evaluated outcomes of rTMS in 13 patients with intractable chronic pain, of which seven patients had CPSP due to thalamic hemorrhage, putaminal hemorrhage, or thalamic infarction. All patients underwent rTMS stimulation over the motor cortex at 1, 5, and 10 Hz, and sham. In the CPSP patients, the 5- and 10-Hz stimulation resulted in significant pain relief immediately after the stimulation, however the durability of the effects was minimal and not present at 90 or 180 min after the stimulation. In the remaining six patients with pain syndromes other than CPSP, the 5- and 10-Hz analgesic effects persisted up to 90 min. Although rTMS in other chronic pain syndromes has shown clinical potential and longer-lasting analgesic effects, it does not seem promising in the treatment of CPSP.

DBS

Alves and Asfora [135] report results of DBS in case of CPSP patient. DBS was targeted to the left centromedian thalamic nuclei and lead to a symptomatic improvement.

Although DBS can provide an excellent control of involuntary movements associated with post-stroke condition, the results of DBS for CPSP are, with some exceptions, disappointing [153]. Indeed, evaluating outcomes of DBS targeting sensory thalamus and the periventricular and periaqueductal gray area (PVG/PAG) in 47 patients with various pain syndromes, Owen and colleagues [154] found that CPSP patients were the most like to fail trial stimulation, as compared to those with phantom-limb pain or pain due to post-brachial plexus injury. A meta-analysis of DBS outcomes in the period between 1966 and 2003 [155], found that the DBS trial was successful in about 50 % of CPSP patients, and about 58 % of those with permanent implantation achieved ongoing pain relief. And better results in CPSP control were reported from the Motor Cortex Stimulation (MCS).

MCS

Tsubokawa and colleagues [153] and Katayama et al. [156] noted that excellent pain control can be achieved in about 50 % of CPSP patients treated with MCS and in some patients, pain relief is accompanied by an improvement of involuntary movements that are a frequent symptom of post-stroke condition. Interestingly, Katayama and colleagues [127] compared analgesic effects of MCS, DBS of the thalamic nucleus ventralis caudalis, and SCS in patients with CPSP. The results from 45 patients indicated that satisfactory pain control was obtained more frequently as the stimulation site was moved to higher levels (7 % by SCS, 25 % by DBS and 48 % by MCS). Indeed, MCS has become the preferred option for neurosurgical management of intractable central neuropatic pain, including post-stroke pain [134, 157, 158]. Tanei and colleagues [134] evaluated outcomes of MCS at 1 month and 6 months after initiation of the treatment in patients with CPSP as compared to other central pain syndromes. Of 11 evaluated patients, 8 were those with CPSP caused either by thalamic hemorrhage or thalamic infarction, 2 patients had postoperative neuropathic pain caused by spinal cord lesions and 1 had facial pain caused by a brainstem lesion due to multiple sclerosis. At 1 month after the implantation, MCS was effective for pain control in six of eight CPSP patients and in all three patients with other central pain. The analgesic efficacy continued for the remaining 6 month observational period.

SCS

Tanei and colleagues [159] retrospectively reviewed effects of SCS in eight CPSP patients. Six of eight patients reported pain relief at least 50 % during the test stimulation, and the benefits continued for about 12 months in five patients without any significant complications.

Facial Neuropathic Pain

Facial neuropathic pain due to cranial neuralgias is debilitating conditions characterized by burning, stabbing pain, and disesthetic sensations in the distribution of the affected nerve. The most common cranial neuralgia known to cause severe morbidity is trigeminal neuralgia. The classification system by Burchiel [160] distinguishes seven diagnostic entities according to the cause of damage to the trigeminal nerve: (1) Trigeminal neuralgia, type 1, (TN1): which is facial pain of spontaneous onset with predominantly episodic pain; (2) Trigeminal neuralgia, type 2, (TN2): facial pain of spontaneous onset with predominantly constant pain; (3) Symptomatic trigeminal neuralgia, (STN): pain resulting from disturbance of trigeminal nerve by a demyelinating plaque in the central pathway of the trigeminal nerve due to multiple sclerosis; (4) Trigeminal neuropathic pain, (TNP): facial pain resulting from unintentional injury to the trigeminal system from facial trauma, oral surgery, ear, nose, and throat (ENT) surgery, root injury from posterior fossa or skull base surgery, stroke, etc.; (5) Trigeminal deafferentation pain, (TDP): facial pain in a region of trigeminal numbness resulting from intentional injury to the trigeminal system from neurectomy, gangliolysis, rhizotomy, nucleotomy, tractotomy, or other neuroablative procedures; (6) Postherpetic neuralgia, (PHN): pain resulting from trigeminal Herpes zoster (shingles) outbreak in the trigeminal distribution. The pain is often described as constant, intense, and unbearable, frequently with presence of allodynia. The Burchiel's classification includes also Atypical facial pain (AFP), which is defined as pain having a substantial psychological component or being psychological rather than of physiological origin. Therefore, the atypical facial pain may or may not include the neuropathic component of the pain.

Treatment Strategies in Facial Neuropathic Pain

Invasive and noninvasive approaches may be used to treat facial neuropathic pain depending on the etiology. It has been more than seven decades since a medication (phenytoin) was first utilized to treat facial pain. New treatments are continually being tried for the treatment of facial neuropathic pain because most pharmacotherapies have a very low success rate and prevalent side effects. There is a wide spectrum of pharmacological agents that can be used for the management of neuropathic facial pain (depending of the etiology) including: anticonvulsants, antidepressants, nonopioid analgesics, benzodiazepine, muscle relaxants, topical agents, and in selected cases opioids as well.

Carbamazepine, has been considered the first-line agent used by most physicians. It decreases the response of trigeminal mechanoreceptive neurons to peripheral stimulation. This drug has been proven to be highly effective, causing pain relief in up to 80 % of patients, both short and long term [161]. Oxcarbazepine, a keto derivative of carbamazepine, it is probably equal or superior to its mother drug due to its very rapid onset, efficacy and better side effect profile [162]. Topiramate, is another anticonvulsant that has been shown to be successful treating refractory trigeminal neuralgia in multiple sclerosis patients [163]. Other medications in the same category that have been used to treat facial neuropathic pain include: valproic acid, lamotrigine, phenytoin (now a second-, or third-line) and gabapentin.

Baclofen, a gamma-aminobutyric acid (GABA) analog, has also been utilized alone or in combination with phenytoin or carbamazepine for the treatment of facial neuropathic pain. Its possible mechanism is the suppression of the response of spinal trigeminal neurons to maxillary nerve stimulation. Clonazepam, a benzodiazepine, has been found to be effective in 65 % of individuals with trigeminal neuralgia, however, side effects such as dizziness and ataxia are prevalent if started at higher dosages [164].

When choosing the medical therapy for this pain syndrome it is recommended to comply with the following recommendations: do not over-treat (reduce dosages if pain remission), be aware that convulsive therapy in the elderly may cause further cognitive deficits, recognize presence of drug resistance over time (adjust dosages accordingly), minimize medications side effects, choose monotherapy over polypharmacy and utilize tolerable and effective medications first (e.g. lamotrigine, gabapentin, topiramate, and oxcarbazepine). Despite the existence of a wide variety of effective medications to treat facial neuropathic pain, many patients do not respond to the treatment or experience side effects that limit the titration of the drug to effective dose, and suffer from refractory pain and severe impairment of function. In those patients, nonpharmacological treatment strategies, including brain stimulation techniques, represent a promising venue to explore. Indeed, a recent study by DaSilva and colleagues [165] confirmed the existence of functional cortical changes in patients with facial neuropathic pain, supporting the rationale for the use of brain stimulation in facial neuropathic pain, and indicating that this patient-population may benefit from brain-stimulation treatment strategies.

Neuromodulation

rTMS and tDCS

Although no rTMS studies targeted exclusively facial-pain population, various rTMS trials in neuropathic pain included patients with neuropathic facial pain as a subpopulation of study samples (total $n = 231$, neuropathic facial pain $n = 74$) [112–114, 116, 166–169]. The main purpose of these trials was to explore various rTMS parameters, target groups, and designs of rTMS in order to maximize its analgesic potential as noninvasive and safer variant to invasive brain stimulation techniques.

A double-blind sham-controlled study by Lefaucheur and colleagues [166] involving seven patients with chronic treatment-resistant trigeminal neuropathy patients and seven patients central pain due to thalamic stroke delivered a single session of real high-frequency (20 Hz) rTMS over the motor cortex and a single session of sham were delivered in a 3-week interval. Notably, individual results in the trigeminal neuropathy group showed a significant pain relief (>30 %) in four of seven patients. This was the first study showing that high frequency (20 Hz) rTMS delivered over the motor cortex in patients with treatment resistant neuropathic pain, including facial pain, can overlast the time of stimulation. Although the pain-relief induced by high frequency rTMS in this study was short-lasting, the findings provided initial evidence for further explorations of stimulation-parameters to optimize rTMS analgesic effects.

Later studies [112, 113] in patients with various types of neuropathic pain (total $n = 96$), including neuropathic facial pain ($n = 30$), suggested that pain origin and site of pain play a role in defining the clinical outcomes: rTMS was significantly less effective in patients with pain due to brainstem stroke as compared with pain due to trigeminal nerve lesion, spinal cord- or brachial plexus lesion, and facial pain yielded better response to the stimulation than pain in upper or lower limb. Other studies [111, 114, 168] in patients with various types of neuropathic pain (total $n = 60$), including neuropathic facial pain ($n = 11$) suggested better analgesic effects and longer duration (up to 1 week) of a single-session high frequency rTMS as compared to low frequency rTMS or sham. Possible prolongation of analgesic effect after five daily sessions of high frequency (20 Hz) rTMS (instead of a single session as delivered in previous studies), as compared to sham was explored by Khedr and colleagues [116] in 24 patients with trigeminal neuralgia and 24 patients with post-stroke pain syndrome. In this study, the set of five real 20 Hz rTMS sessions lead to significantly better pain-improvement than sham and the effect was evident even at the 2-week follow-up after the treatment. Average pain relief of 45 % was reported among TN participants in the active rTMS group, with 79 % of participants acknowledging significant pain relief persisting for the follow-up period of 2 weeks, indicating that repeated rTMS sessions can produce longer-lasting pain relief.

Zaghi and colleagues [169] presented a longitudinal case-report of patient with refractory trigeminal neuralgia treated with high frequency (10 Hz) rTMS over the motor cortex in four treatment periods over 1 year. The treatment periods consisted of 10, 10, 5, and 10 rTMS sessions respectively. The interval between the treatment periods was 4 months, 2 weeks, 3 months, and 1 month respectively. The results showed that although individual treatment periods could result in significant and meaningful pain relief, the observed effects were persistent to about maximum of 4 weeks after the end of stimulation period. This case-study provided valuable evidence that repeated long term application of rTMS is safe and would be beneficial, though costly therapy.

Although up to date there are no findings from randomized sham-controlled studies in patients with neuropathic facial pain yet, open-label tDCS was applied in clinical cases of patients with trigeminal neuralgia and neuropathic facial pain due to surgical disturbance of trigeminal nerve respectively. Figure 15.6 shows a decrease of pain intensity posttreatment and a decrease of consumption of "as needed" pain-medication used to manage break through pain in a patient with trigeminal neuralgia. Five sessions of tDCS at 2 mA were applied on 5 consecutive days.

Although these very preliminary findings indicate clinical usefulness of tDCS in the treatment of facial neuropathic pain, sham-controlled studies in larger samples are warranted.

DBS

The experience with DBS for the management of trigeminal neuropathic pain is based on evaluation of cases reported individually or within large samples of patients with neuropathic pain of various origin [130, 170–173].

Kumar and colleagues [130] reported results of the DBS targeting nucleus ventralis posterior medialis (VPM) in patients with various diagnoses (total $n = 68$), including four patients with trigeminal neuropathy. All four patients with the neuropathic facial pain experienced an excellent pain relief during entire follow-up period that ranged between 12 and 28 months. Similarly, in a case presented by Green and colleagues [170], a patient with a 10-year history of post-herpetic trigeminal neuralgia who underwent a successful treatment with DBS targeting the region of periventricular gray area (PVG) contralateral to the site of pain, and ventral posterior lateral thalamic nucleus (VPL) experienced substantial pain relief. At the 6 months follow-up, the patient remained pain free. Rasche and colleagues [171] observed pain reduction of >25 % up to 100 % by DBS that combined stimulation of VPM and PVG in 4/6 patients with dysesthesia dolorosa in trigeminal nerve region. Cordella and colleagues [173] performed DBS in five patients for the treatment of trigeminal neuralgia due to multiple sclerosis with a goal to assess the efficacy of the DBS on the paroxysmal ophthalmic pain. The patients

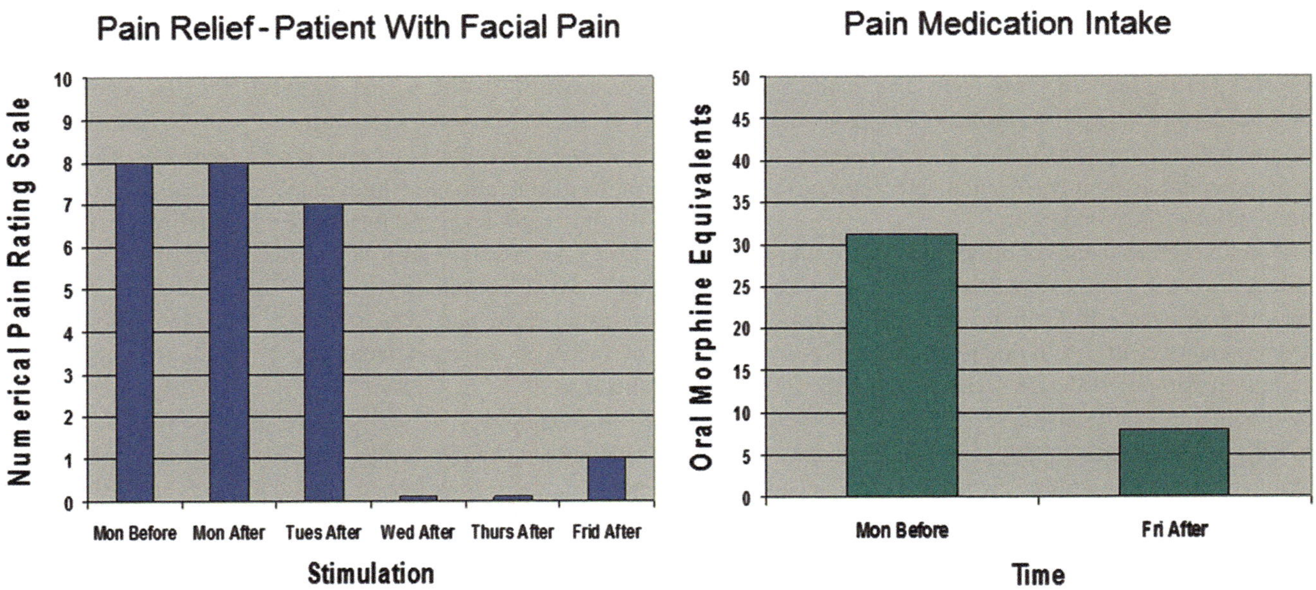

Fig. 15.6 Pain intensity and consumption of "as needed" pain-medication used to manage break through pain in a patient with trigeminal neuralgia after five sessions of tDCS at 2 mA on 5 consecutive days. (From Knotkova et al., 2013; courtesy of the authors [68])

underwent implantation of DBS leads into the hypothalamic posterior nucleus. All five patients reported immediate pain relief, followed by a long-term pain control in the follow-up period up to 4 years, a reduced need for analgesic medication, and improved quality of life. Pain relief specific to ophthalmic branch of trigeminal nerve sustained for the entire follow-up period in all five patients. Pain relief related to second and/or third trigeminal branch was recurrent after 11–28 months. Broggi and colleagues [172] reported results of DBS of posterior thalamus in a mixed sample of patients, including three patients with atypical facial pain, for which DBS was not beneficial.

MCS

There is more experience with MCS than with DBS for the treatment of facial pain of neuropathic origin, with reports emerging since the early 1990s [158, 174–180]. Meyerson and colleagues [174] were the first to report experience with MCS in patients with trigeminal neuropathic pain ($n = 5$) after surgery in the trigeminal territory. MCS in these patients was beneficial, yielding pain relief >50 % in all five patients. In the study by Herregodts and colleagues [175], MCS was performed in seven patients of which six had chronic pain involving facial region: one trigeminal neuralgia, four trigeminal neuropathic pain due to damaged trigeminal nerve after surgery, one pain in the face and upper extremity due to post-stroke central pain syndrome. Follow-up period ranged between 4 and 22 months. Full pain relief was achieved in one patient with TNP; pain relief >50 % was reported in five of the six patients, as one patient with TNP experienced minor temporary pain relief (20 % to 0 in 6 weeks).

Notably, Anderson and colleagues [181] implemented MCS in a patient with neuropathic facial pain that included elements of trigeminal neuralgia, glossopharyngeal neuralgia, and dysphagia. After failing pharmacological and surgical decompressive treatments, the patient underwent a successful MCS trial followed by implantation of a neurostimulation device. During the MCS trial, pain decreased from VAS 10 to 7; after the implantation, pain increased again, but adjustment of stimulation parameters resulted in satisfactory pain relief as well as substantial improvement in swallowing, absence of gagging sensation, and a reduction in episodes of nausea and vomiting. At 2 years, MCS generator was replaced and patient continued to experience benefits from MCS. Improvement of symptoms, namely the improvement of dysphagia had profound positive impact on the patient's functional status.

Overall, evidence on benefits from MCS in patients with facial pain is extensive and supports the use of MCS in facial pain syndromes, with understanding that as an invasive procedure, MCS is reserved for specially selected patients with severe chronic pain that substantially diminishes the patient's function and quality of life and does not respond to noninvasive therapeutic approaches.

Fibromyalgia

Fibromyalgia is a chronic pain syndrome characterized by bilateral pain above and below the waist, axial skeletal pain and at least 11 of 18 discrete tender points. Other symptoms include extreme fatigue, mood disturbances, cognitive disturbances, nonrestorative sleep, and decreased physical function [182]. Although the underlying mechanisms have not yet been fully elucidated, it is thought that fibromyalgia involves imbalance between nociception and normal physiologic pain control, including a pathological decrease of the activity in the inhibitory pain-related pathways [183–186].

It is estimated that fibromyalgia affects 4–10 million individuals in U.S., and about 75–90 % of cases are women (www.fmaware.org, www.wrongdiagnosis.com, [187, 188]).

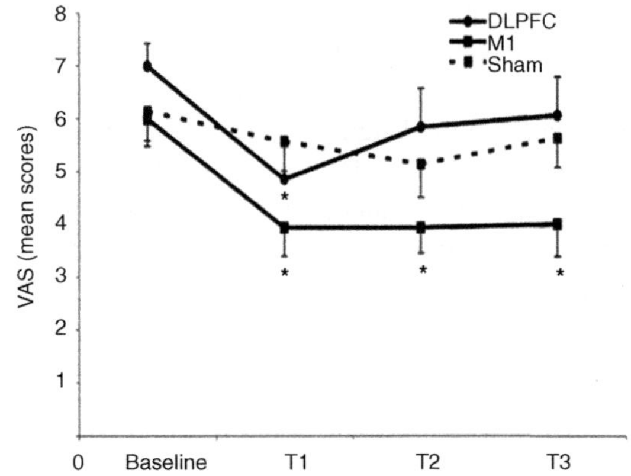

Fig. 15.7 Mean pain scores associated with the three conditions of stimulation: left M1 (primary motor cortex); left DLPFC (dorsolateral prefrontal cortex); and sham tDCS. Pain scores are reported on the Visual Analogue Scale for Pain; 0 = no pain, 10 = worst pain of life. *Asterisk* Indicates statistically significant ($p < 0.05$) as compared with baseline. Each column represents mean score SEM (standard error of mean). *T1*: end of stimulation, *T2*: 30 day follow-up, *T3*: 60 day follow-up. (From Valle et al. 2011; free access article [196])

Treatment Strategies in Fibromyalgia

Pharmacotherapy is considered the first-line of treatment and most commonly used treatment approach in fibromyalgia. However, FDA-approved agents for fibromyalgia, such as pregabalin, duloxetine, and milnacipran have shown high proportion of adverse events and/or patient drop-out from the treatment [182, 189–191]. Therefore, multidisciplinary treatment strategies have been recommended for fibromyalgia, including pharmacotherapy, physical therapy, behavioral interventions, and complementary medicine [192–194]. Despite the combined treatment strategies, many fibromyalgia patients remain with unsatisfactory pain relief, and novel treatment approaches are needed for this difficult-to-treat pain syndrome.

Neuromodulation

Up to date, only noninvasive neuromodulatory approaches, such as rTMS, tDCS, CES, or ECT, have been explored with various degree of success in fibromyalgia.

rTMS

Studies of rTMS in fibromyalgia targeted either the primary motor cortex [195, 196] or the dorsolateral prefrontal cortex (DLPFC) [197–199], which is typically used in the neuromodulatory treatment of depression. Although the stimulation parameters varied, the studies mostly yielded positive results. Notably, the study by Mhalla and colleagues [196] for the first time explored a possibility of a long-term maintenance of rTMS-induced pain relief. The study involved 40 patients randomized to receive either real rTMS or sham applied to the left primary motor cortex. The protocol consisted in total of 14 rTMS sessions: 5 were delivered daily, followed by the maintenance phase of 3 sessions 1 week apart, 3 sessions a fortnight apart and 3 sessions a month apart. The active rTMS significantly reduced pain intensity from day 5 to 1 month after the last delivered rTMS session, and the analgesic effects were associated with a long-term improvement of quality of life.

Overall, the findings from existing rTMS studies support further explorations of rTMS for the treatment of fibromyalgia-related pain in large samples. The evidence up to date suggest that rTMS has a substantial clinical potential in fibromyalgia and may in the future become a valuable therapeutic approach for patients with fibromyalgia.

tDCS

A potential of tDCS to alleviate pain in fibromyalgia has been examined in several studies [200–203], and stimulations of both clinical targets the primary motor cortex and DLPFC have been explored. Notably, more encouraging findings have been yielded by the motor cortex stimulation. For example, Roizenblatt and colleagues [201] reported that the anodal tDCS delivered over the motor cortex to 32 fibromyalgia patients had a positive effect on pain intensity and sleep, leading to a significant decrease of pain intensity, an increase of sleep efficiency by more than 11 % and decreased arousals by 35 %. DLPFC stimulation led to opposite effects and sham stimulation has not induced any significant changes in pain intensity or sleep.

Consequently, Valle and colleagues [203], examined a longer tDCS treatment protocol involving ten daily sessions of anodal tDCS delivered to the left primary motor cortex or DLPFC as compared to sham, in 41 women with chronic medically refractory fibromyalgia. Although both the motor cortex and DLPFC tDCS stimulation lead to improvements of pain scores and quality of life at the end of the 10-session treatment protocol, the long-lasting clinical benefits assessed 30 and 60 days after the end of tDCS treatment were achieved only with the motor-cortex-stimulation protocol (Fig. 15.7).

Notably, a systematic review of literature of rTMS or tDCs studies in patients with fibromyalgia [188] revealed that 80 % of rTMS studies and 100 % tDCs studies that measured pain reported significant decreases. Studies delivering excitatory rTMS or tDCS over M1 showed analogous pain reductions but considerably less side effects compared to medications approved by FDA for fibromyalgia [188]. Therefore, noninvasive neuromodulation with rTMS and tDCS may be beneficial in patients with fibromyalgia, particularly those who are unable to achieve adequate symptom relief with other therapies.

Cranial Electrotherapy Stimulation (CES)

The principles of CES and its analgesic properties in general are described in great detail in another chapter of this Textbook. Overall, it is thought that the CES-induced analgesia is due to its effects on the limbic system, the reticular-activating system (RAS) and/or the hypothalamus [204].

Only few studies exist that evaluated CES in fibromyalgia [204, 205].

For example, a randomized controlled trial by Lichtbroun and colleagues [205] delivered 3-week treatment with CES at 0.5 Hz or sham for 1 h per day in 60 fibromyalgia patients. Patients treated with active CES, but not those receiving sham treatment, experienced a significant improvement in tender-point scores and in self-rated scores of general pain intensity. Published case studies [204] further corroborated positive findings from CES stimulation in fibromyalgia patients.

ECT

Although ECT is known mostly for its use in severe cases of depression, there is some evidence of beneficial effects of ECT on a variety of pain states [206–208].

Usui and colleagues [209] carried out a prospective ECT study to evaluate effects on fibromyalgia pain in 15 patients. All patients received bilateral ECT set at 110 V for 5 s. Twelve patients received six sessions and three patients received only four sessions due to excellent responsiveness to the ECT treatment. ECT resulted in a significant decrease in the tender points and pain intensity 3 days after the last treatment, and the effects appeared to be independent of mood changes. The study also assessed regional cerebral blood flow (rCBF) before and 3 days after the course of ECT. The mean thalamus-to-cerebellum ratio was significantly increased after ECT in comparison to the pretreatment baseline, and the SPECT results suggested that improvement of rCBF in the thalamus may correlate with ECT-induced analgesia. Despite the positive results, a complicating factor of further ECT research in fibromyalgia is the general controversy of this neuromodulatory procedure, and its difficult justification in comparison with other noninvasive neuromodulatory approaches such as rTMS or tDCS that are patient-friendly, easy to use, and show encouraging and growing evidence on safety data.

Headaches

Among various types of primary headaches distinguished by the International Classification of Headache Disorders (2004), migraine and cluster headache were up to date included in the studies exploring effects of neuromodulation in pain management.

Migraine is a chronic neurological disorder characterized by recurrent moderate to severe headaches often in association with a number of autonomic nervous system symptoms [210]. Associated symptoms may include nausea, vomiting, photophobia, and/or phonophobia, blurred vision, nasal stuffiness, diarrhea, frequent urination, pallor, or sweating. Swelling or tenderness of the scalp may occur as can neck stiffness [211]. Up to one-third of people with migraine headaches perceive an aura: a transient visual, sensory, language, or motor disturbance which signals that the headache will soon occur [212, 213]. The exact mechanisms of migraine are not known. It is, however, believed to be a neurovascular disorder [210] involving an increased excitability of the cerebral cortex and abnormal control of pain neurons in the trigeminal nucleus of the brainstem [214]. Typically, the headache is unilateral, throbbing, and moderate to severe in intensity. In more than 40 % of cases however the pain may be bilateral, and neck pain is commonly associated [211] Less commonly pain may occur primarily in the back or top of the head. The is pain usually aggravated by physical activity and lasts 4–72 h in adults, however in young children frequently lasts less than 1 h [215]. The frequency of attacks is variable, from a few in a lifetime to several a week [216].

Cluster headaches are excruciating unilateral headaches of extreme intensity [217]. The duration of the common attack ranges from as short as 15 min to 3 h or more. The onset of an attack is rapid, and most often without the preliminary signs that are characteristic of a migraine [218]. While migraines are diagnosed more often in women, cluster headaches are more prevalent in men. The male-to-female ratio in cluster headache ranges from 4:1 to 7:1, and limited epidemiological studies have suggested prevalence rates of between 56 and 326 people per 100,000 [219].

Cluster headaches occurring in two or more cluster periods lasting from 7 to 365 days with a pain-free remission of 1 month or longer between the clusters are considered episodic. If the attacks occur for more than a year without a pain-free remission of at least 1 month, the condition is considered chronic (IHS Classification).

Cluster headaches have been classified as vascular headaches. The intense pain is caused by the dilation of blood vessels which creates pressure on the trigeminal nerve. While this process is the immediate cause of the pain, the etiology is not fully understood. Among the most widely accepted theories is that cluster headaches are due to an abnormality in the hypothalamus [220]. There is a genetic component to cluster headaches, although no single gene has been identified as the cause [221]. The pain of cluster headaches is remarkably greater than in other headache conditions, including severe migraines. The pain is lancinating or drilling in quality, and is located periorbitally or in the temple, sometimes radiating to the neck or shoulder [222]. The headache is accompanied by at least one of the following autonomic symptoms: ptosis, miosis, conjunctival injection, lacrimation, rhinorrhea, and, less commonly, facial blushing, swelling, or sweating, all appearing on the same side of the head as the pain (IHS classification). The attack is also associated with restlessness, less frequently with photophobia and/or phonophobia. The neck is often stiff or tender in the aftermath of a headache, with jaw or tooth pain sometimes present.

Treatment Approaches to Migraine and Cluster Headache

In migraine, there are three main aspects of treatment: trigger avoidance, acute symptomatic control, and pharmacological prevention [210]. Medications are more effective if used earlier in an attack. Initial recommended management is with simple analgesics such as ibuprofen and acetaminophen (also known as paracetamol) for the headache, an antiemetic for the nausea, and the avoidance of triggers. Specific agents such as triptans or ergotamines may be used by those for whom simple analgesics are not effective [210].

Intravenous metoclopramide and intranasal lidocaine are other potential options. Metoclopramide is the recommended treatment for those who present to the emergency department [223]. It is recommended that opioids and barbiturates not be used [223]. Guidelines are fairly consistent in rating topiramate, divalproex/sodium valproate, propranolol, and metoprolol as having the highest level of evidence for first-line use [224].

Other, nonpharmacological options include acupuncture [225, 226], or chiropractic manipulation, physiotherapy, massage, and relaxation that might be as effective as propranolol or topiramate in the prevention of migraine headaches [227]. There is some tentative evidence of benefit for magnesium, coenzyme Q(10), riboflavin, or vitamin B (12) [228]. Migraine surgery, which involves decompression of certain nerves around the head and neck, may be an option in certain people who do not improve with medications [229]. Medical devices, such as biofeedback may also be helpful in migraine management, mainly when common anti-migraine medications are contraindicated or in case of medication overuse [230, 231].

For the treatment of cluster headaches, medications include prophylactics (preventatives) and abortive. Wide variety of prophylactic medications are available, and patient response to these is highly variable. Current European guidelines suggest the use of the calcium channel blocker verapamil. Steroids, such as prednisolone/prednisone, are also effective, with a high dose given for the first 5 days or longer (in some cases up to 6 months) before tapering down. Methysergide, lithium, and the anticonvulsant topiramate are recommended as alternative treatments [232]. Intravenous magnesium sulfate relieves cluster headaches in about 40 % of patients with low serum ionized magnesium levels [233]. Melatonin has also been demonstrated to bring significant improvement in approximately half of episodic patients; psilocybin, dimethyltryptamine, LSD, and various other tryptamines have shown similar results [234].

Over-the-counter pain medications (such as aspirin, paracetamol, and ibuprofen) typically have no effect on the pain from a cluster headache. In addition, short-term transitional medications (such as steroids) may be used while prophylactic treatment is instituted and adjusted. With abortive treatments often only decreasing the duration of the headache and preventing it from reaching its peak rather than eliminating it entirely, preventive treatment is always indicated for cluster headaches, to be started at the first sign of a new cluster cycle. During the onset of a cluster headache, many people respond to inhalation of 100 % oxygen [235]. When oxygen is used at the onset this can abort the attack in as little as 1 min or as long as 10 min. Once an attack is at its peak, oxygen therapy appears to have little effect so many people keep an oxygen tank close at hand to use at the very first sign of an attack. An alternative first-line treatment is subcutaneous or intranasal administration of sumatriptan [232]. Sumatriptan and zolmitriptan have both been shown to improve symptoms during an attack or indeed abort attacks [236].

Some nonnarcotic treatments that have shown mixed levels of success are botox injections along the occipital nerve [237]. Lithium, melatonin, valproic acid, topiramate as well as gabapentin are medications that can be tried as second line treatment options. Ephedrine hydrochloride 1 % nasal drops can relieve the painful swelling in the nasal passage and sinus on the affected side [238].

Neuromodulation

rTMS

The interest in TMS as a potential treatment for migraine has been triggered by neurophysiological findings showing that pathophysiological mechanisms of migraine involve changes in excitability and neural dynamics in the brain. Recent studies indicated that migraine patients show a sustained state of brain hyperexcitability that is present even between migraine attacks and has a strong inherited basis [239]. Further, during the migraine aura, a wave of excitation followed by a wave of inhibition spreads over the cortex. This spreading inhibition, called Cortical Spreading Depression (CSD), occurs in the occipital cortex, triggering the visual aura. Recent evidence suggests that CSD gives rise to pain by activating trigeminal nociceptors in the meninges [240]. In animal model, single-pulse TMS (sTMS) inhibited CSD, suggesting that sTMS might be an effective acute treatment for migraineurs with aura [241]. Further, it has been thought that perhaps rTMS might be helpful in migraine prevention by producing sustained changes in brain excitability and by modulating neurotransmitter levels [242–244]. Indeed, both types of TMS has been studied in migraine patients: sTMS as an acute treatment and rTMS as a preventive treatment.

In the study by Clarke and colleagues [245], 42 subjects with migraine (5 of those with aura) received either sTMS or sham during the attack. The treatment with active sTMS resulted in 75 % decrease in pain intensity and 32 % reported no further headache over the following 24 h period. Recurrence of headache was decreased by 48 %. Mohammad et al. [246] focused in the double-blind sham-controlled study of sTMS on migraineurs with aura ($n = 42$), who reported t the hospital during an acute attack where two sTMS applications were administered 30 s apart. Two hours after the treatment, 69 % patients receiving the real sTMS reported no or mild pain as compared to 48 % of sham treated patients. Promising results from these studies lead to the development a handheld, lightweight sTMS device for patients' self-treatment at home (for detailed description of the device see Lipton and Pearlman [247]).

Besides sTMS, two small-sample studies ($n = 27$ and 11, respectively) tested the efficacy of rTMS for migraine prevention [248, 249]. Although the treatment in both studies lead to an improvement of pain as compared to baseline, the comparisons of differences between the real TMS and sham rTMS was not significant in either study.

tDCS

Antal and colleagues [250] examined if the inhibitory (cathodal) tDCS can serve as a prophylactic therapy for migraine. tDCS or sham was applied over the visual cortex three times per week for 6 consecutive weeks. For the first 3 weeks, all patients received only sham stimulation, then one group of patients started receiving the real tDCS.

Patients treated with real cathodal tDCS presented with a significant reduction in duration of attacks, the number of migraine days and a decrease of pain intensity as compared to the baseline. However, only the pain intensity decrease was significant as compared to the sham group. The results indicate that the cathodal tDCS delivered over the visual cortex might be a promising prophylactic treatment for migraine-related pain.

DaSilva and colleagues [251] examined the analgesic effects of anodal tDCS/sham delivered over the primary motor cortex in chronic migraine patients at 4-week treatment (Mon, Wed, Fri on weeks 1 and 3, and Tue and Thurs on weeks 2 and 4), and a 4-month follow-up. The results showed a significant interaction time x conditions for pain intensity and length of migraine episodes. Detailed analysis within the active group revealed that there was no change in pain intensity after first 2 weeks of treatment, followed by gradual decrease of pain intensity afterwards at the end of the 4-week treatment and at the follow-up. The pain relief was statistically significant at the end of the follow-up period at 4 months. The findings suggest that tDCS may have delayed effects in chronic migraine. The phenomenon of delayed effects deserves attention in future replication studies and should be thoroughly examined before any definite conclusions are drawn.

DBS

The results of posteromedial hypothalamotomy [252] and the identification of a hypothalamic activation during cluster attacks [253, 254] led to the use of deep brain stimulation (DBS) for refractory CCH. A first series of 16 patients showed excellent results with 13 patients pain free or nearly pain free and three patients improved [255, 256]. Later studies followed consensus criteria for patient selection. In 2008 a review summarized the results of hypothalamic DBS in 38 refractory CCH patients. With a follow-up of between 1 and 4 years, 23 patients (61 %) were pain free or almost pain free [257]. Schoenen and colleagues [258] reported a fatal hemorrhage following DBS implantation due to a previously unnoted cerebral aneurysm. Moreover, in their series of 6 patients, in another patient the procedure had to be stopped due to panic attacks with autonomic disturbances [258]. In DBS pain relief can emerge with a delay of up to 3 months. In a prospective, randomized crossover study of 11 patients receiving DBS electrodes, no difference between active and sham stimulation was observed during the blinded crossover phase, however in the open phase 6 of 11 patients responded to stimulation (decrease in weekly attack frequency of >50 %) [259].

Recently it has been questioned whether stereotactic intervention in these disorders has been targeted at the appropriate locus, and whether this may account for the approximately 40 % of patients with a poor response to DBS [260], since the target data for DBS are derived from positron emission tomography (PET) studies with limited spatial resolution and functional magnetic resonance imaging (fMRI) data which have a better spatial resolution hint at a locus of activation antero-superior to that derived from PET studies [261].

Occipital Nerve Stimulation (ONS)

Occipital nerve stimulation (ONS) had been proposed as a treatment for refractory migraine [262, 263], occipital neuralgia [264–266] and other intractable headache disorders [267]. The role of occipital stimulation in CH was first examined by Burns and colleagues. They published a pilot study of eight patients [268] and a follow-up study of 14 patients [269] on ONS for CCH. In the pilot study six of eight patients and in the follow-up study 10 of 14 patients experienced a reduction in attack frequency. The reduction of attack frequency was more than 40 % in six of eight patients in the pilot study and 6 of 14 patients in the follow-up study. In a study by Magis and colleagues seven of eight patients had a decrease in attack frequency of more than 40 % [270]. Mean attack frequency was decreased by 19, 29, and 80 % in the two studies of Burns and colleagues [268, 269] and the study of Magis and coworkers [270], respectively. In the latter study, on average the ONS to baseline attack ratio per month was 0.65 during the whole follow-up (mean 15.1 months).

SCS

Wolter and colleagues [271] reported a case of a patient with medication refractory cluster headache. A test of cervical SCS electrode was performed as compassionate treatment. The clinical results in this patient in the postoperative course and in the long-term follow-up were quite encouraging [271] and the treatment was applied in other patients with refractory CCH [272]. SCS in that study showed clinical effects comparable to or better than ONS, as SCS in contrast to ONS acts immediately. All of the patients had at least some effect from SCS from the operation day onward. In SCS for CCH, electrodes can also be implanted bilaterally, in the case of side switch of CCH; two patients in the sample actually received a second contralateral electrode, and were able to control head pain on both sides separately [272]. Although being slightly more invasive than ONS, the risks in SCS intervention are minimal. Although there is not enough evidence yet to decide whether SCS might become a first-line treatment for therapy refractory CCH, it can be used as a reserve option in the case of insufficient effects of ONS.

Ganglion Sphenopalatinum Stimulation

The sphenopalatine (pterygopalatine) ganglion (SPG) receives input from the maxillary branch of the trigeminal nerve, parasympathetic fibers originating from the superior salivatory nucleus in the brainstem and sympathetic fibers form the carotid plexus (via the deep petrosal nerve). In the SPG there is a tight anatomical and physiological relationship of sympathetic, parasympathetic, and trigeminal fibers. The SPG plays a pivotal role in driving the parasympathetic features and in sterile meningeal inflammation as substrate for trigeminally mediated head pain, as well as in pain transmission in CH. Consequently the SPG has been targeted in a couple of lesional treatments [273–276]. Moreover, a new study showed that stimulation of the SPG can be effective as an acute treatment for cluster attacks. In six patients, 18 attacks were treated and a complete resolution of symptoms was seen in 11 attacks, a partial resolution of symptoms in three attacks and minimal or no relief in four attacks [277]. Similar results have been reported after SPG stimulation as acute treatment for migraine [278]. SPG stimulation becomes particularly attractive, because it may, in contrast to ONS and SCS, offer the possibility to abort an ongoing attack. Therefore, future studies of stimulation of the SPG are urgently warranted.

Overall invasive neurostimulation has opened promising perspectives for the treatment of refractory CCH. SPG stimulation might in the future become an attractive alternative to ONS and SCS but further clinical studies and observations are warranted.

In conclusion, neurostimulation therapies open a new era in headache management and offer a promising alternative to medications. However, further studies are warranted to provide efficacy and effectiveness data for further development of this novel treatment approach.

Other Chronic Pain Syndromes

There is some evidence of the use of neuromodulatory approaches also in other chronic pain syndromes, such as postherpetic neuralgia (PHN) or low back pain.

Post-herpetic Neuralgia

PHN is a neuropathic-type pain due to nerve damage caused by the varicella zoster virus. Typically, the neuralgia is confined to a dermatomic area of the skin and follows an outbreak of herpes zoster, (commonly known as shingles) in that dermatome. PHN can develop even in herpes zoster patients who have not had acute pain. PHN pain is often described as burning, and can vary from mild discomfort to a chronic pain syndrome that can last for years and cause substantial deterioration in quality of life. The area of previous herpes zoster infection may show evidence of cutaneous scarring with altered sensation in the form of either hypersensitivity or decreased sensation.

The initial choice of pharmacologic treatment should be guided by the side effect profile, drug interactions, patient preference, and comorbidities. Early randomized controlled trials have considered tricyclic antidepressants as first-line therapy for PHN. Subsequently, other therapies including gabapentin, pregabalin, high-concentration capsaicin patch, lidocaine patch 5 %, opioid analgesics, and tramadol have shown to be efficacious in the treatment of PHN [151, 279].

In addition, consensus guidelines for the treatment of neuropathic pain including PHN have been published to guide treating physicians to choose the most appropriate and feasible treatment option [280, 281]. As a general rule, anticonvulsant, neuropathic agents, topical agents, and tramadol are considered first-line treatments for PHN, whereas opioid analgesics and tricyclic antidepressants are more typically second-line treatment due to their side effect profiles, particularly in the elderly. The evidence on efficacy of the different therapies for PHN is limited and they are rarely associated with complete resolution of patients' symptoms.

Besides the traditional pharmacologic treatment, several neurostimulation techniques have been explored for the treatment of PHN including spinal cord stimulators (SCS) [282, 283], peripheral nerve stimulation (PNS) [284–286], or tDCS [68].

A recent study conducted by Yanamoto and Murakawa [282], examined the efficacy of temporary SCS involving the insertion of a quadripolar lead into the epidural space and applied an extracorporeal stimulation generator for several weeks of early PHN from 1 to 6 months of its onset. Thirty-three patients with PHN who had a positive response to epidural block received temporary spinal cord stimulation for 7 days with the analgesic effects measured 1, 3, and 6 months post treatment. Pain relief >50 % was observed in 63.6, 60.6, and 63.6 % of patients at 1, 3, and 6 months, respectively. Another study conducted by Moriyama [283], evaluated the effect of the use of temporary SCS in patients with severe persistent pain of PHN in the thoracic area. Fifty-two patients underwent continuous epidural blocks and 14 also were treated with spinal cord stimulation leads if they had no significant pain reduction with concomitant pharmacotherapy. The overall VAS scores decreased by introducing SCS to the continuous epidural blocks, less epidural analgesia was required leading to a reduction in side effects from neuraxial analgesia. In addition, self-rated satisfaction was higher with SCS than with epidural blocks in all 14 patients. Up to date, evidence suggest that spinal cord stimulation is a promising therapeutic tool for the treatment of PHN, however, controlled large-sample studies are warranted to evaluate its safety and efficacy. Peripheral nerve stimulation has also been attempted but the evidence is limited and based on anecdotal experience [284–286].

Low-Back Pain

Various neurostimulation approaches, such as spinal cord stimulation [287, 288], peripheral field subcutaneous stimulation [289], or tDCS [290] have been explored for the treatment of chronic low-back pain. Currently, the best scientific evidence among these modalities points to spinal cord stimulation as treatment for patients with failed-back surgery syndrome.

A randomized, controlled trial conducted by Kumar et al. [287], demonstrated that SCS can provide better analgesia and improve health-related quality of life and functional capacity when compared to pharmacologic therapy alone. This study evaluated the effectiveness of SCS therapy in addition to conventional medical management (CMM) in 100 patients with failed back surgery syndrome with predominant leg pain of neuropathic etiology. Patients were randomized to receive SCS plus CMM or CMM alone for at least 6 months. At the 6-months follow-up, 24 of the SCS patients (48 %) and 4 of the CMM patients (9 %) ($p < 0.001$) achieved >50 % pain relief in the legs. In addition, the SCS group experienced improved leg and back pain relief, quality of life, and functional capacity, as well as greater treatment satisfaction. Crossover to the SCS group was allowed between 6 and 12 months, and 32 CMM patients crossed to SCS. However, at the 12-month follow-up period, 27 SCS patients (32 %) had experienced device-related complications.

Another randomized, controlled study conducted by North et al. [288], evaluated the outcomes of SCS versus reoperation for patients with persistent radicular pain after lumbosacral surgery. Fifty patients selected for reoperation by standard criteria were followed for 3 years postoperatively and randomized to SCS or reoperation. A successful intervention was based on self-reported pain relief and patient satisfaction. Among 90 % of patients available for follow-up, SCS was more successful than reoperation (9/19 vs. 3/26 patients, $p < 0.01$). Those patients that were initially randomized to SCS were significantly less likely to cross over to the other arm than those randomized to reoperation (5/24 patients vs. 14/26 patients, $p = 0.02$). In addition, patients randomized to reoperation required increased opiate analgesics ($p < 0.025$). These results showed that SCS may be more effective than reoperation in patient with persistent radicular pain after lumbosacral spine surgery.

Transcranial direct current stimulation has also been explored in low-back pain patients, but with no positive results. A recent proof of principle sham-controlled study conducted by O'Connell et al. [290], evaluated the effects of anodal tDCS applied to the motor cortex in eight patients with chronic low back pain. Entered a 15-day experimental period, when they were treated with sham stimulation daily followed by active tDCS. The outcomes of the interest were average pain intensity and unpleasantness in the last 24 h measured using a visual analog scale. No significant differences between the effects of sham and real tDCS were noted. Up to date, this has been the only study published on tDCS for low back pain. Further studies are needed before any definite conclusion can be drawn.

Conclusions

Overall, both invasive and noninvasive neuromodulatory approaches have been explored in various patient populations with difficult-to-treat-chronic pain syndromes. Invasive neuromodulation has been reserved for carefully selected patients who do not respond to conventional pharmacological and nonpharmacological treatments or noninvasive neuromodulation.

Noninvasive neuromodulation with rTMS, tDCS, CES, or Motor imagery represents a patient-friendly, low-risk approach with a great clinical potential for specific chronic pain syndromes and patient populations in need of pain management. The future exploratory work in this field should navigate the development of the method-specific and patient-population specific stimulation protocols and parameters, patient-tailored adjustments for specific cases, as well as the development of evidence-based guidelines for each neuromodulatory technique, in order to facilitate the implementation of neuromodulation to the clinical practice of pain management.

Acknowledgement The authors thank Ms. Evelyn Ouro-Rodrigues and Alexa Riggs for technical support during preparations of this chapter.

References

1. Merskey H, Bogduk N, editors. Classification of chronic pain: descriptions of chronic pain syndromes and definitions of pain terms. Seattle, WA: IASP; 1994. p. 40–3.
2. Allen G, Galer BS, Schwartz L. Epidemiological review of 134 patients with complex regional pain syndrome assessed in a chronic pain clinic. Pain. 1999;80:539–44.
3. Lynch ME. Psychological aspects of regional sympathetic dystrophy: a review of the adult and pediatric literature. Pain. 1992; 49:337.
4. Bennett GJ, Harden RN. Questions concerning the incidence and prevalence of complex regional pain syndrome type I (RSD). Pain. 2003;106(1–2):209–10.
5. Sandroni P, Benrud-Larson LM, Mcclelland RL, et al. Complex regional pain syndrome type I: incidence and prevalence in olmsted county, a population based study. Pain. 2003;103: 199–207.
6. Edston E, Van Hage-Hamsten M. Mast cell tryptase and hemolysis after trauma. Forensic Sci Int. 2003;131:8–13.
7. Huygen FJ, Ramdhani N, Van Toorenenberg A, Klein J, Zijlstra FJ. Mast cells are involved in inflammatory reactions during complex regional pain syndrome type 1. Immunol Lett. 2004;91:147–54.
8. Guo TZ, Offley SC, Boyd EA, Jacobs CR, Kingery WS. Substance P signaling contributes to the vascular and nociceptive abnormalities observed in a tibial fracture rat model of complex regional pain syndrome type 1. Pain. 2004;108:95–107.
9. Droge W. Free radicals in the physiological control of cell function. Physiol Rev. 2002;82:47–95.
10. Coderre TJ, Xanthos DN, Francis L, Bennett GJ. Chronic post-ischemia pain (CPIP): a novel animal model of complex regional pain syndrome-type I (CRPS-I; reflex sympathetic dystrophy) produced by prolonged hindpaw ischemia and reperfusion in the rat. Pain. 2004;112(1–2):94–105.
11. Field J, Protheroe DL, Atkins RM. Algodystrophy after colles fractures is associated with secondary tightness of casts. J Bone Joint Surg Br. 1994;76(6):901–5.
12. Mailis A, Wade J. Profile of caucasian women with possible genetic predisposition to reflex sympathetic dystrophy: a pilot study. Clin J Pain. 1994;10:210–7.
13. Van Hilten JJ, Van De Beek WJ, Roep BO. Multifocal or generalized tonic dystonia of complex regional pain syndrome: a distinct clinical entity associated with HLA DR 13. Ann of Neurol. 2000;48:113–6.
14. Maihöfner C, Handwerker HO, Neundörfer B, Birklein F. Patterns of cortical reorganization in complex regional pain syndrome. Neurology. 2003;61(12):1707–15.
15. Maihöfner C, Handwerker HO, Neundörfer B, Birklein F. Cortical reorganization during recovery from complex regional pain syndrome. Neurology. 2004;63(4):693–701.
16. Maihöfner C, Handwerker HO, Neundorfer B, Birklein F. Mechanical hyperalgesia in complex regional pain syndrome: a role for TNF-alpha? Neurology. 2005;65:311–3.
17. Huygen FJ, De Bruijn AG, De Bruin MT, Groeneweg JG, Klein J, Zijistra FJ. Evidence for local inflammation in complex regional pain syndrome type 1. Mediators Inflamm. 2002;11:47–51.
18. Alexander GM, van Rijn MA, van Hilten JJ, Perreault MJ, Schwartzman RJ. Changes in cerebrospinal fluid levels of pro-inflammatory cytokines in CRPS. Pain. 2005;116:213–9.
19. Allan SM, Tyrrell PJ, Rothwell NJ. Interleukin-1 and neuronal injury. Nat Rev Immunol. 2005;5:629–40.
20. De Mos M, Sturkenboom MC, Huygen FJ. Current understandings on complex regional pain syndrome. Pain Pract. 2009;9:86–99.
21. Woolf CJ, Costigan M. Transcriptional and posttranslational plasticity and the generation of inflammatory pain. Proc Natl Acad Sci U S A. 1999;96:7723–30.
22. Oaklander AL, Rissmiller JG, Gelman LB, Zheng L, Chang Y, Gott R. Evidence of focal small-fiber axonal degeneration in complex regional pain syndrome-1 (Reflex Sympathetic Dystrophy). Pain. 2006;120(3):235–43.
23. Albrecht PJ, Hines S, Eisenberg PE, Pud D, Finlay DR, Connolly MK, Pare M, Davar G, Rice FL. Pathologic alterations of cutaneous innervation and vasculature in affected limbs from patients with complex regional pain syndrome. Pain. 2006;120(3):244–66.
24. Pappagallo M, Knotkova H, DeNardis L. Multifaceted CRPS: emerging mechanisms and pharmacotherapy. Crit Rev Phys Rehab Med. 2006;18(3):257–82.
25. Flor H, Elbert T, Knecht S, Wienbruch C, Pantev C, Birbaumer N, Larbig W, Taub E. Phantom-limb pain as a correlate of cortical reorganization following arm amputation. Nature. 1995;375: 482–4.
26. Birbaumer N, Werner L, Pedro M, Wolfgang L, Klaus U, Stephanie T, Wolfgang G, Edward T, Herta F. Effects of regional

anesthesia on phantom limb pain are mirrored in changes in cortical reorganization. J Neurosci. 1997;17(14):5503–8.
27. Pleger B, Tegenthoff M, Ragert P, Förster AF, Dinse HR, Schwenkreis P, Nicolas V, Maier C. Sensorimotor retuning [corrected] in complex regional pain syndrome parallels pain reduction. Ann Neurol. 2005;57(3):425–9.
28. Pleger B, Ragert P, Schwenkreis P, Förster AF, Wilimzig C, Dinse H, Nicolas V, Maier C, Tegenthoff M. Patterns of cortical reorganization parallel impaired tactile discrimination and pain intensity in complex regional pain syndrome. Neuroimage. 2006;32(2):503–10.
29. Pleger B, Janssen F, Schwenkreis P, Völker B, Maier C, Tegenthoff M. Repetitive transcranial magnetic stimulation of the motor cortex attenuates pain perception in complex regional pain syndrome type I. Neurosci Lett. 2004;356(2):87–90.
30. Shi W, Liu H, Zhang Y, et al. Design, synthesis, and preliminary evaluation of gabapentin-pregabalin mutual prodrugs in relieving neuropathic pain. Arch Pharm. 2005;338:358–64.
31. Mellick GA, Mellicy LB, Mellick LB. Gabapentin in the management of reflex sympathetic dystrophy. J Pain Sympt Manage. 1995;10:265–6.
32. Van de Vusse AC, Stomp-van den Berg SGM, Kessels AHF, Weber WEJ. Randomised controlled trial of gabapentin in complex regional pain syndrome type 1. BMC Neurol. 2004;4:13.
33. Zakrzewska JM, Chaudhry Z, Nurmikko TJ. Lamotrigine (lamictal) in refractory trigeminal neuralgia: results from a double-blind, placebo controlled, crossover trial. Pain. 1997;73: 223–30.
34. Pappagallo M. Preliminary experience with topiramate in the treatment of chronic pain syndromes. San Diego, CA: American Pain Society; 1998.
35. Rowbotham MC, Davies PS, Verkempinck C, et al. Lidocaine patch: double-blind controlled study of a new treatment method for post-herpetic neuralgia. Pain. 1996;65:39–44.
36. Max MB, Lynch SA, Muir J. Effects of desipramine, amitriptyline, and fluoxetine on pain in diabetic neuropathy. N Engl J Med. 1992;326:1250–6.
37. Reuben SS, Sklar J. Intravenous regional anesthesia with clonidine in the management of complex regional pain syndrome of the knee. J Clin Anesth. 2002;14(2):87–91.
38. Khan ZP, Ferguson CN, Jones RM. Alpha-2 and imidazoline receptor agonists: their pharmacology and therapeutic role. Anaesthesia. 1999;54:146–65.
39. Eisenach JC, Rauck RL, Buzzanell C, et al. Epidural clonidine analgesia for intractable cancer pain: phase I. Anesthesiology. 1989;71:647–52.
40. Davis KD, Treede RD, Raja SN. Topical application of clonidine relieves hyperalgesia in patients with sympathetically maintained pain. Pain. 1991;47:309–17.
41. Devers A, Galer BS. Topical lidocaine patch relieves a variety of neuropathic pain conditions: an open-label study. Clin J Pain. 2000;16:205–8.
42. Dellemijn PL, Vanneste JA. Randomised double-blind active-placebo controlled crossover trial of intravenous fentanyl in neuropathic pain. Lancet. 1997;349:753–8.
43. Gimbel JS, Richards P, Portenoy RK. Controlled-release oxycodone for pain in diabetic neuropathy: a randomized controlled trial. Neurology. 2003;60:927–34.
44. Raja SN, Haythornthwaite JA, Pappagallo M, et al. Opioids versus antidepressants in postherpetic neuralgia: a randomized, placebo-controlled trial. Neurology. 2002;59:1015–21.
45. Rowbotham MC, Twilling L, Davies PS. Oral opioid therapy for chronic peripheral and central neuropathic pain. N Engl J Med. 2003;348:1223–32.
46. Watson CP, Babul N. Efficacy of oxycodone in neuropathic pain: a randomized trial in postherpetic neuralgia. Neurology. 1998;50: 1837–41.
47. Rowbotham MC. Pharmacologic management of complex regional pain syndrome. Clin J Pain. 2006;22(5):425–9.
48. Christensen K, Jensen EM, Noer I. The reflex dystrophy syndrome response to treatment with systemic corticosteroids. Acta Chir Scand. 1982;148:653–5.
49. Taskaynatan MA, Ozgul A, Tan AK, Dincer K, Kalyon TA. Bier block with methylprednisolone and lidocaine in CRPS type I: a randomized, double-blinded, placebo-controlled study. Reg Anesth Pain Med. 2004;29(5):408–12.
50. Robinson JN, Sandom J, Chapman PT. Efficacy of pamidronate in complex regional pain syndrome type I. Pain Med. 2004;5 (3):276–80.
51. Kubalek I, Fain O, Paries J, Kettaneh A, Thomas M. Treatment of reflex sympathetic dystrophy with pamidronate: 29 cases. Rheumatology (Oxford). 2001;40(12):1394–7.
52. Varenna M, Zucchi F, Ghiringhelli D, Binelli L, Bevilacqua M, Bettica P, et al. Intravenous clodronate in the treatment of reflex sympathetic dystrophy syndrome. A randomized, double blind, placebo controlled study. J Rheumatol. 2000;27(6):1477–83.
53. Cortet B, Flipo RM, Coquerelle P, Duquesnoy B, Delcambre B. Treatment of severe, recalcitrant reflex sympathetic dystrophy: assessment of efficacy and safety of the second generation bisphosphonate pamidronate. Clin Rheumatol. 1997;16(1):51–6.
54. Manicourt DH, Brasseur JP, Boutsen Y, Depreseux G, Devogelaer JP. Role of alendronate in therapy for posttraumatic complex regional pain syndrome type I of the lower extremity. Arthritis Rheum. 2004;50(11):3690–7.
55. Adami S, Fossaluzza V, Gatti D, Fracassi E, Braga V. Bisphosphonate therapy of reflex sympathetic dystrophy syndrome. Ann Rheum Dis. 1997;56(3):201–4.
56. Gobelet C, Waldburger M, Meier JL. The effect of adding calcitonin to physical treatment on reflex sympathetic dystrophy. Pain. 1992;48(2):171–5.
57. Appelboom T. Calcitonin in reflex sympathetic dystrophy syndrome and other painful conditions. Bone. 2002;30:84S–6.
58. Rajkumar SV, Fonseca R, Witzig TE. Complete resolution of reflex sympathetic dystrophy with thalidomide treatment. Arch Intern Med. 2003;163(12):487–8.
59. Schafers M, Brinkhoff J, Neukirchen S. Combined epineurial therapy with neutralizing antibodies to tumor necrosis factor-alpha and interleukin-1 receptor has an additive effect in reducing neuropathic pain in mice. Neurosci Lett. 2001;310:113–6.
60. Eide PK, Jorum E, Stubhaug A, et al. Relief of post-herpetic neuralgia with the N-methyl-D-aspartic acid receptor antagonist ketamine: a double-blind, crossover comparison with morphine and placebo. Pain. 1994;58:347–54.
61. Nikolajsen L, Hansen CL, Nielsen J. The effect of ketamine on phantom pain: a central neuropathic disorder maintained by peripheral input. Pain. 1996;67:69–77.
62. Correll GE, Maleki J, Gracely EJ, Muir JJ, Harbut RE. Subanesthetic ketamine infusion therapy: a retrospective analysis of a novel therapeutic approach to complex regional pain syndrome. Pain Med. 2004;5(3):263–75.
63. Perez RS, Zuurmond WW, Bezemer PD, Kuik DJ, Van Loenen AC, de Lange JJ, Zuidhof AJ. The treatment of complex regional pain syndrome type I with free radical scavengers: a randomized controlled study. Pain. 2003;102(3):297–307.
64. Zuurmond WW, Langendijk PN, Bezemer PD, Brink HE, de Lange JJ, van Loenen AC. Treatment of acute reflex sympathetic dystrophy with DMSO 50 % in a fatty cream. Acta Anaesthesiol Scand. 1996;40(3):364–7.
65. Reuben SS, Rosenthal EA, Steinberg RB. Surgery on the affected upper extremity of patients with a history of complex regional pain syndrome: a retrospective study of 100 patients. J Hand Surg. 2000;25:1147–51.

66. Stanton-Hicks M, Baron R, Boas R, Gordh T, Harden N, Hendler N, Koltzenburg M, Raj P, Wilder R. Complex regional pain syndromes: guidelines for therapy. Clin J Pain. 1998;14(2): 155–66.
67. Picarelli H, Teixeira MJ, de Andrade DC, Myczkowski ML, Luvisotto TB, Yeng LT, Fonoff ET, Pridmore S, Marcolin MA. Repetitive transcranial magnetic stimulation is efficacious as an add-on to pharmacological therapy in complex regional pain syndrome (CRPS) type I. J Pain. 2010;11(11):1203–10.
68. Knotkova H, Soto E, Leuschner Z, Greenberg A, Stock V, Cruciani RA. Transcranial direct current stimulation (tDCS) for the treatment of chronic pain. J Pain. 2013;14(4):S64.
69. Cruciani RA, Esteban S, Sibirceva U, Knotkova H. Non-invasive brain stimulation therapy for the management of complex regional pain syndrome (CRPS). J Pain Manag. 2009;2(3):277–85. Special issue on "Brain stimulation for treatment of pain".
70. Knotkova H, Homel P, Cruciani RA. Cathodal tDCS over the somatosensory cortex relieved chronic neuropathic pain in a patient with complex regional pain syndrome (CRPS/RSD): case report. J Pain Manag. 2009;2(3):365–8. Special issue on "Brain stimulation for treatment of pain".
71. Lagueux E, Charest J, Lefrançois-Caron E, Mauger ME, Mercier E, Savard K, Tousignant-Laflamme Y. Modified graded motor imagery for complex regional pain syndrome type 1 of the upper extremity in the acute phase: a patient series. Int J Rehabil Res. 2012;35(2):138–45.
72. Walz AD, Usichenko T, Moseley GL, Lotze M. Graded motor imagery and the impact on pain processing in a case of CRPS. Clin J Pain. 2013;29(3):276–9.
73. Johnson S, Hall J, Barnett S, Draper M, Derbyshire G, Haynes L, Rooney C, Cameron H, Moseley GL, de C Williams AC, McCabe C, Goebel A. Using graded motor imagery for complex regional pain syndrome in clinical practice: failure to improve pain. Eur J Pain. 2012;16(4):550–61.
74. Fonoff ET, Hamani C, Ciampi de Andrade D, Yeng LT, Marcolin MA, Jacobsen Teixeira M. Pain relief and functional recovery in patients with complex regional pain syndrome after motor cortex stimulation. Stereotact Funct Neurosurg. 2011;89(3):167–72.
75. Velasco F, Carrillo-Ruiz JD, Castro G, Argüelles C, Velasco AL, Kassian A, Guevara U. Motor cortex electrical stimulation applied to patients with complex regional pain syndrome. Pain. 2009;147 (1–3):91–8.
76. Son UC, Kim MC, Moon DE, Kang JK. Motor cortex stimulation in a patient with intractable complex regional pain syndrome type II with hemibody involvement: case report. J Neurosurg. 2003;98 (1):175–9.
77. Van Eijs F, Geurts JW, Van Zundert J, Faber CG, Kessels AG, Joosten EA, van Kleef M. Spinal cord stimulation in complex regional pain syndrome type I of less than 12-month duration. Neuromodulation. 2012;15(2):144–50. Discussion 150.
78. Taylor RS. Spinal cord stimulation in complex regional pain syndrome and refractory neuropathic back and leg pain/failed back surgery syndrome: results of a systematic review and meta-analysis. J Pain Symptom Manage. 2006;31(4 Suppl):S13–9.
79. Kemler MA, Furneer CA. Economic evaluation of spinal cord stimulation for chronic reflex sympathetic dystrophy. Neurology. 2002;59(8):1203–9.
80. Pahapill PA, Zhang W. Restoration of altered somatosensory cortical representation with spinal cord stimulation therapy in a patient with complex regional pain syndrome: a magnetoencephalography case study. Neuromodulation. 2013;17:22–6.
81. Sears NC, Machado AG, Nagel SJ, Deogaonkar M, Stanton-Hicks M, Rezai AR, Henderson JM. Long-term outcomes of spinal cord stimulation with paddle leads in the treatment of complex regional pain syndrome and failed back surgery syndrome. Neuromodulation. 2011;14(4):312–8. Discussion 318.
82. Kooijman CM, Dijkstra PU, Geertzen JHB, Elzinga A, Van Der Schans CP. Phantom pain and phantom sensation in upper limb amputees: an epidemiological study. Pain. 2000;87(1):33–41.
83. Jensen TS, Krebs B, Nielsen J, Rasmussen P. Non-painful phantom limb phenomena in amputees: incidence, clinical characteristics and temporal course. Acta Neurol Scand. 1984;70:407–14.
84. Nikolajsen L, Jensen TS. Phantom limb pain. Br J Anaesth. 2001;87:107–16.
84. Nikolajsen L, Finnerup NB, Kramp S, Vimtrup AS, Keller J, Jensen TS. A randomized study of the effects of gabapentin on postamputation pain. Anesthesiology. 2006;105(5):1008–15.
85. Subedi B, Grossberg GT. Phantom limb pain: mechanisms and treatment approaches. Pain Res Treat. 2011;2011:861605.
86. Cohen LG, Bandinelli S, Findley TW, Hallett M. Motor reorganization after upper limb amputation in man: a study with focal magnetic stimulation. Brain. 1991;114:615–27.
87. Wolpaw JR, Tennissen A. Activity-dependent spinal cord plasticity in health and disease. Annu Rev Neurosci. 2001;24:807–43.
88. Buonomano DV, Merzenich M. Cortical plasticity: from synapse to maps. Annu Rev Neurosci. 1998;21:149–86.
89. Robinson LR, Czerniecki JM, Ehde DM, et al. Trial of amitriptyline for relief of pain in amputees: results of a randomized controlled study. Arch Phys Med Rehabil. 2004;85(1):1–6.
90. Wilder-Smith CH, Hill LT, Laurent S. Postamputation pain and sensory changes in treatment-naive patients: characteristics and responses to treatment with tramadol, amitriptyline, and placebo. Anesthesiology. 2005;103(3):619–28.
91. Spiegel DR, Lappinen E, Gottlieb M. A presumed case of phantom limb pain treated successfully with duloxetine and pregabalin. Gen Hosp Psychiatry. 2010;32(2):228. e5–7.
92. Kuiken TA, Schechtman L, Harden RN. Phantom limb pain treatment with mirtazapine: a case series. Pain Pract. 2005;5 (4):356–60.
93. Sato K, Higuchi H, Hishikawa Y. Management of phantom limb pain and sensation with milnacipran. J Neuropsychiatry Clin Neurosci. 2008;20(3):368.
94. Hackworth RJ, Tokarz KA, Fowler IM, Wallace SC, Stedje-Larsen ET. Profound pain reduction after induction of memantine treatment in two patients with severe phantom limb pain. Anesth Analg. 2008;107(4):1377–9.
95. Schley M, Topfner S, Wiech K, et al. Continuous brachial plexus blockade in combination with the NMDA receptor antagonist memantine prevents phantom pain in acute traumatic upper limb amputees. Eur J Pain. 2007;11(3):299–308.
96. Zuniga RE, Schlicht CR, Abram SE. Intrathecal baclofen is analgesic in patients with chronic pain. Anesthesiology. 2000;92 (3):876–80.
97. Omote K, Ohmori H, Kawamata M, Matsumoto M, Namiki A. Intrathecal buprenorphine in the treatment of phantom limb pain. Anesth Analg. 1995;80:1030–2.
98. Knotkova H, Cruciani RA, Tronnier VM, Rasche D. Current and future options for the management of phantom-limb pain. J Pain Res. 2012;5:39–49.
99. Borghi B, D'Addabbo M, White PF, Gallerani P, et al. The use of prolonged peripheral neural blockade after lower extremity amputation: the effect on symptoms associated with phantom limb syndrome. Anesth Analg. 2010;111:1308–15.
100. Karanikolas M, Aretha D, Tsolakis I, Monantera G, et al. Optimized perioperative analgesia reduces chronic phantom limb pain intensity, prevalence, and frequency: a prospective, randomized, clinical trial. Anesthesiology. 2011;114(5):1144–54.
101. Hayes C, Armstrong-Brown A, Burstal R. Perioperative intravenous ketamine infusion for the prevention of persistent post-amputation pain: a randomized, controlled trial. Anaesth Intens Care. 2004;32(3):330–8.

102. Wilson JA, Nimmo AF, Fleetwood-Walker SM, Colvin LA. A randomized double blind trial of the effect of preemptive epidural ketamine on persistent pain after lower limb amputation. Pain. 2008;135(1–2):108–18.
103. Bishnu S, George TG. Phantom limb pain: mechanisms and treatment approaches. Pain Res Treat. 2011;2011:1–8.
104. Walsh NE, Rogers JN. Injection procedures. In: DeLisa JA, Gans BM, Walsh NE, editors. Physical medicine and rehabilitation principles and practice, vol. 1. Philadelphia, PA: Lippincott-Williams & Wilkins; 2005. p. 311–61.
105. Siegfried J, Cetinalp E. Neurosurgical treatment of phantom limb pain. In: Siegfried J, Zimmermann M, editors. Phantom and stump pain. Berlin: Springer; 1981.
106. Ulger O. Effectiveness of phantom excercises for phantom limb pain: a pilot study. J Rehab Med. 2009;41(7):582–4.
107. Brown CA, Lido C. Reflexology treatment for patients with lower limb amputations and phantom limb pain: an exploratory pilot study. Complement Ther Clin Pract. 2008;14(2):124–31.
108. DeRoos C, Veenstra AC, DeJongh A, DenHollander-Gijsman M, Van Der Wee NJ, Zitman FG, VanRood YR. Treatment of chronic phantom limb pain using a trauma focused psychological approach. Pain Res Manag. 2010;15(2):65–71.
109. Canavero S, Bonicalzi V, Dotta M, Vighetti S, Asteggiano G, Cocito D. Transcranial magnetic cortical stimulation relieves central pain. Stereotact Funct Neurosurg. 2002;78:192–6.
110. Canavero S, Bonicalzi V. Therapeutic extradural cortical stimulation for central and neuropathic pain: a review. Clin J Pain. 2002;18(1):48–55.
111. Andre-Obadia N, Peyron R, Mertens P, Mauguiere F, Laurent B, Garcia-Larea L. Transcranial magnetic stimulation for pain control: double-blind study of different frequencies against placebo, and correlation with motor cortex stimulation efficacy. Clin Neurophysiol. 2006;7:1536–44.
112. Lefaucheur J, Hatem S, Nineb A, Menard-Lefaucheur I, Wendling S, Karavel Y, Nguyen J. Somatotopic organization of the analgesic effects of motor cortex rTMS in neuropathic pain. Neurology. 2006;F67:1998–2004.
113. Lefaucheur JP, Drouot X, Menard-Lefaucheur I, Zerah F, Bendib B, Cesaro P, Keravel Y, Nguyen JP. Neurogenic pain relief by repetitive transcranial magnetic cortical stimulation depends on the origin and the site of pain. J Neurol Neurosurg Psychiatry. 2004;75:612–6.
114. Hirayama A, Saitoh Y, Kishima H, Shimokawa T, Oshino S, Hirata M, Kato A, Yoshimine T. Reduction of intractable deafferentation pain by navigation-guided repetitive transcranial magnetic stimulation of the primary motor cortex. Pain. 2006;122:22–7.
115. Topper R, Foltys H, Meister IG, Sparing R, Boroojerdi B. Repetitive transcranial magnetic stimulation of the parietal cortex transiently ameliorates phantom limb pain-like syndrome. Clin Neurophysiol. 2003;114:1521–30.
116. Khedr EM, Kotb H, Kamel NF, Ahmed MA, Sadek R, Rothwell JC. Longlasting antalgic effects of daily sessions of repetitive transcranial magnetic stimulation in central and peripheral neuropathic pain. J Neurol Neurosurg Psychiatry. 2005;76:833–8.
117. DiRollo A, Pallanti S. Phantom limb pain: low frequency repetitive transcranial magnetic stimulation in unaffected hemisphere. Case Report Med. 2011;2011:130751.
118. Ahmed MA, Mohamed SA, Sayed D. Long-term antalgic effects of repetitive transcranial magnetic stimulation of motor cortex and serum beta-endorphin in patients with phantom pain. Neurol Res. 2011;33(9):953–8.
119. Giummarra MJ, Gibson SJ, Georgiou-Karistianis N, Bradshaw JL. Central mechanisms in phantom limb perception: the past, present, and future. Brain Res Rev. 2007;54(1):219–32.
120. Decety J. Do executed and imagined movements share the same central structures? Cogn Brain Res. 1996;3:87–93.
121. MacIver K, Lloyd DM, Kelly S, Roberts N, Nurmikko T. Phantom limb pain, cortical reorganization and the therapeutic effects of mental imagery. Brain. 2008;131:2181–91.
122. MacLachlan M, McDonald D, Waloch J. Mirror treatment of lower limb phantom pain: a case study. Disabil Rehabil. 2004;26:901–4.
123. Brodie EE, Whyte A, Niven CA. Analgesia through the looking-glass? a randomized controlled trial investigating the effect of viewing a "virtual" limb upon phantom limb pain, sensation and movement. Euro J Pain. 2007;11:428–36.
124. Moseley GL, Gallace A, Spence C. Is mirror therapy all it is cracked up to be? current evidence and future directions. Pain. 2008;138:7–10.
125. Chan BL, Heilman KM, Tsao JW. Mirror therapy for phantom limb pain. N Engl J Med. 2007;357:2006–7.
126. Nguyen JP, Nizard J, Keravel Y, Lefaucheur JP. Invasive brain stimulation for the treatment of neuropathic pain. Nat Rev Neurol. 2011;7:699–709.
127. Katayama Y, Yamamoto T, Kobayashi K, Kasai M, Oshima H, Fukaya C. Motor cortex stimulation for phantom limb pain: comprehensive therapy with spinal cord and thalamic stimulation. Stereotact Funct Neurosurg. 2002;77(1–4):159–62.
128. Lima MC, Fregni F. Motor cortex stimulation for chronic pain: systematic review and meta-analysis of the literature. Neurology. 2008;70(24):2329–37.
129. Fontaine D, Hamani C, Lozano A. Efficacy and safety of motor cortex stimulation for chronic neuropathic pain: critical review of the literature. J Neurosurg. 2009;110:251–6.
130. Kumar K, Toth C, Nath RK. Deep brain stimulation for intractable pain: a 15-year experience. Neurosurgery. 1997;4:736–47.
131. Viswanathan A. Use of spinal cord stimulation in the treatment of phantom limb pain: case series and review of literature. Pain Pract. 2010;10(5):479–84.
132. Krainick JU, Thoder U. Spinal cord stimulation in post-amputation pain. In: Siegfried J, Zimmerman M, editors. Phantom and stump pain. Berlin, Germany: Springer; 2002. p. 527–35.
133. Nandi D, Yianni J, Humphreys J, Wang S, O'sullivan V, Shepstone B, Stein JF, Aziz TZ. Phantom limb pain relieved with different modalities of central nervous system stimulation: a clinical and functional imaging case report of two patients. Neuromodulation. 2004;7(3):176–83.
134. Tanei T, Nakahara N, Takebayashi S, Ito M, Hashizume Y, Wakabayashi T. Primary angiitis of the central nervous system mimicking tumor-like lesion: case report. Neurol Med Chir (Tokyo). 2011;51(1):56–9.
135. Alves RV, Asfora WT. Deep brain stimulation for Dejerine-Roussy syndrome: case report. Minim Invasive Neurosurg. 2011;54(4):183–6.
136. Klit H, Finnerup NB, Jensen TS. Central post-stroke pain: clinical characteristics, pathophysiology, and management. Lancet Neurol. 2009;8(9):857–68.
137. Leijon G, Boivie J. Central post-stroke pain: a controlled trial of amitriptyline and carbamazepine. Pain. 1989;36:27–36.
138. Lampl C, Yazdi K, Roper C. Amitriptyline in the prophylaxis of central post-stroke pain: preliminary results of 39 patients in a placebo-controlled, long-term study. Stroke. 2002;33(12):3030–2.
139. Vestergaard K, Andersen G, Gottrup H, et al. Lamotrigine for central post-stroke pain: a randomized controlled trial. Neurology. 2001;56(2):184–90.
140. Awerbuch G, Sandyk R. Mexiletine for thalamic pain syndrome. Int J Neurosci. 1990;55:129–33.
141. Edmonson EA, Simpson Jr RK, Stubler DK, et al. Systemic lidocaine therapy poststroke pain. South Med J. 1993;86 (10):1093–6.
142. Kvarnstrom A, Karlsten R, Quiding H, et al. The analgesic effect of intravenous ketamine and lidocaine on pain after spinal cord injury. Acta Anaesthesiol Scand. 2004;48(4):498–506.

143. Crisologo PA, Neal B, Brown R, et al. Lidocaine-induced spinal block can relieve central post-stroke pain: role of the block in chronic pain diagnosis. Anesthesiology. 1991;74(1):184–5.
144. Canavero S, Bonicalzi V, Pagni CA, et al. Propofol analgesia in central pain: preliminary clinical observations. J Neurol. 1995;242 (9):561–7.
145. Morley JS, Bridson J, Nash TP, et al. Low-dose methadone has an analgesic effect in neuropathic pain: a double-blind randomized controlled crossover trial. Palliat Med. 2003;17(7):576–87.
146. Mailis A, Amani N, Umana M, et al. Effect of intravenous sodium amytal on cutaneous sensory abnormalities, spontaneous pain and algometric pain pressure thresholds in neuropathic pain patients: a placebo-controlled study. Pain. 1997;70(1):69–81.
147. Arner S, Meyerson BA. Lack of analgesic effect of opioids on neuropathic and idiopathic forms of pain. Pain. 1988;33(1):11–23.
148. Backonja M, Arndt G, Gombar KA, et al. Response of chronic neuropathic pain syndromes to ketamine: a preliminary study. Pain. 1994;56(1):51–7.
149. McQuay HJ, Carroll D, Jadad AR, et al. Dextromethorphan for the treatment of neuropathic pain: a double-blind randomised controlled crossover trial with integral n-of-1 design. Pain. 1994;59 (1):127–33.
150. Dworkin RH, O'Connor AB, Backonja M, et al. Pharmacological management of neuropathic pain: evidence-based recommendations. Pain. 2007;132:237–51.
151. Finnerup NB, Otto M, McQuay HJ, et al. Algorithm for neuropathic pain treatment: an evidence based proposal. Pain. 2005;118:289–305.
152. Saitoh Y, Hirayama A, Kishima H, Shimokawa T, Oshino S, Hirata M, Tani N, Kato A, Yoshimine T. Reduction of intractable deafferentation pain due to spinal cord or peripheral lesion by high-frequency repetitive transcranial magnetic stimulation of the primary motor cortex. J Neurosurg. 2007;107(3):555–9.
153. Tsubokawa T, Katayama Y, Yamamoto T, Hirayama T, Koyama S. Chronic motor cortex stimulation in patients with thalamic pain. J Neurosurg. 1993;78(3):393–401.
154. Owen SL, Green AL, Nandi DD, Bittar RG, Wang S, Aziz TZ. Deep brain stimulation for neuropathic pain. Acta Neurochir Suppl. 2007;97(Pt 2):111–6.
155. Bittar RG, Kar-Purkayastha I, Owen SL, Bear RE, Green A, Wang S, Aziz TZ. Deep brain stimulation for pain relief: a meta-analysis. J Clin Neurosci. 2005;12(5):515.
156. Katayama Y, Fukaya C, Yamamoto T. Poststroke pain control by chronic motor cortex stimulation: neurological characteristics predicting a favorable response. J Neurosurg. 1998;89(4):585–91.
157. Brown JA, Barbaro NM. Motor cortex stimulation for central and neuropathic pain: current status. Pain. 2003;104(3):431–5.
158. Nguyen JP, Lefaucher JP, Le Guerinel C, Eizenbaum JF, Nakano N, Carpentier A, Brugières P, Pollin B, Rostaing S, Keravel Y. Motor cortex stimulation in the treatment of central and neuropathic pain. Arch Med Res. 2000;31(3):263–5.
159. Tanei T, Nakahara N, Takebayashi S, Hirano M, Kajita Y, Wakabayashi T. Dual lead spinal cord stimulation using octad lead for central post-stroke pain. No Shinkei Geka. 2012;40 (4):325–9.
160. Burchiel KJ. A new classification for facial pain. Neurosurgery. 2003;53(5):1164–6. Discussion 1166–7.
161. Nicol CF. A four year double-blind study of tegretol in facial pain. Headache. 1969;9(1):54–7.
162. Magenta P, Arghetti S, Di Palma F, et al. Oxcarbazepine is effective and safe in the treatment of neuropathic pain: pooled analysis of seven clinical studies. Neurol Sci. 2005;26(4):218–26.
163. Din MU, Zvartan-Hind M, Gilari A, Lisak R, Khan OA. Topiramate relieved refractory trigeminal neuralgia in multiple sclerosis patients. Neurology. 2000;53(1):216–8.
164. Court JE, Kase CS. Treatment of tic douloureux with a new anticonvulsant (clonazepam). J Neurol Neurosurg Psychiatry. 1976;39(3):297–9.
165. DaSilva AF, Becerra L, Pendse G, Chizh B, Tully S, Borsook D. Colocalized structural and functional changes in the cortex of patients with trigeminal neuropathic pain. PLoS One. 2008;3 (10):e3396.
166. Lefaucheur JP, Drouot X, Nguyen JP. Interventional neurophysiology for pain control: duration of pain relief following repetitive transcranial magnetic stimulation of the motor cortex. Neurophysiol Clin. 2001;31(4):247–52.
167. Rollnik JD, Wüstefeld S, Däuper J, Karst M, Fink M, Kossev A, Dengler R. Repetitive transcranial magnetic stimulation for the treatment of chronic pain: a pilot study. Eur Neurol. 2002;48 (1):6–10.
168. André-Obadia N, Mertens P, Gueguen A, Peyron R, Garcia-Larrea L. Pain relief by rTMS: differential effect of current flow but no specific action on pain subtypes. Neurology. 2008;71(11):833–40.
169. Zaghi S, DaSilva AF, Acar M, Lopes M, Fregni F. One-year rTMS treatment for refractory trigeminal neuralgia. J Pain Symptom Manage. 2009;38(4):e1–5.
170. Green AL, Nandi D, Armstrong G, Carter H, Aziz T. Post-herpetic trigeminal neuralgia treated with deep brain stimulation. J Clin Neurosci. 2003;4:512–4.
171. Rasche D, Rinaldi PC, Young RF, Tronnier VM. Deep brain stimulation for the treatment of various chronic pain syndromes. Neurosurg Focus. 2006;21(6):E8.
172. Broggi G, Franzini A, Leone M, Bussone G. Update on neurosurgical treatment of chronic trigeminal autonomic cephalalgias and atypical facial pain with deep brain stimulation of posterior hypothalamus: results and comments. Neurol Sci. 2007;28 Suppl 2: S138–45.
173. Cordella R, Franzini A, La Mantia L, Marras C, Erbetta A, Broggi G. Hypothalamic stimulation for trigeminal neuralgia in multiple sclerosis patients: efficacy on the paroxysmal ophthalmic pain. Mult Scler. 2009;11:1322–8.
174. Meyerson B, Lindblom U, Linderoth B, Lind G, Herregodts P. Motor cortex stimulation as treatment of trigeminal neuropathic pain. Acta Neurochir Suppl. 1993;58:150–3.
175. Herregodts P, Stadnik T, De Ridder F, D'Haens J. Cortical stimulation of central neuropathic pain: 3-D surface MRI for easy determination of the motor cortex. Acta Neurochir Suppl. 1995;64:132–5.
176. Ebel H, Rust D, Tronnier V, Böker D, Kunze S. Chronic precentral stimulation in trigeminal neuropathic pain. Acta Neurochir. 1996;138:1300–6.
177. Rainov N, Heidecke V. Motor cortex stimulation for neuropathic facial pain. Neurol Res. 2003;25:157–61.
178. Brown J, Pilitsis J. Motor cortex stimulation for central and neuropathic facial pain: a prospective study of 10 patients and observation of enhanced sensory and motor function during stimulation. Neurosurgery. 2005;56:290–7.
179. Rasche D, Ruppolt M, Stippich C, Unterberg A, Tronnier V. Motor cortex stimulation for long-term relief of chronic neuropathic pain: a 10 year experience. Pain. 2006;121:43–52.
180. Lefaucheur JP, Drouot X, Cunin P, Bruckert R, Lepetit H, Créange A, Wolkenstein P, Maison P, Keravel Y, Nguyen JP. Motor cortex stimulation for the treatment of refractory peripheral neuropathic pain. Brain. 2009;132:1463–71.
181. Anderson W, Kiyofuji S, Conway J, Busch C, North R, Garonzik I. Dysphagia and neuropathic facial pain treated with motor cortex stimulation case report. Neurosurgery. 2009;65:E626.
182. Arnold LM, Bradley LA, Clauw DJ, Glass JM, Goldenberg DL. Multidisciplinary care and stepwise treatment for fibromyalgia. J Clin Psychiatry. 2008;69(12):e35.

183. Gracely RH, Petzke F, Wolf JM, Clauw DJ. Functional magnetic resonance imaging evidence of augmented pain processing in fibromyalgia. Arthritis Rheum. 2002;46(5):1333–43.
184. Montoya P, Sitges C, García-Herrera M, Izquierdo R, Truyols M, Collado D. Considerations on alterations in brain activity in patients with fibromyalgia. Reumatol Clin. 2006;2(5):251–60.
185. Cook DB, Stegner AJ, McLoughlin MJ. Imaging pain of fibromyalgia. Curr Pain Headache Rep. 2007;11(3):190–200.
186. Diers M, Koeppe C, Yilmaz P, Thieme K, Markela-Lerenc J, Schiltenwolf M, van Ackern K, Flor H. Pain ratings and somatosensory evoked responses to repetitive intramuscular and intracutaneous stimulation in fibromyalgia syndrome. J Clin Neurophysiol. 2008;25(3):153–60.
187. Wolfe F. Fibromyalgia. Rheum Dis Clin North Am. 1990;16 (3):681–98.
188. Marlow NM, Bonilha HS, Short EB. Efficacy of transcranial direct current stimulation and repetitive transcranial magnetic stimulation for treating fibromyalgia syndrome: a systematic review. Pain Pract. 2013;13(2):131–45.
189. Zhao Y, Sun P, Watson P, Mitchell B, Swindle R. Comparison of medication adherence and healthcare costs between duloxetine and pregabalin initiators among patients with fibromyalgia. Pain Pract. 2011;11(3):204–16.
190. Clauw DJ. Pharmacotherapy for patients with fibromyalgia. J Clin Psychiatry. 2008;69 Suppl 2:25–9.
191. Mease PJ, Russell IJ, Kajdasz DK, Wiltse CG, Detke MJ, Wohlreich MM, Walker DJ, Chappell AS. Long-term safety, tolerability, and efficacy of duloxetine in the treatment of fibromyalgia. Semin Arthritis Rheum. 2010;39(6):454–64.
192. Guymer EK, Littlejohn GO. Fibromyalgia. Diagnosis and management. Australas Chiropr Osteopathy. 2002;10(2):81–4.
193. Sumpton JE, Moulin DE. Fibromyalgia: presentation and management with a focus on pharmacological treatment. Pain Res Manag. 2008;13(6):477–83.
194. Häuser W, Petzke F, Sommer C. Comparative efficacy and harms of duloxetine, milnacipran, and pregabalin in fibromyalgia syndrome. J Pain. 2010;11(6):505–21.
195. Passard A, Attal N, Benadhira R, Brasseur L, Saba G, Sichere P, Perrot S, Januel D, Bouhassira D. Effects of unilateral repetitive transcranial magnetic stimulation of the motor cortex on chronic widespread pain in fibromyalgia. Brain. 2007;130(Pt 10): 2661–70.
196. Mhalla A, Baudic S, de Ciampi Andrade D, Gautron M, Perrot S, Teixeira MJ, Attal N, Bouhassira D. Long-term maintenance of the analgesic effects of transcranial magnetic stimulation in fibromyalgia. Pain. 2011;152(7):1478–85.
197. Sampson SM, Rome JD, Rummans TA. Slow-frequency rTMS reduces fibromyalgia pain. Pain Med. 2006;7(2):115–8.
198. Carretero B, Martín MJ, Juan A, Pradana ML, Martín B, Carral M, Jimeno T, Pareja A, Montoya P, Aguirre I, Salva J, Roca M, Gili M, Garcia-Toro M. Low-frequency transcranial magnetic stimulation in patients with fibromyalgia and major depression. Pain Med. 2009;10(4):748–53.
199. Short EB, Borckardt JJ, Anderson BS, Frohman H, Beam W, Reeves ST, George MS. Ten sessions of adjunctive left prefrontal rTMS significantly reduces fibromyalgia pain: a randomized, controlled pilot study. Pain. 2011;152(11):2477–84. doi:10.1016/j.pain.2011.05.033.
200. Fregni F, Gimenes R, Valle AC, Ferreira MJ, Rocha RR, Natalle L, Bravo R, Rigonatti SP, Freedman SD, Nitsche MA, Pascual-Leone A, Boggio PS. A randomized, sham-controlled, proof of principle study of transcranial direct current stimulation for the treatment of pain in fibromyalgia. Arthritis Rheum. 2006;54 (12):3988–98.
201. Roizenblatt S, Fregni F, Gimenez R, Wetzel T, Rigonatti SP, Tufik S, Boggio PS, Valle AC. Site-specific effects of transcranial direct current stimulation on sleep and pain in fibromyalgia: a randomized, sham-controlled study. Pain Pract. 2007;7(4): 297–306.
202. Riberto M, Marcon Alfieri F, Monteiro de Benedetto Pacheco K, Dini Leite V, Nemoto Kaihami H, Fregni F, Rizzo Battistella L. Efficacy of transcranial direct current stimulation coupled with a multidisciplinary rehabilitation program for the treatment of fibromyalgia. Open Rheumatol J. 2011;5:45–50.
203. Valle A, Roizenblatt S, Botte S, Zaghi S, Riberto M, Tufik S, Boggio PS, Fregni F. Efficacy of anodal transcranial direct current stimulation (tDCS) for the treatment of fibromyalgia: results of a randomized, sham-controlled longitudinal clinical trial. J Pain Manag. 2009;2(3):353–61.
204. Gilula MF. Cranial electrotherapy stimulation and fibromyalgia. Expert Rev Med Devices. 2007;4(4):489–95.
205. Lichtbroun AS, Raicer MM, Smith RB. The treatment of fibromyalgia with cranial electrotherapy stimulation. J Clin Rheumatol. 2001;7(2):72–8. Discussion 78.
206. Hsieh JC, Belfrage M, Stone-Elander S, Hansson P, Ingvar M. Central representation of chronic ongoing neuropathic pain studied by positron emission tomography. Pain. 1995;63 (2):225–36.
207. Fukui S, Shigemori S, Nosaka S. Central pain associated with low thalamic blood flow treated by electroconvulsive therapy. J Anesth. 2002;16(3):255–7.
208. Fukui S, Shigemori S, Yoshimura A, Nosaka S. Chronic pain with beneficial response to electroconvulsive therapy and regional cerebral blood flow changes assessed by single photon emission computed tomography. Reg Anesth Pain Med. 2002;27(2):211–3.
209. Usui C, Doi N, Nishioka M, Komatsu H, Yamamoto R, Ohkubo T, et al. Electroconvulsive therapy improves severe pain associated with fibromyalgia. Pain. 2006;121(3):276–80.
210. Bartleson JD, Cutrer FM. Migraine update: diagnosis and treatment. Minn Med. 2010;93(5):36–41.
211. Lay CL, Broner SW. Migraine in women. Neurol Clin. 2009;27 (2):503–11.
212. Rossi P, Ambrosini A, Buzzi MG. Prodromes and predictors of migraine attack. Funct Neurol. 2005;20(4):185–91.
213. Buzzi MG, Cologno D, Formisano R, Rossi P. Prodromes and the early phase of the migraine attack: therapeutic relevance. Funct Neurol. 2005;20(4):179–83.
214. Dodick DW, Gargus JJ. Why migraines strike. Sci Am. 2008;299 (2):56–63.
215. Bigal ME, Arruda MA. Migraine in the pediatric population: evolving concepts. Headache. 2010;50(7):1130–43.
216. Olesen J, Goadsby PJ. Synthesis of migraine mechanisms. In: Olesen J, Goadsby PJ, Ramadan NM, Tfelt-Hansen P, Welch KMA, editors. The headaches. Philadelphia, PA: Lippincott Williams & Wilkins; 2006. p. 383–98.
217. Capobianco DJ, Dodick DW. Diagnosis and treatment of cluster headache. Semin Neurol. 2006;26(2):242–59.
218. Meyer EL, Laurell K, Artto V, Bendtsen L, Linde M, Kallela M, Tronvik E, Zwart JA, Jensen RM, Hagen K. Lateralization in cluster headache: a nordic multicenter study. J Headache Pain. 2009;10(4):259–63.
219. Torelli P, Castellini P, Cucurachi L, Devetak M, Lambru G, Manzoni G. Cluster headache prevalence: methodological considerations a review of the literature. Acta Biomed Ateneo Parmense. 2006;77(1):4–9.
220. Stillman MJ. Testosterone replacement therapy for treatment refractory cluster headache. Headache. 2006;46(6):925–33.
221. Pinessi L, Rainero I, Rivoiro C, Rubino E, Gallone S. Genetics of cluster headache: an update. J Headache Pain. 2005;6(4):234–6.
222. Matharu M, Goadsby P. Pract Neurol. 2001;1(1):42–9.
223. Gilmore B, Michael M. Treatment of acute migraine headache. Am Fam Physician. 2011;83(3):271–80.

224. Loder E, Burch R, Rizzoli P. The 2012 AHS/AAN guidelines for prevention of episodic migraine: a summary and comparison with other recent clinical practice guidelines. Headache. 2012;52 (6):930–45.
225. Lee MS, Ernst E. Acupuncture for pain: an overview of cochrane reviews. Chin J Integr Med. 2011;17(3):187–9.
226. Linde K, Allais G, Brinkhaus B, Manheimer E, Vickers A, White AR. Acupuncture for migraine prophylaxis. Cochrane Database Syst Rev. 2009;1, CD001218. doi:10.1002/14651858.CD001218.pub2.
227. Chaibi A, Tuchin PJ, Russell MB. Manual therapies for migraine: a systematic review. J Headache Pain. 2011;12(2):127–33.
228. Bianchi A, Salomone S, Caraci F, Pizza V, Bernardini R, Damato C. Role of magnesium, coenzyme Q10, riboflavin, and vitamin B12 in migraine prophylaxis. Vitam Horm. 2010;69:297–312.
229. Kung TA, Guyuron B, Cederna PS. Migraine surgery: a plastic surgery solution for refractory migraine headache. Plast Reconstr Surg. 2011;127(1):181–9.
230. Nestoriuc Y, Martin A. Efficacy of biofeedback for migraine: a meta-analysis. Pain. 2007;128(1–2):111–27.
231. Nestoriuc Y, Martin A, Rief W, Andrasik F. Biofeedback treatment for headache disorders: a comprehensive efficacy review. Appl Psychophysiol Biofeedback. 2008;33(3):125–40.
232. May A, Leone M, Afra J, Linde M, Sándor P, Evers S, Goadsby P. EFNS guidelines on the treatment of cluster headache and other trigeminal-autonomic cephalalgias. Eur J Neurol. 2006;13(10): 1066–77.
233. Mauskop A, Altura BT, Cracco RQ, Altura BM. Intravenous magnesium sulfate relieves cluster headaches in patients with low serum ionized magnesium levels. Headache. 1995;35 (10):597–600.
234. Leone M, et al. Melatonin versus placebo in the prophylaxis of cluster headache: a double-blind pilot study with parallel groups. Cephalalgia. 1995;16(7):494–6.
235. Cohen AS, Burns B, Goadsby PJ. High-flow oxygen for treatment of cluster headache: a randomized trial. JAMA. 2009;302(22): 2451–7.
236. Law S, Derry S, Moore RA. Triptans for acute cluster headache. Cochrane Database Syst Rev. 2013;7:CD008042.
237. Sostak P, Krause P, Förderreuther S, Reinisch V, Straube A. Botulinum toxin type-A therapy in cluster headache: an open study. J Headache Pain. 2007;8(4):236–41.
238. Kittrelle JP, Grouse DS, Seybold ME. Cluster headache: local anesthetic abortive agents. Arch Neurol. 1985;42(5):496–8.
239. de Vries B, Frants RR, Ferrari MD, van den Maagdenberg AM. Molecular genetics of migraine. Hum Genet. 2009;126(1):115–32.
240. Bolay H, Reuter U, Dunn AK, Huang Z, Boas DA, Moskowitz MA. Intrinsic brain activity triggers trigeminal meningeal afferents in a migraine model. Nat Med. 2002;8(2):136–42.
241. Holland PR. Modulation of trigeminovascular processing: novel insights into primary headache disorders. Cephalalgia. 2009;29 Suppl 3:1–6.
242. Keck ME, Welt T, Müller MB, Erhardt A, Ohl F, Toschi N, Holsboer F, Sillaber I. Repetitive transcranial magnetic stimulation increases the release of dopamine in the mesolimbic and mesostriatal system. Neuropharmacology. 2002;43(1):101–9.
243. Strafella AP, Paus T, Barrett J, Dagher A. Repetitive transcranial magnetic stimulation of the human prefrontal cortex induces dopamine release in the caudate nucleus. J Neurosci. 2001;21 (15):RC157.
244. Michael N, Gösling M, Reutemann M, Kersting A, Heindel W, Arolt V, Pfleiderer B. Metabolic changes after repetitive transcranial magnetic stimulation (rTMS) of the left prefrontal cortex: a sham-controlled proton magnetic resonance spectroscopy (1H MRS) study of healthy brain. Eur J Neurosci. 2003;17 (11):2462–8.
245. Clarke BM, Upton AR, Kamath MV, Al-Harbi T, Castellanos CM. Transcranial magnetic stimulation for migraine: clinical effects. J Headache Pain. 2006;7(5):341–6. Epub 2006 Oct 25.
246. Mohammad TM, Hughes G, Nkrumah M, et al. Self-Administered transcranial magnetic stimulation (TMS) during the aura phase improved and aborts headache. Headache. 2006;46:857.
247. Lipton RB, Pearlman SH. Transcranial magnetic simulation in the treatment of migraine. Neurotherapeutics. 2010;7(2):204–12.
248. Brighina F, Piazza A, Vitello G, Aloisio A, Palermo A, Daniele O, Fierro B. rTMS of the prefrontal cortex in the treatment of chronic migraine: a pilot study. J Neurol Sci. 2004;227(1):67–71.
249. Teepker M, Hötzel J, Timmesfeld N, Reis J, Mylius V, Haag A, Oertel WH, Rosenow F, Schepelmann K. Low-frequency rTMS of the vertex in the prophylactic treatment of migraine. Cephalalgia. 2010;30(2):137–44.
250. Antal A, Kriener N, Lang N, Boros K, Paulus W. Cathodal transcranial direct current stimulation of the visual cortex in the prophylactic treatment of migraine. Cephalalgia. 2011;31 (7):820–8.
251. DaSilva AF, Mendonca ME, Zaghi S, Lopes M, Dossantos MF, Spierings EL, Bajwa Z, Datta A, Bikson M, Fregni F. tDCS-induced analgesia and electrical fields in pain-related neural networks in chronic migraine. Headache. 2012;52(8):1283–95.
252. Sano K, Mayanagi Y, Sekino H, Ogashiwa M, Ishijima B. Results of stimulation and destruction of the posterior hypothalamus in man. J Neurosurg. 1970;33:689–707.
253. May A, Bahra A, Buchel C, Frackowiak RS, Goadsby PJ. Hypothalamic activation in cluster headache attacks. Lancet. 1998;352: 275–8.
254. Sprenger T, Boecker H, Tolle TR, Bussone G, May A, Leone M. Specific hypothalamic activation during a spontaneous cluster headache attack. Neurology. 2004;62:516–7.
255. Franzini A, Ferroli P, Leone M, Broggi G. Stimulation of the posterior hypothalamus for treatment of chronic intractable cluster headaches: first reported series. Neurosurgery. 2003;52:1095–9. Discussion 1099–1101.
256. Leone M. Deep brain stimulation in headache. Lancet Neurol. 2006;5:873–7.
257. Leone M, Proietti Cecchini A, Franzini A, Broggi G, Cortelli P, Montagna P, et al. Lessons from 8 years experience of hypothalamic stimulation in cluster headache. Cephalalgia. 2008;28: 787–97. Discussion 798.
258. Schoenen J, Di Clemente L, Vandenheede M, Fumal A, De Pasqua V, Mouchamps M, et al. Hypothalamic stimulation in chronic cluster headache: a pilot study of efficacy and mode of action. Brain. 2005;128:940–7.
259. Fontaine D, Lazorthes Y, Mertens P, Blond S, Geraud G, Fabre N, et al. Safety and efficacy of deep brain stimulation in refractory cluster headache: a randomized placebo-controlled double-blind trial followed by a 1-year open extension. J Headache Pain. 2010;11:23–31.
260. Matharu MS, Zrinzo L. Deep brain stimulation in cluster headache. Expert Rev Neurother. 2011;11:473–5.
261. Matharu MS, Zrinzo L. Deep brain stimulation in cluster headache: hypothalamus or midbrain tegmentum? Curr Pain Headache Rep. 2010;14:151–9.
262. Matharu MS, Bartsch T, Ward N, Frackowiak RS, Weiner R, Goadsby PJ. Central neuromodulation in chronic migraine patients with suboccipital stimulators: a PET study. Brain. 2004;127:220–30.
263. Popeney CA, Alo KM. Peripheral neurostimulation for the treatment of chronic, disabling transformed migraine. Headache. 2003;43:369–75.
264. Johnstone C, Sundaraj R. Occipital nerve stimulation for the treatment of occipital neuralgia: eight case studies. Neuromodulation. 2006;9:41–7.

265. Kapural L, Mekhail N, Hayek SM, Stanton-Hicks M, Malak O. Occipital nerve electrical stimulation via the midline approach and subcutaneous surgical leads for treatment of severe occipital neuralgia: a pilot study. Anesth Analg. 2005;101:71–174.
266. Slavin KV, Nersesyan H, Wess C. Peripheral neurostimulation for treatment of intractable occipital neuralgia. Neurosurgery. 2006;58:112–9. Discussion 112–119.
267. Weiner RL, Reed KL. Peripheral neurostimulation for control of intractable occipital neuralgia. Neuromodulation. 1999;2:217–21.
268. Burns B, Watkins L, Goadsby PJ. Treatment of medically intractable cluster headache by occipital nerve stimulation: long-term follow-up of eight patients. Lancet Neurol. 2007;369:1099–106.
269. Burns B, Watkins L, Goadsby PJ. Treatment of intractable chronic cluster headache by occipital nerve stimulation in 14 patients. Neurology. 2009;72:341–5.
270. Magis D, Allena M, Bolla M, De Pasqua V, Remacle JM, Schoenen J. Occipital nerve stimulation for drug-resistant chronic cluster headache: a prospective pilot study. Lancet Neurol. 2007;6:314–21.
271. Wolter T, Kaube H, Mohadjer M. High cervical epidural neurostimulation for cluster headache: case report and review of the literature. Cephalalgia. 2008;28:1091–4.
272. Wolter T, Kiemen A, Kaube H. High cervical spinal cord stimulation for chronic cluster headache. Cephalalgia. 2011;31:1170–80.
273. Felisati G, Arnone F, Lozza P, Leone M, Curone M, Bussone G. Sphenopalatine endoscopic ganglion block: a revision of a traditional technique for cluster headache. Laryngoscope. 2006;116:1447–50.
274. Lad SP, Lipani JD, Gibbs IC, Chang SD, Adler Jr JR, Henderson JM. Cyberknife targeting the pterygopalatine ganglion for the treatment of chronic cluster headaches. Neurosurgery. 2007;60:E580–1. Discussion E581.
275. Sanders M, Zuurmond WW. Efficacy of sphenopalatine ganglion blockade in 66 patients suffering from cluster headache: a 12- to 70-month follow-up evaluation. J Neurosurg. 1997;87:876–80.
276. Solomon S, Apfelbaum RI. Surgical decompression of the facial nerve in the treatment of chronic cluster headache. Arch Neurol. 1986;43:479–82.
277. Ansarinia M, Rezai A, Tepper SJ, Steiner CP, Stump J, Stanton-Hicks M, et al. Electrical stimulation of sphenopalatine ganglion for acute treatment of cluster headaches. Headache. 2010;50: 1164–74.
278. Tepper SJ, Rezai A, Narouze S, Steiner C, Mohajer P, Ansarinia M. Acute treatment of intractable migraine with sphenopalatine ganglion electrical stimulation. Headache. 2009;49:983–9.
279. Dworkin RH, Backonja M, Rowbotham MC, et al. Advances in neuropathic pain: diagnosis, mechanisms, and treatment recommendations. Arch Neurol. 2003;60:1525–34.
280. Attal N, Brasseur L, Parker F, et al. Effects of gabapentin on different components of neuropathic syndromes: a pilot study. Eur J Neurol. 1998;40:191–200.
281. Attal N, Cruccu G, Haanpaa M, et al. EFNS guidelines on pharmacological treatment of neuropathic pain. Eur J Neurol. 2006;13:1153–69.
282. Yanamoto F, Murakawa K. The effects of temporary spinal cord stimulation (or spinal nerve root stimulation) on the management of early postherpetic neuralgia from one to six months of its onset. Neuromodulation. 2012;15(2):151–4.
283. Moriyama K. Effect of temporary spinal cord stimulation on postherpetic neuralgia in the thoracic nerve area. Neuromodulation. 2009;12(1):39–43.
284. Lynch PJ, McJunkin T, Eross E, Gooch S, Maloney J. Case report: successful epiradicular peripheral nerve stimulation of the C2 dorsal root ganglion for postherpetic neuralgia. Neuromodulation. 2011;14(1):58–61.
285. Dunteman E. Peripheral nerve stimulation for unremitting ophthalmic postherpetic neuralgia. Neuromodulation. 2002;5(1):32–7.
286. Yakovlev AE, Peterson AT. Peripheral nerve stimulation in treatment of intractable postherpetic neuralgia. Neuromodulation. 2007;10(4):373–5.
287. Kumar K, Taylor RS, Jacques L. Spinal cord stimulation versus conservative medical management for neuropathic pain a multicenter randomized control trial in patients with failed back surgery syndrome. Pain. 2007;132(1–2):179–88.
288. North RB, Kidd DH, Farrokhi F, Piantadosi SA. Spinal cord stimulation versus repeated lumbosacral spine surgery for chronic pain: a randomized, controlled trial. Neurosurgery. 2005;56(1):98–106.
289. Reverberi C, Dario A, Barolat G. Spinal cord stimulation (SCS) in conjunction with peripheral nerve field stimulation (PNfS) for the treatment of complex pain in failed back surgery syndrome (FBSS). Neuromodulation. 2013;16(1):78–82.
290. O'Connell NE, Cossar J, Marston L, Wand BM, Bunce D, De Souza LH, Maskill DW, Sharp A, Moseley GL. Transcranial direct current stimulation of the motor cortex in the treatment of chronic nonspecific low back pain: a randomized, double-blind exploratory study. Clin J Pain. 2013;29(1):26–34.

Applications of Neuromodulation in Neurology and Neurorehabilitation

16

Nam-Jong Paik

Movement Disorders

The term "movement disorders" has been coined for diseases characterized by abnormal or excessive movements occurring in conscious patients [1]. A useful definition of movement disorders is that they are neurologic syndromes in which there is either an excess of movement or a paucity of voluntary and automatic movements, unrelated to weakness or spasticity [2]. The excessive movements are commonly referred to as hyperkinesias and the paucity of movement is referred to as hypokinesia. Fahn et al. suggested a modern classification based on these two major types of abnormal movements (Table 16.1) [3]. Because review of all these movement disorders is beyond the scope of this chapter, we focused on the type of movement disorders that have the history of using neuromodulatory approaches as a therapeutic tool. Those include akinesia or bradykinesia in hypokinesias, and dystonia, tremor, tics, and chorea in hyperkinesias.

Parkinson's Disease

Parkinson's disease (PD) is the most common cause of Parkinsonism and is generally thought to affect approximately 0.3 % of the general population, with about five million people with PD worldwide [4, 5]. Although the pathophysiology of PD is still not understood completely, recent advances suggest that dopamine depletion from the basal ganglia and disruptions in the pathway to the thalamus and motor cortex may be the cause of parkinsonian symptoms. The syndrome is manifested by typical motor symptoms, abbreviated as TRAP: rest Tremor, Rigidity, Akinesia (or bradykinesia), and Postural instability. Nonmotor symptoms such as cognitive dysfunction, behavioral changes, and sleep dysfunction are now also recognized as important manifestations of PD to be controlled. The main strategy for the treatment of PD is pharmacologic management with rehabilitation such as physical, occupational, and speech therapy. Neuromodulatory approaches in selected people with PD have shown promising results in treating PD.

The American Academy of Neurology (AAN) suggested a useful algorithm for the treatment of PD (Fig. 16.1) [6].

Pharmacologic Treatment in PD

The timing of initiating symptomatic pharmacologic therapy in patients with PD can be determined by the degree of functional impairment and is influenced by some factors, including the following [6]: whether PD affects the dominant or nondominant hand, whether symptoms of PD influence the ability to work, presence of more disabling parkinsonian features such as bradykinesia or gait disturbance, or treatment philosophy of patient and physician.

The main categories of the drugs used for symptomatic therapy include levodopa, monoamine oxidase (MAO) B inhibitors, dopamine agonists, catechol-*O*-methyl transferase (COMT) inhibitors, anticholinergic agents, and amantadine.

Levodopa (L-dopa) is the most effective anti-parkinsonian drug [7], particularly for the management of bradykinesia. It is thought that L-dopa in early PD should be reserved until it is required for symptomatic control during therapy with a dopamine agonist.

Among MAO B inhibitors, selegiline (Eldepryl) is the most studied drug to control the symptoms of PD. Although some studies reported the possible benefits of selegiline to treat PD as a monotherapy [8] or adjunct therapy [9], the relative risks and benefits of MAO B inhibitors are still uncertain [10, 11].

Bromocriptine, pramipexole, opinirole, rotigotine, and injectable apomorphine are the dopamine agonists currently

N.-J. Paik (✉)
Department of Rehabilitation Medicine, Seoul National University College of Medicine, Seoul National University Bundang Hospital, 173-82 Gumi-Ro Bundang-Gu, Seongnam 463-707, Republic of Korea
e-mail: njpaik@snu.ac.kr

H. Knotkova and D. Rasche (eds.), *Textbook of Neuromodulation*,
DOI 10.1007/978-1-4939-1408-1_16, © Springer Science+Business Media, LLC 2015

Table 16.1 A classification of movement disorders

I. Hypokinesis
Akinesia/bradykinesia (parkinsonism)
Apraxia
Blocking (holding) tics
Cataplexy and drop attacks
Catatonia, psychomotor depression, and obsessional slowness
Freezing phenomenon
Hesitant gaits
Hypothyroid slowness
Rigidity
Stiff Muscles
II. Hyperkinesias
Abdominal dyskinesias
Akathitic movements
Ataxia/asynergia/dysmetria
Athetosis
Ballism
Chorea
Dystonia
Hemifacial spasm
Hyperekplexia
Hypnogenic dyskinesias
Jumping disorders
Jumpy stumps
Moving toes and fingers
Myoclonus
Myokymia and synkinesis
Myorhythmia
Paroxysmal dyskinesias
Periodic movements in sleep
SEM sleep behavior disorder
Restless legs
Stereotypy
Tics
Tremor

From [3]; with permission

approved by the United States Food and Drug Administration. These are the first-line therapeutic agents as initial therapy or adjunct to L-dopa in both early and advanced PD [7].

Tolcapone (Tasmar) and entacapone (Comtan) are useful COMT inhibitors as L-dopa extenders [12]. They have less effect in monotherapy but they can prolong and potentiate the L-dopa effect. This reduces off-time and increases on-time in PD treated with L-dopa to minimize the motor fluctuations.

Anticholinergics can compensate the cholinergic sensitivity induced by dopamine depletion in PD and can improve the parkinsonian symptoms [13]. Trihexyphenidyl and benztropine, biperiden, orphenadrine, and procylidine are examples of anticholinergics. The symptomatic efficacy of anticholinergics is less than that observed with L-dopa or other dopaminergic compounds [7]. It has been suggested that anticholinergics can improve the rigidity and tremor but have little effect on bradykinesia [14].

Amantadine has mild antiparkinsonian activity although its mechanism is not well understood [15]. Possibly amantadine can increase dopamine release, stimulate dopamine receptors and inhibit dopamine reuptake. Clinical studies suggest that it can be tried as a short-term monotherapy in early PD, particularly for bradykinesia and rigidity [15, 16].

Non-pharmacologic Management of PD

PD is a chronic progressive disorder, which causes various kinds of impairments and disabilities. It requires a wide-range of non-pharmacologic management including education, support, nutrition, and rehabilitation such as physical, occupational, and speech therapy.

Many patients and their caregivers are frightened after knowing that they have PD, known to be a chronic and progressive disease causing substantial disabilities. Education for general aspects of PD is required to help them understand and control over the disease and should be individualized according to patient's severity and symptoms of PD.

PD places a great burden on patients and their caregivers. Emotional or psychological support for them is very important [17]. Referral to the psychologist or counseling for legal or financial problems may be needed according to the individuals.

Because patients with PD are usually elderly and gastrointestinal symptoms including dysphagia are commonly occurred during the disease course, therefore nutritional status should be monitored [18, 19]. According to the nutritional status and combined gastrointestinal symptoms, nutritional supplementation or diet modification may be required.

Rehabilitation in PD

The American Academy of Neurology suggests that some exercise modalities may be effective to improve functional outcomes in patients with PD, including the following [20]:

1. Multidisciplinary rehabilitation with standard physical and occupational therapy
2. Treadmill training with body weight support
3. Balance training and high-intensity resistance exercise
4. Cued exercise with visual (mirror), auditory (metronome), and tactile feedback
5. Active muscle therapy

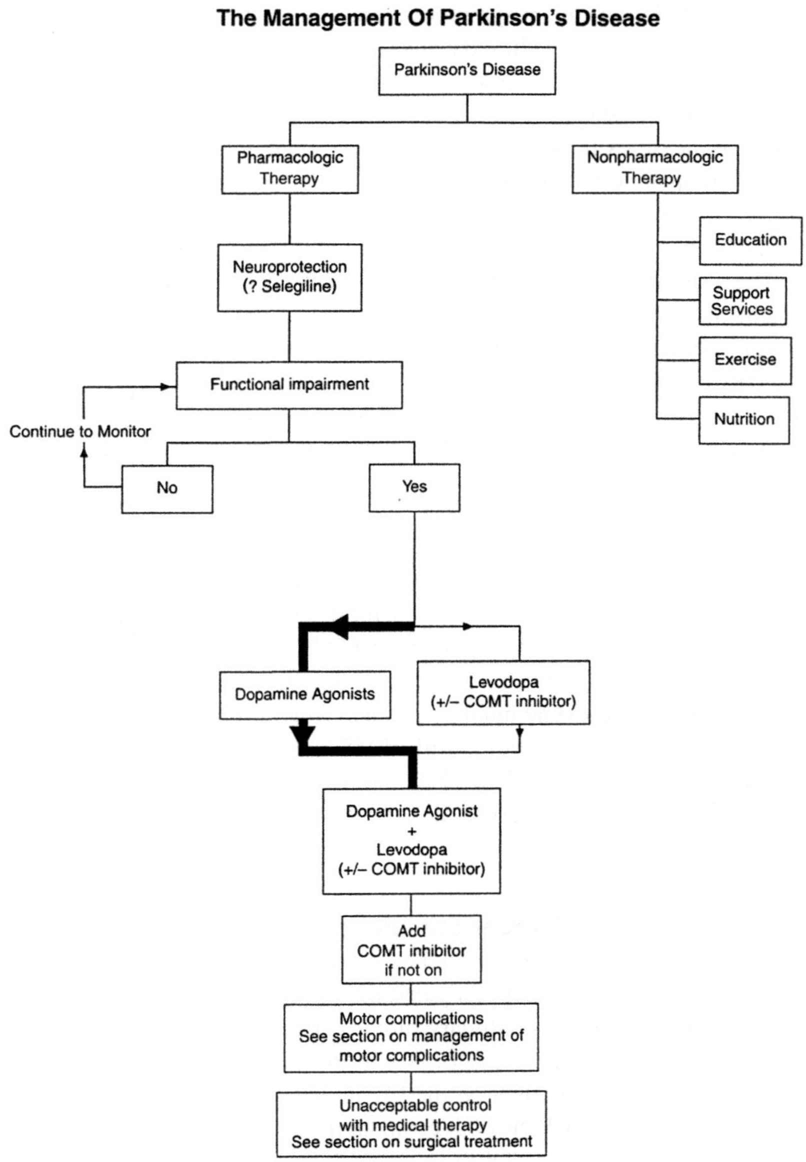

Fig. 16.1 Algorithm for the treatment of PD. From [6]; with permission

Although speech therapy for dysarthria and hypophonia in PD is known to be helpful to improve speech volume [20], the efficacy of speech therapy is not clear [21].

Neuromodulatory Approaches for the PD

Electroconvulsive Therapy (ECT)

Electroconvulsive therapy has been applied in psychiatric disorders and there is increasing evidence supporting the positive effects in patients with PD [22]. ECT has beneficial effects on cardinal motor symptoms of PD and the common psychiatric comorbidities such as depression [23]. Among several possible mechanisms of action, a neurochemical one is the most widely accepted explanation [22]. ECT can have significant effects on dopaminergic, noradrenergic, and serotonergic transmission [24]. Despite these possible positive effects of ECT in PD, the current neurological guidelines have not mentioned this as a useful treatment tool [6] and well-designed clinical studies have not been reported yet. Possible side effects of ECT are delirium, dyskinesia, worsening parkinsonian symptoms, transient agitation, and psychotic symptoms such as hallucinations and delusions [22].

Repetitive Transcranial Magnetic Stimulation (rTMS)

Repetitive transcranial magnetic stimulation (rTMS) has been known to modulate the dopamine release and normalize abnormal cortical excitability or network activity in PD [25]. Through this action, rTMS can have beneficial effects on motor and non-motor symptoms of PD [26, 27]. For the effect of rTMS on motor symptoms, Elahi et al. recently systematically reviewed the controlled clinical trials [26]. From this systematic review with meta-analysis which included ten prospective controlled clinical studies with outcome measures for motor function, they found a benefit of high-frequency rTMS on motor signs in PD with effect size of −0.58 in Unified Parkinson's Disease Rating Scale (UPDRS) but little effect of low-frequency rTMS [26].

The Movement Disorder Society recently reviewed treatments for the non-motor symptoms of PD and included rTMS as one treatment modality [27]. For depression, there is a lack of well-designed studies and the society concluded that there is insufficient evidence for rTMS to be rated for the treatment of depression in PD [27]. With regards to the other non-motor symptoms such as psychosis and sleep disorder, there was also insufficient evidence for the effect of rTMS.

rTMS has been found to be generally safe with minimal adverse events in PD. The problem of most concern is the occurrence of seizure during and after rTMS. Under the guidelines for the safety of rTMS [28–30], the literature contains reports on several hundred patients with movement disorders who have been studied with rTMS, with no reports of accidental seizures [25]. No study has revealed aggravating of functional scores in patients with movement disorder after rTMS [25].

Transcranial Direct Current Stimulation (tDCS)

There have been few clinical studies about the effect of tDCS on PD. Fregni et al. investigated the motor effects of single session tDCS to the primary motor cortex (M1) and dorsolateral prefrontal cortex (DLPFC) in PD patients with OFF state [31]. Anodal tDCS on the M1 improved a motor function measured by UPDRS but cathodal tDCS on the M1 and anodal tDCS on the DLPFC showed no significant improvement. Boggio et al. studied the effects of tDCS on working memory in patients with PD and there was a significant improvement in working memory measured by task accuracy after anodal tDCS on the left DLPFC [31]. Benninger et al. conducted a randomized, double-blinded, sham-controlled trial of eight sessions of anodal tDCS applied to the motor and prefrontal cortices over 2.5 weeks in 25 patients with PD [32]. tDCS improved gait in some measures for a short time and improved bradykinesia in both the on and off states for longer than 3 months, but changes in UPDRS, reaction time, physical and mental well-being, and self-assessed mobility did not differ between the tDCS and sham interventions [32]. Shill et al. reported the negative results of tDCS measured by UPDRS and several depression scales in patients with early PD [33]. Therefore, role of tDCS on PD is not conclusive to date, although it seems to induce some beneficial effects. Further studies are needed to investigate the differing effects of intensity, duration, mode, stimulation site of tDCS, and to determine the duration of effects, and to assess effects under different clinical situations: on versus off medication, motor versus non-motor symptom.

Deep Brain Stimulation (DBS)

Deep brain stimulation (DBS) was introduced by Benabid and colleagues in the year of 1987. Many patients with PD have undergone implantation of DBS electrodes to control their motor or non-motor symptoms to date [34]. DBS is the most investigated therapy among various kinds of neuromodulation and was approved by the Food and Drug Administration (FDA) in 2002 "as an adjunctive therapy in reducing some of the symptoms of advanced, levodopa-responsive PD that are not adequately controlled by medication" [35]. DBS is a surgical procedure in which one or more electrodes are implanted in specific sites of the brain and electrodes are connected to an impulse generator that delivers electrical stimuli to brain tissue to modulate or disrupt the patterns of neural signaling within a targeted region (Fig. 16.2) [35]. The most common targets of DBS in PD are subthalamic nucleus and the internal segment of the globus pallidus.

DBS usually inhibits the cells and excites fibers around the implanted electrodes to influence multiple pathways (e.g., thalamocortical circuits, downstream pathways) and other brain structures [35]. DBS can modulate the neuronal excitability in the basal ganglia, and induce the neurotransmitter release such as adenosine and glutamate [36], and increase blood flow and neurogenesis [37]. Through the action of these mechanisms, DBS can influence a broad neural network beyond the local stimulation site of the brain and is thought to control the symptoms in PD.

There have been four randomized, controlled clinical trials of DBS. Deuschl et al. reported the improvement in quality of life measured by Parkinson's Disease Questionnaire (PDQ-39) and motor symptoms assessed by UPDRS-III at 6 months after bilateral DBS of the subthalamic nucleus [38]. In a trial by Williams et al., a DBS group showed better PDQ-39 score than the medical therapy group at 1-year follow-up [39]. Weaver et al. found that the group with DBS of the subthalamic nucleus or globus pallidus gained more "on" time period compared to the medical therapy group at 6 months of follow-up [40] and Okun et al. reported similar results [41].

Patients for DBS are selected based on the patient's symptoms and the likelihood of a response to therapy. Tremor, on–off fluctuations, dyskinesia and levodopa-responsive symptoms are expected to improve after DBS, whereas gait, balance and speech problems are less likely to improve [35]. After all possible medication therapies have

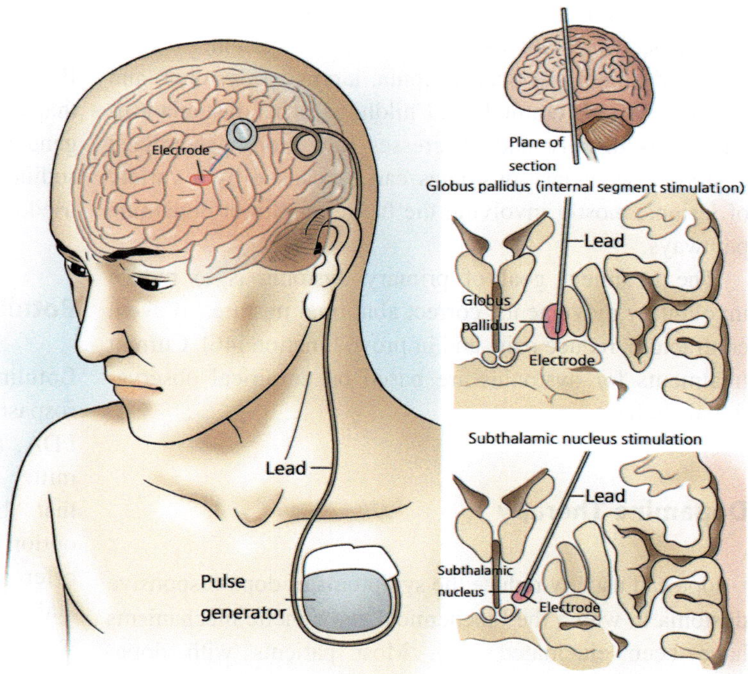

Fig. 16.2 Electrode implantation for deep brain stimulation. From [35]; with permission

been failed, DBS should be considered an adjuvant therapy. Characteristics of potential candidates for DBS in PD are summarized in Table 16.2 [35].

The two adverse events of most concerned after implanting the leads for DBS are infection and intracranial hemorrhage. The rates of infection requiring further surgery range from 1.2 to 15.2 % [35]. One large case series reported that the total incidence of hemorrhage of image-guided DBS was 0.9 % [42]. Estimated occurrence of post DBS seizures was 2.4 % from one review article [43]. Hardware-related problems such as lead fractures are possible complications after DBS [44]. A wide range of neurologic (e.g., cognitive impairment, memory difficulties, speech problems, disequilibrium, dysphagia, motor and sensory disturbances) and neuropsychological adverse effects (e.g., mania, depression, apathy, laughter, crying, panic, fear, anxiety, suicidal ideation) can occur after DBS and these adverse effects are related to device implantation or electrical stimulation [35]. Electrode relocation, adjustment of device programming or discontinuation of therapy may be required according to the cause of adverse effects.

Table 16.2 Characteristics of potential candidates for deep brain stimulation in Parkinson's disease

Good candidates
• Adequate response to dopaminergic therapy
• Presence of on–off fluctuations
• Dyskinesia impaing quality of life
• Medication-resistant tremor
• Reasonable cognitive function
Borderline candidates[a]
• Severe dyskinesias with a poor on–off dopaminergic response
• On–off fluctuations with moderate cognitive function
• On–off fluctuations with a poor on–off dopaminergic response
• Medication-resistant tremor with moderate cognitive dysfunction
• Medication-resistant tremor with poor on–off dopaminergic response
Poor candidates
• Severe dementia
• Severe autonomic dysfunction
• Poor dopaminergic response
• Atypical parkinsonism (e.g., corticobasal ganglionic degeneration, progressive supranuclear palsy, multiple system atrophy, and dementia with Lewy bodies)
• Unstable psychiatric disease
• Absence of a dedicated caregiver

[a]For borderline candidates, the risks and benefits of DBS must be carefully weighed by a multidisciplinary team
Adapted from [35]; with permission

Dystonia

Dystonia is characterized by abnormalities in the control of movement with involuntary muscle contractions causing twisting movements or abnormal postures, and is the third most common movement disorder [45]. Dystonia can be classified as primary (childhood-onset, adult onset and mixed phenotype) and secondary dystonias. The most common dystonic disorders are the adult-onset idiopathic dystonias, which are usually focal or segmental, such as cranial dystonia, cervical dystonia, laryngeal dystonia, and dystonic writer's cramp [46]. Childhood-onset dystonia usually starts distally and progresses into more generalized dystonia. Secondary dystonias can be caused by a variety of lesions, mostly involving the basal ganglia or dopamine pathways.

The treatment goal of primary dystonia is to reduce involuntary movements, correct abnormal postures, prevent contracture, reduce pain, and improve function [46]. Current treatments for dystonias are based on empirical observational studies.

Dopamine Therapy

L-dopa can usually reduce the symptoms of dopa-responsive dystonia in which the biochemical and genetic mechanisms have been elucidated [47]. Most patients with dopa-responsive dystonia improve dramatically, even with small doses of L-dopa (100 mg of L-dopa with 25 mg of decarboxylase inhibitor), but some may require doses of L-dopa as high as 1,000 mg/day [47]. L-dopa can be discontinued if there is no clinical improvement after 3 months of L-dopa therapy.

Antidopaminergic Therapy

Antidopaminergic drugs might have potential benefits for the dystonia but limited use due to the possibility of side effects [46]. However, tetrabenazine, dopamine-depleting drugs, have been found useful in some patients with dystonia, particularly in those with tardive dystonia [47].

Anticholinergic Therapy

Anticholinergics such as trihexyphenidyl are most useful in the treatment of generalized and segmental dystonia [48]. Common adverse events of anticholinergics are dry mouth, urinary retention, drowsiness or confusion and these side effects should be monitored during the therapy.

Anticonvulsants

Anticonvulsants such as carbamazepine and phenytoin can control the attacks of kinesigenic paroxysmal dystonia [46].

Other Pharmacologic Agents

Benzodiazepines, tizanidine, cyclobenzaprine and baclofen that act as muscle relaxants can be used in patients with generalized dystonia [46]. Slow release morphine sulfate, sodium oxybate, levitiracetam, and zonisamide can also be used in the treatment of dystonia.

Botulinum Toxin

Botulinum toxin was approved for the treatment of blepharospasm, hemifacial spasm, and cervical dystonia by the FDA. The Therapeutics and Technology Assessment Committee of the American Academy of Neurology concluded that "botulinum toxin should be offered as a treatment option for cervical dystonia (level A evidence); can be offered for blepharospasm, focal upper extremity dystonia, adductor laryngeal dystonia, and upper extremity essential tremor (level B); and can be considered for hemifacial spasm, focal lower limb dystonia and motor tics (level C)" [46, 49].

Surgical Procedures Except DBS

In selected cases of dystonia, peripheral surgical denervation (e.g., posterior ramisectomy, anterior cervical rhizotomy, microvascular decompression of the spinal accessory nerve), myectomy and stereotatic surgery (e.g., thlamotomy, pallidotomy) can be tried [50].

Neuromodulatory Approaches for Dystonia

Noninvasive neuromodulations such as rTMS and tDCS are still in experimental stages but several studies have reported possible beneficial effects of these neuromodulatory approaches. Further studies are required to clarify the optimal stimulation targets and protocols of noninvasive neuromodulation based on pathophysiology of dystonia, which can result in significant and lasting improvement of symptoms in dystonia.

Repetitive Transcranial Magnetic Stimulation (rTMS)

There have been several studies which investigated the effect of rTMS on dystonia. Murase et al. investigated the effect of low-frequency sub-threshold-intensity rTMS over the primary motor cortex, premotor cortex and supplementary motor area on writer's cramp [51]. There was an improvement of handwriting only after premotor cortex stimulation. Borich et al. also reported that low-frequency rTMS on premotor cortex could improve the handwriting in patients with focal hand dystonia [52]. Siebner et al. demonstrated that low-frequency rTMS over the motor cortex in patients with writer's cramp can reinforce deficient intracortical inhibition and may improve handwriting temporarily [53]. In one case study, low-frequency rTMS on the left premotor cortex improved the neck dystonia but improvement of limb dystonia was not observed [54].

There have been efforts to demonstrate the effects of sensory modulation by rTMS on dystonia. Low-frequency rTMS over the primary somatosensory cortex can improve the writer's cramp while increasing the cortical activity in both hemispheres [55]. Low-frequency rTMS over the anterior cingulated cortex in patients with benign essential blepharospasm was also found to improve the blink frequency, time of eye closure and the number of sustained blinks [55].

Transcranial Direct Current Stimulation (tDCS)

Previous studies of tDCS in dystonia were only focused to focal hand dystonia. In one randomized, double-blind, sham-controlled study, the effect of cathodal stimulation to the contralateral motor cortex was investigated [56]. Cathodal tDCS failed to show favorable effects and to restore normal handwriting kinematics and cortical inhibition. In a case-series study, cathodal tDCS on the primary motor cortex had no beneficial effect on fine motor control in professional guitarists with musician's dystonia [57]. In a placebo-controlled, double-blinded study with nine professional pianists with focal hand dystonia, there were no beneficial effects of single session tDCS-supported sensorimotor retraining on fine motor control in all three tDCS protocols (anodal, cathodal, and sham stimulation) [58].

Deep Brain Stimulation (DBS)

In a randomized, double-blind, sham-controlled trial, the effect of bilateral pallidal DBS in primary segmental or generalized dystonia was investigated. After 3 months of DBS there was significant improvement of symptoms in dystonia measured by the Burke-Fahn-Marsden Dystonia Rating Scale (BMFMDRS) [59]. Another randomized controlled trial also reported similar effects of bilateral pallidal DBS [60].

For the focal dystonia, effect of pallidal DBS on cervical dystonia or cranio-cervical dystonia has been reported. One prospective, single-blind, multicenter study reported that bilateral pallidal DBS improved the Toronto Western Spasmodic Torticollis Rating Scale (TWSTRS) after 12 months of stimulation in patients with cervical dystonia [61]. In a multicenter case series study in patients with Meige syndrome, pallidal DBS showed improvement of symptoms measured by BMFMDRS at mean follow-up of 4.4 and 38.8 months after stimulation [62]. In another case series studied on Meige syndrome, pallidal DBS showed similar favorable outcomes to control the symptoms [63, 64].

There have been few studies regarding the effect of DBS on sites other than the pallidum. Among the several studies about the DBS on the subthalamic nucleus [65–67], Ostrem et al. reported improvement of TWSTRS total score at 12 months after bilateral subthalamic nucleus DBS without marked side effects in patients with primary cervical dystonia [65]. In one case series in patients with medically intractable primary generalized dystonia, two out of a series of three patients showed mild to moderate improvement in limb dystonia after DBS on posterior part of the ventrolateral thalamic nucleus [68].

The adverse event rate after DBS in patients with dystonia is similar with those in PD. The potential long-term adverse effects of DBS in dystonia are unknown [50]. Several factors have been suggested as predictors for favorable outcomes in dystonia: young age, short disease duration, and mutation in DYT1 gene [50].

Essential Tremor

Essential tremor (ET) is the most common neurologic disorder. It induces postural or action tremor. ET is a heterogeneous disorder that varies in character, aggravating factors and association with other neurological impairments [69]. The most commonly involved body parts of ET are hands and arms. But head, voice, trunk, and legs can also be involved. ET can be aggravated by anxiety or other adrenergic mechanisms, and can be reduced by intake of alcohol. Diagnostic core and secondary criteria for ET suggested by Bain et al. are the following [70]:

1. Core criteria: bilateral action tremor of the hands and forearms (but not rest tremor), absence of other neurologic signs, with the exception of cogwheel phenomenon, may have isolated head tremor with no signs of dystonia.
2. Secondary criteria: long duration (>3 years), positive family history, beneficial response to alcohol.

Conventional treatment for ET includes the pharmacological therapy (beta blockers, anticonvulsants, benzodiazepines) and botulinum toxin injection.

Neuromodulatory approaches for ET are promising but still investigatory. Finding an effective noninvasive brain stimulation treatment for ET is challenging as the optimal stimulation parameters are not known yet and there are numerous permutations of stimulus parameters that can be tested [71].

Beta Blockers

Among beta blockers, propranolol is the most investigated agent to date. AAN guidelines concluded that 60–320 mg/day of propranolol is effective for the treatment of limb tremor and probably reduces head tremor [72]. Adverse events of propranolol are fatigue, bradycardia, impotence and lightheadedness, and propranolol is contraindicated in the presence of heart block and asthma.

Anticonvulsants

AAN guidelines suggested that primidone is effective for the treatment of limb tremor in ET. The starting dose of primidone is 25 mg before sleep and dose can be increased carefully over several weeks while observing the tolerance and therapeutic response [72]. Adverse events associated with primidone are drowsiness, vomiting, dizziness, fatigue, and acute toxic reactions.

One randomized controlled trial showed that 1,200 mg/day of gabapentin can reduce the symptoms in ET [73]. Topiramate was also known to be effective in limb tremor associated with ET, but have high rate of side effects such as nausea, paresthesia, and concentration difficulty [72].

Benzodiazepines

Because of concern with abuse and withdrawal symptoms, benzodiazepines are considered a second-line choice for treatment of chronic ET. AAN guidelines suggest that alprazolam is probably effective and clonazepam is possibly effective for limb tremor [72].

Botulinum Toxin

AAN guidelines concluded that botulinum toxin type A injection has a modest effect for the treatment of limb tremor in ET and shows dose-dependent hand weakness [72]. Although the evidence is limited, botulinum toxin type A injection can be effective for the treatment of head and voice tremor in ET with accompanying possible side effects such as breathiness, hoarseness, and swallowing difficulty [72].

Neuromodulatory Approaches for ET

Electroconvulsive Therapy

To date, only one case study reported the transient improvement of ET during ECT [74]. There is still lack of evidence and further study is needed to assess the effect of ECT in ET.

Repetitive Transcranial Magnetic Stimulation (rTMS)

There are several trials using rTMS to treat the ET but the research is still limited. Hellriegel et al. demonstrated that continuous theta burst stimulation (cTBS) reduced tremor amplitude subclinically when assessed with accelerometry, although there were no significant changes in clinical rating after stimulation [75]. A recent open label trial showed that bilateral low-frequency rTMS on the posterior cerebellar cortex can improve clinical scores on tremor, drawing, functional, disability, and reduce tremor amplitude [76]. In a double-blind, crossover, placebo-controlled study, low frequency rTMS over the cerebellum improved the Tremor Clinical Rating Scale and accelerometric values [77].

Deep Brain Stimulation (DBS)

In DBS for the treatment of ET, the usual target brain site is thalamic ventral intermediate nucleus [78]. However, research targeting thalamic is limited.

Two prospective studies reported the possible beneficial effect of thalamic DBS on limb tremor [79]. Although it was reported that bilateral thalamic DBS is more effective than unilateral DBS to control the appendicular tremors in ET, bilateral DBS had a higher occurrence of adverse events [80]. To date, it seems that DBS on thalamic ventral intermediate nucleus to control the limb tremor in ET has limited evidence [72].

DBS has been also tried to control the voice and head tremor associated with ET. In two case-series studies, beneficial effects of thalamic DBS on voice or head tremor were observed [81, 82]. In a multicenter prospective study, thalamic DBS reduced head tremor but had no effect on voice tremor [83]. Ondo et al. reported that unilateral thalamic DBS was not beneficial for the head tremor associated with ET [84]. Although compared to the other surgical therapy such as thalamotomy, DBS seems to have less adverse events [72], there are still limited studies for the effect of DBS on ET and further studies are required.

Tics or Tourette's Syndrome

A tic is a brief, rapid, repetitive, and seemingly purposeless stereotyped action that may involve a single muscle or multiple muscle groups [85]. Motor tics can affect any part of the body but they typically begin in the eyelids or face and, over time, involve other muscle groups, spreading to the neck, shoulders, trunk, legs, and feet with an apparent rostro-caudal migration [85]. Tics are voluntarily suppressible for variable periods, but this usually occurs at the expense of mounting inner tension and an irresistible need to perform the tic, followed by a rebound burst of tics [46]. Tics can be transient but many patients with childhood onset evolve to Tourette's syndrome, a genetic disorder with additional behavior disorders such as obsessive-compulsive disorder, attention deficit hyperactivity disorder, anxiety disorder or other behavioral disturbances.

Although pharmacological approach is considered a first-line therapy, some neuromodulatory approaches have shown positive effects on controlling the tic.

Dopamine Antagonists

Dopamine receptor blockers such as fluphenazine, pimozide, and tetrabenazine have been used to control the tics and appear to be effective [86, 87].

Dopamine Agonists

Ropinirole, a selective nonergoline dopamine agonist, has a beneficial effect in reducing the symptoms of Tourette's syndrome [88].

Other Drugs

Topiramate was found safe and effective for the treatment of moderately severe Tourette's syndrome [89]. Other drugs known to be effective in the treatment of tics include clonazepam, flutamide, ondansetron, baclofen, donepezil, and nicotine [46].

Botulinum Toxin Injection

In a randomized, double-blind, controlled clinical trial, botulinum toxin injection reduced tic frequency and the urge [90]. AAN also concluded that botulinum toxin injection as a treatment for tics have a level C evidence [49].

Neuromodulatory Approaches for Tics and Tourette's Syndrome

Electroconvulsive Therapy (ECT)

In a few case reports, there was significant improvement of tic symptoms following ECT. However, to date, there is no study to provide high-level evidence [91].

Repetitive Transcranial Magnetic Stimulation (rTMS)

There is limited evidence for the effect of rTMS on tics. Kwon et al. reported that low-frequency rTMS over the supplementary motor area in children with Tourette's syndrome reduced the tic symptoms without side effects [92]. However, in a single-blinded, placebo-controlled trial, there was no significant improvement of tic symptoms after low frequency rTMS on motor or premotor cortex [93]. Orth et al. found no significant effect of low-frequency rTMS over premotor cortex with subthreshold intensity in patients with Gilles de la Tourette syndrome [94]. Further studies to find out the effective protocols of rTMS to control tics are still required.

Deep Brain Stimulation (DBS)

DBS improved tics in a single case study and in small series, although long-term benefit is unclear [95]. Potential targets of stimulation include midline thalamic centromedian-parafascicular nuclei, the ventralis oralis complex of the thalamus, motor, and limbic globus pallidus pars interna, and the anterior limb of the internal capsule [95]. Okun et al. also demonstrated that scheduled DBS on the bilateral centromedian thalamic region in patients with Tourette's syndrome could improve motor and vocal tics in their preliminary small-size clinical trial [96]. Porta et al. reported their long-term follow-up results after bilateral thalamic DBS in patients with severe and refractory Tourette's syndrome [97], showing a significant reduction in tic severity at 5–6 years follow-up.

Chorea

Chorea is a rapid, involuntary, non-repetitive or arrhythmic movement involving the face, trunk, and limbs that flows randomly from one part of the body to another [46]. Huntington's disease (HD) is an autosomal-dominant neurodegenerative disorder characterized clinically by abnormal movements, cognitive decline, behavioral disturbances, and progressive functional deterioration with typical motor symptom of chorea [98].

Although pharmacologic therapy can be applied first to control the chorea, the beginning of pharmacologic therapy should be determined prudently to avoid worsening of other symptoms of HD by pharmacologic therapy, if chorea is not severe to interfere with function. Because chorea can be influenced by mood or posture, providing a calm, predictable environment or assistive devices should precede the pharmacologic treatment.

For pharmacologic treatment, tetrabenazine, a dopamine receptor antagonist, was effective to control chorea in patients with HD in recent systematic review [99]. Neuroleptics are also able to control the chorea by the action of blocking dopamine transmission [98]. Anti-glutamatergic agents such as riluzole, amantadine, remacemide, and lamotrigine have demonstrated anti-choreic effects [98].

Neuromodulatory Approaches for Chorea

Neuromodulatory approaches including ECT, rTMS, and DBS have limited evidence to treat chorea to the date.

Electroconvulsive Therapy

There is very limited evidence of ECT in chorea, because only one case study reported a possible effect of ECT controlling chorea [100].

Repetitive Transcranial Magnetic Stimulation (rTMS)

The data of rTMS in chorea treatment is also very limited despite its potential benefit considering involvement of neuronal circuit including basal ganglia [101]. In a single case study, continuous theta burst stimulation over the left-hand motor area improved the symptoms of hemichorea [102]. In one case series study including four patients with HD, low-frequency rTMS over the supplementary motor area reduced the symptoms of chorea [103].

Deep Brain Stimulation (DBS)

In a recent review, there were only single case studies for the effect of DBS in patients with chorea [104–107]. Although Edward et al. suggested that DBS may be a useful treatment option in well-selected patients with choreiform disorders [104], there is limited evidence to date and a well-designed controlled study should be conducted in the future.

Neurodegenerative Disorders

Alzheimer's Disease

Dementia is a syndrome of gradual and progressive cognitive decline due to a variety of underlying pathologies. Alzheimer's disease (AD) is the most common cause of dementia, although it is now recognized that up to half of all cases of AD demonstrate mixed pathologies on autopsy, such as vascular components [108]. Alzheimer's disease affects an estimated 15 million people worldwide and is the leading cause of dementia in elderly people. With the proportion of elderly in the population increasing steadily, the burden of the disease, both to caregivers and national economies, is expected to become substantially greater over the next 2–3 decades [109, 110]. Alzheimer's disease is a progressive neurodegenerative disorder with a mean duration of around 8.5 years between onset of clinical symptoms and death. Brain regions that are associated with higher mental functions, particularly the neocortex and hippocampus, are those most affected by the characteristic pathology of Alzheimer's disease. This includes the extracellular deposits of beta-amyloid (derived from amyloid precursor protein; APP) in senile plaques, intracellular formation of neurofibrillary tangles (containing an abnormally phosphorylated form of a microtubule associated protein, tau), and the loss of neuronal synapses and pyramidal neurons. These changes result in the development of the typical symptomatology of Alzheimer's disease characterized by gross and progressive impairments of cognitive function and often accompanied by behavioral disturbances such as aggression, depression, and wandering. Carers find these features the most difficult to cope with and they often lead to the need for institutionalization of the patient [110].

The clinical presentation and progression of dementia symptoms varies considerably among people with the same underlying level of pathology. Although two people may have the same amount of dementia-related brain damage, one may experience debilitating effects while the other demonstrates few symptoms. The observation of this phenomenon led to the conceptualization of cognitive reserve: the hypothetical ability of the brain, at varying individual capacities, to withstand a certain level of injury before the clinical manifestation of dementia [111]. The level of cognitive reserve capacity depends on both innate protective effects and the ability of the brain to actively compensate for injury [112]. It is believed that some compensatory mechanisms are able to counteract symptoms until this ability is overwhelmed [113]. In this model, once an individual reaches his or her maximal premorbid cognitive ability, different factors are at play, which either support maintenance of cognition or impair cognitive ability. The plasticity of the brain is thought to be a factor that contributes significantly to the ability to build cognitive reserve [112]. Reserve includes both passive and active processes that modify risk for the clinical expression of disease. Passive reserve is accounted for by brain size and synapse density [111]. Individuals with larger brains and greater synapse density can tolerate more extensive pathology before they reach the threshold at which symptoms become clinically evident. Active reserve refers to the efficiency with which an individual can use alternate networks or cognitive strategies to cope with the brain pathology. Cognitive reserve is related to the brain's metabolic activity and can be modified by mental activity. Brain reserve and cognitive reserve are not mutually exclusive. Mental activity is a strong signal for the generation of neurons and synapses. Individuals are thought to possess innate cognitive reserve that allows dementia-related pathology to accumulate before symptoms appear, but also have the ability to actively build reserve as a compensatory mechanism for brain damage. Although individuals with higher cognitive reserve take longer to exhibit dementia symptoms, ongoing damage will eventually exhaust the brain's protective and compensatory abilities, leading to dementia manifestation and progression [114].

Pharmacologic Treatment

While no drug has been shown to completely protect neurons, agents that inhibit the degradation of acetylcholine within the synapses are the mainstay of treatment for Alzheimer's disease. Cholinesterase/acetylcholinesterase inhibitors are the only agents approved by the United States Food and Drug Administration for the treatment of Alzheimer's disease. Other drugs have been studied, but their use remains controversial.

A number of organizations have proposed guidelines for the treatment of dementia [115], and many insurers and managed-care organizations have developed criteria for the use of acetylcholinesterase inhibitors. All of the guidelines stress the importance of adherence to therapy, and many recommend the use of instruments to monitor response to treatment. Because of cost, most organizations recommend discontinuing therapy when dementia is severe.

Acetylcholinesterase Inhibitors

The cholinesterase inhibitor tacrine (Cognex) is used rarely because of potential liver toxicity and the need for frequent laboratory monitoring. The acetylcholinesterase inhibitors donepezil (Aricept), rivastigmine (Exelon), and galantamine (Reminyl) have proved effective in clinical trials.

All three drugs have a low risk of serious reactions, but they commonly have cholinergic side effects such as nausea, anorexia, vomiting, and diarrhea. Tolerance to these side effects often develops. However, if therapy with an acetylcholinesterase inhibitor is interrupted for more than several days, the drug should be restarted at the lowest dosage and retitrated, because of renewed susceptibility to side effects. Instruments that measure cognition, behavior, and functional ability have shown that acetylcholinesterase inhibitors are beneficial in patients with Alzheimer's disease.

Although clinical trials have shown that treatment with acetylcholinesterase inhibitors delays nursing home placement and improves cognition and functional ability, these benefits may not apply to all patients with Alzheimer's disease. Nonetheless, it is safe to conclude that patients who tolerate and respond to acetylcholinesterase inhibitors will experience modest cognitive improvements. In fact, deterioration of cognition will be delayed by 1 year in about 20 % of treated patients [116].

Neuromodulatory Approaches for the AD

Electroconvulsive Therapy (ECT)

ECT is a well-established and effective treatment for depression in the elderly; it is currently an overlooked treatment option in the elderly with dementia and depression [117, 118]. In healthy non-geriatric patients, ECT occasionally results in reversible cognitive side effects such as reduced concentration, sustained disorientation, and retrograde memory loss but the effects in dementia are currently greatly unknown [118]. Most of what has been prospectively studied and published on the performance of ECT in dementia applies to patients with either mild dementia (MMSE > 21 points) or moderately mild dementia (MMSE, 15–20). This is of great relevance to all published results because Nelson and Rosenberg [119] concluded that post-ECT confusion scores correlated with the degree of dementia ($P < 0.01$), and Hausner et al. [118] found that the extent of pre-ECT cognitive deficits was the best predictor of MMSE score decline from baseline to follow-up 6 weeks after the last ECT treatment ($P = 0.007$). This suggests that moderate to severe dementia might result in more adverse effects after ECT than in individuals without dementia. From a clinical perspective, cognitive testing and monitoring are recommended before, during, and after ECT in patients with dementia with depression. It is essential to inform both the family and the patients about possible risks and benefits of the treatment.

Repetitive Transcranial Magnetic Stimulation (rTMS)

A recent meta-analysis of publications searching for the effects of rTMS on cognitive functions found convincing data supporting improvement in several cognitive functions, including executive functions, learning, and memory [120]. It has been demonstrated in elderly subjects that rTMS induces a transient improvement in the associative memory task and that it is associated with recruitment of right prefrontal and bilateral posterior cortical regions [121].

Three studies have been carried out to assess the effects of rTMS on naming and language performance in patients with probable AD.

In two crossover, sham-controlled, single-session studies rTMS was applied to the dorsolateral prefrontal cortex (DLPFC) during the execution of naming tasks. In the first study, a significantly improved accuracy in action naming, but not in object naming, was found following high-frequency rTMS of either left or right DLPFC in each of the 15 examined patients [122]. In the second study, the effect of rTMS applied to the DLPFC on picture naming was assessed in 24 AD patients with different degrees of cognitive decline. The results of the previous study were replicated only in mild AD patients (MMSE $\geq$ 17/30); in contrast, in patients with moderate to severe AD (MMSE $<$ 17/30), both action and object naming were facilitated after both left and right rTMS to DLPFC. The lack of effects of rTMS on object naming in early-stage AD might be related to a "ceiling" effect. The rTMS effect was bilateral both in mild and severe AD patients. The bilateral facilitation effect could be attributed to the presence of compensatory mechanisms based on the recruitment of right hemispheric resources to support the residual naming performance [123].

In a recent study, Cotelli et al. aimed to investigate whether the application of high-frequency rTMS to the left DLPFC leads to significant facilitation of language production or comprehension in patients with moderate AD [124]. Ten patients were randomly assigned to one of two groups. The first group underwent a 4-week real rTMS stimulation protocol, while the second underwent a 2-week placebo treatment, followed by 2 weeks of real rTMS stimulation. No significant effects were observed on naming performance. However, a significant effect was observed on auditory sentence comprehension after 2 weeks of real rTMS sessions, as compared to sham. Two additional weeks of daily rTMS sessions resulted in no further improvements, but a significant benefit on auditory sentence comprehension was still detected 8 weeks after the end of the rTMS intervention. An important finding was the absence of any effects on memory and executive functions. Therefore, these results were thought to be specific to the language network, and not due to a general, nonspecific effect on cognitive processing. None of these three studies reports any side effects of the rTMS applications.

In another study, Ahmed et al. [125] aimed to compare the long-term efficacy of high- versus low-frequency rTMS, applied bilaterally over the DLPFC, on cortical excitability and cognitive function of AD patients. The high-frequency rTMS group improved significantly more than the low frequency and sham groups in all assessed rating scales (MMSE, Instrumental Daily Living Activity Scale and the Geriatric Depression Scale) after treatment. The improvement was maintained for 3 months. The authors thus concluded that high-frequency rTMS may be a useful addition to therapy for the treatment of patients with mild to moderate degree of AD.

Since cognitive training may improve cognitive functions in AD, in a recent study Bentwich et al. [126] aimed to obtain a synergistic effect of rTMS interlaced with cognitive training in patients with AD. Eight patients with mild to moderate probable AD were subjected to daily rTMS-cognitive training sessions (5/week) for 6 weeks, followed by maintenance sessions (2/week) for additional 6 months. The following six regions, located individually by MRI, were stimulated: Broca and Wernicke (language functions), right and left DLPFC (judgment, executive functions, and long-term memory), and right and left parietal somatosensory association cortex (spatial and topographical orientation and praxias). Cognitive trainings were developed to fit these regions. Alzheimer Disease Assessment Scale-Cognitive (ADAS-cog) improved by approximately 4 points after both 6 weeks and 4.5 months of treatment, and Clinical Global Impression of Change (CGIC) by 1.0 points and 1.6 points, respectively. MMSE, the ADAS-Activities of Daily Living (ADAS-ADL) and Hamilton Depression Scale (HAMILTON) improved, but without statistical significance, while Neuropsychiatric Inventory (NPI) did not change. These findings provide direct evidence that rTMS is helpful in restoring brain functions and could reflect rTMS potential to recruit compensatory networks that underlie the memory-encoding and the other cognitive functions [125].

Transcranial Direct Current Stimulation (tDCS)

According to in vitro studies, neuronal depolarization is frequently altered in AD, and AD patients sometimes reveal temporoparietal hypoactivity (as characterized by focal slow wave activity in magnetoencephalography). Therefore increasing cortical excitability is a useful tool in AD. Anodal tDCS could increase cortical excitability and promoting neuronal depolarization in AD patients.

Otherwise, motor cortex and global cortical hyperexcitability is found in AD, correlating with cognitive severity in a TMS study. As cathodal tDCS led to reduced cortical excitability caused by neuronal hyperpolarization, it might also be beneficial in AD by lowering its somewhat increased cortical excitability.

This non-synaptic mechanisms based on changes in the membrane potential underlying the after-effects of anodal and cathodal tDCS might be responsible for modulating cognitive function in AD [127, 128].

The effect of anodal tDCS over the left temporal cortex and dorsolateral prefrontal cortex (DLPFC) was investigated on recognition and working memory in 10 AD patients, revealing enhancement in a visual recognition memory task after anodal tDCS of the DLPFC and left temporal cortex. In another study, an improvement in a word-recognition memory in ten patients with probable AD was proven after anodal tDCS to the temporoparietal areas. In contrast, cathodal tDCS lead to decreased word-recognition memory [129]. The effect of anodal tDCS persisted up to 30 min after stimulation, indicating a long-lasting increase in brain excitability. Long-term enhancement of visual recognition memory for up to 4 weeks after therapy was found after anodal tDCS in 15 AD patients [130].

Deep Brain Stimulation (DBS)

Hamani et al. [131] reported memory improvement in a patient who underwent fornix/hypothalamus DBS for obesity. These findings led Laxton et al. [132] to develop a phase I trial of fornix/hypothalamus DBS in six patients with mild AD. The researchers used positron emission tomography to measure pre- and postoperative cerebral glucose utilization as an indicator of quantitative effects of DBS. Increased glucose metabolism was observed in the temporal and parietal cortical areas at 1 month in all patients and was sustained in most of the affected areas at 1-year follow-up. Cognitive assessments suggested improvement or slowing of anticipated decline at 6 and 12 months after DBS. No conclusions regarding the efficacy of DBS in AD can yet be drawn from this phase I study. However, given the unrelenting and destructive nature of AD, any advances in treatment options should be explored [133].

Neurodegenerative Disorder Associated With Human Immunodeficiency Virus (HIV) Infection

Clinically obvious signs and symptoms of at least mild neurologic disease are found in approximately 50 % of individuals with AIDS and about 30 % of asymptomatic HIV-positive individuals. The typical presentation of HIV dementia includes cognitive, behavioral, and motor dysfunction, and has been characterized as a subcortical dementia. The initial symptoms of HIV dementia can be subtle and overlooked, or misdiagnosed as depression. In the early stages, memory loss, mental slowing, reading and comprehension difficulties, and apathy are frequent complaints [134]. The typical cognitive deficits of HIV dementia are characterized primarily by memory loss that is selective for impaired retrieval; impaired ability to manipulate acquired knowledge; personality changes that are characterized by apathy, inertia, and irritability; and general slowing of all thought processes. However, considerable individual variability in presentation has been reported [135].

The cause of HIV associated neurologic problems has not been precisely determined. It has been hypothesized that neuronal cell death may be associated with later stage HIV, but there is also evidence of more subtle injury to neurons. Degradation of neurons, together with cell death, may represent different stages of neurodegeneration. For example, HIV in the central nervous system may directly or indirectly increase oxidative stress or reduce trophic factors resulting in neural injury such as dendritic simplification or loss of synapses in the neural networks [136].

HIV enters the brain early in the disease process and continued replication occurs within the macrophages. The invasion of HIV into the brain can cause neurodegeneration in multiple brain areas. There is a loss of neurons in the frontal cortex of HIV-infected individuals and the degree of neurodegeneration in this region is associated with severity of cognitive difficulties prior to death. HIV also shows an affinity for the basal ganglia, and high viral loads have been found in this region among individuals with HIV dementia. Moreover, one study noted an "extensive loss" of MAP2-immunoreactive neurons and dendrites in the basal ganglia of individuals with HIV encephalitis [137]. Finally, there is neuropathological evidence that hippocampal neurons are affected in HIV disease. In the presence of HIV, hippocampal neurons are particularly susceptible to protein-Tat induced apoptosis, are found to be sites of increased gliosis and chemokine expression, and have shorter terminals and decreased dendritic spine density [138].

Conventional Treatment in HIV

Zidovudine

Only one placebo-controlled clinical trial of antiretroviral therapy with zidovudine for HIV dementia in adults has been published. Despite the paucity of information from controlled clinical trials, in fact a substantial amount of evidence has accumulated to indicate that HIV dementia is treatable and its deficits and functional impact are reversible in a proportion of patients. Early studies with high dose (greater than 1,200 mg) zidovudine suggested that the incidence of HIV dementia was significantly lower in zidovudine recipients than in patients receiving no treatment and that the effect might be dose-related. The original licensing trial of zidovudine showed significant improvements in neuropsychological performance for individuals with advanced

HIV infection; however, this trial excluded those with severe dementia [139]. Recently, Chiesi et al. [140] showed a 40 % reduction in risk of HIV dementia after AIDS with zidovudine. These results have not been confirmed by large US observational analyses, possibly reflecting the influence of zidovudine dose on neuroprotection. It appears that neuroprotective effects of antiretroviral monotherapy, at currently used doses, are relatively limited.

Antiretroviral Agents

A widespread assumption up to now is that effective HIV dementia antiretroviral therapy must include agents with good CNS penetration. Suppression of systemic infection may reduce further CNS seeding, and thus even a "non-penetrating" protease inhibitor may have some effect. The non-nucleoside reverse transcriptase inhibitor, nevirapine (Viramune), apparently has good CSF penetration, and might be considered in antiretroviral protocols for HIV dementia. Sacktor et al. [141] reported on the antiretroviral agents which are either in development or already in clinical trial.

Immune-Based and Neuroprotective Therapies

Dewhurst et al. [142] discuss the role of a number of candidate neurotoxins which may be important in causation of HIV dementia, triggering neuronal damage through common pathways involving the induction of oxidative stress and excitotoxicity.

Neuromodulatory Approaches for the HIV

In several randomized controlled studies utilizing 2- or 4-week tDCS treatment protocols, tDCS delivered over the dorsolateral prefrontal cortex (DLPFC) was shown to safely relieve Major Depressive Disorder (MDD) in the general population [143]. Although the mechanisms of tDCS antidepressant effect are not fully understood, it is reasonable to assume that tDCS might have induced a change in the DLPFC activity, which is highly relevant to alterations of mood-related neuronal networks [144]. Knotkova H et al. found beneficial effect of tDCS for HIV associated MDD in pilot feasibility study [309].

Post-stroke Rehabilitation

Stroke is defined as a sudden, focal neurological deficit due to a cerebrovascular abnormality and this can be caused by an obstruction in the blood flow (cerebral infarction), or the rupture of an artery that feeds the brain (cerebral hemorrhage).

Ischemic stroke could be further classified as (1) large-artery atherosclerosis, (2) cardioembolism, (3) small-vessel occlusion, (4) stroke of other determined etiology, and (5) stroke of undetermined etiology depending on etiology in TOAST classification [145] or as (1) total anterior circulation infarction, (2) partial anterior circulation infarct, (3) lacunar infarction or (4) posterior circulation infarction depending on extent and affected area of the brain in The Oxford Community Stroke Project classification (also known as the Bamford or Oxford classification) [146].

Stroke is the leading cause of long-term disability in most of countries [147], and about 15–30 % of stroke victim is suffering from a permanent disability and requires assistance for walking or activities of daily living (ADL) [148].

Depending on the affected area of the brain, many symptoms are seen after stroke including motor weakness, sensory loss, coordination and balance problem, apraxia, neglect, aphasia, dysarthria, dysphasia, central pain, shoulder pain, depression, cognitive problems, and behavioral problems.

Although acute stroke management such as acute thrombolysis has been developed recently most post-stroke care relies on rehabilitative intervention to overcome disability and impairments [149, 150].

In the literature, neuromodulation techniques in stroke patients were usually tested in ischemic stroke patients although some studies also included hemorrhagic strokes. It is a general concept that ischemic and hemorrhagic stroke might have different mechanisms of recovery, and hemorrhagic stroke has better functional prognosis than ischemic stroke [151]. In terms of chronicity, neuromodulation technique has been used during acute, subacute and chronic stage. Although application of neuromodulation in the acute stage of stroke might result in an increased risk of seizure, theoretically it is more beneficial to apply neuromodulation earlier than later because this period is an active period of brain reorganization, and could have a greater benefit than at the chronic stage.

Early rehabilitative intervention is important to enhance recovery after neurologic deficits including motor impairment, aphasia, visuospatial neglect, dysphagia [152, 153], and neural reorganization, brain plasticity, plays a major role during this period [154, 155]. The changes of brain network activities after an injury or rehabilitative interventions can be visualized using neuroimaging techniques, such as positron emission tomography (PET) or functional magnetic resonance imaging (fMRI), and such findings give useful information on the clinical application of noninvasive brain stimulation for neurorehabilitation.

Noninvasive brain stimulation, in the form of repetitive transcranial magnetic stimulation (rTMS) or transcranial direct current stimulation (tDCS), provides the means to modulate brain activity in a specific brain region and to induce plasticity at the network level [156].

Modern concept of functional recovery after stroke is essentially a re-learning process with a partially disrupted neural network [157]. Theoretically we can specifically assist this re-learning process by inhibiting competing maladaptive regions or facilitating local activity to promote change during practice using after-effects of brain neuromodulation.

Recent bench to bedside research demonstrated that brain stimulation alone or in combination with routine rehabilitative training have shown promising results on stroke recovery. We can potentially facilitate motor, cognitive and language recovery after brain injury, and brain neuromodulation could be applied as an adjuvant therapy for rehabilitative training after stroke. However, the clinically beneficial effect of noninvasive brain stimulation is still modest according to previous proof-of-concept studies and optimal stimulation protocol of these modalities in terms of optimal target population, delivery timing, and stimulation parameters should further be pursued [158]. Up to now, only the rTMS device by NeuroStar TMS Therapy® (Neuronetics, a Malvern, Pennsylvania) has won US FDA's approval for treatment of depression in patients that do not respond to drug therapy in October 2008 [159]. Other applications for stroke are off label, and current proof-of-concept studies should be followed by large scale phase III clinical trials, with eventually proof of effectiveness in a meta-analysis study.

Motor Recovery

Despite recently acute stroke therapies such as tPA and mechanical thrombolysis that promote brain reperfusion within golden time have been developed, half of stroke patients still suffer from residual motor weakness [160].

To improve motor recovery in these patients, many exercises featuring task-oriented high-intensity repetitive training are being applied in clinics [149]. Constraint-induced Movement Therapy (CIMT), robotic interactive therapy, neuromuscular electrical stimulation, virtual reality training for upper limb and body weight-supported treadmill training are such examples. These methods make patients avoid "learned disuse" and to "forced use" of an impaired extremity [161]. Constraint-induced Movement Therapy (CIMT) [162] is a core example with the concept of avoiding disuse and forced use principle. In classical CIMT, patients' intact upper limbs are constrained for 90 % of waking hours using a sling or mitt, and trained in functionally oriented activities using hand-over-hand skilled guidance ("shaping exercise") with only the paretic arm for 6 or more hours per day over 2 weeks. The Extremity Constraint Induced Therapy Evaluation (EXCITE) Trial [163] was a multicenter single-blind randomized controlled trial comparing CIMT to customary care in chronic stage of stroke patients. At 1 year, the CIMT group performed better on a series of timed, functional tasks. This EXCITE trial was the first neuroplasticity therapy with multicenter evidence.

Some pharmacological interventions, usually catecholaminergic medications such as D-amphetamine and levodopa, are coupled with customary rehabilitative training to improve motor function but results are still mixed, still waiting further approval [164].

There are many small placebo controlled trials that investigated the clinical effects of rTMS or tDCS applied to the motor scalp area. These studies demonstrated a change of cortical excitability or improvement of motor performance after stimulation. The application of these noninvasive brain stimulations for motor recovery after stroke is mainly based on the concept of inter-hemispheric competition or rivalry [165–167].

In the inter-hemispheric rivalry theory, the activities of motor cortexes from bilateral hemispheres are balanced by transcallosal interhemispheric inhibitory projections for motor execution in normal condition. However, transcallosal interhemispheric inhibitory projections from the unaffected motor cortex to the affected motor cortex is elevated compared to inhibitory tone from affected to unaffected motor cortex after stroke, leading to over-inhibition of affected motor cortex and impeding motor execution of paretic hand and motor recovery [167, 168]. Therefore, inhibiting the motor cortical activities of the unaffected hemisphere could restore the excitability of affected hemisphere [167].

Another simple strategy to improve motor recovery after stroke is to simply reactivate the affected motor cortical excitability. Trans-cranial induction of either (1) facilitation of affected motor cortex M1 (using high frequency rTMS, intermittent theta burst stimulation, iTBS or anodal tDCS) or inhibition of M1 of the unaffected hemisphere (using low frequency rTMS, continuous theta burst stimulation, iTBS or cathodal tDCS) has been shown to improve motor function of the paretic side (Fig. 16.3).

Several detailed studies are available in the literature [169, 170]. In rTMS research, the inhibition of the unaffected M1 cortical excitability using 1 Hz inhibitory protocols [171–173] or facilitation of affected M1 cortical excitability using 3–20 Hz of excitatory protocols [174–176] have been shown to promote recovery of motor function of the paretic hand after stroke. Stimulation intensity was measured with resting motor threshold (rMT), and ranged between 80 and 130 %.

The use of 1 Hz rTMS has been proven effective for motor improvement using various measuring tools [174–176]. In the neuroimaging study, it was found that neural activity over the affected hemisphere was increased following inhibitory rTMS over unaffected hemisphere, justifying the strategy to use inhibitory rTMS over

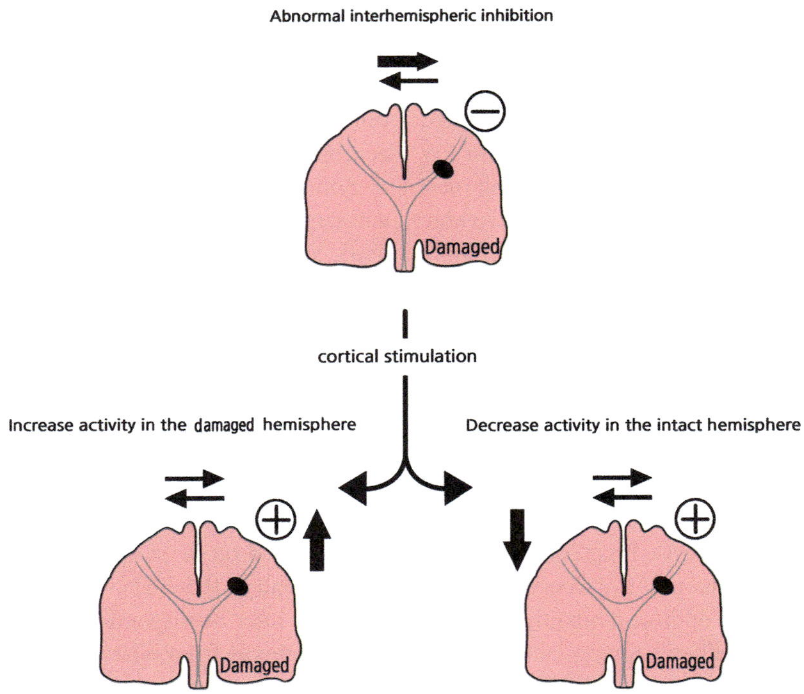

Fig. 16.3 Strategy to improve motor function after stroke. After stroke, transcallosal interhemispheric inhibitory projections from the unaffected motor cortex to affected motor cortex is elevated compared to inhibitory tone from affected to unaffected motor cortex after stroke. Therefore, either (1) facilitation of affected motor cortex (using high frequency rTMS, intermittent theta burst stimulation, iTBS or anodal tDCS) or inhibition of motor cortex of the unaffected hemisphere (using low frequency rTMS, continuous theta burst stimulation, iTBS or cathodal tDCS) could be a strategy to improve motor function of paretic upper limb (Adapted from [167])

unaffected hemisphere [177]. Recently, Kakuda et al. [178] performed a multi-center study in 214 chronic post-stroke patients and demonstrated that multiple sessions (average 22 sessions) of 1 Hz rTMS over the unaffected motor cortex combined with customary occupational therapy had a beneficial effect on improvement of motor recovery, and effects were maintained up to 4 weeks after the intervention. Although this study was a one-arm study without sham control, this study demonstrated the therapeutic value of repeated sessions of low frequency rTMS applied to the unaffected motor cortex as an adjuvant therapy in stroke neurorehabilitation.

However, in one study rTMS over the unaffected hemisphere demonstrated decreased performance in complex motor task [157] in some patients, questioning the general applicability of the unaffected hemisphere approach.

Application of high-frequency rTMS on the affected hemisphere demonstrated inconsistent results [174–176]. Besides, high frequency rTMS has more safety concerns than low frequency rTMS due to its potential to induce seizure.

In one group's studies [174, 175], 3 Hz rTMS applied to the affected hemisphere was safe and induced long-term beneficial effect up to 1 year. However, in Takeuchi et al.'s study [179] comparing high frequency rTMS to the affected hemisphere and low frequency to unaffected hemisphere, high frequency stimulation showed negative results, contrary to positive results of low frequency stimulation. Khedr et al. also reported that 1 Hz stimulation on unaffected hemisphere elicited greater motor improvement than 3 Hz stimulation [180].

According to current literature review, low-frequency rTMS on unaffected hemisphere produces better effects than high-frequency rTMS on affected hemisphere [179–181]. This phenomenon is postulated the finding that low-frequency rTMS induces bilateral cortical excitability changes at the same time, whereas high-frequency rTMS induces excitability changes only on the affected cortex [172].

Low frequency rTMS also has been shown to be effective for spasticity control [178]. This effect is considered a secondary effect of increased descending inhibitory control over the motor neuron pool from the affected motor cortex.

The intensity of the stimulation is also important. Subthreshold stimulation may exert only local effect on the stimulated area, but suprathreshold stimulation may affect not only the stimulated cortex but also the contralateral homogenous motor cortex and related motor network [171, 172, 174, 175].

For greater and longer lasting effects, theta burst stimulation (TBS), a modified patterned stimulation of conventional rTMS has also been attempted at the compensation of the increased risk of seizure. In TBS, intermittent TBS (iTBS) corresponds to high frequency rTMS, and continuous TBS (cTBS) low frequency rTMS [182].

Talelli et al. [183] and Ackerley et al. [184] applied iTBS over the affected motor cortex and cTBS over the unaffected motor cortex in chronic stroke patients and found some positive results.

Sometimes, priming protocol was applied hoping to enhance the rTMS effect. Carey et al. [185] and Kakuda et al. [186] applied 6 Hz priming rTMS prior to 1 Hz rTMS to enhance the effect of 1 Hz rTMS applied to unaffected hemisphere in stroke. This concept of "meta-plasticity" and "homeostatic plasticity" effect, that is, changes in brain activity can induce subsequent change in brain activity has been shown in normal subjects using rTMS and tDCS and produced the idea of priming stimulation [187]. Table 16.3 summarizes the rTMS protocol for post-stroke motor recovery [169].

Along with rTMS, tDCS can also be applied as an adjuvant therapy for motor neurorehabilitation. Single or multiple sessions of either facilitatory anodal tDCS applied to affected M1 [167, 188] or inhibitory cathodal tDCS to unaffected M1 [189, 190] can also enhance paretic hand motor function beyond the stimulation period.

tDCS and rTMS have their own advantages and disadvantages [191]. tDCS is easy to administer and relatively inexpensive as compared to rTMS and it can be administered in combination with various rehabilitative training.

If repeated sessions of stimulation are applied, there is a possibility to have a longer lasting after-effect [172]. Reis et al. [192] demonstrated that repeated sessions of anodal tDCS facilitated long-term retention and consolidation of acquired skills as compared to sham stimulation in healthy subjects.

Although first positive results for improvement of motor performance came out from anodal tDCS protocol, anodal protocol over affected M1 is reported to produce less beneficial effects than cathodal tDCS protocol over unaffected M1 according to recent literatures [193, 194]. Kim et al. [193] tested whether multiple sessions of tDCS combined with occupational therapy could elicit more improvement in motor function of the paretic upper limb than sham stimulation (occupational therapy alone) in patients with subacute stroke. They recruited 18 patients with hand motor impairment and randomly assigned them to one of the three 10-day sessions of intervention; anodal tDCS over the affected motor cortex, cathodal tDCS over the unaffected motor cortex, or sham stimulation. They observed that only cathodal tDCS led to a greater improvement in paretic hand function assessed with Fugl-Meyer score than the sham procedure at 6-month follow-up whereas anodal tDCS showed trends towards improvement.

Sometimes bihemispheric tDCS combining anodal tDCS to affected hemisphere and cathodal tDCS to unaffected hemisphere has been attempted in healthy subjects [195, 196] and stroke patients [197, 198] hoping to enhance motor improvement. Kang and Paik [195] compared unilateral versus bilateral tDCS application when performing a motor learning task in 11 healthy subjects, and found that there was no significant difference between applications in terms of induced implicit motor sequence learning, although two applications were more effective than sham stimulation. Likewise in stroke patients, it is not clear whether bilateral tDCS application is more effective in terms of enhancing motor recovery than unilateral application.

Peripheral nerve stimulation or somatosensory stimulation is also known to increase cortical excitability and to enhance motor function of a paretic hand in patients with subacute and chronic stroke [199, 200].

Somatosensory stimulation can be coupled with TMS in a synchronous manner in paired association stimulation (PAS) protocol. When ascending volley of somatosensory stimulation is coupled with TMS descending volley in a synchronous manner, it can increase the cortical excitability and enhance motor performance in healthy subject [201]. Previous studies showed that this protocol also induces changes in cortical excitability [202, 203] and improves motor function in stroke patients [204].

Celnik and Paik et al. tested whether combining somatosensory stimulation and tDCS induces larger or longer lasting after effects than stimulating somatosensory stimulation or tDCS alone [205]. They combined peripheral nerve stimulation to the paretic hand with anodal tDCS to the ipsilesional M1, and found that combined stimulation resulted in a greater improvement in the number of correct key presses relative to either stimulation alone or sham stimulation, and this improvement was maintained until 6 days after the end of the training.

Recent failure in multicenter phase III clinical trial on cortical epidural stimulation to promote motor recovery after stroke provoked important caveats in applying noninvasive cortical stimulation to stroke patients [206].

In a phase II feasibility trial, epidural stimulation guided by functional MRI for the optimal stimulation site in chronic stroke patients was successful [207]. However, in a phase III trial only a limited number of patients (less than 20 % of participants) showed motor evoked responses, and this was one of main factors that led to unexpected failure of the trial. Later post hoc subgroup analysis revealed significant improvements in those patients with evoked motor responses. When we consider that functional recovery after stroke is essentially motor learning with a partially disrupted neural network [157], at least cortico-spinal output has to be adequate to allow functional recovery of motor function.

Table 16.3 rTMS protocol for post-stroke motor recovery

Source	Design	Size	Lesion site	Time after stroke	Frequency, intensity, pulse number and duration	Stimulated area	Outcome measures	Results
Khedr et al. 2005 [174]	RCT	26 real, 26 sham*	MCA territory (24 RH, 28 LH)	Real: 7.1 ± 1.4 days Sham: 7.3 ± 1.5 days	3 Hz, 120 % RMT, 3,000 pulses, 10 sessions	AH	Scandinavian stroke scale, NIHSS, Barthel index	Improvement of motor function
Khedr et al. 2010 [175]	RCT	16 real 3 Hz, 16 real 10 Hz, 16 sham	MCA (21 RH, 27 LH)	3 Hz: 8.0 ± 5.1 day 10 Hz: 6.0 ± 2.8 days Sham: 6.2 ± 1.5 days	3 Hz, 130 % RMT, 750 pulses, 5 sessions 10 Hz, 100 % RMT, 750 pulses, 5 sessions	AH	Muscle strength, NIHSS, mRS	Improvement of motor function over 1 year
Fregni et al. 2006 [172]	RCT	10 real, 5 sham	Various lesions (3 RH, 12 LH)	Real: 3.5 ± 2.9 years Sham: 4.0 ± 2.6 years	1 Hz, 100 % MT, 1,200 pulses, 5 sessions	UH	Jebsen-Taylor hand function test, simple reaction time, choice reaction time, Purdue pegboard, MMSE, digit span, Stroop test	Improvement of motor function only in the affected hand over 2 weeks
Takeuchi et al. 2005 [171]	RCT	10 real, 10 sham	Subcortex (12 RH, 8 LH)	28.7 ± 16.7 months	1 Hz, 90 % RMT, 1,500 pulses, 1 session	UH	Pinch force, acceleration	Improvement of motor function
Emara et al. 2010 [181]	RCT	20 real 1 Hz, 20 real 5 Hz, 20 sham	29 RH, 31 LH	1 Hz: 6.5 months 5 Hz: 2.5 months Sham: 3.5 months	1 Hz, 110–120 % MT, 1 500 pulses, 10 sessions, 5 Hz, 80–90 % MT, 7 500 pulses, 10 sessions	1 Hz: UH, 5 Hz: AH	Thumb-index finger tapping test, activity index, mRS	Improvement of motor function over 12 weeks in 1 Hz and 5 Hz and 5 Hz rTMS
Khedr et al. 2009 [180]	RCT	12 real 1 Hz, 12 real 3 Hz, 12 sham	MCA (23 RH, 13 LH)	1 Hz: 16.3 ± 3.6 days 3 Hz: 17.2 ± 3.6 days Sham: 17.7 ± 3.8 days	1 Hz, 130 % RMT, 900 pulses, 5 sessions 3 Hz, 130 % RMT, 900 pulses, 5 sessions	1 Hz: UH, 3 Hz: AH	Grip strength, keyboard tapping, pegboard task, NIHSS, Barthel index	Improvement of motor function over 3 months (1 Hz rTMS was better than 3 Hz rTMS)
Liepert et al. 2007 [173]	RCT	12	10 subcortex, 2 pons	7.3 ± 4.5 days	1 Hz, 90 % RMT, 1 200 pulses, 2 sessions (crossover: real and sham)	UH	Grip strength, nine hold peg test	Improvement of dexterity of only affected hand
Takeuchi et al. 2009 [179]	RCT	10 AH, 10 UH, 10 bilateral	Subcortex (12 RH, 18 LH)	AH: 35.6 ± 38.7 months, UH: 24.7 ± 28.9 months Bilateral: 26.1 ± 28.0 month	AH: 10 Hz, 90 % RMT, 1,000 pulses, 1 session UH: 1 Hz, 90 % RMT, 1,000 pulses, 1 session bilateral: alternating	AH, UH, bilateral	Pinch force, acceleration	AH: no effect UH, bilateral: improvement of acceleration, bilateral > UH
Malcolm et al. 2007 [176]	RCT	9 real, 10 sham	10 RH, 10 LH	Real: 3.9 ± 3.1 years Sham: 3.8 ± 3.7 years	20 Hz, 90 % MT, 2 000 pulses, 10 sessions	AH (homologue to the hand area of the UH)	Wolf motor function test, motor activity log, box and block test	No improvement of motor function

Ackerley et al. 2010 [184]	RCT	10 patients	Subcortex (4 RH, 6 LH)	28.9 ± 25.0 month	Continuous TBS: 90 % AMT, 600 pulses, 1 session; intermittent TBS: 90 % AMT, 600 pulses, 1 session; sham TBS (crossover)	Continous TBS:UH, intermittent TBS, AH	Grip-lift kinetics, action research arm test	Improvement of grip-lift kinetics with real TBS, decrement of action research arm test with continuous TBS
Talelli et al. 2007 [183]		6 patients	MCA (1 RH, 5 LH)	31.0 ± 37.9 months	Continuous TBS: 5 Hz, burst of 3 pulses at 50 Hz, 80 % AMT, 300 pulses, 1 session; intermittent TBS: 5 Hz, 20 bursts of 10 pulses at 50 Hz, every 8 s, 80 % AMT, 600 pulses, 1 session; sham TBS	Continous TBS:UH, intermittent TBS, AH	Simple reaction time and grip strength, choice reaction time, fatigue, attention	Improvement of simple reaction time only by intermittent TBS over 20 min

rTMS repetitive transcranial magnetic stimulation, *RCT* randomized controlled trial, *AH* affected hemisphere, *UH* unaffected hemisphere, *RH* right hemisphere, *LH* left hemisphere, *MCA* middle cerebral artery, *TBS* theta burst stimulation, *MT* motor threshold, *RMT* resting motor threshold, *AMT* active motor threshold, *MMSE* Mini-Mental State Examination, *NIHSS* National Institute of Health Stroke Scale, *mRS* modified Rankin Scale, *VMC* voluntary muscle contraction

"Real" group received real rTMS while "sham" group received rTMS applied with coil angled away from the head to reproduce the noise of the stimulation as well as some local sensation

From [169]; with permission

Therefore, cortico-spinal descending pathways should be checked for their integrity using TMS or tractography before applying brain stimulation.

It is also important to determine the exact location of stimulation considering the potentially variable lesion geometry, mechanism and stage of stroke recovery, and to deliver the patient-specific neuromodulation protocol.

Recently, Bashir et al. and Kim et al. compared applying neuronavigated rTMS over conventional rTMS in terms of physiologic and behavioral effects of low-frequency rTMS in healthy subjects, and found that navigated rTMS leads to more robust neuromodulation resulting in greater physiologic and behavioral effects. Neuronavigational rTMS can maximize accuracy in targeting a given cortical therefore, study results have implications for future therapeutic applications of neuromodulation [208, 209].

Recently, it was found that response to rTMS is modulated by a common polymorphism of the brain-derived neurotrophic factor gene (BDNF). The BDNF is known to influence synaptic plasticity, and response to rTMS in BDNF Val66Met carriers was different from that of Val66Val individuals, suggesting that polymorphism may be one factor that influences the response to neuromodulation [210].

According to current knowledge, brain neuromodulation appears to be a safe and promising intervention for brain rehabilitation and has a potential to be used as an adjuvant therapy for neurorehabilitation when appropriately combined with classical behavioral therapy. However, improvement of function after brain neuromodulation is still modest, and at least network should be partially preserved for the after-effects to occur. More studies are needed to assess its long-term benefits on a large scale of patients [211].

It is unlikely that brain neuromodulation alone makes the brain form appropriate connections needed for recovery. Maybe brain neuromodulation works by strengthening existing connections or assisting the brain to form new connection. Therefore, brain neuromodulation techniques should always be accompanied by behavioral training.

Further fine establishment of stimulation protocols maximizing the beneficial effect of interventions, in terms of parameters showing better effect and duration, optimal patient and time selection for intervention and individualized localization depending on the pattern of reorganization should be pursued. Location, extent, time since injury, geography of delivered stimulation is different from patient to patient [212].

Visuospatial Neglect

Neglect is defined as an impaired or lost ability to respond to sensory stimuli presented from the contralesional hemisphere in a patient with neurological damage [213]. Visuospatial neglect is a common problem after stroke, estimated to occur in about 82 % of right cerebral hemisphere strokes and 65 % of left cerebral hemisphere strokes [214]. Neglect is an important impairment to overcome in stroke rehabilitation, because it is associated with poor functional outcomes [215].

Various rehabilitation techniques for neglect have been tried. Visual scanning therapy was initially applied to treat neglect and was reported to have some beneficial effect [216] but it could improve only the neglect for visual tasks and is quite time consuming [217]. To reduce the theoretically right ward deviation in a patient with neglect, optokinetic stimulation, neck muscle vibration, caloric- or galvanic-vestibular stimulation, and prism adaptation have also been applied as therapeutic tools and some studies reported a positive effect, although a well-designed randomized controlled trial with sufficient sample size is lacking to date [218–222]. There is no convincing evidence for the pharmacologic treatment in neglect [223].

Because previous treatments for neglect have shown limited effect, need for a new modality has been suggested. Recently, noninvasive brain stimulation has emerged as a possible treatment tool for neglect. The rational for application of noninvasive brain stimulation for visual spatial neglect after brain injury is also based on the concept of inter-hemispheric rivalry. Usually a right hemispheric lesion after stroke causes the attentional vector generated by the right hemisphere to be weaker and results in the reduction of inhibition on the left hemisphere [224]. This disinhibition supposed to lead to hyperexcitability of the intact left hemisphere and right ward deviation of visual field [224].

Therefore, the purpose of noninvasive brain stimulation for neglect is to reduce the hyperexcitability of intact left hemisphere or to increase the excitability of damaged right hemisphere, which is expected to neutralize the right ward deviation. Several studies for rTMS and a couple of studies for tDCS have been published up to now [225, 226]. The initial study of rTMS for visuospatial neglect applied 25 Hz high frequency stimulation to the unaffected parietal cortex and demonstrated improvement in the bisected lines length judgment test [227]. Thereafter, all studies have used the rMTS protocol to inhibit the unaffected parietal or posterior parietal cortex to treat neglect after stroke.

Studies with low-frequency rTMS over the posterior parietal cortex demonstrated the long-term effect on neglect [228–230]. Lim et al. tested whether multiple sessions of inhibitory 1 Hz rTMS applied to the left parietal cortex can improve hemispatial neglect after stroke with an open-label design [231]. They recruited seven consecutive patients with hemispatial neglect and compared with seven retrospectively recruited historical control patients. rTMS was applied to the left parietal area immediately prior to occupational therapy for 10 days whereas historical control patients

Table 16.4 rTMS protocol for post-stroke hemispatial neglect (From Shin J, Yang EJ, Cho K, et al. Clinical application of repetitive transcranial magnetic stimulation in stroke rehabilitation. Neural Regen Res 2012; 7: 627–34) [169]

Source	Design	Size	Lesion site	Time after stroke	Frequency, intensity, pulse number and duration	Stimulated area	Outcome measures	Results
Oliveri et al., 2001 [227]	Case study	7 patients	5 RH, 2 LH	15.1 ± 19.1 week	25 Hz, 115 % MT, 10 pulses, 1 session	UH (P5 or P6)	Length judgment of bisected line	Improvement of visuospatial neglect
Koch et al., 2008 [233]	Case study	12 patients	RH	Patients: 32–172 days; neglect (-) patients: 31–158 days	1 Hz, 90 % RMT, 600 pulses, 1 session	UH	Naming of visual chimeric objects	Improvement of visuospatial neglect
Song et al., 2009 [230]	RCT	7 rTMS, 7 rTMS (−)	RH	rTMS: 38.4 ± 15.2 days; rTMS (−): 31.6 ± 11.5 days	0.5 Hz, 90 % MT, 450 pulses, 20 sessions (P3)	UH (P3)	Line cancellation, line bisection	Improvement of visuospatial neglect
Lim et al., 2010 [231]	Case study	7 rTMS, 7 rTMS (−)	RH	rTMS: 61.9 ± 111.1 day; rTMS (−): 139.0 ± 194.8 days	1 Hz, 90 % MT, 900 pulses, 10 sessions	UH	Line bisection, Albert test	Improvement of line bisection test, but not of Albert test
Shindo et al., 2006 [229]	Case study	2 patients	RH	180.5 ± 7.8 days	0.9 Hz, 95 % MT, 900 pulses, 6 sessions	UH (P5)	Behavioral inattention test, MMSE or Revised Hasegawa dementia scale, Brunnstrom recovery stage, Barthel index	Improvement of visuospatial neglect unti 5 weeks after rTMS
Brighina et al., 2003 [228]	Case study	3 patients	RH	3–5 months	1 Hz, 90 % MT, 900 pulses, 7 sessions	UH (P5)	Line bisection test, clock drawing	Improvement of visuospatial neglect until 15 days after rTMS
Nyffeler et al., 2009 [232]	Case study	11 patients 5 2 × TBS, 5 4 × TBS, 5 sham, 5 control*	RH	7.1 ± 13.0 month	Continuous TBS: 30 Hz, burst of 3 pulses, every 100 msec, 100 % RMT, 801 pulses, 2 or 4 trains	UH (P3)	Subtask of Vienna test system	Improvement of visuospatial neglect, lasting effect of neglect: 4 TBS trains showed longer effect than 2 TBS trains

RCT randomized controlled trial, *TBS* theta burst stimulation, *MT* motor threshold, *RMT* resting motor threshold, *P3/P5* left parietal cortex according to the International 10–20 EEG coordinate system, *P6* right parietal cortex according to the International 10–20 EEG coordinate system, *MMSE* Mini-Mental State Examination

Four experiments were performed, and each experiment included five patients. Therefore, three patients participated in two experiments and three patients in three experiments

received only behavioral therapy. After treatment, rTMS group showed a greater improvement in the line bisection test than did the control group.

Two studies applied continuous theta burst stimulation (cTBS) [226, 232]. Nyffeler et al. reported that continuous inhibitory TBS over the unaffected posterior parietal cortex showed more improvement for left-sided targets and reaction time in a visuospatial task compared to sham stimulation [232]. Koch et al. demonstrated the effect of multiple sessions of continuous TBS on neglect [226]. Ten sessions of continuous TBS of the posterior parietal cortex over 2 weeks showed more improvement in behavioral inattention test compared to the sham stimulation. Table 16.4 summarizes the rTMS protocol for post-stroke hemispatial neglect [169].

In summary for rTMS for neglect, although previous studies have shown the promising perspectives, the evidence is still lacking. Long-term after-effects of rTMS should be investigated in the future study. Considering the brain network for visuospatial perception and theory of interhemispheric rivalry, we need further study with excitatory rTMS over the affected hemisphere or other different stimulation sites and modes to find out the most effective rTMS protocol for neglect.

With regard to the tDCS, only two studies have reported an effect on neglect after stroke. One study applied one session of anodal tDCS with 2 mA over the affected posterior parietal cortex. Compared to sham tDCS, the percent deviation score of the line bisection test and the omissions for the shape unstructured cancellation test improved more immediately after anodal tDCS [234]. In another study, researchers investigated the effect of anodal tDCS over the affected posterior parietal cortex and cathodal tDCS over the unaffected posterior parietal cortex in ten patients with neglect after stroke [235]. Both anodal tDCS over the affected hemisphere and cathodal tDCS over the unaffected hemisphere improved some in the clinical test compared to the effect of sham tDCS. Based on these two studies, the expected increase of excitability on the affected hemisphere after anodal tDCS seems to improve the clinical symptoms of neglect in stroke patients. Because randomized controlled trials have not been tried, convincing evidence for tDCS on neglect is currently lacking.

Aphasia

Aphasia is defined as an acquired loss or impairment of the language system after brain damage [236]. About 24–30 % of the patients suffer from various types of aphasia following stroke and degree of recovery varies among patients [237, 238]. Aphasia is not only an important disability in daily life but also a key prognostic factor for functional outcome after stroke [239]. Therefore, there have been efforts to treat the aphasia in order to improve functional outcome and quality of life in patients with stroke.

Speech and language therapy is usually the primary therapeutic approach in rehabilitation of aphasia after stroke [240]. A comprehensive review on speech and language therapy for aphasia following stroke was recently published [241]. In this review, speech language therapy showed better functional communication outcomes in receptive and expressive language compared with no therapy. However, when the speech language therapy is compared to social support and stimulation, they found no evidence of a difference in functional communication. Although they also compared the effects of experimental (e.g., constraint-induced language therapy), intensive and group speech language therapies with a conventional one, no significant difference was found. In summary, there is some evidence of the effectiveness of speech language therapy with aphasia following stroke but evidence is insufficient to draw any conclusion regarding the effectiveness of any one specific speech language therapy approach over another [241].

Compared to lesion-deficit approach, the recent development of neuroimaging makes it possible to investigate brain connectivity in language function and plastic changes after stroke. Recovery from aphasia is associated with a process of reorganization and plasticity in this complex language network [242, 243]. Noninvasive brain stimulation is expected to modulate the excitability of cortical regions that are associated with specific language networks involved in aphasia after stroke, then to enhance the cortical reorganization that leads to good recovery [244]. To date, some studies with rTMS and tDCS have reported promising results in patients with aphasia.

Usually noninvasive stimulation for aphasia treatment has been based on the concept that considered hyperexcitability of the homologous area in the unaffected hemisphere to the damaged brain after stroke as a maladaptation [245], part of the concept of interhemispheric rivalry. Therefore more studies of rTMS or tDCS for aphasia have used the protocol of inhibiting the right unaffected hemisphere or exciting the left affected hemisphere, which can lead to increasing the excitability of damaged brain regions in the left hemisphere.

Some studies have reported that low frequency rTMS over the unaffected right inferior frontal gyrus improved aphasia but they did not use a control group and only investigated the effect of rTMS in non-fluent aphasia [246–252]. Barwood et al. demonstrated that ten sessions of low-frequency rTMS over the right pars triangularis improved the speech language performance in Boston diagnostic aphasia examination in their sham-controlled study with non-fluent aphasia after stroke. Weiduschat et al. also conducted a randomized controlled pilot study in heterogeneous group of aphasia (five Wernicke's, two Broca's and one amnestic aphasia) to investigate the effect of low-frequency rTMS over the right pars triangularis on aphasia [253]. There was an improvement of speech performance in Aachen aphasia test after real rTMS compared to sham stimulation. Recently, one randomized, double blind, sham controlled study did not find the significant effect of low frequency rTMS over the right inferior frontal gyrus on the recovery from aphasia in acute stage ischemic stroke [254]. However, the rTMS subgroup with a lesion including the anterior part of language area showed greater improvement primarily in naming reaction time 15 weeks after completion of the therapeutic treatment in the additional analyses.

Intermittent theta-burst stimulation (iTBS), high-frequency rTMS, and anodal tDCS over the left hemisphere were also tried to directly increase the excitability of damaged left hemisphere, which are expected to restore the perilesional neuronal activity. Application of up regulating intermittent TBS over the left Broca's area localized through fMRI study in aphasic patients with chronic stroke showed improvement in semantic fluency, coinciding with an increase in left fronto-temporo-parietal language networks in fMRI mapping [255]. In one small case study including three patients with aphasia, high-frequency rTMS over the left dorsolateral prefrontal cortex improved object naming. Table 16.5 summarizes the rTMS protocol for post-stroke aphasia [169].

There have been several studies of tDCS. In a cross-over design with sham control, five sessions of anodal tDCS over

Table 16.5 rTMS protocol for post-stroke aphasia

Source	Design	Size	Type of aphasia	Time after stroke	Frequency, intensity, pulse number and duration	Stimulated area	Neuro-navigation	Outcome measures	Results
Naeser et al. 2005 [248]	Case study	4	Global, motor, conduction aphasia	5–11 years	1 Hz, 90 % MT, 1,200 pulses, 10 sessions	Right Broca's homologue	Yes	Snodgrass and Vanderwart picture naming BNT, Boston diagnostic aphasia exam	Improvement of picture naming over 8 months in ¾ patients
Martin et al. 2004 [246]	Case study	2	Motor aphasia	10.2 years	1 Hz, 90 % MT, 600 pulses, 10 sessions	Right pars triangularis	Yes	BNT	Improvement of naming in ½ patients
Martin et al. 2009 [249]	Case study	4	Motor aphasia	5–11 years	1 Hz, 90 % MT, 1,200 pulses, 10 sessions	Right Brodman area 45	Yes	BNT, Boston diagnostic aphasia exam	Improvement of picture naming over 2 months
Hamilton et al. 2010 [250]	Case study	1	Motor aphasia	5 years	1 Hz, 90 % MT, 1,200 pulses, 10 sessions	Right pars trangularis	Yes	WAB, Cooke theft picture description, naming	Improvement of naming, picture description, spontaneous speech
Kakuda et al. 2010 [256]	Case study	2	Sensory aphasia	7.8 months	1 Hz, 90 % MT, 1,200 pulses, 10 sessions for a week and weekly for 3 months	Wernicke's area	No	Token test, auditory comprehension of standard language test of aphasia	Improvement of auditory and visual comprehension, sponataneous speech, writing, repetition and naming
Winhuisen et al. 2005 [257]	Case study	11	Global, motor, sensory aphasia	2 weeks	4 Hz, 20 % max output (2.1 T), 40 pulses	Right or left IFG (activated region in PET)	No	Aachen aphasia test battery	Improvement of verb generation (left IFG > right IFG)
Kakuda et al. 2010 [258]	Case study	4	Motor aphasia	13.8 ± 10.7 months	1 Hz, 90 % MT, 1,200 pulses, 10 sessions	Homologous to activated region in fMRI during word repetition task	No	WAB, Standard language test of aphasia	Improvement of naming, spontaneous speech, writing and repetition

From [169]; with permission

the left hemispheric area that was activated during an overt naming task in fMRI demonstrated improvement in naming task [259]. Another study demonstrated that five sessions of anodal tDCS over the left inferior frontal gyrus improved aphasia. In a recent double-blind, sham-controlled study, anodal tDCS was applied to the left perilesional brain regions that showed the greatest activation on a pre-tDCS fMRI during overt picture naming [260]. Anodal tDCS over the affected left hemisphere reduced reaction time during naming until 3 weeks after treatment. However, Monti et al. did not prove the effect of anodal tDCS over the left frontotemporal area on aphasia with single session [261].

Some studies investigated the effect of inhibitory cathodal tDCS of the right hemisphere on aphasia. Kang et al. evaluated whether inhibitory cathodal tDCS, applied over a healthy right Broca's homologue area could improve picture naming in patients with post-stroke aphasia [262]. Ten right-handed patients received an intervention of cathodal tDCS (2 mA for 20 min) and of sham tDCS (2 mA for 1 min) daily for five consecutive days in a crossover design combined with simultaneous conventional speech therapy. Improved picture naming was observed following the last tDCS treatment session, but no changes were observed after sham tDCS. They further investigated the factors associated with good responses to tDCS combined with speech therapy in 37 aphasic patients after stroke [263]. All patients received ten sessions of speech therapy for 30 min over 2–3 weeks while the cathodal tDCS was applied to Broca's homologous area in unaffected hemisphere with 1 mA for 20 min. After tDCS intervention, Aphasia Quotient significantly improved, and improvement was greater in patients with less severe, fluent type of aphasia. Initial severity over 10 % in AQ was favorable for improvement in statistical analysis.

By stimulating more specific targeted areas, the therapeutic effect of noninvasive brain stimulation could be maximized. One study with a neuro-navigational system suggested that TMS suppression of the right pars triangularis, but not the pars opercularis, improves naming in aphasia, indicating the need to specify the stimulation site within the selected gyrus level, such as inferior frontal gyrus [251]. Kim et al. also reported that neuronavigated rTMS leads to more robust neuromodulation of Broca's area, resulting in delayed verbal reaction time in healthy virtual lesioning study [209].

Therefore, using a neuro-navigational system could be a solution for this question. The target area for activation or deactivation can be visualized using functional neuroimaging such as functional MRI or PET [255, 264, 265] and these target areas can be specified by a neuro-navigation system. This technique may be particularly important with an attempt to directly excite the perilesional left hemispheric area by rTMS in aphasia, because the stimulation can be applied to the damaged, non-excitable tissue when using the conventional technique.

Epidural cortical stimulation has been tried as an adjunctive therapy for aphasia in some previous studies [266, 267]. In one preliminary study, four stroke patients with chronic non-fluent aphasia underwent functional MRI guided surgical implantation of an epidural stimulation device which was activated only during intensive speech therapy [266]. They found that there was no adverse event related to the implantation of device and cortical stimulation except the transient tingling around the implanted stimulator, and suggested that epidural stimulation of the ipsilesional premotor cortex may augment the effect of speech therapy.

Dysphagia

Dysphagia is a commonly documented morbidity after stroke, but its reported frequencies are widely discrepant, ranging between 19 and 81 % depending definition, time and tool of evaluation [268]. The presence of dysphagia has been associated with an increased risk for aspiration pneumonia and mortality [269]. There is emerging evidence that early detection of dysphagia in patients with acute stroke reduces not only these risks but also reduces the length of hospital stay and overall healthcare expenditures [270].

Current treatment for dysphagia includes prevention of aspiration in the form of diet and fluid modifications, compensatory maneuvers, position changes and rehabilitation exercises [271]. Diet modification is a common treatment for dysphagia. In general, thin liquids are the most difficult to control and are more likely to be aspirated because they can leak into the pharynx before swallowing is triggered. Hence, thickened liquids and soft cohesive solids are generally those with the safest consistency.

A variety of behavioral techniques are used, including modifications in posture, head position and respiration, as well as specific swallowing maneuvers. Oral sensory stimulation involving altered temperature and taste may be considered therapy because it can alter the timing of swallowing by reducing both the oral onset time and pharyngeal delay time. Therapeutic exercises are used to improve the patient's oral motor range of motion, strength and coordination of oral, pharyngeal and respiratory muscles for swallowing.

Neuromuscular electrical stimulation is a widely used treatment for oropharyngeal dysphagia. It involves passing a small electrical current transcutaneously to create a muscle contraction or to deliver somatosensory input [272, 273].

When safe feeding is not possible, a pharyngeal bypass measured may be employed to eliminate the need for oropharyngeal swallowing and provide nutrition and hydration.

There are no specific "medication for dysphagia," though some symptoms may be managed with medication. Anticholinergic drugs and botulin toxin injections can reduce salivary flow in individuals with aspiration of oral secretions [274].

It has been known that the swallowing motor cortex is reorganized after stroke and associated with recovery from dysphagia [275]. Noninvasive brain stimulation is expected to modulate the brain plasticity during the recovery phase of dysphagia after stroke. Some studies of rTMS or tDCS have investigated the role of noninvasive stimulation on the recovery of dysphagia.

Recent reports have identified positive treatment effects in swallowing functions subsequent to rTMS highlighting its therapeutic potential as a treatment for dysphagia [276]. Khedr et al. [277] recruited 26 post-stroke dysphagic patients in a 5–10-day post-stroke onset. The experimental group received repetitive trains of 3-Hz stimulation on the esophageal cortical area of the affected hemisphere for 5 days. Improvement in the dysphagia rating was observed only in the experimental group but not in the sham group at 2 months post-stimulation. Abo-Elfetoh et al. [276, 278] also investigated rTMS effect on 22 acute ischemic stroke patients with bulbar symptoms. The experimental group received repetitive trains of 3-Hz stimulation on the esophageal cortical area of both hemispheres for five consecutive days and significant improvement in swallowing function was observed. Although both studies showed improvement in swallowing functions after rTMS, both used only a four-point rating scale to describe the general swallowing functions based on clinical examination. Verin et al. [276] conducted a pilot study using rTMS to stimulate the mylohyoid cortical area in seven post-stroke dysphagic patients. The patients had improvement in swallowing functions up to 3 weeks after stimulation when

Table 16.6 rTMS protocol for post-stroke dysphagia

Source	Design	Size	Lesion site	Time after stroke	Frequency, intensity, pulse number and duration	Stimulated area	Outcome measures	Results
Khedr et al. 2009 [277]	RCT	12 real, 14 sham*	12 RH, 14 LH	5–10 days	3 Hz, 120 % RMT, 300 pulses, 5 sessions	Esophageal motor cortex of AH	Dysphagia outcome and severity scale, Barthel index, grip strength	Improvement of dysphagia and motor disability over 2 months
Khedr and Elfetoh 2012 [278]	RCT	11 real, 11 sham	11 lateral medulla, 11 brain stem	1–3 months	3 Hz, 130 % RMT, 300 pulses, 5 sessions	Esophageal motor cortex of bilateral hemispheres	Dysphagia outcome and severity scale, Barthel index, NIHSS, grip strength	Improvement of swallowing coordination and aspiration

RCT randomized controlled trial, *AH* affected hemisphere, *UH* unaffected hemisphere, *RH* right hemisphere, *LH* left hemisphere, *RMT* resting motor threshold, *MT* motor threshold, *NIHSS* National Institute of Health Stroke Scale

"Real" group received real rTMS while "sham" group received rTMS applied with coil angled away from the head to reproduce the noise of the stimulation as well as some local sensation

From [169]; with permission

measured with videofluoroscopic swallowing study. However, their study did not include any control group. Further studies that include both active and sham rTMS groups and using various swallowing assessment tools (e.g., clinical examination, videofluoroscopic swallowing studies, swallowing-specific quality of life questionnaires) are needed to better understand the effect of rTMS on swallowing functions. Table 16.6 summarizes the rTMS protocol for post-stroke dysphagia [169].

One small pilot study reported transient improvement of swallowing function after anodal tDCS to the sensorimotor cortical representation of swallowing muscles in the unaffected hemisphere over the course of five consecutive days with concurrent standardized swallowing maneuvers in fourteen patients with subacute unilateral hemispheric infarction [279]. Jafferson et al. [280] demonstrated that anodal tDCS increases pharyngeal motor cortex excitability in an intensity-dependent manner, with little evidence of transcallosal spread.

Yang et al. also investigate the effects of tDCS combined with swallowing training on post-stroke dysphagia [281]. Sixteen patients with post-stroke dysphagia received anodal tDCS (1 mA for 20 min) or sham (1 mA for 30 s) over the pharyngeal motor cortex of the affected hemisphere during 30 min of conventional swallowing training for 10 days. Three months after the intervention, anodal tDCS elicited greater improvement compared to the sham group after controlling for age, initial stroke severity, lesion size, baseline dysphagia score, and time from stroke onset.

Cognitive Decline

Recently, in the field of rehabilitation for cognitive impairment after stroke, noninvasive brain stimulation has been investigated as a new therapeutic modality. Wassermann et al. [28] found that rTMS to parasagittal areas improved the performance on story recall on the Wechsler Memory Scale. Evers et al. [282] systematically investigated a potential enhancing effect of rTMS on cognitive processing operationalized by behavioral and neurophysiological measurements. High-frequency rTMS at 20 Hz over the left prefrontal cortex significantly decreased reaction times as well as the latency of the P 300 component in a choice reaction task. Improvement of performance by high-frequency TMS has also been shown after stimulation of Wernicke's area for tasks of reasoning and picture naming [283].

Low-frequency stimulation seems to deteriorate cognitive functioning in lieu of having improving effects. Two studies report no worsening cognitive effects [284], and one study by Trojano et al. [285] noted a selective deterioration of functioning directly and after 10 min of 1-Hz stimulation.

Kang et al. [286] demonstrated that anodal tDCS applied to the left DLPFC was found to improve attention versus sham stimulation in stroke patients, which suggests that noninvasive cortical intervention could potentially be used during rehabilitative training to improve attention.

Post-amputation Rehabilitation

Neuromodulatory Approaches for the Amputation

Peripheral, spinal, and cerebral neuronal mechanisms may generate and maintain phantom limb pain, including plastic changes occurring in the primary somatosensory cortex [287, 288]. Similar plastic changes may occur in the primary motor cortex (M1), as shown after nerve transections in animals [289–291]. In humans, cortical plastic changes could be shown by using an ischemic nerve block as a model for a transient deafferentation [292], and studying the cortical representation of proximal stump muscles after amputation by transcranial magnetic stimulation (TMS) mapping [293, 294] or positron emission tomography [295].

The physiopathology of the phantom limb pain is still an open field between various hypotheses. The two major research streams on the painful phantom limb are focused on the pivotal influence of the periphery and of the spinal cord, while the other is focused on the fundamental role of supra-segmental structures and of the cortex. These two streams seem to be more complementary than in opposition. Roricht et al. [296, 297] observed higher excitability of the motor cortex contralateral to the intact arm in some patients with upper arm amputation, and higher excitability of the motor cortex contralateral to the amputated limb in other patients. Roricht says that variability in excitability in two hemispheres could depend on the site of amputation and on the time since amputation. The hypothesis of interhemispheric balance contrasts with Schwenkreis and colleagues [298], who found a significant reduction of intracortical inhibition in forearm amputees and an enhancement of intracortical facilitation in upper arm amputees on the affected side, revealing a hyperexcitability of phantom limb hemisphere. Others studies, with EEG or with single-pulse and paired-pulse TMS investigations, are necessary to evaluate excitability of the non-phantom limb hemisphere and of phantom limb hemisphere and its modification with treatment, to understand the role of excitability in phantom limb pain.

Conversely, the electrical stimulation of the primary motor cortex (M1) has proved to be an effective treatment for intractable deafferentation pain. Cortical stimulation can be performed noninvasively by transcranial magnetic stimulation. A number of studies have shown that a single session of repetitive transcranial magnetic stimulation can relieve pain transiently in some patients with chronic neuropathic pain [299–301]. In contrast, one study failed to show any long-term therapeutic effect of 3 weeks daily parietal cortex rTMS in two patients with phantom limb pain [302]. The majority of studies apply >1 frequencies with pulses below motor threshold on motor cortical area corresponding to the hand of the painful side. M1 stimulation at high frequency was shown to reduce pain scores by 20–45 % after active stimulation and by less than 10 % after sham stimulation. Application of rTMS at high frequency is more effective than applications of rTMS at low frequency (≤ 1) in this area of stimulation [299]. However, the effect of stimulation in the unaffected hemisphere for phantom limb pain is unexplored.

The mechanism for the analgesic effect of noninvasive brain stimulation is that it can induce plastic changes in the brain or modulates plastic changes associated with chronic pain. Initial evidence suggests that rTMS affects central neurotransmitters activity in other neurological disease. Other studies also indicate the possible role of endogenous opioid secretions triggered by long-term motor cortex stimulation. Maarrawi et al. [303] reported that motor cortex stimulation may induce release of endogenous opioids in brain structures involved in the processing of acute and chronic pain. Analgesic effects of rTMS in phantom pain were delivered by increase in the endogenous beta-endorphin release. Topper et al. [302] found that opiate antagonist naloxone abolished the rTMS-induced pain relief which was taken as evidence that the analgesic effect of rTMS acted via the release of endorphins. Borckardt et al. also found that a single session of high-frequency rTMS applied at 10 Hz over the left DLPFC for a total of 4,000 pulses immediately after gastric bypass surgery was associated with a 40 % reduction in total morphine use during the first 2 days after surgery.

As for other explanation, Raij et al. [304] suggested that in chronic pain defective inhibition of M1 led to pain perception and 20 Hz rTMS restored these defective mechanism and analgesia. In fact chronic motor cortex stimulation using implanted electrodes is an effective treatment of drug-resistant pain [305, 306].

The low frequency rTMS is known to reduce the excitability of the stimulated motor cortex. The therapeutic applications of rTMS in pain syndromes are limited by the short duration of the induced effects, but prolonged pain relief can be obtained by repeating rTMS sessions every day for several weeks. This can increase the excitability of the contralateral motor cortex via transcallosal pathways, and so it can have analgesic effects in a way similar to the epidural motor cortex stimulation and to the high frequency rTMS of motor cortex.

Some hypotheses resulted from electrophysiological and PET studies [306, 307]. In these studies, cerebral blood flow was found to increase in thalamus ipsilateral to the stimulated motor cortex, in the orbitofrontal and anterior cingulated gyri, the anterior insula and upper brainstem near the periaqueductal gray matter. Cingulate and orbitofrontal activation should participate in a modulation of affective or emotional component of pain, while descending activation of the brainstem should inhibit the transmission of discriminative noxious information [306–308]. Naloxone injection significantly decreased the analgesic effects of rTMS of motor cortex stimulation, but did not change the effects of rTMS of the dorsolateral prefrontal cortex [308]. The differential effects of naloxone on motor cortex and dorsolateral prefrontal cortex stimulation suggest that the analgesic effects induced by the stimulation of these two cortical sites are mediated by differential mechanisms [308].

Conclusion

Neuromodulation is the promising field in neurology and neurorehabilitation. Deep brain stimulation in selected patients with some movement disorders is widely accepted as the proven therapeutic modality. Many literatures also support the beneficial effect of noninvasive cortical stimulation methods such as rTMS and tDCS on the various impairments in movement disorders, neurodegenerative diseases and stroke. These neuromodulation therapies seem to have its role along with conventional therapeutics in neurorehabilitation.

However, it is not yet clear how to use the neuromodulation in the clinical setting of neurology and neurorehabilitation. It should be determined that what parameters in neuromodulation (e.g., frequency, intensity, stimulation site) can maximize the beneficial effect in various clinical situations. Best candidates for specific neuromodulation therapies need to be determined. The investigation for the effect of combined treatment with other therapeutics such as medications, conventional rehabilitation is also important. Furthermore, the basic mechanism of action of various neuromodulation methods is not well understood and this should be clarified.

The research field of neuromodulation in neurology and neurorehabilitation is gradually growing to answer the questions raised as above. Along with these efforts I hope we can further understand the mechanism of the actions in neuromodulation and can suggest better neuromodulation protocol to treat the patients with neurological disorders.

References

1. Ajit Kumar DBC. Approach to the patient with a movement disorder and overview of movement disorders. In: Watts RL, Koller WC, editors. Movement disorders: neurologic principles and practice. 2nd ed. New York, NY: McGraw-Hills Companies Inc.; 2004. p. 3–16.
2. Fahn S. Classification of movement disorders. Mov Disord. 2011;26(6):947–57.
3. Fahn S, Jankovic J, Hallett M. Principles and practice of movement disorders. 2nd ed. Philadelphia, PA: Elsevier; 2011.
4. de Lau LM, Breteler MM. Epidemiology of Parkinson's disease. Lancet Neurol. 2006;5(6):525–35.
5. Scherzer CR, Eklund AC, Morse LJ, Liao Z, Locascio JJ, Fefer D, Schwarzschild MA, Schlossmacher MG, Hauser MA, Vance JM, Sudarsky LR, Standaert DG, Growdon JH, Jensen RV, Gullans SR. Molecular markers of early Parkinson's disease based on gene expression in blood. Proc Natl Acad Sci U S A. 2007;104(3): 955–60.
6. Olanow CW, Watts RL, Koller WC. An algorithm (decision tree) for the management of Parkinson's disease (2001): treatment guidelines. Neurology. 2001;56(11 Suppl 5):S1–88.
7. Poewe W, Granata R, Geser F. Pharmacologic treatment of Parkinson's disease. In: Watts RL, Koller WC, editors. Movement disorders: neurologic principles and practice. New York, NY: McGraw-Hill Companies, Inc.; 2004. p. 247–71.
8. Palhagen S, Heinonen EH, Hagglund J, Kaugesaar T, Kontants H, Maki-Ikola O, Palm R, Turunen J. Selegiline delays the onset of disability in de novo Parkinsonian patients. Swedish Parkinson Study Group. Neurology. 1998;51(2):520–5.
9. Golbe LI, Lieberman AN, Muenter MD, Ahlskog JE, Gopinathan G, Neophytides AN, Foo SH, Duvoisin RC. Deprenyl in the treatment of symptom fluctuations in advanced Parkinson's disease. Clin Neuropharmacol. 1988;11(1):45–55.
10. Ives NJ, Stowe RL, Marro J, Counsell C, Macleod A, Clarke CE, Gray R, Wheatley K. Monoamine oxidase type B inhibitors in early Parkinson's disease: meta-analysis of 17 randomised trials involving 3525 patients. BMJ. 2004;329(7466):593.
11. Caslake R, Macleod A, Ives N, Stowe R, Counsell C. Monoamine oxidase B inhibitors versus other dopaminergic agents in early Parkinson's disease. Cochrane Database Syst Rev 2009; (4): CD006661.
12. Nutt JG. Catechol-O-methyltransferase inhibitors for treatment of Parkinson's disease. Lancet. 1998;351(9111):1221–2.
13. Katzenschlager R, Sampaio C, Costa J, Lees A. Anticholinergics for symptomatic management of Parkinson's disease. Cochrane Database Syst Rev 2003; (2): CD003735.
14. Rascol O, Goetz C, Koller W, Poewe W, Sampaio C. Treatment interventions for Parkinson's disease: an evidence based assessment. Lancet. 2002;359(9317):1589–98.
15. Schwab RS, Poskanzer DC, England Jr AC, Young RR. Amantadine in Parkinson's disease. Review of more than two years' experience. JAMA. 1972;222(7):792–5.
16. Parkes JD, Baxter RC, Marsden CD, Rees JE. Comparative trial of benzhexol, amantadine, and levodopa in the treatment of Parkinson's disease. J Neurol Neurosurg Psychiatry. 1974;37(4): 422–6.
17. Carter JH, Stewart BJ, Archbold PG, Inoue I, Jaglin J, Lannon M, Rost-Ruffner E, Tennis M, McDermott MP, Amyot D, Barter R, Cornelius L, Demong C, Dobson J, Duff J, Erickson J, Gardiner N, Gauger L, Gray P, Kanigan B, Kiryluk B, Lewis P, Mistura K, Malapira T, Zoog K, et al. Living with a person who has Parkinson's disease: the spouse's perspective by stage of disease. Parkinson's Study Group. Mov Disord. 1998;13(1):20–8.
18. Pfeiffer RF. Gastrointestinal dysfunction in Parkinson's disease. Parkinsonism Relat Disord. 2011;17(1):10–5.
19. Salat-Foix D, Suchowersky O. The management of gastrointestinal symptoms in Parkinson's disease. Expert Rev Neurother. 2012;12(2):239–48.
20. Suchowersky O, Gronseth G, Perlmutter J, Reich S, Zesiewicz T, Weiner WJ. Practice parameter: neuroprotective strategies and alternative therapies for Parkinson disease (an evidence-based review): report of the Quality Standards Subcommittee of the American Academy of Neurology. Neurology. 2006;66(7): 976–82.
21. Herd CP, Tomlinson CL, Deane KH, Brady MC, Smith CH, Sackley CM, Clarke CE. Speech and language therapy versus placebo or no intervention for speech problems in Parkinson's disease. Cochrane Database Syst Rev 2012; (8): CD002812.
22. Kennedy R, Mittal D, O'Jile J. Electroconvulsive therapy in movement disorders: an update. J Neuropsychiatry Clin Neurosci. 2003;15(4):407–21.
23. Popeo D, Kellner CH. ECT for Parkinson's disease. Med Hypotheses. 2009;73(4):468–9.
24. Fochtmann L. A mechanism for the efficacy of ECT in Parkinson's disease. Convuls Ther. 1988;4(4):321–7.
25. Wu AD, Fregni F, Simon DK, Deblieck C, Pascual-Leone A. Noninvasive brain stimulation for Parkinson's disease and dystonia. Neurotherapeutics. 2008;5(2):345–61.

26. Elahi B, Chen R. Effect of transcranial magnetic stimulation on Parkinson motor function – systematic review of controlled clinical trials. Mov Disord. 2009;24(3):357–63.
27. Seppi K, Weintraub D, Coelho M, Perez-Lloret S, Fox SH, Katzenschlager R, Hametner EM, Poewe W, Rascol O, Goetz CG, Sampaio C. The movement disorder society evidence-based medicine review update: treatments for the non-motor symptoms of Parkinson's disease. Mov Disord. 2011;26 Suppl 3:S42–80.
28. Wassermann EM. Risk and safety of repetitive transcranial magnetic stimulation: report and suggested guidelines from the International Workshop on the Safety of Repetitive Transcranial Magnetic Stimulation, June 5-7, 1996. Electroencephalogr Clin Neurophysiol. 1998;108(1):1–16.
29. Belmaker B, Fitzgerald P, George MS, Lisanby SH, Pascual-Leone A, Schlaepfer TE, Wassermann E. Managing the risks of repetitive transcranial stimulation. CNS Spectr. 2003;8(7):489.
30. Machii K, Cohen D, Ramos-Estebanez C, Pascual-Leone A. Safety of rTMS to non-motor cortical areas in healthy participants and patients. Clin Neurophysiol. 2006;117(2):455–71.
31. Fregni F, Boggio PS, Santos MC, Lima M, Vieira AL, Rigonatti SP, Silva MT, Barbosa ER, Nitsche MA, Pascual-Leone A. Noninvasive cortical stimulation with transcranial direct current stimulation in Parkinson's disease. Mov Disord. 2006;21(10): 1693–702.
32. Benninger DH, Lomarev M, Lopez G, Wassermann EM, Li X, Considine E, Hallett M. Transcranial direct current stimulation for the treatment of Parkinson's disease. J Neurol Neurosurg Psychiatry. 2010;81(10):1105–11.
33. Shill HA, Obradov S, Katsnelson Y, Pizinger R. A randomized, double-blind trial of transcranial electrostimulation in early Parkinson's disease. Mov Disord. 2011;26(8):1477–80.
34. Shipton EA. Movement disorders and neuromodulation. Neurol Res Int. 2012;2012:309431.
35. Okun MS. Deep-brain stimulation for Parkinson's disease. N Engl J Med. 2012;367(16):1529–38.
36. Lee KH, Chang SY, Roberts DW, Kim U. Neurotransmitter release from high-frequency stimulation of the subthalamic nucleus. J Neurosurg. 2004;101(3):511–7.
37. Vedam-Mai V, van Battum EY, Kamphuis W, Feenstra MG, Denys D, Reynolds BA, Okun MS, Hol EM. Deep brain stimulation and the role of astrocytes. Mol Psychiatry. 2012;17(2): 124–31. 115.
38. Deuschl G, Schade-Brittinger C, Krack P, Volkmann J, Schafer H, Botzel K, Daniels C, Deutschlander A, Dillmann U, Eisner W, Gruber D, Hamel W, Herzog J, Hilker R, Klebe S, Kloss M, Koy J, Krause M, Kupsch A, Lorenz D, Lorenzl S, Mehdorn HM, Moringlane JR, Oertel W, Pinsker MO, Reichmann H, Reuss A, Schneider GH, Schnitzler A, Steude U, Sturm V, Timmermann L, Tronnier V, Trottenberg T, Wojtecki L, Wolf E, Poewe W, Voges J. A randomized trial of deep-brain stimulation for Parkinson's disease. N Engl J Med. 2006;355(9):896–908.
39. Williams A, Gill S, Varma T, Jenkinson C, Quinn N, Mitchell R, Scott R, Ives N, Rick C, Daniels J, Patel S, Wheatley K. Deep brain stimulation plus best medical therapy versus best medical therapy alone for advanced Parkinson's disease (PD SURG trial): a randomised, open-label trial. Lancet Neurol. 2010;9(6):581–91.
40. Weaver FM, Follett K, Stern M, Hur K, Harris C, Marks Jr WJ, Rothlind J, Sagher O, Reda D, Moy CS, Pahwa R, Burchiel K, Hogarth P, Lai EC, Duda JE, Holloway K, Samii A, Horn S, Bronstein J, Stoner G, Heemskerk J, Huang GD. Bilateral deep brain stimulation vs best medical therapy for patients with advanced Parkinson disease: a randomized controlled trial. JAMA. 2009;301(1):63–73.
41. Okun MS, Fernandez HH, Wu SS, Kirsch-Darrow L, Bowers D, Bova F, Suelter M, Jacobson CET, Wang X, Gordon Jr CW, Zeilman P, Romrell J, Martin P, Ward H, Rodriguez RL, Foote KD. Cognition and mood in Parkinson's disease in subthalamic nucleus versus globus pallidus interna deep brain stimulation: the COMPARE trial. Ann Neurol. 2009;65(5):586–95.
42. Zrinzo L, Foltynie T, Limousin P, Hariz MI. Reducing hemorrhagic complications in functional neurosurgery: a large case series and systematic literature review. J Neurosurg. 2012;116 (1): 84–94.
43. Coley E, Farhadi R, Lewis S, Whittle IR. The incidence of seizures following Deep Brain Stimulating electrode implantation for movement disorders, pain and psychiatric conditions. Br J Neurosurg. 2009;23(2):179–83.
44. Falowski S, Ooi YC, Smith A, Verhargen Metman L, Bakay RA. An evaluation of hardware and surgical complications with deep brain stimulation based on diagnosis and lead location. Stereotact Funct Neurosurg. 2012;90(3):173–80.
45. Breakefield XO, Blood AJ, Li Y, Hallett M, Hanson PI, Standaert DG. The pathophysiological basis of dystonias. Nat Rev Neurosci. 2008;9(3):222–34.
46. Jankovic J. Treatment of hyperkinetic movement disorders. Lancet Neurol. 2009;8(9):844–56.
47. Jankovic J. Treatment of dystonia. In: Watts RL, Koller WC, editors. Movement disorders: neurologic principles and practice. New York, NY: McGraw-Hill Companies, Inc.; 2004. p. 247–71.
48. Burke RE, Fahn S, Marsden CD. Torsion dystonia: a double-blind, prospective trial of high-dosage trihexyphenidyl. Neurology. 1986;36(2):160–4.
49. Simpson DM, Blitzer A, Brashear A, Comella C, Dubinsky R, Hallett M, Jankovic J, Karp B, Ludlow CL, Miyasaki JM, Naumann M, So Y. Assessment: botulinum neurotoxin for the treatment of movement disorders (an evidence-based review): report of the Therapeutics and Technology Assessment Subcommittee of the American Academy of Neurology. Neurology. 2008;70(19):1699–706.
50. Delnooz CC, van de Warrenburg BP. Current and future medical treatment in primary dystonia. Ther Adv Neurol Disord. 2012;5 (4):221–40.
51. Murase N, Rothwell JC, Kaji R, Urushihara R, Nakamura K, Murayama N, Igasaki T, Sakata-Igasaki M, Mima T, Ikeda A, Shibasaki H. Subthreshold low-frequency repetitive transcranial magnetic stimulation over the premotor cortex modulates writer's cramp. Brain. 2005;128(Pt 1):104–15.
52. Borich M, Arora S, Kimberley TJ. Lasting effects of repeated rTMS application in focal hand dystonia. Restor Neurol Neurosci. 2009;27(1):55–65.
53. Siebner HR, Tormos JM, Ceballos-Baumann AO, Auer C, Catala MD, Conrad B, Pascual-Leone A. Low-frequency repetitive transcranial magnetic stimulation of the motor cortex in writer's cramp. Neurology. 1999;52(3):529–37.
54. Allam N, Brasil-Neto JP, Brandao P, Weiler F, Barros Filho J, Tomaz C. Relief of primary cervical dystonia symptoms by low frequency transcranial magnetic stimulation of the premotor cortex: case report. Arquivos De Neuro-Psiquiatria. 2007;65(3A): 697–9.
55. Havrankova P, Jech R, Walker ND, Operto G, Tauchmanova J, Vymazal J, Dusek P, Hromcik M, Ruzicka E. Repetitive TMS of the somatosensory cortex improves writer's cramp and enhances cortical activity. Neuro Endocrinol Lett. 2010;31(1):73–86.
56. Benninger DH, Lomarev M, Lopez G, Pal N, Luckenbaugh DA, Hallett M. Transcranial direct current stimulation for the treatment of focal hand dystonia. Mov Disord. 2011;26(9):1698–702.
57. Buttkus F, Weidenmuller M, Schneider S, Jabusch HC, Nitsche MA, Paulus W, Altenmuller E. Failure of cathodal direct current stimulation to improve fine motor control in musician's dystonia. Mov Disord. 2010;25(3):389–94.
58. Buttkus F, Baur V, Jabusch HC, de la Cruz Gomez-Pellin M, Paulus W, Nitsche MA, Altenmuller E. Single-session tDCS-supported retraining does not improve fine motor control in musician's dystonia. Restor Neurol Neurosci. 2011;29(2):85–90.

59. Kupsch A, Benecke R, Muller J, Trottenberg T, Schneider GH, Poewe W, Eisner W, Wolters A, Muller JU, Deuschl G, Pinsker MO, Skogseid IM, Roeste GK, Vollmer-Haase J, Brentrup A, Krause M, Tronnier V, Schnitzler A, Voges J, Nikkhah G, Vesper J, Naumann M, Volkmann J. Pallidal deep-brain stimulation in primary generalized or segmental dystonia. N Engl J Med. 2006;355(19):1978–90.
60. Vidailhet M, Vercueil L, Houeto JL, Krystkowiak P, Benabid AL, Cornu P, Lagrange C, Tezenas du Montcel S, Dormont D, Grand S, Blond S, Detante O, Pillon B, Ardouin C, Agid Y, Destee A, Pollak P. Bilateral deep-brain stimulation of the globus pallidus in primary generalized dystonia. N Engl J Med. 2005;352(5):459–67.
61. Kiss ZH, Doig-Beyaert K, Eliasziw M, Tsui J, Haffenden A, Suchowersky O. The Canadian multicentre study of deep brain stimulation for cervical dystonia. Brain. 2007;130(Pt 11): 2879–86.
62. Reese R, Gruber D, Schoenecker T, Bazner H, Blahak C, Capelle HH, Falk D, Herzog J, Pinsker MO, Schneider GH, Schrader C, Deuschl G, Mehdorn HM, Kupsch A, Volkmann J, Krauss JK. Long-term clinical outcome in Meige syndrome treated with internal pallidum deep brain stimulation. Mov Disord. 2011;26 (4):691–8.
63. Ostrem JL, Marks Jr WJ, Volz MM, Heath SL, Starr PA. Pallidal deep brain stimulation in patients with cranial-cervical dystonia (Meige syndrome). Mov Disord. 2007;22(13):1885–91.
64. Ghang JY, Lee MK, Jun SM, Ghang CG. Outcome of pallidal deep brain stimulation in Meige syndrome. J Kr Neurosurg Soc. 2010;48(2):134–8.
65. Ostrem JL, Racine CA, Glass GA, Grace JK, Volz MM, Heath SL, Starr PA. Subthalamic nucleus deep brain stimulation in primary cervical dystonia. Neurology. 2011;76(10):870–8.
66. Pahapill PA, O'Connell B. Long-term follow-up study of chronic deep brain stimulation of the subthalamic nucleus for cervical dystonia. Neuromodulation. 2010;13(1):26–30.
67. Allert N, Kelm D, Blahak C, Capelle HH, Krauss JK. Stuttering induced by thalamic deep brain stimulation for dystonia. J Neural Transm. 2010;117(5):617–20.
68. Vercueil L, Pollak P, Fraix V, Caputo E, Moro E, Benazzouz A, Xie J, Koudsie A, Benabid AL. Deep brain stimulation in the treatment of severe dystonia. J Neurol. 2001;248(8):695–700.
69. Jankovic J. Essential tremor: a heterogenous disorder. Mov Disord. 2002;17(4):638–44.
70. Bain P, Brin M, Deuschl G, Elble R, Jankovic J, Findley L, Koller WC, Pahwa R. Criteria for the diagnosis of essential tremor. Neurology. 2000;54(11 Suppl 4):S7.
71. Chen R. Repetitive transcranial magnetic stimulation as a treatment for essential tremor? Clin Neurophysiol. 2012;123(5):850–1.
72. Zesiewicz TA, Elble RJ, Louis ED, Gronseth GS, Ondo WG, Dewey Jr RB, Okun MS, Sullivan KL, Weiner WJ. Evidence-based guideline update: treatment of essential tremor: report of the Quality Standards subcommittee of the American Academy of Neurology. Neurology. 2011;77(19):1752–5.
73. Gironell A, Kulisevsky J, Barbanoj M, Lopez-Villegas D, Hernandez G, Pascual-Sedano B. A randomized placebo-controlled comparative trial of gabapentin and propranolol in essential tremor. Arch Neurol. 1999;56(4):475–80.
74. Kushner SA, Prudic J, Louis ED. Transient improvement of essential tremor during electroconvulsive therapy. J ECT. 2007;23(2):99–102.
75. Hellriegel H, Schulz EM, Siebner HR, Deuschl G, Raethjen JH. Continuous theta-burst stimulation of the primary motor cortex in essential tremor. Clin Neurophysiol. 2012;123(5):1010–5.
76. Popa T, Russo M, Vidailhet M, Roze E, Lehericy S, Bonnet C, Apartis E, Legrand AP, Marais L, Meunier S, Gallea C. Cerebellar rTMS stimulation may induce prolonged clinical benefits in essential tremor, and subjacent changes in functional connectivity: an open label trial. Brain Stimul. 2013;6(2):175–9.
77. Gironell A, Kulisevsky J, Lorenzo J, Barbanoj M, Pascual-Sedano B, Otermin P. Transcranial magnetic stimulation of the cerebellum in essential tremor: a controlled study. Arch Neurol. 2002;59 (3):413–7.
78. Flora ED, Perera CL, Cameron AL, Maddern GJ. Deep brain stimulation for essential tremor: a systematic review. Mov Disord. 2010;25(11):1550–9.
79. Koller W, Pahwa R, Busenbark K, Hubble J, Wilkinson S, Lang A, Tuite P, Sime E, Lazano A, Hauser R, Malapira T, Smith D, Tarsy D, Miyawaki E, Norregaard T, Kormos T, Olanow CW. High-frequency unilateral thalamic stimulation in the treatment of essential and Parkinsonian tremor. Ann Neurol. 1997;42(3): 292–9.
80. Ondo W, Almaguer M, Jankovic J, Simpson RK. Thalamic deep brain stimulation: comparison between unilateral and bilateral placement. Arch Neurol. 2001;58(2):218–22.
81. Carpenter MA, Pahwa R, Miyawaki KL, Wilkinson SB, Searl JP, Koller WC. Reduction in voice tremor under thalamic stimulation. Neurology. 1998;50(3):796–8.
82. Taha JM, Janszen MA, Favre J. Thalamic deep brain stimulation for the treatment of head, voice, and bilateral limb tremor. J Neurosurg. 1999;91(1):68–72.
83. Limousin P, Speelman JD, Gielen F, Janssens M. Multicentre European study of thalamic stimulation in Parkinsonian and essential tremor. J Neurol Neurosurg Psychiatry. 1999;66(3):289–96.
84. Ondo W, Jankovic J, Schwartz K, Almaguer M, Simpson RK. Unilateral thalamic deep brain stimulation for refractory essential tremor and Parkinson's disease tremor. Neurology. 1998;51(4): 1063–9.
85. Juncos J. Pathophysiology and differential diagnosis of tics. In: Watts RL, Koller WC, editors. Movement disorders: neurologic principles and practice. New York, NY: McGraw-Hill Companies, Inc.; 2004. p. 693–704.
86. Pringsheim T, Marras C. Pimozide for tics in Tourette's syndrome. Cochrane Database Syst Rev 2009; (2): CD006996.
87. Kenney C, Jankovic J. Tetrabenazine in the treatment of hyperkinetic movement disorders. Expert Rev Neurother. 2006;6(1):7–17.
88. Anca MH, Giladi N, Korczyn AD. Ropinirole in Gilles de la Tourette syndrome. Neurology. 2004;62(9):1626–7.
89. Jankovic J, Jimenez-Shahed J, Brown LW. A randomised, double-blind, placebo-controlled study of topiramate in the treatment of Tourette syndrome. J Neurol Neurosurg Psychiatry. 2010;81(1): 70–3.
90. Marras C, Andrews D, Sime E, Lang AE. Botulinum toxin for simple motor tics: a randomized, double-blind, controlled clinical trial. Neurology. 2001;56(5):605–10.
91. Bloch MH. Emerging treatments for Tourette's disorder. Curr Psychiatry Rep. 2008;10(4):323–30.
92. Kwon HJ, Lim WS, Lim MH, Lee SJ, Hyun JK, Chae JH, Paik KC. 1-Hz low frequency repetitive transcranial magnetic stimulation in children with Tourette's syndrome. Neurosci Lett. 2011;492(1):1–4.
93. Munchau A, Bloem BR, Thilo KV, Trimble MR, Rothwell JC, Robertson MM. Repetitive transcranial magnetic stimulation for Tourette syndrome. Neurology. 2002;59(11):1789–91.
94. Orth M, Kirby R, Richardson MP, Snijders AH, Rothwell JC, Trimble MR, Robertson MM, Munchau A. Subthreshold rTMS over pre-motor cortex has no effect on tics in patients with Gilles de la Tourette syndrome. Clin Neurophysiol. 2005;116(4): 764–8.
95. Galvez-Jimenez N. Tics and Tourette syndrome: an adult perspective. Cleve Clin J Med. 2012;79 Suppl 2:S35–9.
96. Okun MS, Foote KD, Wu SS, Ward HE, Bowers D, Rodriguez RL, Malaty IA, Goodman WK, Gilbert DM, Walker HC, Mink JW, Merritt S, Morishita T, Sanchez JC. A trial of scheduled deep brain stimulation for Tourette syndrome: moving away from continuous

deep brain stimulation paradigms. Arch Neurol. 2012;70(1): 85–94.
97. Porta M, Servello D, Zanaboni C, Anasetti F, Menghetti C, Sassi M, Robertson MM. Deep brain stimulation for treatment of refractory Tourette syndrome: long-term follow-up. Acta Neurochir. 2012;154(11):2029–41.
98. Fj M. Clinical features and treatment of Huntington's disease. In: Watts RL, Koller WC, editors. Movement disorders: neurologic principles and practice. New York, NY: McGraw-Hill Companies, Inc.; 2004. p. 589–601.
99. Mestre T, Ferreira J, Coelho MM, Rosa M, Sampaio C. Therapeutic interventions for symptomatic treatment in Huntington's disease. Cochrane Database Syst Rev 2009; (3): CD006456.
100. Beale MD, Kellner CH, Gurecki P, Pritchett JT. ECT for the treatment of Huntington's disease: a case study. Convuls Ther. 1997;13(2):108–12.
101. Lee MS, Marsden CD. Movement disorders following lesions of the thalamus or subthalamic region. Mov Disord. 1994;9(5): 493–507.
102. Di Lazzaro V, Dileone M, Pilato F, Contarino MF, Musumeci G, Bentivoglio AR, Tonali PA, Rothwell JC. Repetitive transcranial magnetic stimulation of the motor cortex for hemichorea. J Neurol Neurosurg Psychiatry. 2006;77(9):1095–7.
103. Brusa L, Versace V, Koch G, Bernardi G, Iani C, Stanzione P, Centonze D. Improvement of choreic movements by 1 Hz repetitive transcranial magnetic stimulation in Huntington's disease patients. Ann Neurol. 2005;58(4):655–6.
104. Edwards TC, Zrinzo L, Limousin P, Foltynie T. Deep brain stimulation in the treatment of chorea. Mov Disord. 2012;27(3): 357–63.
105. Kefalopoulou Z, Zrinzo L, Aviles-Olmos I, Bhatia K, Jarman P, Jahanshahi M, Limousin P, Hariz M, Foltynie T. Deep brain stimulation as a treatment for chorea-acanthocytosis. J Neurol. 2013;260(1):303–5.
106. Shin H, Ki CS, Cho AR, Lee JI, Ahn JY, Lee JH, Cho JW. Globus pallidus interna deep brain stimulation improves chorea and functional status in a patient with chorea-acanthocytosis. Stereotact Funct Neurosurg. 2012;90(4):273–7.
107. Spielberger S, Hotter A, Wolf E, Eisner W, Muller J, Poewe W, Seppi K. Deep brain stimulation in Huntington's disease: a 4-year follow-up case report. Mov Disord. 2012;27(6):806–7. author reply 07–8.
108. Schneider JA, Arvanitakis Z, Leurgans SE, Bennett DA. The neuropathology of probable Alzheimer disease and mild cognitive impairment. Ann Neurol. 2009;66(2):200–8.
109. Francis PT, Palmer AM, Snape M, Wilcock GK. The cholinergic hypothesis of Alzheimer's disease: a review of progress. J Neurol Neurosurg Psychiatry. 1999;66(2):137–47.
110. Esiri MM. The basis for behavioural disturbances in dementia. J Neurol Neurosurg Psychiatry. 1996;61(2):127–30.
111. Stern Y. What is cognitive reserve? Theory and research application of the reserve concept. J Int Neuropsychol Soc. 2002;8(3): 448–60.
112. Stern Y. Cognitive reserve and Alzheimer disease. Alzheimer Dis Assoc Disord. 2006;20(3 Suppl 2):S69–74.
113. Palop JJ, Chin J, Mucke L. A network dysfunction perspective on neurodegenerative diseases. Nature. 2006;443(7113):768–73.
114. Desmurget M, Bonnetblanc F, Duffau H. Contrasting acute and slow-growing lesions: a new door to brain plasticity. Brain. 2007;130(Pt 4):898–914.
115. DeLaGarza VW. Pharmacologic treatment of Alzheimer's disease: an update. Am Fam Physician. 2003;68(7):1365–72.
116. Feldman H, Gauthier S, Hecker J, Vellas B, Subbiah P, Whalen E. A 24-week, randomized, double-blind study of donepezil in moderate to severe Alzheimer's disease. Neurology. 2001;57(4):613–20.
117. Gaspar D, Samarasinghe LA. ECT in psychogeriatric practice – a study of risk factors, indications and outcome. Compr Psychiatry. 1982;23(2):170–5.
118. Hausner L, Damian M, Sartorius A, Frolich L. Efficacy and cognitive side effects of electroconvulsive therapy (ECT) in depressed elderly inpatients with coexisting mild cognitive impairment or dementia. J Clin Psychiatry. 2011;72(1):91–7.
119. Nelson JP, Rosenberg DR. ECT treatment of demented elderly patients with major depression: a retrospective study of efficacy and safety. Convuls Ther. 1991;7(3):157–65.
120. Guse B, Falkai P, Wobrock T. Cognitive effects of high-frequency repetitive transcranial magnetic stimulation: a systematic review. J Neural Transm. 2010;117(1):105–22.
121. Sole-Padulles C, Bartres-Faz D, Junque C, Clemente IC, Molinuevo JL, Bargallo N, Sanchez-Aldeguer J, Bosch B, Falcon C, Valls-Sole J. Repetitive transcranial magnetic stimulation effects on brain function and cognition among elders with memory dysfunction. A randomized sham-controlled study. Cereb Cortex. 2006;16(10):1487–93.
122. Cotelli M, Manenti R, Cappa SF, Geroldi C, Zanetti O, Rossini PM, Miniussi C. Effect of transcranial magnetic stimulation on action naming in patients with Alzheimer disease. Arch Neurol. 2006;63(11):1602–4.
123. Cotelli M, Manenti R, Cappa SF, Zanetti O, Miniussi C. Transcranial magnetic stimulation improves naming in Alzheimer disease patients at different stages of cognitive decline. Eur J Neurol. 2008;15(12):1286–92.
124. Cotelli M, Calabria M, Manenti R, Rosini S, Zanetti O, Cappa SF, Miniussi C. Improved language performance in Alzheimer disease following brain stimulation. J Neurol Neurosurg Psychiatry. 2011;82(7):794–7.
125. Nardone R, Bergmann J, Christova M, Caleri F, Tezzon F, Ladurner G, Trinka E, Golaszewski S. Effect of transcranial brain stimulation for the treatment of Alzheimer disease: a review. Int J Alzheimers Dis. 2012;2012:687909.
126. Bentwich J, Dobronevsky E, Aichenbaum S, Shorer R, Peretz R, Khaigrekht M, Marton RG, Rabey JM. Beneficial effect of repetitive transcranial magnetic stimulation combined with cognitive training for the treatment of Alzheimer's disease: a proof of concept study. J Neural Transm. 2011;118(3):463–71.
127. Fernandez A, Maestu F, Amo C, Gil P, Fehr T, Wienbruch C, Rockstroh B, Elbert T, Ortiz T. Focal temporoparietal slow activity in Alzheimer's disease revealed by magnetoencephalography. Biol Psychiatry. 2002;52(7):764–70.
128. Ardolino G, Bossi B, Barbieri S, Priori A. Non-synaptic mechanisms underlie the after-effects of cathodal transcutaneous direct current stimulation of the human brain. J Physiol. 2005;568 (Pt 2):653–63.
129. Ferrucci R, Mameli F, Guidi I, Mrakic-Sposta S, Vergari M, Marceglia S, Cogiamanian F, Barbieri S, Scarpini E, Priori A. Transcranial direct current stimulation improves recognition memory in Alzheimer disease. Neurology. 2008;71(7):493–8.
130. Boggio PS, Valasek CA, Campanha C, Giglio AC, Baptista NI, Lapenta OM, Fregni F. Non-invasive brain stimulation to assess and modulate neuroplasticity in Alzheimer's disease. Neuropsychol Rehabil. 2011;21(5):703–16.
131. Hamani C, McAndrews MP, Cohn M, Oh M, Zumsteg D, Shapiro CM, Wennberg RA, Lozano AM. Memory enhancement induced by hypothalamic/fornix deep brain stimulation. Ann Neurol. 2008;63(1):119–23.
132. Laxton AW, Tang-Wai DF, McAndrews MP, Zumsteg D, Wennberg R, Keren R, Wherrett J, Naglie G, Hamani C, Smith GS, Lozano AM. A phase I trial of deep brain stimulation of memory circuits in Alzheimer's disease. Ann Neurol. 2010;68 (4):521–34.

133. Lyons MK. Deep brain stimulation: current and future clinical applications. Mayo Clin Proc. 2011;86(7):662–72.
134. Moore DJ, Masliah E, Rippeth JD, Gonzalez R, Carey CL, Cherner M, Ellis RJ, Achim CL, Marcotte TD, Heaton RK, Grant I. Cortical and subcortical neurodegeneration is associated with HIV neurocognitive impairment. AIDS. 2006;20(6):879–87.
135. Navia BA, Dafni U, Simpson D, Tucker T, Singer E, McArthur JC, Yiannoutsos C, Zaborski L, Lipton SA. A phase I/II trial of nimodipine for HIV-related neurologic complications. Neurology. 1998;51(1):221–8.
136. Nath A, Geiger J. Neurobiological aspects of human immunodeficiency virus infection: neurotoxic mechanisms. Prog Neurobiol. 1998;54(1):19–33.
137. Masliah E, Ge N, Achim CL, DeTeresa R, Wiley CA. Patterns of neurodegeneration in HIV encephalitis. J NeuroAIDS. 1996;1 (1):161–73.
138. Sa MJ, Madeira MD, Ruela C, Volk B, Mota-Miranda A, Paula-Barbosa MM. Dendritic changes in the hippocampal formation of AIDS patients: a quantitative Golgi study. Acta Neuropathol. 2004;107(2):97–110.
139. Portegies P, de Gans J, Lange JM, Derix MM, Speelman H, Bakker M, Danner SA, Goudsmit J. Declining incidence of AIDS dementia complex after introduction of zidovudine treatment. BMJ. 1989;299(6703):819–21.
140. Cinque P, Vago L, Brytting M, Castagna A, Accordini A, Sundqvist VA, Zanchetta N, Monforte AD, Wahren B, Lazzarin A, et al. Cytomegalovirus infection of the central nervous system in patients with AIDS: diagnosis by DNA amplification from cerebrospinal fluid. J Infect Dis. 1992;166(6):1408–11.
141. Sacktor N, McArthur J. Prospects for therapy of HIV-associated neurologic diseases. J Neurovirol. 1997;3(2):89–101.
142. Dewhurst S, Gelbard HA, Fine SM. Neuropathogenesis of AIDS. Mol Med Today. 1996;2(1):16–23.
143. Fregni F, Boggio PS, Nitsche MA, Marcolin MA, Rigonatti SP, Pascual-Leone A. Treatment of major depression with transcranial direct current stimulation. Bipolar Disord. 2006;8(2):203–4.
144. Boggio PS, Rigonatti SP, Ribeiro RB, Myczkowski ML, Nitsche MA, Pascual-Leone A, Fregni F. A randomized, double-blind clinical trial on the efficacy of cortical direct current stimulation for the treatment of major depression. Int J Neuropsychopharmacol. 2008;11(2):249–54.
145. Adams Jr HP, Bendixen BH, Kappelle LJ, Biller J, Love BB, Gordon DL, Marsh 3rd EE. Classification of subtype of acute ischemic stroke. Definitions for use in a multicenter clinical trial. TOAST. Trial of Org 10172 in Acute Stroke Treatment. Stroke. 1993;24(1):35–41.
146. Bamford J, Sandercock P, Dennis M, Burn J, Warlow C. Classification and natural history of clinically identifiable subtypes of cerebral infarction. Lancet. 1991;337(8756):1521–6.
147. Hoyert DL, Kochanek KD, Murphy SL. Deaths: final data for 1997. National vital statistics reports. Hyattsville, MD: National Center for Health Statistics; 1999.
148. Association AH. Heart and stroke statistical update. Dallas, TX: American Heart Association; 2008.
149. Langhorne P, Bernhardt J, Kwakkel G. Stroke rehabilitation. Lancet. 2011;377(9778):1693–702.
150. Langhorne P, Sandercock P, Prasad K. Evidence-based practice for stroke. Lancet Neurol. 2009;8(4):308–9.
151. Paolucci S, Antonucci G, Grasso MG, Bragoni M, Coiro P, De Angelis D, Fusco FR, Morelli D, Venturiero V, Troisi E, Pratesi L. Functional outcome of ischemic and hemorrhagic stroke patients after inpatient rehabilitation: a matched comparison. Stroke. 2003;34(12):2861–5.
152. Maulden SA, Gassaway J, Horn SD, Smout RJ, DeJong G. Timing of initiation of rehabilitation after stroke. Arch Phys Med Rehabil. 2005;86(12 Suppl 2):S34–40.
153. Johansson BB. Brain plasticity and stroke rehabilitation. The Willis lecture. Stroke. 2000;31(1):223–30.
154. Calautti C, Baron JC. Functional neuroimaging studies of motor recovery after stroke in adults: a review. Stroke. 2003;34(6): 1553–66.
155. Ward NS. Plasticity and the functional reorganization of the human brain. Int J Psychophysiol. 2005;58(2–3):158–61.
156. Pascual-Leone A, Amedi A, Fregni F, Merabet LB. The plastic human brain cortex. Annu Rev Neurosci. 2005;28:377–401.
157. Hikosaka O, Nakamura K, Sakai K, Nakahara H. Central mechanisms of motor skill learning. Curr Opin Neurobiol. 2002;12(2):217–22.
158. Hiscock A, Miller S, Rothwell J, Tallis RC, Pomeroy VM. Informing dose-finding studies of repetitive transcranial magnetic stimulation to enhance motor function: a qualitative systematic review. Neurorehabil Neural Repair. 2008;22(3):228–49.
159. Schonfeldt-Lecuona C, Cardenas-Morales L, Freudenmann RW, Kammer T, Herwig U. Transcranial magnetic stimulation in depression – lessons from the multicentre trials. Restor Neurol Neurosci. 2010;28(4):569–76.
160. Thom T, Haase N, Rosamond W, Howard VJ, Rumsfeld J, Manolio T, Zheng ZJ, Flegal K, O'Donnell C, Kittner S, Lloyd-Jones D, Goff Jr DC, Hong Y, Adams R, Friday G, Furie K, Gorelick P, Kissela B, Marler J, Meigs J, Roger V, Sidney S, Sorlie P, Steinberger J, Wasserthiel-Smoller S, Wilson M, Wolf P. Heart disease and stroke statistics – 2006 update: a report from the American Heart Association Statistics Committee and Stroke Statistics Subcommittee. Circulation. 2006;113(6):e85–151.
161. O'Dell MW, Lin CC, Harrison V. Stroke rehabilitation: strategies to enhance motor recovery. Annu Rev Med. 2009;60:55–68.
162. Wolf SL, Winstein CJ, Miller JP, Thompson PA, Taub E, Uswatte G, Morris D, Blanton S, Nichols-Larsen D, Clark PC. Retention of upper limb function in stroke survivors who have received constraint-induced movement therapy: the EXCITE randomised trial. Lancet Neurol. 2008;7(1):33–40.
163. Wolf SL, Winstein CJ, Miller JP, Taub E, Uswatte G, Morris D, Giuliani C, Light KE, Nichols-Larsen D. Effect of constraint-induced movement therapy on upper extremity function 3 to 9 months after stroke: the EXCITE randomized clinical trial. JAMA. 2006;296(17):2095–104.
164. Martinsson L, Hardemark H, Eksborg S. Amphetamines for improving recovery after stroke. Cochrane Database Syst Rev 2007; (1): CD002090.
165. Hummel F, Cohen LG. Improvement of motor function with noninvasive cortical stimulation in a patient with chronic stroke. Neurorehabil Neural Repair. 2005;19(1):14–9.
166. Nowak DA, Grefkes C, Ameli M, Fink GR. Interhemispheric competition after stroke: brain stimulation to enhance recovery of function of the affected hand. Neurorehabil Neural Repair. 2009;23(7):641–56.
167. Hummel FC, Cohen LG. Non-invasive brain stimulation: a new strategy to improve neurorehabilitation after stroke? Lancet Neurol. 2006;5(8):708–12.
168. Murase N, Duque J, Mazzocchio R, Cohen LG. Influence of interhemispheric interactions on motor function in chronic stroke. Ann Neurol. 2004;55(3):400–9.
169. Shin J, Yang EJ, Cho K, Barcenas CL, Kim WJ, Min Y, Paik NJ. Clinical application of repetitive transcranial magnetic stimulation in stroke rehabilitation. Neural Regen Res. 2012;7(8):627–34.
170. Ayache SS, Farhat WH, Zouari HG, Hosseini H, Mylius V, Lefaucheur JP. Stroke rehabilitation using noninvasive cortical stimulation: motor deficit. Expert Rev Neurother. 2012;12(8):949–72.
171. Takeuchi N, Chuma T, Matsuo Y, Watanabe I, Ikoma K. Repetitive transcranial magnetic stimulation of contralesional primary motor cortex improves hand function after stroke. Stroke. 2005;36 (12):2681–6.

172. Fregni F, Boggio PS, Valle AC, Rocha RR, Duarte J, Ferreira MJ, Wagner T, Fecteau S, Rigonatti SP, Riberto M, Freedman SD, Pascual-Leone A. A sham-controlled trial of a 5-day course of repetitive transcranial magnetic stimulation of the unaffected hemisphere in stroke patients. Stroke. 2006;37(8):2115–22.
173. Liepert J, Zittel S, Weiller C. Improvement of dexterity by single session low-frequency repetitive transcranial magnetic stimulation over the contralesional motor cortex in acute stroke: a double-blind placebo-controlled crossover trial. Restor Neurol Neurosci. 2007;25(5–6):461–5.
174. Khedr EM, Ahmed MA, Fathy N, Rothwell JC. Therapeutic trial of repetitive transcranial magnetic stimulation after acute ischemic stroke. Neurology. 2005;65(3):466–8.
175. Khedr EM, Etraby AE, Hemeda M, Nasef AM, Razek AA. Long-term effect of repetitive transcranial magnetic stimulation on motor function recovery after acute ischemic stroke. Acta Neurol Scand. 2010;121(1):30–7.
176. Malcolm MP, Triggs WJ, Light KE, Gonzalez Rothi LJ, Wu S, Reid K, Nadeau SE. Repetitive transcranial magnetic stimulation as an adjunct to constraint-induced therapy: an exploratory randomized controlled trial. Am J Phys Med Rehabil. 2007;86 (9):707–15.
177. Grefkes C, Nowak DA, Wang LE, Dafotakis M, Eickhoff SB, Fink GR. Modulating cortical connectivity in stroke patients by rTMS assessed with fMRI and dynamic causal modeling. Neuroimage. 2010;50(1):233–42.
178. Kakuda W, Abo M, Shimizu M, Sasanuma J, Okamoto T, Yokoi A, Taguchi K, Mitani S, Harashima H, Urushidani N, Urashima M. A multi-center study on low-frequency rTMS combined with intensive occupational therapy for upper limb hemiparesis in post-stroke patients. J Neuroeng Rehabil. 2012;9(1):4.
179. Takeuchi N, Tada T, Toshima M, Matsuo Y, Ikoma K. Repetitive transcranial magnetic stimulation over bilateral hemispheres enhances motor function and training effect of paretic hand in patients after stroke. J Rehabil Med. 2009;41(13):1049–54.
180. Khedr EM, Abdel-Fadeil MR, Farghali A, Qaid M. Role of 1 and 3 Hz repetitive transcranial magnetic stimulation on motor function recovery after acute ischaemic stroke. Eur J Neurol. 2009;16 (12):1323–30.
181. Emara TH, Moustafa RR, Elnahas NM, Elganzoury AM, Abdo TA, Mohamed SA, Eletribi MA. Repetitive transcranial magnetic stimulation at 1Hz and 5Hz produces sustained improvement in motor function and disability after ischaemic stroke. Eur J Neurol. 2010;17(9):1203–9.
182. Huang YZ, Edwards MJ, Rounis E, Bhatia KP, Rothwell JC. Theta burst stimulation of the human motor cortex. Neuron. 2005;45 (2):201–6.
183. Talelli P, Greenwood RJ, Rothwell JC. Exploring Theta Burst Stimulation as an intervention to improve motor recovery in chronic stroke. Clin Neurophysiol. 2007;118(2):333–42.
184. Ackerley SJ, Stinear CM, Barber PA, Byblow WD. Combining theta burst stimulation with training after subcortical stroke. Stroke. 2010;41(7):1568–72.
185. Carey JR, Anderson DC, Gillick BT, Whitford M, Pascual-Leone A. 6-Hz primed low-frequency rTMS to contralesional M1 in two cases with middle cerebral artery stroke. Neurosci Lett. 2010;469 (3):338–42.
186. Kakuda W, Abo M, Kobayashi K, Momosaki R, Yokoi A, Fukuda A, Umemori T. Application of combined 6-Hz primed low-frequency rTMS and intensive occupational therapy for upper limb hemiparesis after stroke. NeuroRehabilitation. 2011;29(4):365–71.
187. Lang N, Siebner HR, Ernst D, Nitsche MA, Paulus W, Lemon RN, Rothwell JC. Preconditioning with transcranial direct current stimulation sensitizes the motor cortex to rapid-rate transcranial magnetic stimulation and controls the direction of after-effects. Biol Psychiatry. 2004;56(9):634–9.
188. Hummel FC, Voller B, Celnik P, Floel A, Giraux P, Gerloff C, Cohen LG. Effects of brain polarization on reaction times and pinch force in chronic stroke. BMC Neurosci. 2006;7:73.
189. Fregni F, Boggio PS, Mansur CG, Wagner T, Ferreira MJ, Lima MC, Rigonatti SP, Marcolin MA, Freedman SD, Nitsche MA, Pascual-Leone A. Transcranial direct current stimulation of the unaffected hemisphere in stroke patients. Neuroreport. 2005;16 (14):1551–5.
190. Boggio PS, Nunes A, Rigonatti SP, Nitsche MA, Pascual-Leone A, Fregni F. Repeated sessions of noninvasive brain DC stimulation is associated with motor function improvement in stroke patients. Restor Neurol Neurosci. 2007;25(2):123–9.
191. Gandiga PC, Hummel FC, Cohen LG. Transcranial DC stimulation (tDCS): a tool for double-blind sham-controlled clinical studies in brain stimulation. Clin Neurophysiol. 2006;117(4):845–50.
192. Reis J, Schambra HM, Cohen LG, Buch ER, Fritsch B, Zarahn E, Celnik PA, Krakauer JW. Noninvasive cortical stimulation enhances motor skill acquisition over multiple days through an effect on consolidation. Proc Natl Acad Sci U S A. 2009;106(5): 1590–5.
193. Kim DY, Lim JY, Kang EK, You DS, Oh MK, Oh BM, Paik NJ. Effect of transcranial direct current stimulation on motor recovery in patients with subacute stroke. Am J Phys Med Rehabil. 2010;89 (11):879–86.
194. Rossi C, Sallustio F, Di Legge S, Stanzione P, Koch G. Transcranial direct current stimulation of the affected hemisphere does not accelerate recovery of acute stroke patients. Eur J Neurol. 2013;20(1):202–4.
195. Kang EK, Paik NJ. Effect of a tDCS electrode montage on implicit motor sequence learning in healthy subjects. Exp Trans Stroke Med. 2011;3(1):4.
196. Vines BW, Cerruti C, Schlaug G. Dual-hemisphere tDCS facilitates greater improvements for healthy subjects' non-dominant hand compared to uni-hemisphere stimulation. BMC Neurosci. 2008;9:103.
197. Lindenberg R, Renga V, Zhu LL, Nair D, Schlaug G. Bihemispheric brain stimulation facilitates motor recovery in chronic stroke patients. Neurology. 2010;75(24):2176–84.
198. Mahmoudi H, Borhani Haghighi A, Petramfar P, Jahanshahi S, Salehi Z, Fregni F. Transcranial direct current stimulation: electrode montage in stroke. Disabil Rehabil. 2011;33(15–16): 1383–8.
199. Conforto AB, Kaelin-Lang A, Cohen LG. Increase in hand muscle strength of stroke patients after somatosensory stimulation. Ann Neurol. 2002;51(1):122–5.
200. Chang CW, Shieh SF, Li CM, Wu WT, Chang KF. Measurement of motor nerve conduction velocity of the sciatic nerve in patients with piriformis syndrome: a magnetic stimulation study. Arch Phys Med Rehabil. 2006;87(10):1371–5.
201. Stefan K, Kunesch E, Cohen LG, Benecke R, Classen J. Induction of plasticity in the human motor cortex by paired associative stimulation. Brain. 2000;123(Pt 3):572–84.
202. Castel-Lacanal E, Marque P, Tardy J, de Boissezon X, Guiraud V, Chollet F, Loubinoux I, Moreau MS. Induction of cortical plastic changes in wrist muscles by paired associative stimulation in the recovery phase of stroke patients. Neurorehabil Neural Repair. 2009;23(4):366–72.
203. Rogers LM, Brown DA, Stinear JW. The effects of paired associative stimulation on knee extensor motor excitability of individuals post-stroke: a pilot study. Clin Neurophysiol. 2011;122(6):1211–8.
204. Uy J, Ridding MC, Hillier S, Thompson PD, Miles TS. Does induction of plastic change in motor cortex improve leg function after stroke? Neurology. 2003;61(7):982–4.
205. Celnik P, Paik NJ, Vandermeeren Y, Dimyan M, Cohen LG. Effects of combined peripheral nerve stimulation and brain

polarization on performance of a motor sequence task after chronic stroke. Stroke. 2009;40(5):1764–71.
206. Plow EB, Carey JR, Nudo RJ, Pascual-Leone A. Invasive cortical stimulation to promote recovery of function after stroke: a critical appraisal. Stroke. 2009;40(5):1926–31.
207. Brown JA, Lutsep HL, Weinand M, Cramer SC. Motor cortex stimulation for the enhancement of recovery from stroke: a prospective, multicenter safety study. Neurosurgery. 2006;58 (3):464–73.
208. Bashir S, Edwards D, Pascual-Leone A. Neuronavigation increases the physiologic and behavioral effects of low-frequency rTMS of primary motor cortex in healthy subjects. Brain Topogr. 2011;24(1):54–64.
209. Kim WJ, Min YS, Yang EJ, Paik NJ. Neuronavigated versus Conventional Repetitive Transcranial Magnetic Stimulation Method for Virtual Lesioning on the Broca's area. Neuromodulation. 2014;17(1):16–21.
210. Cheeran B, Talelli P, Mori F, Koch G, Suppa A, Edwards M, Houlden H, Bhatia K, Greenwood R, Rothwell JC. A common polymorphism in the brain-derived neurotrophic factor gene (BDNF) modulates human cortical plasticity and the response to rTMS. J Physiol. 2008;586(Pt 23):5717–25.
211. Talelli P, Rothwell J. Does brain stimulation after stroke have a future? Curr Opin Neurol. 2006;19(6):543–50.
212. Wagner T, Fregni F, Eden U, Ramos-Estebanez C, Grodzinsky A, Zahn M, Pascual-Leone A. Transcranial magnetic stimulation and stroke: a computer-based human model study. Neuroimage. 2006;30(3):857–70.
213. Kerkhoff G. Spatial hemineglect in humans. Prog Neurobiol. 2001;63(1):1–27.
214. Stone SP, Halligan PW, Greenwood RJ. The incidence of neglect phenomena and related disorders in patients with an acute right or left hemisphere stroke. Age Ageing. 1993;22(1):46–52.
215. Meijer R, Ihnenfeldt DS, de Groot IJ, van Limbeek J, Vermeulen M, de Haan RJ. Prognostic factors for ambulation and activities of daily living in the subacute phase after stroke. A systematic review of the literature. Clin Rehabil. 2003;17(2):119–29.
216. Antonucci G, Guariglia C, Judica A, Magnotti L, Paolucci S, Pizzamiglio L, Zoccolotti P. Effectiveness of neglect rehabilitation in a randomized group study. J Clin Exp Neuropsychol. 1995;17(3):383–9.
217. Kerkhoff G, Schenk T. Rehabilitation of neglect: an update. Neuropsychologia. 2012;50(6):1072–9.
218. Keller I, Lefin-Rank G, Losch J, Kerkhoff G. Combination of pursuit eye movement training with prism adaptation and arm movements in neglect therapy: a pilot study. Neurorehabil Neural Repair. 2009;23(1):58–66.
219. Schindler I, Kerkhoff G, Karnath HO, Keller I, Goldenberg G. Neck muscle vibration induces lasting recovery in spatial neglect. J Neurol Neurosurg Psychiatry. 2002;73(4):412–9.
220. Rode G, Tiliket C, Charlopain P, Boisson D. Postural asymmetry reduction by vestibular caloric stimulation in left hemiparetic patients. Scand J Rehabil Med. 1998;30(1):9–14.
221. Kerkhoff G, Hildebrandt H, Reinhart S, Kardinal M, Dimova V, Utz KS. A long-lasting improvement of tactile extinction after galvanic vestibular stimulation: two Sham-stimulation controlled case studies. Neuropsychologia. 2011;49(2):186–95.
222. Serino A, Barbiani M, Rinaldesi ML, Ladavas E. Effectiveness of prism adaptation in neglect rehabilitation: a controlled trial study. Stroke. 2009;40(4):1392–8.
223. Coulthard E, Singh-Curry V, Husain M. Treatment of attention deficits in neurological disorders. Curr Opin Neurol. 2006;19 (6):613–8.
224. Koch G, Veniero D, Caltagirone C. To the other side of the neglected brain: the hyperexcitability of the left intact hemisphere. Neuroscientist. 2013;19(2):208–17.
225. Mylius V, Ayache SS, Zouari HG, Aoun-Sebaiti M, Farhat WH, Lefaucheur JP. Stroke rehabilitation using noninvasive cortical stimulation: hemispatial neglect. Expert Rev Neurother. 2012;12 (8):983–91.
226. Koch G, Bonni S, Giacobbe V, Bucchi G, Basile B, Lupo F, Versace V, Bozzali M, Caltagirone C. Theta-burst stimulation of the left hemisphere accelerates recovery of hemispatial neglect. Neurology. 2012;78(1):24–30.
227. Oliveri M, Bisiach E, Brighina F, Piazza A, La Bua V, Buffa D, Fierro B. rTMS of the unaffected hemisphere transiently reduces contralesional visuospatial hemineglect. Neurology. 2001;57 (7):1338–40.
228. Brighina F, Bisiach E, Oliveri M, Piazza A, La Bua V, Daniele O, Fierro B. 1 Hz repetitive transcranial magnetic stimulation of the unaffected hemisphere ameliorates contralesional visuospatial neglect in humans. Neurosci Lett. 2003;336(2):131–3.
229. Shindo K, Sugiyama K, Huabao L, Nishijima K, Kondo T, Izumi S. Long-term effect of low-frequency repetitive transcranial magnetic stimulation over the unaffected posterior parietal cortex in patients with unilateral spatial neglect. J Rehabil Med. 2006;38(1): 65–7.
230. Song W, Du B, Xu Q, Hu J, Wang M, Luo Y. Low-frequency transcranial magnetic stimulation for visual spatial neglect: a pilot study. J Rehabil Med. 2009;41(3):162–5.
231. Lim JY, Kang EK, Paik NJ. Repetitive transcranial magnetic stimulation to hemispatial neglect in patients after stroke: an open-label pilot study. J Rehabil Med. 2010;42(5):447–52.
232. Nyffeler T, Cazzoli D, Hess CW, Muri RM. One session of repeated parietal theta burst stimulation trains induces long-lasting improvement of visual neglect. Stroke. 2009;40(8):2791–6.
233. Koch G, Oliveri M, Cheeran B, Ruge D, Lo Gerfo E, Salerno S, Torriero S, Marconi B, Mori F, Driver J, Rothwell JC, Caltagirone C. Hyperexcitability of parietal-motor functional connections in the intact left-hemisphere of patients with neglect. Brain. 2008;131(Pt 12):3147–55.
234. Ko MH, Han SH, Park SH, Seo JH, Kim YH. Improvement of visual scanning after DC brain polarization of parietal cortex in stroke patients with spatial neglect. Neurosci Lett. 2008;448(2):171–4.
235. Sparing R, Thimm M, Hesse MD, Kust J, Karbe H, Fink GR. Bidirectional alterations of interhemispheric parietal balance by non-invasive cortical stimulation. Brain. 2009;132(Pt 11): 3011–20.
236. Benson DF, Ardila A. Aphasia: a clinical perspective. New York, NY: Oxford University Press; 1996.
237. Engelter ST, Gostynski M, Papa S, Frei M, Born C, Ajdacic-Gross V, Gutzwiller F, Lyrer PA. Epidemiology of aphasia attributable to first ischemic stroke: incidence, severity, fluency, etiology, and thrombolysis. Stroke. 2006;37(6):1379–84.
238. Laska AC, Hellblom A, Murray V, Kahan T, Von Arbin M. Aphasia in acute stroke and relation to outcome. J Intern Med. 2001;249(5):413–22.
239. Gialanella B. Aphasia assessment and functional outcome prediction in patients with aphasia after stroke. J Neurol. 2011;258(2): 343–9.
240. Bhogal SK, Teasell R, Speechley M. Intensity of aphasia therapy, impact on recovery. Stroke. 2003;34(4):987–93.
241. Brady MC, Kelly H, Godwin J, Enderby P. Speech and language therapy for aphasia following stroke. Cochrane Database Syst Rev 2012; (5): CD000425.
242. Saur D, Lange R, Baumgaertner A, Schraknepper V, Willmes K, Rijntjes M, Weiller C. Dynamics of language reorganization after stroke. Brain. 2006;129(Pt 6):1371–84.
243. Turkeltaub PE, Messing S, Norise C, Hamilton RH. Are networks for residual language function and recovery consistent across aphasic patients? Neurology. 2011;76(20):1726–34.
244. Mylius V, Zouari HG, Ayache SS, Farhat WH, Lefaucheur JP. Stroke rehabilitation using noninvasive cortical stimulation: aphasia. Expert Rev Neurother. 2012;12(8):973–82.

245. Winhuisen L, Thiel A, Schumacher B, Kessler J, Rudolf J, Haupt WF, Heiss WD. The right inferior frontal gyrus and poststroke aphasia: a follow-up investigation. Stroke. 2007;38 (4):1286–92.
246. Martin PI, Naeser MA, Theoret H, Tormos JM, Nicholas M, Kurland J, Fregni F, Seekins H, Doron K, Pascual-Leone A. Transcranial magnetic stimulation as a complementary treatment for aphasia. Semin Speech Lang. 2004;25(2):181–91.
247. Naeser MA, Martin PI, Nicholas M, Baker EH, Seekins H, Kobayashi M, Theoret H, Fregni F, Maria-Tormos J, Kurland J, Doron KW, Pascual-Leone A. Improved picture naming in chronic aphasia after TMS to part of right Broca's area: an open-protocol study. Brain Lang. 2005;93(1):95–105.
248. Naeser MA, Martin PI, Nicholas M, Baker EH, Seekins H, Helm-Estabrooks N, Cayer-Meade C, Kobayashi M, Theoret H, Fregni F, Tormos JM, Kurland J, Doron KW, Pascual-Leone A. Improved naming after TMS treatments in a chronic, global aphasia patient – case report. Neurocase. 2005;11(3):182–93.
249. Martin PI, Naeser MA, Ho M, Doron KW, Kurland J, Kaplan J, Wang Y, Nicholas M, Baker EH, Alonso M, Fregni F, Pascual-Leone A. Overt naming fMRI pre- and post-TMS: two nonfluent aphasia patients, with and without improved naming post-TMS. Brain Lang. 2009;111(1):20–35.
250. Hamilton RH, Sanders L, Benson J, Faseyitan O, Norise C, Naeser M, Martin P, Coslett HB. Stimulating conversation: enhancement of elicited propositional speech in a patient with chronic non-fluent aphasia following transcranial magnetic stimulation. Brain Lang. 2010;113(1):45–50.
251. Naeser MA, Martin PI, Theoret H, Kobayashi M, Fregni F, Nicholas M, Tormos JM, Steven MS, Baker EH, Pascual-Leone A. TMS suppression of right pars triangularis, but not pars opercularis, improves naming in aphasia. Brain Lang. 2011;119 (3):206–13.
252. Medina J, Norise C, Faseyitan O, Coslett HB, Turkeltaub PE, Hamilton RH. Finding the right words: transcranial magnetic stimulation improves discourse productivity in non-fluent aphasia after stroke. Aphasiology. 2012;26(9):1153–68.
253. Weiduschat N, Thiel A, Rubi-Fessen I, Hartmann A, Kessler J, Merl P, Kracht L, Rommel T, Heiss WD. Effects of repetitive transcranial magnetic stimulation in aphasic stroke: a randomized controlled pilot study. Stroke. 2011;42(2):409–15.
254. Waldowski K, Seniow J, Lesniak M, Iwanski S, Czlonkowska A. Effect of low-frequency repetitive transcranial magnetic stimulation on naming abilities in early-stroke aphasic patients: a prospective, randomized, double-blind sham-controlled study. ScientificWorldJournal. 2012;2012:518568.
255. Szaflarski JP, Vannest J, Wu SW, DiFrancesco MW, Banks C, Gilbert DL. Excitatory repetitive transcranial magnetic stimulation induces improvements in chronic post-stroke aphasia. Med Sci Monit. 2011;17(3):CR132–9.
256. Kakuda W, Abo M, Uruma G, Kaito N, Watanabe M. Low-frequency rTMS with language therapy over a 3-month period for sensory-dominant aphasia: case series of two post-stroke Japanese patients. Brain Inj. 2010;24(9):1113–7.
257. Winhuisen L, Thiel A, Schumacher B, Kessler J, Rudolf J, Haupt WF, Heiss WD. Role of the contralateral inferior frontal gyrus in recovery of language function in poststroke aphasia: a combined repetitive transcranial magnetic stimulation and positron emission tomography study. Stroke. 2005;36(8):1759–63.
258. Kakuda W, Abo M, Kaito N, Watanabe M, Senoo A. Functional MRI-based therapeutic rTMS strategy for aphasic stroke patients: a case series pilot study. Int J Neurosci. 2010;120 (1):60–6.
259. Baker JM, Rorden C, Fridriksson J. Using transcranial direct-current stimulation to treat stroke patients with aphasia. Stroke. 2010;41(6):1229–36.
260. Fridriksson J, Richardson JD, Baker JM, Rorden C. Transcranial direct current stimulation improves naming reaction time in fluent aphasia: a double-blind, sham-controlled study. Stroke. 2011;42 (3):819–21.
261. Monti A, Cogiamanian F, Marceglia S, Ferrucci R, Mameli F, Mrakic-Sposta S, Vergari M, Zago S, Priori A. Improved naming after transcranial direct current stimulation in aphasia. J Neurol Neurosurg Psychiatry. 2008;79(4):451–3.
262. Kang EK, Kim YK, Sohn HM, Cohen LG, Paik NJ. Improved picture naming in aphasia patients treated with cathodal tDCS to inhibit the right Broca's homologue area. Restor Neurol Neurosci. 2011;29(3):141–52.
263. Jung IY, Lim JY, Kang EK, Sohn HM, Paik NJ. The factors associated with good responses to speech therapy combined with transcranial direct current stimulation in post-stroke aphasic patients. Ann Rehab Med. 2011;35(4):460–9.
264. Menke R, Meinzer M, Kugel H, Deppe M, Baumgartner A, Schiffbauer H, Thomas M, Kramer K, Lohmann H, Floel A, Knecht S, Breitenstein C. Imaging short- and long-term training success in chronic aphasia. BMC Neurosci. 2009;10:118.
265. Abo M, Kakuda W, Watanabe M, Morooka A, Kawakami K, Senoo A. Effectiveness of low-frequency rTMS and intensive speech therapy in poststroke patients with aphasia: a pilot study based on evaluation by fMRI in relation to type of aphasia. Eur Neurol. 2012;68(4):199–208.
266. Cherney LR, Erickson RK, Small SL. Epidural cortical stimulation as adjunctive treatment for non-fluent aphasia: preliminary findings. J Neurol Neurosurg Psychiatry. 2010;81(9):1014–21.
267. Balossier A, Etard O, Descat C, Vivien D, Emery E. Epidural electrical stimulation for the treatment of chronic poststroke aphasia: still compulsory 6 years later! Br J Neurosurg. 2013;27(2):246–8.
268. Barer DH. The natural history and functional consequences of dysphagia after hemispheric stroke. J Neurol Neurosurg Psychiatry. 1989;52(2):236–41.
269. Sharma JC, Fletcher S, Vassallo M, Ross I. What influences outcome of stroke – pyrexia or dysphagia? Int J Clin Pract. 2001;55(1):17–20.
270. Martino R, Pron G, Diamant N. Screening for oropharyngeal dysphagia in stroke: insufficient evidence for guidelines. Dysphagia. 2000;15(1):19–30.
271. Geeganage C, Beavan J, Ellender S, Bath PM. Interventions for dysphagia and nutritional support in acute and subacute stroke. Cochrane Database Syst Rev 2012; (10): CD000323.
272. Tippett DC. Clinical challenges in the evaluation and treatment of individuals with poststroke dysphagia. Top Stroke Rehabil. 2011;18(2):120–33.
273. Cecconi E, Di Piero V. Dysphagia – pathophysiology, diagnosis and treatment. Front Neurol Neurosci. 2012;30:86–9.
274. Perez I, Smithard DG, Davies H, Kalra L. Pharmacological treatment of dysphagia in stroke. Dysphagia. 1998;13(1):12–6.
275. Hamdy S, Rothwell JC, Aziz Q, Thompson DG. Organization and reorganization of human swallowing motor cortex: implications for recovery after stroke. Clin Sci. 2000;99(2):151–7.
276. Verin E, Leroi AM. Poststroke dysphagia rehabilitation by repetitive transcranial magnetic stimulation: a noncontrolled pilot study. Dysphagia. 2009;24(2):204–10.
277. Khedr EM, Abo-Elfetoh N, Rothwell JC. Treatment of post-stroke dysphagia with repetitive transcranial magnetic stimulation. Acta Neurol Scand. 2009;119(3):155–61.
278. Khedr EM, Abo-Elfetoh N. Therapeutic role of rTMS on recovery of dysphagia in patients with lateral medullary syndrome and brainstem infarction. J Neurol Neurosurg Psychiatry. 2010;81 (5):495–9.
279. Kumar S, Wagner CW, Frayne C, Zhu L, Selim M, Feng W, Schlaug G. Noninvasive brain stimulation may improve stroke-related dysphagia: a pilot study. Stroke. 2011;42(4):1035–40.

280. Jefferson S, Mistry S, Singh S, Rothwell J, Hamdy S. Characterizing the application of transcranial direct current stimulation in human pharyngeal motor cortex. Am J Physiol Gastrointest Liver Physiol. 2009;297(6):G1035–40.
281. Yang EJ, Baek SR, Shin J, Lim JY, Jang HJ, Kim YK, Paik NJ. Effects of transcranial direct current stimulation (tDCS) on post-stroke dysphagia. Restor Neurol Neurosci. 2012;30(4):303–11.
282. Evers S, Bockermann I, Nyhuis PW. The impact of transcranial magnetic stimulation on cognitive processing: an event-related potential study. Neuroreport. 2001;12(13):2915–8.
283. Topper R, Mottaghy FM, Brugmann M, Noth J, Huber W. Facilitation of picture naming by focal transcranial magnetic stimulation of Wernicke's area. Exp Brain Res. 1998;121(4):371–8.
284. Fitzgerald PB, Benitez J, Daskalakis JZ, Brown TL, Marston NA, de Castella A, Kulkarni J. A double-blind sham-controlled trial of repetitive transcranial magnetic stimulation in the treatment of refractory auditory hallucinations. J Clin Psychopharmacol. 2005;25(4):358–62.
285. Trojano L, Conson M, Maffei R, Grossi D. Categorical and coordinate spatial processing in the imagery domain investigated by rTMS. Neuropsychologia. 2006;44(9):1569–74.
286. Kang EK, Baek MJ, Kim S, Paik NJ. Non-invasive cortical stimulation improves post-stroke attention decline. Restor Neurol Neurosci. 2009;27(6):645–50.
287. Flor H, Elbert T, Knecht S, Wienbruch C, Pantev C, Birbaumer N, Larbig W, Taub E. Phantom-limb pain as a perceptual correlate of cortical reorganization following arm amputation. Nature. 1995;375(6531):482–4.
288. Flor H, Elbert T, Muhlnickel W, Pantev C, Wienbruch C, Taub E. Cortical reorganization and phantom phenomena in congenital and traumatic upper-extremity amputees. Exp Brain Res. 1998;119(2):205–12.
289. Sanes JN, Suner S, Lando JF, Donoghue JP. Rapid reorganization of adult rat motor cortex somatic representation patterns after motor nerve injury. Proc Natl Acad Sci U S A. 1988;85(6):2003–7.
290. Sanes JN, Suner S, Donoghue JP. Dynamic organization of primary motor cortex output to target muscles in adult rats. I. Long-term patterns of reorganization following motor or mixed peripheral nerve lesions. Exp Brain Res. 1990;79(3):479–91.
291. Donoghue JP, Suner S, Sanes JN. Dynamic organization of primary motor cortex output to target muscles in adult rats. II. Rapid reorganization following motor nerve lesions. Exp Brain Res. 1990;79(3):492–503.
292. Brasil-Neto JP, Valls-Sole J, Pascual-Leone A, Cammarota A, Amassian VE, Cracco R, Maccabee P, Cracco J, Hallett M, Cohen LG. Rapid modulation of human cortical motor outputs following ischaemic nerve block. Brain. 1993;116(Pt 3):511–25.
293. Cohen LG, Bandinelli S, Findley TW, Hallett M. Motor reorganization after upper limb amputation in man. A study with focal magnetic stimulation. Brain. 1991;114(Pt 1B):615–27.
294. Pascual-Leone A, Peris M, Tormos JM, Pascual AP, Catala MD. Reorganization of human cortical motor output maps following traumatic forearm amputation. Neuroreport. 1996;7(13):2068–70.
295. Kew JJ, Ridding MC, Rothwell JC, Passingham RE, Leigh PN, Sooriakumaran S, Frackowiak RS, Brooks DJ. Reorganization of cortical blood flow and transcranial magnetic stimulation maps in human subjects after upper limb amputation. J Neurophysiol. 1994;72(5):2517–24.
296. Casale R, Alaa L, Mallick M, Ring H. Phantom limb related phenomena and their rehabilitation after lower limb amputation. Eur J Phys Rehabil Med. 2009;45(4):559–66.
297. Roricht S, Meyer BU, Niehaus L, Brandt SA. Long-term reorganization of motor cortex outputs after arm amputation. Neurology. 1999;53(1):106–11.
298. Schwenkreis P, Witscher K, Janssen F, Dertwinkel R, Zenz M, Malin JP, Tegenthoff M. Changes of cortical excitability in patients with upper limb amputation. Neurosci Lett. 2000;293(2):143–6.
299. Lefaucheur JP, Drouot X, Keravel Y, Nguyen JP. Pain relief induced by repetitive transcranial magnetic stimulation of precentral cortex. Neuroreport. 2001;12(13):2963–5.
300. Lefaucheur JP, Drouot X, Menard-Lefaucheur I, Zerah F, Bendib B, Cesaro P, Keravel Y, Nguyen JP. Neurogenic pain relief by repetitive transcranial magnetic cortical stimulation depends on the origin and the site of pain. J Neurol Neurosurg Psychiatry. 2004;75(4):612–6.
301. Pleger B, Janssen F, Schwenkreis P, Volker B, Maier C, Tegenthoff M. Repetitive transcranial magnetic stimulation of the motor cortex attenuates pain perception in complex regional pain syndrome type I. Neurosci Lett. 2004;356(2):87–90.
302. Topper R, Foltys H, Meister IG, Sparing R, Boroojerdi B. Repetitive transcranial magnetic stimulation of the parietal cortex transiently ameliorates phantom limb pain-like syndrome. Clin Neurophysiol. 2003;114(8):1521–30.
303. Maarrawi J, Peyron R, Mertens P, Costes N, Magnin M, Sindou M, Laurent B, Garcia-Larrea L. Motor cortex stimulation for pain control induces changes in the endogenous opioid system. Neurology. 2007;69(9):827–34.
304. Raij TT, Forss N, Stancak A, Hari R. Modulation of motor-cortex oscillatory activity by painful Adelta- and C-fiber stimuli. Neuroimage. 2004;23(2):569–73.
305. Tsubokawa T, Katayama Y, Yamamoto T, Hirayama T, Koyama S. Chronic motor cortex stimulation for the treatment of central pain. Acta Neurochir Suppl. 1991;52:137–9.
306. Garcia-Larrea L, Peyron R, Mertens P, Gregoire MC, Lavenne F, Le Bars D, Convers P, Mauguiere F, Sindou M, Laurent B. Electrical stimulation of motor cortex for pain control: a combined PET-scan and electrophysiological study. Pain. 1999;83(2):259–73.
307. Peyron R, Laurent B, Garcia-Larrea L. Functional imaging of brain responses to pain. A review and meta-analysis. Clin Neurophysiol. 2000;30(5):263–88.
308. de Andrade DC, Mhalla A, Adam F, Texeira MJ, Bouhassira D. Neuropharmacological basis of rTMS-induced analgesia: the role of endogenous opioids. Pain. 2011;152(2):320–6.
309. Knotkova H, Rosedale M, Strauss SM, Horne J, Soto E, Cruciani RA, Malaspina D, Malamud D. Using transcranial direct current stimulation to treat depression in HIV-infected persons: the outcomes of a feasibility study. Front Psychiatry. 2012;3:59.

Neuromodulation for Addiction

17

Jens Kuhn, Michaela Möller, Doris Lenartz, Christian P. Bührle, and Veerle Visser-Vandewalle

Introduction

The colloquially used term "addiction" denotes a large variety of heterogeneous disorders. It comprises substance-related addictions (as, for instance, to alcohol, nicotine, and opioids; ICD-10: substance-related disorders; DSM-IV: "Mental and Behavioural Disorders due to Psychoactive Substance Use"; DSM-5: "Substance Use Disorder"), but also substance-unrelated disorders like compulsive shopping, media addiction, or pathological gambling. However, in the context of this chapter we will exclusively refer to substance-related addictions. Both classification systems (ICD-10 and DSM IV/DSM-5) use specific diagnostic criteria like a strong desire to obtain and administer the substance, difficulties in controlling substance consumption behavior, a physiological withdrawal state, evidence of tolerance, progressive neglect of alternative amenities or interests, increased amount of time necessary to obtain or use the substance or to recover from its effects, and persevering with substance use despite clear evidence of overtly harmful consequences. Not all but at least two or more of these criteria have to be present together at any given time during the previous year to establish diagnosis (ICD-10 and DSM IV/DSM-5).

J. Kuhn (✉) • M. Möller
Department of Psychiatry and Psychotherapy, University of Cologne, Kerpener Str. 62, Cologne, Germany
e-mail: jens.kuhn@uk-koeln.de; michaela.moeller_@uk-koeln.de

D. Lenartz • C.P. Bührle • V. Visser-Vandewalle
Department of Stereotaxy and Functional Nuerosurgery, University of Cologne, Cologne, Germany
e-mail: doris.lenartz@uk-koeln.de; christian.buehrle@uk-koeln.de; veerle.visser-vandewalle@uk-koeln.de

Epidemiological Significance

Substance-related addictions constitute the most frequently occurring psychiatric disease category [1]. Approximately 25 % of all deaths in the Western industrial nations are caused directly or indirectly by consuming psychotropic substances. About five million deaths may be linked directly or indirectly to nicotine abuse. According to statistical data provided by Procter this number will presumably double on a global scale until the year 2025 [2].

Half of the world population consumes alcohol. A large number of this group meets the World Health Organization (WHO) criteria for high-risk consumption. The WHO expects that as many as 2.5 million fatalities are caused by alcoholism per year (WHO, 2011). Apart from that, about 4 % of the overall economic burden of disease is attributed to alcohol consumption, and increased alcohol consumption is causally linked to more than 60 diseases or medical conditions [3, 4].

The worldwide number of consumers of illicit substances is estimated at 200 million people. Here, the most frequently used drug is cannabis. Hall and Degenhard assume that globally 125–203 million persons between the age of 15 and 65 consume cannabis of whom a high percentage is actually addicted to the substance [5].

Estimations of the United Nations Office on Drugs and Crime (UNODC) World drug report in 2010 account that globally more than 15 million persons consume opioids. Within this substance category, heroin is the drug most frequently abused (UNODC World drug report 2010).

Neurobiology of Reward and Addiction

The etiology of addiction due to psychoactive substances is multifactorial to a very high extent. Among others, these factors include social and environmental influences, a person's individual biography, as well as specific personality traits. Genetic predispositions are of prime importance as far

H. Knotkova and D. Rasche (eds.), *Textbook of Neuromodulation*,
DOI 10.1007/978-1-4939-1408-1_17, © Springer Science+Business Media, LLC 2015

as the susceptibility to substance dependence is concerned. However, from a neuropathophysiological point of view, addiction is considered a chronic disease of the brain resulting from a dysregulation, viz. a suboptimal or lacking function of neural circuits still largely unknown, which is closely linked to the abovementioned diagnostic criteria. In particular, this condition is specifically characterized by craving and a high relapse risk [6]. As regards the latter, three principal mechanisms which cause craving and are ultimately responsible for relapse are discussed, notably a stressful conduct of life, an environmental stimulus previously associated with drug abuse (drug cues), and re-exposure to the drug itself (priming) [7]. Three slightly different but considerably overlapping sub-networks of the intrinsic reward system are believed to be responsible for cue-, drug-, and stress-induced relapse. In each of these cases, a dysfunction of the nucleus accumbens, being a key structure within the reward system, apparently plays a pivotal role. As an essential part of the ventral striatum—the main entry structure of the basal ganglia—the nucleus accumbens probably fulfils an important integrative or mediating function in discriminating between the different inputs, e.g., limbic and frontocortical projections. This putative regulative function of the nucleus accumbens is pertinent to several psychiatric disorders and depends not only on interactions between D_1 and D_2 receptor activation, e.g., by way of the dopaminergic projections from the ventral tegmental area (VTA) [8], but also on a D_1-associated co-activation of *N*-methyl-D-aspartate (NMDA) receptors, thus also involving the glutamatergic system [9]. Furthermore, the differential involvement of receptor types and the interaction of tonic and phasic burst activity levels of the dopaminergic projections add to the complexity of this issue. The consumption of psychotropic substances appears to induce a functionally detrimental alteration of synaptic plasticity, which, in turn, would cause an irregular mode of operation of this delicate integrative system following repeated or chronic drug consumption.

Effects of Therapeutic Neurosurgical Lesions on Addictive Behavior

From the 1960s onwards, as a result of emerging concepts that substance-related addiction may be a chronically recurrent disease of the brain engendered by a substance-induced malfunction of the brain reward system, addiction was tried to be treated by different stereotactic lesions in addicts [10].

One approach, which was carried out in several studies on more than 400 patients suffering from diverse addictive disorders, is based on performing bilateral anterior cingulotomy, for instance by thermocoagulation [11]. In this setting, the attempt to alleviate the obsessive and compulsive components associated with addictive disorders played a significant role [12–14]. As the optimum result, an abstinence rate of 45 % in 348 heroin-addicted patients treated by bilateral cingulotomy was reported after an observation period of 2 years [15].

Dieckmann et al. carried out hypothalamotomy in patients suffering from substance dependence and reported positive effects in a quite small sample of patients [16]. Furthermore, an alternative approach chosen was stereotactic ablation of the nucleus accumbens (NAc). This led to maintenance of abstinence in 11 out of 28 heroin-addicted patients in a study by Gao et al. over 6 months [17]. Wu et al. reported with the same approach maintenance of abstinence in 9 out of 12 alcohol-addicted patients also for a period of 6 months. However, the documentation of negative effects such as changes in personality traits and memory problems which have been observed in 19.2 % of cases in the study of Gao was inconsistent between the two studies, since Wu et al. did not observe any untoward effects [18].

Commonly, stereotactic lesional approaches of the early years were criticized because of the absence of control groups, insufficient progress documentation, and rather unsystematic recording of significant side effects. Moreover, general efficiency of lesional procedures—especially concerning addictive disorders—has been challenged on the basis of a current meta-analysis [19]. Nevertheless, recent experimental work in animals describes potential effects of lesional procedures addressing addictive behavior. Thus, Baunez et al. were able to show that rats with lesions in the nucleus subthalamicus (STN) exhibit a diminished desire to obtain cocaine reward, while, by contrast to that, their motivation for food gratification was enhanced [20].

Based on observations in patients presenting with changes in smoking behavior following ischemic stroke in the insular cortex [21], Canadian researchers launched a study in rats, where a reversible inactivation of the granular insular cortex by means of a baclofen/muscimol mixture injection was used in order to elucidate possible influences of this subsystem on craving behavior for nicotine. Indeed, inactivation of the granular insular cortex resulted in decreased nicotine consumption. Furthermore, after a so-called deletion phase relapse prevention was observed [22].

Noninvasive Neuromodulatory Techniques and Addiction

Considering the presented data and reflections on the potential benefit of DBS in addiction, it seemed to be worthwhile to also assess the respective virtues of other neuromodulatory techniques such as transcranial magnet simulation (TMS) or transcranial direct current stimulation (tDCS) as alternative or supplementary therapeutic strategies for addiction diseases. Although using procedures less invasive than DBS may be considered advantageous, the actions of tDCS or TMS are, nevertheless, often only transient and merely affect areas on brain surface or immediately beneath, i.e., in the cortex, without being able to influence deep brain structures. Accordingly, the studies outlined below primarily focus on comparatively short-term effects, for instance on the amelioration of craving. Long-term effects, e.g., those furthering the persistence of abstinence, have not yet been satisfactorily studied. Hence, TMS and tDCS currently are of only medial relevance for treating addictive behavior.

Transcranial direct current stimulation (tDCS) is a noninvasive, simple, and rather unspecific technique for neuromodulation. Deplorably, its mode of action is still far from being understood. Since, however, tDCS presumably alters spontaneous cortical neuronal activity [23], the notion that this technique may, among many other actions, also influence cognitive processing must not be ejected from the outset.

Along with related techniques (TMS) this method is therefore explored as a therapeutic alternative in different types of dependency or addiction-related fields like smoking cessation, as well as drug and food craving. With this type of noninvasive stimulation techniques, the dorsolateral prefrontal cortex (DLPFC) is the major target. In a randomized sham-controlled study Boggio et al. investigated whether tDCS of the DLPFC modified craving in patients suffering from alcohol addiction while being exposed to alcohol-associated cues. Thirteen subjects received sham and active bilateral tDCS in DLPFC. For evoking craving, alcohol-associated cues were presented in a video. The results showed that active tDCS decreased alcohol craving compared to sham stimulation [24]. In addition, Boggio et al. investigated whether tDCS may be a useful tool to modify stimulus processing associated with cue-induced nicotine craving [25]. They observed the consequences of repeated tDCS sessions on craving behavior in a randomized, parallel, sham-controlled, crossover trial in humans. Twenty-seven subjects were randomly assigned to two groups and subsequently exposed to either tDCS or sham stimulation of the left dorsolateral prefrontal cortex for 5 days. In the group of being actively stimulated, smoking cues had an attenuated effect on craving after stimulation as compared to sham stimulation. Additionally, the number of cigarettes smoked decreased in the stimulated group. A third study by Boggio et al. also claims that tDCS might have a specific effect on craving behavior. The authors assessed the impact of tDCS of the dorsolateral prefrontal cortex upon marijuana craving in humans. They observed that right anodal/left cathodal tDCS of DLPFC diminishes craving for marijuana [26]. In a randomized, blinded, crossover study Goldmann et al. examined the effect of prefrontal tDCS on food craving and self-reported ability to resist the urge of food in 19 healthy individuals who had reported frequent craving for food [27]. Pictures of food were shown to the test persons and visual analogue scales were used to rate food cravings and inability to resist foods before, during, and after receiving either real or sham tDCS. The findings show on the one hand a reduction in craving ratings and an inability to resist food from pre- to post-stimulation whether stimulation was active or sham. On the other hand, the percent change from pre- to post-stimulation was greater for real stimulation than for sham. We also attempted to gauge the efficiency of TMS relating to addictive behavior, but the current body of observations is rather unclear and inconsistent. However, there are also indications that TMS could have an effect on addictive disease. Thus a group from India observed the effects of TMS on craving in a placebo-controlled trial in alcohol-addicted humans [28]. The results show that right dorsolateral prefrontal high-frequency rTMS apparently had effects on craving for alcohol.

Taken together, the previously described data give the assumption that the effects of tDCS and TMS on craving might be related to a modulation of neural circuits associated with reward and decision making. Nevertheless, further research would be required for supporting this allegation.

The Scientific Rationale Behind Deep Brain Stimulation for Treating Addiction

The consideration to treat severe substance-related addictions with DBS rests on five principal aspects:

- Since the first application of "deep brain stimulation" (DBS) in the late 1980s, the electrical stimulation of basal ganglia has become a routine treatment in movement disorders. Up to this day, DBS has been performed in more than 100,000 individuals suffering from idiopathic Parkinson's disease, essential tremor, and dystonia, respectively [29–31]. Outcome studies have demonstrated marked beneficiary effects, but overall few and well-tolerated side effects. Since the year 2000, DBS has been applied and evaluated in psychiatric disorders at stages refractory to standard treatments [32, 33]. So far, a considerable number of investigations have demonstrated beneficial clinical effects of DBS in depression, obsessive-compulsive disorder (OCD), and Tourette's syndrome, respectively. Hence, DBS has become a viable treatment option in OCD under the humanitarian device exemption, and current discussions aim at extending the therapeutic scope of this technique even further [34], including the substance-related addictions discussed here.
- The assumption that substance-related addictions are consequential to dysfunctions of the brain's reward

system resulting from chronic exposure to psychoactive substances is increasingly underscored by recent studies. A better understanding of neural pathways being affected in addiction has created a new range of treatment options that directly target and attempt to reconstitute the compromised functions of a variety of brain circuits, e.g., by deep brain stimulation.

- This notion is supported by preliminary findings concerning the application of DBS in mental disorders distinct from addiction in which positive influences on comorbid addictive consumption patterns have been observed [35, 36]. In 2007, we communicated the case history of a patient who, as an unintended side effect, was able to discontinue his long-term alcohol consumption during DBS treatment of the NAc. Here, the primary therapeutic objective of DBS, i.e., the attempt to alleviate an anxiety disorder having proved refractory to several treatment approaches, was not attained. We also retrospectively examined the extent of tobacco use in nicotine addicts who already were being stimulated in the NAc in an attempt to ameliorate psychiatric disorders other than substance addiction-associated ones. The evaluated sample comprised ten patients with refractory anxiety disease and obsessive-compulsive disorder, as well as treatment-resistant Tourette's syndrome [37]. Three of ten patients experienced a long-lasting remission of their nicotine addiction during NAc stimulation. This abstinence rate of 30 % attained by DBS which was stable during a follow-up period of several years is obviously larger than the voluntary abstinence rate within the general population being estimated as 9 % [38]. A similar observation was described by Mantione et al. Here, a patient who had undergone DBS of the NAc for addressing severe obsessive-compulsive disorder also quit tobacco use after having smoked for many years before the intervention, with previous attempts to quit this habit having failed on a regular basis [36].
- In contrast to former lesional neurosurgical procedures which inflict permanent damage to the brain, DBS as a stereotactic neurosurgical approach is a less invasive, reversible, and adjustable procedure of neuromodulation. As a consequence, a lower side effect profile but also an increased efficiency may be expected. As an addition, the entire body of findings derived from earlier neurosurgical procedures may now be used as a knowledge base and developed to good effect.
- By mimicking different aspects of addiction, translational animal research may likewise be able to indicate that stimulation of important structures of the reward system has a significant positive impact on related behavioral patterns. The data pertinent thereto will be discussed in detail on the following pages.

DBS to Treat Addictive Patterns in Animal Models

A comprehensive database of experimental work in animals is already being collected and listed in the following, being categorized according to the effects of various classes of psychotropic substances.

Cocaine

In 2005, Rouaud et al. reported that high-frequency STN stimulation in rats reduced cocaine craving, while the motivation to consume cocaine increased again immediately after STN stimulation had been stopped [39].

Levy et al. were able to show that stimulation of the medial prefrontal cortices in rats induced a change in addictive behavior. Stimulation at 100 or 200 Hz reduced cocaine craving while no effects on sugar consumption were observed [40].

Another research group around Friedman et al. observed in cocaine-addicted rats a markedly reduced self-administration of this drug under a combined stimulation paradigm in the lateral habenula (high frequency: 100 Hz; low frequency: 10 Hz—stimulation phases). Remarkably, the effect vanished, when either stimulation frequency, i.e., 10 or 100 Hz, was not applied in combination but separately. High-frequency stimulation maximally lasted for 4 s, followed by a 20-s pause between subsequent stimulation episodes. The duration of low-frequency stimulation was between 15 and 60 s [41].

Vassoler et al. investigated short-lasting DBS of the NAc shell region in rats.

This represents a noteworthy difference when compared with studies in patients. We should therefore like to put particular emphasis on this peculiarity. During stimulation, an absence of priming-induced cocaine relapse was observed. At the same time, influence of DBS on food ingestion was not altered [42].

Taken together, the alluded data in animal studies document a stimulation-based influence on different cocaine consumption patterns in four areas of the brain: the STN, the medial prefrontal cortex, the lateral habenula, and the nucleus accumbens. All regions are assumed to be integral parts of the intrinsic reward circuit. However, these findings do not permit drawing any conclusions relating to the presumably most promising key structure for treating cocaine addiction in humans.

Ethyl Alcohol

Animal studies on alcohol addiction are, as a rule, confounded by the problem that rats—a frequently used species in DBS studies—usually tend to dislike and reject alcohol. For coping with this inborn tendency, Henderson et al. used a specially bred rat species, which indeed rather likes the taste of alcohol, the so-called alcohol-preferring rat. They demonstrated that high-frequency stimulation of the NAc not only was effective in reducing the amount of ethanol consumption in this rat strain, but also reduced preference for alcohol and the quantity consumed after a phase of abstinence [43].

Knapp et al. also observed the effects of DBS in ethanol consumption. They administered a saccharin-ethanol mixture to rats, within which the concentartion of saccharin was continuously diminished over 5–7 weeks for both familiarizing these rodents with the taste of alcohol and establishing a stable and reproducible consumption pattern with regard to a 10 % ethanol solution. After the onset of NAc stimulation, ethanol consumption was reduced noticeably. However, this effect ceased when stimulation was discontinued [44]. Both animal studies mentioned provide also some insight into the nature and degree of DBS side effects. One may be concerned whether stimulating the reward system may exert unintended and unforeseen influences on vital and substantial functions, such as reproduction and water intake. At least the latter issue was excluded in these two animal experiments. Both studies showed that DBS had a beneficiary effect on alcohol intake, while water consumption stayed stable or even increased [43, 44].

Opioids

Liu et al. stereotactically implanted DBS electrodes unilaterally into the core of the NAc and connected them to implantable pulse generators, which were fastened to the rat skull. For assessing the effects of stimulation, a 900-second conditioned place preference (CPP) paradigm was used. Their data show that chronic stimulation of the rat NAc significantly attenuates the time that rats spent in the drug-paired side in CPP and the morphine reinforcement of treated rats as compared with a non-stimulated control group [45].

Recent research by Guo et al. explored NAc stimulation on heroin-seeking behavior in self-administering rats. DBS was performed either bilaterally or unilaterally within the NAc core of the animals and attenuated cue- and heroin-induced reinstatement of drug seeking. Furthermore, it was observed that the effects of unilateral DBS in the right NAc were almost equivalent to those of bilateral neurostimulation [46].

In conclusion, cross-study comparisons, where epistemologically justifiable, appear to provide some indication that high-frequency NAc stimulation might generally be suitable for markedly ameliorating pathological consumption patterns with respect to various classes of psychotropic substances, e.g., cocaine, alcohol, morphine, and heroin in animal models.

DBS for Influencing Substance Dependencies in Humans

Initial observations in humans indicating putative positive effects of DBS on addictive behavioral stereotypes were either incidental [35, 36] or retrospective [37]. Based on such reports and supported by data derived from animal experimentation as well as by recent advances in partially understanding neurobiological mechanisms responsible for addiction, a small number of pilot patients suffering from severe substance dependencies have been treated with DBS in the NAc.

Müller et al. reported about two of three alcohol-addicted patients who remained abstinent for at least 1 year during DBS in the NAc. The third patient was able to markedly reduce his alcohol intake [41]. Corresponding observations were made in a further, likewise severely alcohol-addicted patient during DBS by our group [48]. Significant amelioration of alcohol abuse and associated craving was attained by therapeutic DBS of the NAc.

Furthermore, in the latter study [48], an event-related potential, the so-called error-related negativity (ERN), was recorded. ERN is believed to be generated in the anterior cingulate zone in response to errors. Remarkably, the amplitude of the ERN depended on the stimulation status ("stimulation on"/"stimulation off") with higher amplitudes in the "on." Hence, it could be shown that NAc stimulation at least evokes a functional influence on an associated cortical structure, in particular the anterior cingulate cortex. A purely speculative assumption might imply that the observed higher amplitude in the "on" status reflects a better error and decision processing [48]. This hypothesis is supported by findings of the Magdeburg group. They observed a less risky, more careful choice behavior in one patient with active compared to inactive DBS [49].

Zhou's group observed the effects of DBS on substance abuse in a heroin-addicted patient. This is a particularly interesting case, since heroin is the psychotropic substance with arguably the highest level of addiction potential. An anesthesiologically supported opioid detoxification was followed by stereotactic electrode implantation and subsequent chronic NAc stimulation. In the course of 6 years, the patient did not relapse to heroin abuse and additionally reduced nicotine consumption. Abstinence even persisted when the entire DBS system was removed for more than 12 months [50].

These observations allow—with all due caution—to infer that NAc stimulation in some cases not only may alleviate substance-induced dysfunctions of the intrinsic brain reward system, but also possibly modify the state of this system from a drug-related dysfunctional one to an improved condition with augmented or partially restored capabilities. As a result of the extreme complexity of both DBS mode of action and the still rather poorly understood reward system, plausible mechanisms underlying functional improvements remain—as yet—elusive. The question whether neuroplastic changes, e.g., by way of long-term potentiation (LTP) or depression (LDP), are involved here may only be speculated on, given the substantially limited understanding of these phenomena. For obtaining a solid knowledge base, the entire field certainly merits further study not only in the clinical domain, but especially in animal experimentation, i.e., in the basic sciences.

A research group around Denys described effective DBS treatment in a patient suffering from therapy-resistant heroin addiction. During NAc stimulation he was able to reduce heroin consumption until attaining abstinence for more than 6 months at the time of this writing, with the exception of a 14-day relapse. The patient reported that renewed heroin intake was solely motivated by his curiosity concerning treatment effects, but not triggered by or associated with craving. Beyond that, the ability to reduce heroin consumption critically depended on the proper adjustment of stimulation parameters. In contrast to stimulation of the middle contact points (1 and 2) of the electrode which led to an increase in heroin use and reported craving, stimulation of the ventral contact points (0 and 1) only resulted in a limited reduction in drug use and craving. However, stimulation of the two dorsal contact points (2 and 3), being positioned at the border between internal capsule and NAc, caused a significant reduction of heroin usage and craving under optimized stimulation conditions (3.5V amplitude at contacts 2 and 3, 90 μs pulse width, and 180 Hz frequency) [51]. Our own research group reported on two long-term, therapy-resistant heroin-addicted patients who had been treated by a protracted opiate replacement therapy with a constant dose of levomethadone. A 10-point visual analog scale (VAS), ranging from 1 (no craving) to 10 (intense craving), was used to estimate the patients' subjective level of craving. If VAS score was lower than 5 gradual reduction of patient-blinded administration of levomethadone had to be performed. Except for a single incident of heroin consumption a few weeks after surgery, both patients achieved total withdrawal in the course of NAc stimulation for more than 1 and in excess of 2 years, respectively, until the time of this writing. Both patients reported that the incident of drug consumption under stimulation was motivated by mere curiosity, whereas in comparison to the preoperative status, psychotropic effects had been experienced less intensive [52].

Hypotheses Pertinent to the Effects of DBS on Addiction, viz. Substance Addiction

Although observations of the effects of DBS on addictive behavior have been increasing in number over recent years, and this technique is now being applied to a growing number of neurological and even psychiatric disorders, the mechanisms underlying its actions are still highly controversial and far from understood. Accordingly, the following remarks about possible underlying effects of DBS relating to dependency disorders have to be considered only as preliminary and tentative attempts at explanation.

For quite some time, a rather simplistic model for explaining the mode of action of DBS was used. A reversible functional, i.e., bioelectrical, blockade of impulse propagation within the stimulated target was assumed. Assessing the partially positive modification of addictive behavior by stereotactic lesions in animal studies or in stereotactic ablation of the NAc in humans as mentioned above, such a concept appears to be plausible. Nevertheless, many other aspects like sustained or temporally delayed effects which were observed in clinical studies of various psychiatric disorders cannot fully be accounted for by such an approach.

Different studies on alcoholism indicate that acute and chronic administration of ethanol induces an alteration of striatal transmission and produces long-lasting changes in synaptic output [53–56]. For instance, Adermark et al. evaluated changes in striatal neurotransmission induced by long-term self-administration of ethanol in male Wistar rats and concluded that the dorsolateral striatum might be a key brain region involved in the initiation of neuronal adaptations provoked by ethanol consumption [57]. According to these and other related findings it seems reasonable to postulate a modifying effect of DBS at both neurochemical and neuronal levels. The current state of knowledge about DBS effects appears to indicate that DBS possibly brings about certain structural and functional changes, not only within the stimulated target structure itself, but also of remote neuronal circuits linked to the stimulation site by way of efferent or reciprocal projections. This phenomenon is denominated "neuromodulation" [58]. Animal studies indicate that DBS of the NAc which, on neuroanatomical and neurochemical grounds, we believe to be the currently most promising target for addictive disorders caused changes in the firing patterns of thalamic and frontal cortical areas being connected to the NAc via reciprocal projections. These alleged influences on temporospatial firing patterns in networks remote from the NAc might alter the degree of neuronal synchronism, i.e., the levels of entropy in various interconnected neuronal networks [59]. Denys et al. recently investigated a monosynaptic "top-down" synchronism between the medioventral frontal cortex and the NAc in OCD patients who had undergone DBS. The authors suggested that DBS of the NAc may retrogradely influence neuroelectric activity of superior cortical structures [60].

On the neurochemical scale, the ability to alter local levels of the most essential transmitter, dopamine, seems especially interesting within the framework of the reward system [61]. In this setting the "dopamine hypothesis" is based on the assumption that DBS exerts its effect by modulating cerebral dopamine transmission. In line with this, animal models could indicate that psychotropic substances (e.g., cocaine) promote rather immediate changes of synaptic plasticity in D_1-expressing neurons of the NAc, which may be reversed by inhibitory stimulation of limbic afferents [9]. Further support for the "dopamine hypothesis" is derived from neuroimaging where DBS of thalamic seed regions in Tourette patients was found to be associated with a reduction of thalamic dopamine release [62]. However, other groups found an increased dopamine release during DBS [63].

Still, it is quite unclear whether the observed positive effects may be generalized to other forms of addiction caused by misuse of psychoactive substances. Observations of abstinence-sustaining effects of DBS pertaining to nicotine and alcohol in humans [35, 37] as well as animal studies on alcohol and cocaine indicating alterations in addictive behavior after DBS favor this idea [39]. However, the fact that, e.g., in patients with successfully treated heroin addiction by means of DBS concomitant consumption of drugs from other categories did not decline, so that no abstinence could be achieved for these substances, seems to speak against the validity of an overall extension to all forms of substance addiction [52]. Observations described by Koo and colleagues add a new aspect to basic aspects of heroin addiction which also influence present hypotheses concerning the putative mechanism of DBS. The authors observed that BDNF reduces morphine reward (i.e., opposed to its effects on cocaine) at the site of the VTA terminals in the NAc via activation of D_1 receptors [64]. From their findings in general, it may be inferred that addiction-inducing and -maintaining mechanisms are not the same for all psychotropic substances and therefore, modern therapy strategies (e.g., DBS) cannot be universalized to different categories of substance addiction. In addition, they could show that the BDNF-associated effects could be mediated by optogenetic stimulation of VTA neurons. Thus, when considering the mechanisms underlying the effects of DBS in addiction, its influence on the modulating effect of BDNF must be accounted for.

In summary, on one hand, translational research prompts speculation whether DBS of the NAc and other target structures not mentioned here in further detail are potential tools for treating addiction. On the other hand, this requires extensive further research and thorough cross-validation as well as confirmation of the results obtained.

Conclusion

Addiction due to psychoactive substances is among the mental disorders known as the one with the most unfavorable prognosis. Current medications or other therapeutic regimens are characterized by high relapse rates, failed detoxifications, and non-responses and lead to large numbers of long-time addicted patients. Thus, new treatment strategies are urgently needed.

At the same time, animal studies, incidental findings in humans, and initial case reports about beneficial treatment results of DBS within the NAc in alcohol, heroin, and nicotine addiction appear to be promising. Even techniques like tDCS and TMS might alter addictive behavior, most probably, only on a short-term basis. Relying on the scientific evidence supporting a compromised operation of the intrinsic reward system induced by substance abuse, neurostimulation of this dysfunctional network might have positive effects. However clinical studies with larger samples are needed to further support the hypothesis.

References

1. McGinnis JM, Foege WH. Actual causes of death in the United States. JAMA. 1993;270:2207–12.
2. Proctor RN. The global smoking epidemic: a history and status report. Clin Lung Cancer. 2004;5:371–6.
3. Room R, Babor T, Rehm J. Alcohol and public health. Lancet. 2005;365:519–30.
4. Rehm J, Mathers C, Popova S, Thavorncharoensap M, Teerawattananon Y, Patra J. Global burden of disease and injury and economic cost attributable to alcohol use and alcohol-use disorders. Lancet. 2009;373:2223–33.
5. Degenhardt L, Hall W. Extent of illicit drug use and dependence, and their contribution to the global burden of disease. Lancet. 2012;379:55–70.
6. Adinoff B. Neurobiologic processes in drug reward and addiction. Harv Rev Psychiatry. 2004;12:305–20.
7. Schmidt HD, Anderson SM, Famous KR, Kumaresan V, Pierce RC. Anatomy and pharmacology of cocaine priming-induced reinstatement of drug seeking. Eur J Pharmacol. 2005;526:65–76.
8. Goto Y, Otani S, Grace AA. The Yin and Yang of dopamine release: a new perspective. Neuropharmacology. 2007;53:583–7.
9. Pascoli V, Turiault M, Lüscher C. Reversal of cocaine-evoked synaptic potentiation resets drug-induced adaptive behaviour. Nature. 2011;481(7379):71–5.
10. Cosgrove GR, Rauch SL. Stereotactic cingulotomy. Neurosurg Clin N Am. 2003;14:225–35.
11. Stelten BM, Noblesse LH, Ackermans L, Temel Y, Visser-Vandewalle V. The neurosurgical treatment of addiction. Neurosurg Focus. 2008;25:E5.
12. Cosgrove GR. Surgery for psychiatric disorders. CNS Spectr. 2000;5:43–52.
13. Ballantine Jr HT, Cassidy WL, Flanagan NB, Marino Jr R. Stereotaxic anterior cingulotomy for neuropsychiatric illness and intractable pain. J Neurosurg. 1967;26:488–95.
14. Ballantine Jr HT, Bouckoms AJ, Thomas EK, Giriunas IE. Treatment of psychiatric illness by stereotactic cingulotomy. Biol Psychiatry. 1987;22:807–19.
15. Medvedev SV, Anichkov AD, Poliakov II. Physiological mechanisms of the effectiveness of bilateral stereotactic cingulotomy in treatment of strong psychological dependence in drug addiction. Fiziol Cheloveka. 2003;29:117–23.

16. Dieckmann G, Schneider H. Influence of stereotactic hypothalamotomy on alcohol and drug addiction. Appl Neurophysiol. 1978;41:93–8.
17. Gao G, Wang X, He S, Li W, Wang Q, Liang Q, et al. Clinical study for alleviating opiate drug psychological dependence by a method of ablating the nucleus accumbens with stereotactic surgery. Stereotact Funct Neurosurg. 2003;81:96–104.
18. Wu HM, Wang XL, Chang CW, Li N, Gao L, Geng N, et al. Preliminary findings in ablating the nucleus accumbens using stereotactic surgery for alleviating psychological dependence on alcohol. Neurosci Lett. 2010;473:77–81.
19. Leiphart JW, Valone 3rd FH. Stereotactic lesions for the treatment of psychiatric disorders. J Neurosurg. 2010;113:1204–11.
20. Baunez C, Dias C, Cador M, Amalric M. The subthalamic nucleus exerts opposite control on cocaine and 'natural' rewards. Nat Neurosci. 2005;8:484–9.
21. Naqvi NH, Rudrauf D, Damasio H, Bechara A. Damage to the insula disrupts addiction to cigarette smoking. Science. 2007;315:531–4.
22. Forget B, Pushparaj A, Le Foll B. Granular insular cortex inactivation as a novel therapeutic strategy for nicotine addiction. Biol Psychiatry. 2010;68:265–71.
23. Bindman LJ, Lippold OC, Redfearn JW. The action of brief polarizing currents on the cerebral cortex of the rat (1) during current flow and (2) in the production of long-lasting after-effects. J Physiol. 1964;172:369–82.
24. Boggio PS, Sultani N, Fecteau S, Merabet L, Mecca T, Pascual-Leone A, et al. Prefrontal cortex modulation using transcranial DC stimulation reduces alcohol craving: a double-blind, sham-controlled study. Drug Alcohol Depend. 2008;92:55–60.
25. Boggio PS, Liguori P, Sultani N, Rezende L, Fecteau S, Fregni F. Cumulative priming effects of cortical stimulation on smoking cue-induced craving. Neurosci Lett. 2009;463:82–6.
26. Boggio PS, Zaghi S, Villani AB, Fecteau S, Pascual-Leone A, Fregni F. Modulation of risk-taking in marijuana users by transcranial direct current stimulation (tDCS) of the dorsolateral prefrontal cortex (DLPFC). Drug Alcohol Depend. 2010;112:220–5.
27. Goldman RL, Borckardt JJ, Frohman HA, O'Neil PM, Madan A, Campbell LK, et al. Prefrontal cortex transcranial direct current stimulation (tDCS) temporarily reduces food cravings and increases the self-reported ability to resist food in adults with frequent food craving. Appetite. 2011;56:741–6.
28. Mishra BR, Nizamie SH, Das B, Praharaj SK. Efficacy of repetitive transcranial magnetic stimulation in alcohol dependence: a sham-controlled study. Addiction. 2010;105:49–55.
29. Deuschl G, Schade-Brittinger C, Krack P, Volkmann J, Schäfer H, Bötzel K, et al. A randomized trial of deep-brain stimulation for Parkinson's disease. N Engl J Med. 2006;355:896–908.
30. Kupsch A, Benecke R, Müller J, Trottenberg T, Schneider GH, Poewe W, et al. Pallidal deep-brain stimulation in primary generalized or segmental dystonia. N Engl J Med. 2006;355:1978–90.
31. Schuurman PR, Bosch DA, Bossuyt PM, Bonsel GJ, van Someren EJ, de Bie RM, et al. A comparison of continuous thalamic stimulation and thalamotomy for suppression of severe tremor. N Engl J Med. 2000;342:461–8.
32. Nuttin B, Cosyns P, Demeulemeester H, Gybels J, Meyerson B. Electrical stimulation in anterior limbs of internal capsules in patients with obsessive-compulsive disorder. Lancet. 1999;354:1526.
33. Vandewalle V, van der Linden C, Groenewegen HJ, Caemaert J. Stereotactic treatment of Gilles de la Tourette syndrome by high frequency stimulation of thalamus. Lancet. 1999;353:724.
34. Kuhn J, Grundler TO, Lenartz D, Sturm V, Klosterkotter J, Huff W. Deep brain stimulation for psychiatric disorders. Dtsch Arztebl Int. 2010;107:105–13.
35. Kuhn J, Lenartz D, Huff W, Lee SH, Koulousakis A, Klosterkoetter J, Sturm V. Remission of alcohol dependency following deep brain stimulation of the nucleus accumbens: valuable therapeutic implications? J Neurol Neurosurg Psychiatry. 2007;78:1152–3.
36. Mantione M, van de Brink W, Schuurman PR, Denys D. Smoking cessation and weight loss after chronic deep brain stimulation of the nucleus accumbens: therapeutic and research implications: case report. Neurosurgery. 2010;66:E218. discussion E218.
37. Kuhn J, Bauer R, Pohl S, Lenartz D, Huff W, Kim EH, et al. Observations on unaided smoking cessation after deep brain stimulation of the nucleus accumbens. Eur Addict Res. 2009;15:196–201.
38. Meyer C, Rumpf HJ, Schumann A, Hapke U, John U. Intentionally reduced smoking among untreated general population smokers: prevalence, stability, prediction of smoking behaviour change and differences between subjects choosing either reduction or abstinence. Addiction. 2003;98:1101–10.
39. Rouaud T, Lardeux S, Panayotis N, Paleressompoulle D, Cador M, Baunez C. Reducing the desire for cocaine with subthalamic nucleus deep brain stimulation. Proc Natl Acad Sci U S A. 2010;107:1196–200.
40. Levy D, Shabat-Simon M, Shalev U, Barnea-Ygael N, Cooper A, Zangen A. Repeated electrical stimulation of reward-related brain regions affects cocaine but not "natural" reinforcement. J Neurosci. 2007;27:14179–89.
41. Friedman A, Lax E, Dikshtein Y, Abraham L, Flaumenhaft Y, Sudai E, et al. Electrical stimulation of the lateral habenula produces enduring inhibitory effect on cocaine seeking behavior. Neuropharmacology. 2010;59:452–9.
42. Vassoler FM, Schmidt HD, Gerard ME, Famous KR, Ciraulo DA, Kometsky C, et al. Deep brain stimulation of the nucleus accumbens shell attenuates cocaine priming-induced reinstatement of drug seeking in rats. J Neurosci. 2008;28:8735–9.
43. Henderson MB, Green AI, Bradford PS, Chau DT, Roberts DW, Leiter JC. Deep brain stimulation of the nucleus accumbens reduces alcohol intake in alcohol-preferring rats. Neurosurg Focus. 2010;29:E12.
44. Knapp CM, Tozier L, Pak A, Ciraulo DA, Kornetsky C. Deep brain stimulation of the nucleus accumbens reduces ethanol consumption in rats. Pharmacol Biochem Behav. 2009;92:474–9.
45. Liu HY, Jin J, Tang JS, Sun WX, Jia H, Yang XP, et al. Chronic deep brain stimulation in the rat nucleus accumbens and its effect on morphine reinforcement. Addict Biol. 2008;13:40–6.
46. Guo L, Zhou H, Wang R, Xu J, Zhou W, Zhang F, et al. DBS of nucleus accumbens on heroin seeking behaviors in self-administering rats. Drug Alcohol Depend. 2013;129:70–81.
47. Muller UJ, Sturm V, Voges J, Heinze HJ, Galazky I, Heldmann M, et al. Successful treatment of chronic resistant alcoholism by deep brain stimulation of nucleus accumbens: first experience with three cases. Pharmacopsychiatry. 2009;42:288–91.
48. Kuhn J, Grundler TO, Bauer R, Huff W, Fischer AG, Lenartz D, et al. Successful deep brain stimulation of the nucleus accumbens in severe alcohol dependence is associated with changed performance monitoring. Addict Biol. 2011;16:620–3.
49. Munte TF, Heldmann M, Hinrichs H, Marco-Pallares J, Krämer UM, Sturm V, Heinze HJ. Nucleus accumbens is involved in human action monitoring: evidence from invasive electrophysiological recordings. Front Hum Neurosci. 2007;1:11.
50. Zhou H, Xu J, Jiang J. Deep brain stimulation of nucleus accumbens on heroin-seeking behaviors: a case report. Biol Psychiatry. 2011;69:e41–2.
51. Valencia-Alfonso CE, Luigjes J, Smolders R, Cohen MX, Levar N, Mazaheri A, et al. Effective deep brain stimulation in heroin addiction: a case report with complementary intracranial electroencephalogram. Biol Psychiatry. 2012;71:e35–7.
52. Kuhn J, Moller M, Treppmann JF, Bartsch C, Lenartz D, Gruendler TO, et al. Deep brain stimulation of the nucleus accumbens and its

usefulness in severe opioid addiction. Mol Psychiatry. 2014;19 (2):145–6.

53. Adermark L, Clarke RB, Soderpalm B, Ericson M. Ethanol-induced modulation of synaptic output from the dorsolateral striatum in rat is regulated by cholinergic interneurons. Neurochem Int. 2011;58:693–9.
54. Adermark L, Jonsson S, Ericson M, Soderpalm B. Intermittent ethanol consumption depresses endocannabinoid-signaling in the dorsolateral striatum of rat. Neuropharmacology. 2011;61:1160–5.
55. Gerdeman GL, Partridge JG, Lupica CR, Lovinger DM. It could be habit forming: drugs of abuse and striatal synaptic plasticity. Trends Neurosci. 2003;26:184–92.
56. Vengeliene V, Bilbao A, Molander A, Spanagel R. Neuropharmacology of alcohol addiction. Br J Pharmacol. 2008;154:299–315.
57. Adermark L, Jonsson S, Soderpalm B, Ericson M. Region-specific depression of striatal activity in Wistar rat by modest ethanol consumption over a ten-month period. Alcohol. 2013;47:289–98.
58. Kringelbach ML, Jenkinson N, Owen SL, Aziz TZ. Translational principles of deep brain stimulation. Nat Rev Neurosci. 2007;8:623–35.
59. McCracken CB, Grace AA. Nucleus accumbens deep brain stimulation produces region-specific alterations in local field potential oscillations and evoked responses in vivo. J Neurosci. 2009;29:5354–63.
60. Cohen MX, Bour L, Mantione M, Figee M, Vink M, Tijssen MA, et al. Top-down-directed synchrony from medial frontal cortex to nucleus accumbens during reward anticipation. Hum Brain Mapp. 2012;33:24–52.
61. Gardner EL. Addiction and brain reward and antireward pathways. Adv Psychosom Med. 2011;30:22–60.
62. Kuhn J, Janouschek H, Raptis M, Rex S, Lenartz D, Neuner I, et al. In vivo evidence of deep brain stimulation-induced dopaminergic modulation in Tourette's syndrome. Biol Psychiatry. 2012;71:e11–3.
63. van Dijk A, Klompmakers AA, Feenstra MG, Denys D. Deep brain stimulation of the accumbens increases dopamine, serotonin, and noradrenaline in the prefrontal cortex. J Neurochem. 2012;123:897–903.
64. Koo JW, Mazei-Robison MS, Chaudhury D, Chaudhury D, Juarez B, LaPlant Q, et al. BDNF is a negative modulator of morphine action. Science. 2012;338:124–8.

Enhancement of Sensory and Cognitive Functions in Healthy Subjects 18

Tal Sela and Michal Lavidor

Introduction

Sensory and cognitive enhancement is already in widespread use, but not always recognized as such. The automated spelling software in the word processor, the smart phone, and the tweets are all part of our cognitive enhancement infrastructure that helps us produce, receive, retrieve, and transfer information. The brain stimulation kinds of enhancement described in this chapter may appear unusual, futuristic, risky, or problematic but will likely in time become as prosaic and accepted as the others.

Cognitive enhancement may be defined as the amplification or extension of core capacities of the mind by improving or augmenting internal or external information processing system [1, 2]. Cognition can be defined as the processes an organism uses to organize information. This includes acquiring information (sensation and perception), selecting (attention), communicating (language), representing (understanding), and retaining (memory) information, and using it to guide behavior (reasoning and coordination of motor outputs).

Interventions to improve cognitive function may be directed at any one of these core faculties. An intervention that is aimed at correcting a specific pathology or defect of a cognitive subsystem may be characterized as therapeutic. An enhancement is an intervention that improves a subsystem in some way other than repairing something that is broken or remedying a specific dysfunction. In practice, the distinction between therapy and enhancement is often difficult to discern, and it could be argued that it lacks practical significance.

The aim of the present chapter is to introduce up-to-date brain stimulation tools that were successful in enhancing cognitive functions in healthy individuals. This review mainly focuses on major advances in functions such as language, cognitive control, planning, learning and memory among healthy individuals by using Transcranial Magnetic Stimulation (TMS), transcranial direct current stimulation (tDCS), and transcranial alternating current stimulation (tACS). After presenting findings from various cognitive domains, we provide the reader with a methodological section that specifies the different considerations that one should consider when designing and evaluating a brain stimulation experiment in the context of cognitive research. Finally, we will conclude and describe future directions in the field.

Transcranial Magnetic Stimulation (TMS)

Transcranial Magnetic Stimulation (TMS) is now a standard lab tool for investigating perceptual and cognitive functions [3]. TMS has the ability to interfere with brain processes at well-defined spatial locations at a temporal precision of single milliseconds (Table 18.1). This combination of reasonable spatial resolution and excellent temporal resolution is unique to TMS.

TMS: Modes of Operation

When TMS was first developed [4], it served to stimulate the motor cortex. Later developments led to its applications in language studies and other domains of cognition and perception. Amassian and colleagues [8] were the first to demonstrate suppression of visual perception with TMS; participants were unable to identify visually presented letters when a TMS pulse was given over the occipital pole between 80 and 100 ms after the letters were briefly presented.

The ability to impair performance such as inducing (temporary and reversible) stuttering in healthy subjects with TMS was termed the "virtual lesion" mode [5] and

T. Sela (✉) • M. Lavidor
Department of Psychology, Bar-Ilan University, 1 Max ve-Anna Webb Street, Ramat Gan 5290002, Israel
e-mail: Tal9.sela@gmail.com

H. Knotkova and D. Rasche (eds.), *Textbook of Neuromodulation*,
DOI 10.1007/978-1-4939-1408-1_18, © Springer Science+Business Media, LLC 2015

Table 18.1 TMS principles

• During transcranial magnetic stimulation (TMS; see also [3]) a focal electric current is induced in the cortex by a magnetic pulse which undergoes minimal attenuation by the intervening soft tissue and bone.
• The magnetic pulse is generated after a brief current is discharged from a capacitor into a circular or figure-of-eight shaped coil, which is held above the subject's scalp. The induced electric field is strongest near the coil and typically stimulates a cortical area of a few centimeters in diameter.
• TMS pulses cause coherent firing of neurons in the stimulated area as well as changes in firing due to synaptic input. At the microscopic level, the electric field affects the neurons' transmembrane voltage and thereby the voltage-sensitive ion channels.
• Brain imaging tools can be used to detect the associated electrical currents and changes in blood flow of metabolism. In motor cortex stimulation, peripheral effects can be observed as muscle activity with surface electromyography (EMG). Moreover, there may be behavioral changes, for instance, stuttering when TMS is applied over Broca's area of healthy subjects.

was employed to map cognitive functions of cortical areas. Since performance under TMS can be compared to a control condition which could be sham, placebo, a different site and/or a different timing stimulation, a within-subjects experimental design overcomes the known problems of real lesion studies. The concept of the "virtual lesion" mode therefore captures the unique nature of inhibition-induced TMS studies which make it possible to establish (heuristically sound and replicable) causal relationships between brain regions and cognitive functions.

More recent technological developments resulted in another TMS mode designed to explore connectivity between cortical networks. The combination of TMS with brain imaging techniques (e.g., PET, fMRI) allows researchers to examine functional connections between neural processes [6]. For example, TMS effects have been shown to induce changes in brain activity locally (in the cortex beneath the TMS coil) and in distant cortical areas interconnected to the stimulated site. Rounis et al. [7] showed that rTMS over the primary motor cortex induced changes in the motor cortex and also in the cerebellum. It is clear now that the effects induced by TMS are not restricted to the stimulated site but also induce different functional changes in remote interconnected sites.

TMS Protocols

In essence, three main stimulation protocols are available: single pulse, event-related protocol, and offline protocols.

The single pulse protocol has the best temporal resolution and can reveal critical processing times of cognitive stimuli. In this protocol, a single pulse is applied at different predefined points in time when subjects are engaged in their task. The prototype of this protocol is the seminal work by Amassian et al. [8] that induced errors in identifying letters only when the TMS pulse was applied over the primary visual cortex at around 80 ms following the letters. Using the same stimulation at other time points (for example 120 ms following letter presentation) did not affect letter identification accuracy. Töpper et al. [9] induced longer response latencies to picture naming when the single pulse TMS was applied over Wernicke's region 80 ms following the to-be-named picture, but not when applied at other time points.

Event-related online protocols apply a train of pulses synchronized with stimuli presentation. The number of pulses given depends on frequency and duration; for example, a common protocol of 10 Hz for 500 ms translates that subjects receive a train of five pulses for 500 ms. Pobric et al. [10], for example, applied such a protocol coupled with word pair presentation in a semantic decision task. Any protocol that applies trains of magnetic pulses is called repetitive TMS (rTMS), and can be interwoven with stimuli presentation in an online protocol, or applied before or after stimuli presentation in an offline protocol.

Offline protocols are a train of pulses applied before stimuli presentation, so that subjects' pre-TMS and post-TMS responses can be compared. There are two typical frequencies that are used in offline rTMS protocols: one that uses 1 Hz frequency for 5–20 min, at a rate of one pulse per second. The newer offline rTMS protocol is set at 50 Hz, where 300 pulses are applied within 20 s [11]. Many previous studies have established the 1 Hz protocol as inhibitory; for example, Oliveri et al. [12] reported slower RTs and poorer accuracy in idiom comprehension following 5-min 1 Hz rTMS over Wernicke's area. Knecht et al. [13] showed that the inhibitory effect of the 1 Hz protocol lasts about half the stimulation time; i.e., 10-min stimulation will affect behavior for about 5 min.

There are fewer cognitive studies using the 50 Hz protocol (also known as Theta burst [11]) compared to the 1 Hz, though the few published studies report consistent inhibition effects that last about an hour. Vallesi et al. [14], for example, showed how 50 Hz rTMS over the right dorsolateral prefrontal cortex (rDLPFC) impaired temporal processing.

TMS and Cognitive Enhancement

Andoh et al. [15, 16] applied rTMS over Wernicke's area and reported a facilitation effect on auditory language processing. They interpreted the observed effects as a change in activity in brain regions engaged during the language task (e.g., bilateral middle temporal gyrus, left superior temporal gyrus, and inferior frontal gyrus). Moreover, they also showed that rTMS could have differential effects on language processing depending on the stimulation frequency used, namely, 1 Hz-rTMS facilitated detection of the native language, whereas 50 Hz-bursts of rTMS facilitated detection of foreign languages [16]. These results suggest that rTMS could induce changes in cortical excitability and connectivity depending on the *intensity* of the "virtual lesion" induced in the stimulated area.

Repetitive TMS of the same area, e.g., Broca's area, can induce opposite effects depending on the information processes tapped by the task. For instance, high frequency rTMS (5–10 Hz) over Broca's area has been associated with the facilitation of phonological and syntactic performance on the one hand, and impaired semantic performance on the other (e.g., [17]). Similarly, low-frequency rTMS (1 Hz) over Wernicke's area has been documented to have no effect during a picture-naming task [18], but to induce facilitative effects when performing a speech fragment-detection task in the native language [15].

Recently, TMS applied over motor or cognitive functions has highlighted a mechanism that may underlie performance changes by providing experimental support for the hypothesis that some brain functions operate in a state of interhemispheric compensation, i.e., TMS may reflect use of adaptive plasticity in the nondominant hemisphere for function recovery [19]. These plastic-adapting changes of the intact hemisphere could intervene rapidly and be specific to functions that are normally mediated by the perturbed area [20]. For example, Kobayashi et al. [21] observed that rTMS applied over the left motor cortex during a motor task facilitated performance with the ipsilateral hand (decreased RT in the left hand). According to this author, given that the left hemisphere controls the right hand, low-frequency rTMS over the left motor cortex could lead to the disinhibition of the contralateral right motor cortex [21]—presumably through the suppression of transcallosal inhibition [22]—and thus to subsequently better performance with the ipsilateral left hand. Hilgetag et al. [23] reported that right hemispheric parietal stimulation improved the ipsilateral detection of visual stimuli. They suggested that the inhibition induced at the site of stimulation was matched by increased excitability in the contralateral hemisphere, resulting in measurable behavioral enhancement.

The idea of interhemispheric compensation might explain some of the contrasting TMS effects found in TMS studies and thus elucidate mechanisms of interhemispheric collaboration during language processing. The idea that TMS of one region may disinhibit the homologous regions in the contralateral hemisphere [24] suggests for instance that the stimulation of the Wernicke's area in the LH causes an inhibitory effect of this region on the homologous right area, resulting in faster processing of some semantic tasks (for example [10]). This hypothesis is supported by Oliveri et al. [12] who reported that stimulation over the right temporal lobe improved performance via disinhibition of the LH in a semantic task of processing idioms. According to this explanation, LH semantic processing mechanisms may interfere with the ability of the RH to carry out semantic processing. The nature of the semantic processing in each hemisphere might be qualitatively different than LH processes (for example, the coarser vs. finer modes [25]).

Transcallosal disinhibition was directly demonstrated in healthy subjects by applying rTMS at a frequency of 4 Hz over the left IFG, while simultaneously measuring language activity with positron emission tomography [26]. Repetitive TMS decreased left IFG activity and increased right IFG activity, showing a rightward shift of language activity caused by a virtual brain lesion, thus further supporting the hypothesis that right homologous activations may be linked to a disinhibition phenomenon [27].

How can performance enhancement be achieved via remote stimulation? There are some examples of TMS studies of Aphasia that have led to behavioral improvement. These improvements are thought to be due to selective disinhibition in structures connected to the lesion site. In fact lesions may form new sets of excitatory and inhibitory interactions, and facilitation could be related to the reduction or suppression of interference effects [28]. In line with this hypothesis, authors of PET studies of patients with focal cerebral lesions have noted that mechanisms underlying functional facilitation have been related to paradoxical increases in blood flow in structures distal but connected to the lesion site [29]. This increase in CBF has been interpreted as a functional disinhibition of structures that are connected by interhemispheric or intrahemispheric pathways to the critical lesion site.

TMS: Major Caveats

While TMS appears to be quite versatile, its potential for future broad public use is questionable. First, the user experience might be aversive as the magnetic stimulation is noisy and explicit. Second, patients need to arrive to a TMS Clinique, as the TMS system is not easily mobile. Furthermore, additional complementary expensive systems are required to position the TMS coil in a specific cortical location. These reasons and others imply that it is still doubtful whether TMS will ever be a practically useful enhancement method. Another stimulation method, namely, transcranial direct current stimulation (tDCS) may overcome these caveats—it is cheap, light-weight, mobile, quite, safe, and painless. The unique advantage of tDCS will be reviewed in the following section.

Table 18.2 tDCS principles

• In transcranial direct current stimulation (tDCS), a weak direct current (1–2 mA) is being delivered through two electrodes, an anode and a cathode, that are fixed on the scalp throughout the stimulation.
• The current enters the brain from the anode, passes through neuronal tissue, and exits out of the cathode.
• tDCS induces stimulation polarity-dependent cortical activity and excitability enhancements or reductions, which emerge during stimulation, but can remain for 1 h after stimulation [62, 117, 118].
• The primary mechanism of tDCS is thought to be a modulation of resting membrane potential, by which tDCS affects spontaneous cortical activity, with anodal tDCS causing neural depolarization and thus enhancing cortical excitability, and cathodal tDCS causing neural hyperpolarization and decreased cortical excitability [62, 118].
• The physiological effects of tDCS have been linked with neurophysiological mechanisms of long-term potentiation and depression [117]. tDCS to the motor cortex has proven to be a powerful method in modulating excitability and has been suggested to be related to long-term potentiation (LTP-like: anodal tDCS), and long-term depression (LTD-like: cathodal tDCS) [117, 119]; see also [98] for a comprehensive review regarding the physiological basis of tDCS).
• This method affords a highly reliable sham condition [120] in which the stimulation is turned on and off over a relatively short period of time, with the participants being unable to distinguish this condition from real stimulation.

Electrical Brain Stimulation: tDCS

Behaviorally, tDCS studies have examined cognitive performance across a number of task domains including working memory [30], visual recognition memory [31], probabilistic classification [32], and probabilistic guessing [33]. The idea is that anodal tDCS may promote upregulation while cathodal advance downregulation, as found and replicated in motor or visual domains (Table 18.2). This idea has been questioned with respect to cathodal tDCS effects on cognition as shown by a recent meta-analysis [34]. Nonetheless, some studies showed cathodal effects on performance in cognitive tasks (e.g., [35, 36]).

Other forms of transcranial electrical brain stimulation such as transcranial alternating current stimulation (tACS) and transcranial random noise stimulation (tRNS) [37, 38] are assumed to modulate specifically oscillatory cortical activity, depending on stimulation frequency. However, so far only few studies have been conducted showing how the usage of these techniques alters perception and cognition (e.g., [37, 39]).

The different techniques of electrical brain stimulation have been introduced for several main purposes. Mainly, these methods may be capable of improving cognition under certain preconditions. The different methods can help to identify areas and interactions between them which are causally involved in cognitive functions, and the specific physiological mechanisms involved [40]. Next, several lines of study will be introduced covering advances achieved with tDCS in diverse domains such as cognitive control, language, memory, and learning.

Enhancing Language with tDCS

The modern endeavor to understand the basics of language and its neural substrate, which started with the seminal work of Broca [41] and Wernicke [42], may benefit from the (re) constitution of the realm of brain stimulation, which provides tools that allow to make strong causal inference (see [43]) regarding the hallmark of brain functions—the language system.

To date, several tDCS studies explored naming, picture naming and verbal fluency. Naming is a basic, fundamental capacity of the human brain that requires a number of cognitive processes that involve perception of the visual stimuli, the semantic and lexical processing of its features, the selection and retrieval of relevant information, and finally the articulation of a target concept. Several studies used tDCS in order to improve performance, utilizing the facilitatory mode of anodal tDCS. For example, Iyer and colleagues study [44] produced the first direct evidence for a cognitive enhancement in the context of language production by showing that it is possible to change transiently human verbal fluency capacity by means of electrical stimulation, and showed that this effect depended on intensity. Iyer and colleagues [44] investigated the effects of tDCS on prefrontal cortex related functions. There were no significant effects on performance with 1 mA DC. However, with 2 mA, verbal fluency was improved during anodal stimulation, and there were no effects on a variety of other tasks.

In another study, Sparing and colleagues [45] explored whether tDCS could enhance visual picture naming. Fifteen healthy participants performed the task before, during, and after tDCS was applied over the posterior perisylvian region (PPR). This position corresponds with the location of Wernicke's area, including the posterior part of the left superior temporal gyrus (STG), and has been used previously in a number of TMS studies (e.g., [46]). Using a double-blind, within subjects design, the participants underwent four different 2 mA stimulation sessions: anodal and cathodal stimulation of left PPR as the main target stimulation and anodal stimulation of the homologous region of the right hemisphere and sham stimulation as control conditions. Results showed that the participants responded significantly faster following anodal tDCS to the left PPR. This significant decrease of naming latency was found directly at the end of anodal tDCS to the left PPR, and was not evident during stimulation, nor did the facilitation effect extract its influence after 5 and 10 min post stimulation.

In essence, anodal DC produced small yet consistent and significant differences in the studies reviewed above. Interestingly, although different regions of interest were used (PPR and DLPFC), naming/verbal fluency performance was improved, suggesting that DC can directly improve the neural mechanism which underlies the function (PPR for example) or a remote terminal that is a part of the network that underlies the function (e.g., DLPFC). This seems reasonable given the idea that picture naming and word generation involves a massive activation of temporal and frontal regions [47].

Another major contribution into the study of naming by means of tDCS arrived from Ross and colleagues [48] who investigated whether stimulation of the anterior temporal lobes (ATL) would be effective in modulating the memory of known people's proper names. The results showed that anodal stimulation to the right ATL significantly improved face naming accuracy for people but not landmarks. The Ross et al. [48] study should be noted for implanting a control condition (landmarks), a design that provided a selective and specific effect, thus significantly enhancing the study's validity.

Neural Underpinning of DC Effects

Behavioral changes which occur due to tDCS manipulation are vital, and should be considered as the foremost criteria by which to decide whether a particular set of stimulation parameters (e.g., electrodes position and size, stimulation intensity and length) create a transient change in behavior. Neuroimaging and electroencephalography methods can aid in revealing the nature of changes that occur after anodal or cathodal stimulation.

Holland and colleagues [49] tested whether tDCS over the left inferior frontal cortex can be used to increase spoken picture-naming performance in neurologically unimpaired individuals. For all participants, the anodal was placed over the left inferior frontal cortex (IFC) with the cathode placed over the contralateral frontopolar cortex. The results showed a significant effect of left anodal tDCS on naming latency responses when compared to sham responses. The fMRI measures showed that left anodal tDCS significantly reduced BOLD signal in the left frontal cortex, including Broca's area, compared to sham responses. The imaging data also showed a regionally specific effect. Within the stimulated frontal cortex, not all regions were equally affected; Broca's area, but not other regions (e.g., precentral or anterior insular cortices), were modulated by anodal tDCS. Holland and colleagues suggested that the reduction of BOLD signal in Broca's area might be analogous to the neural priming effects that is seen when utilizing behavioral priming paradigms.

Enhancing Cognitive Control With tDCS

A common feature of human existence is the ability to reverse decisions after they are made but before they are implemented. This cognitive control process, termed response inhibition, allows individuals to recover from potentially harmful situations before it is too late—for example, avoiding touching a hot stove when realizing it is too hot, or not commenting negatively about a coworker who suddenly appears. Cognitive control in general, and response inhibition in particular, are impaired in several neuropsychiatric disorders, such as attention deficit hyperactivity disorder (ADHD; [50]), and appears to be critically dependent upon intact function of the right Inferior Frontal Gyrus (rIFG; [51]).

Response inhibition can be evaluated by the Stop-Signal task (SST; [52]). In the SST there are two types of trials: "*go*" trials and "*stop*" trials. In the "*go*" trials, subjects are required to make a simple discrimination task within a prespecified time window; the "*go*" trials are more frequent, thus setting up a prepotent response tendency. The "*stop*" trials are less frequent, and require subjects to refrain from making the response when a stop signal is randomly presented following the go signal [52].

Cognitive control processes, in general, are attributed mainly to the prefrontal cortex (PFC). Response inhibition has been localized more specifically to the right Inferior Frontal Gyrus (rIFG), based upon both functional brain imaging and lesion based approaches. For example, in a recent fMRI study, Li et al. [53] showed that successful inhibition was associated with greater activation of multiple cortical areas, among other the right inferior and middle frontal gyri. Rubia et al. [54] also showed common activation foci across different stop task versions in bilateral, but predominantly right hemispheric inferior prefrontal cortex. Studies employing temporary deactivation using TMS over the rIFG indeed found impaired inhibitory control [55] supporting the potential role of the rIFG in response inhibition. However, although TMS was successful in establishing interference stimulation protocol that impaired cognitive control [56], its use also raised some concerns. The same repetitive stimulation protocol resulted in facilitative effects in several reported studies [57, 58]. The inconsistent effects and other practical limitations of TMS such as mobility and subjects comfort mean that it might not be the ideal tool for developing enhancement stimulation protocols. Up-to-date there are two teams that employed tDCS to affect SST task, using different sites, as described below.

Jacobson et al. [59] demonstrated that anodal stimulation applied over the rIFG led to significant improvement in the SST performance, but not on response time in a control task that used SST stimuli but did not employ the response inhibition task. In addition, stimulation over rAG, an area known to be without involvement in the SST [55] did not affect response inhibition, demonstrating regional selectivity of the effect. Jacobson et al. [59] results (see Fig. 18.1a–c) both support theories of brain mechanisms underlying response inhibition, and provide a potential method for behavioral modification.

A different research team targeted a different area. Other cortical areas are also involved in the cognitive control network. Li et al. [60] systematically investigated the neural correlates of motor inhibition with the stop-signal task and found a linear correlation between the BOLD activation of pre-supplementary motor area (Pre-SMA) and SSRTs. Therefore Hsu et al. [61] conducted a tDCS SST study in order to investigate the functional role of the Pre-SMA in motor inhibition. Three tDCS conditions were employed: Pre-SMA anodal/left cheek cathodal, left cheek anodal/Pre-SMA cathodal, and a control group with no tDCS stimulation. Current intensity was set to 1.5 mA for 10 min. Hsu et al. [61] found that the effects of inhibitory (cathodal) tDCS replicated previous TMS findings by impairing performance on the task. The pattern was similar to TMS findings in the sense that there was marked failure to inhibit responses when a stop signal was presented (an elevated noncancelled rate). Additionally, facilitatory effects were observed as a consequence of applying excitatory (anodal) tDCS over the Pre-SMA. Decreased noncancelled rates suggested improvement in inhibiting responses when a stop signal was presented. Such improvement or decrement in noncancelled rates implied that neuronal excitability was modulated by tDCS, as many studies have suggested [62]. These findings also suggest a critical role for Pre-SMA in suppressing unwanted actions and facilitating desired ones as seen in a recent microstimulation study [63]. Together, such effects on noncancelled rates provide direct evidence showing that the region containing Pre-SMA is also important in inhibitory control.

Whether pre-SMA or the right IFG, the SST studies demonstrated clearly a potential clinical tDCS intervention for individuals exhibiting difficulties with inhibitory control. However, further research is required to understand the nature of the neuronal changes following tDCS that allow modification of cognitive control (here as measured by SST performance). Jacobson et al. [64] have reported an EEG-tDCS study that suggested a possible neuronal mechanism for tDCS effects in the SST. They found that the right IFG stimulation protocol applied in their behavioral SST study [34] generated a significant and selective diminution of the power of theta band (4–7 Hz). The theta diminution was observed in the rIFG area (represented the anode electrode), and was not found in the lOFC area (represented the cathode electrode). A significant effect was observed only in the theta but not in other bands. Since there is evidence that the electrophysiological activity associated with behavioral inhibition is theta band activity [65, 66], these results may explain the improvement in behavioral inhibition following tDCS over the rIFG (see Fig. 18.1d–f).

Enhancing Other PFC-Related Functions

tDCS has already shown to improve high-order cognitive functions, PFC supported, in different domains such as decision-making [33], risk taking [67, 68] and probabilistic classification [32]. The explicit postulation is that even with respect to relatively complex functions that underlie different types of process it is possible that facilitation (or inhibition), by using basic designs of tDCS, would modify performance.

To date, some studies have tried to target executive control regulation with the usage of tDCS. For example, Sela et al. [69] used tDCS to test the hypothesis that a prefrontal cognitive control network is involved in directing semantic decisions that is required for the comprehension of idioms. Recent conceptualization argues in favor of a broad role of the PFC in figurative language comprehension [70, 71]; see also meta-analysis by [72], and proposed that prefrontal regions are responsible for suppression of alternative interpretations and response monitoring during figurative comprehension.

Sela et al. [73] used a double-blind, sham controlled mix design in order to explore this “PFC regulation hypothesis.” Participants were randomly allocated to one of two stimulation groups (left DLPFC anodal/Right DLPFC cathodal or left DLPFC cathodal anodal/Right DLPFC anodal). The stimulation lasted 15 min, with intensity of 1.5 mA. Over a 1-week interval, the participants were tested twice, completing a semantic decision task and a control task (a spoonerism task, which assesses phonological awareness [74]) after either receiving active or sham stimulation. The semantic decision task required the participants to judge the relatedness of an idiom and a target word, with the idiom being predictable or not. Targets were figuratively related, literally related, or unrelated to the idiom. The results showed that after DC stimulation, a general deceleration (around 10 %) in reaction times to targets was found. In addition, the results indicated that the neural enhancement of a left lateralized prefrontal network (left DLPFC anodal/right DLPFC cathodal) improved performance when the participants had to make decisions when it came to figurative targets of highly predictable idioms, whereas the neural enhancement of the opposite network (left DLPFC cathodal anodal/Right DLPFC anodal) improved the participants’ performance in literal targets of unpredictable idioms (see Fig. 18.2). These effects were quite robust, explaining 28 % and 23 % of the variance, respectively. Finally, the results showed no difference with respect to performance in the control task.

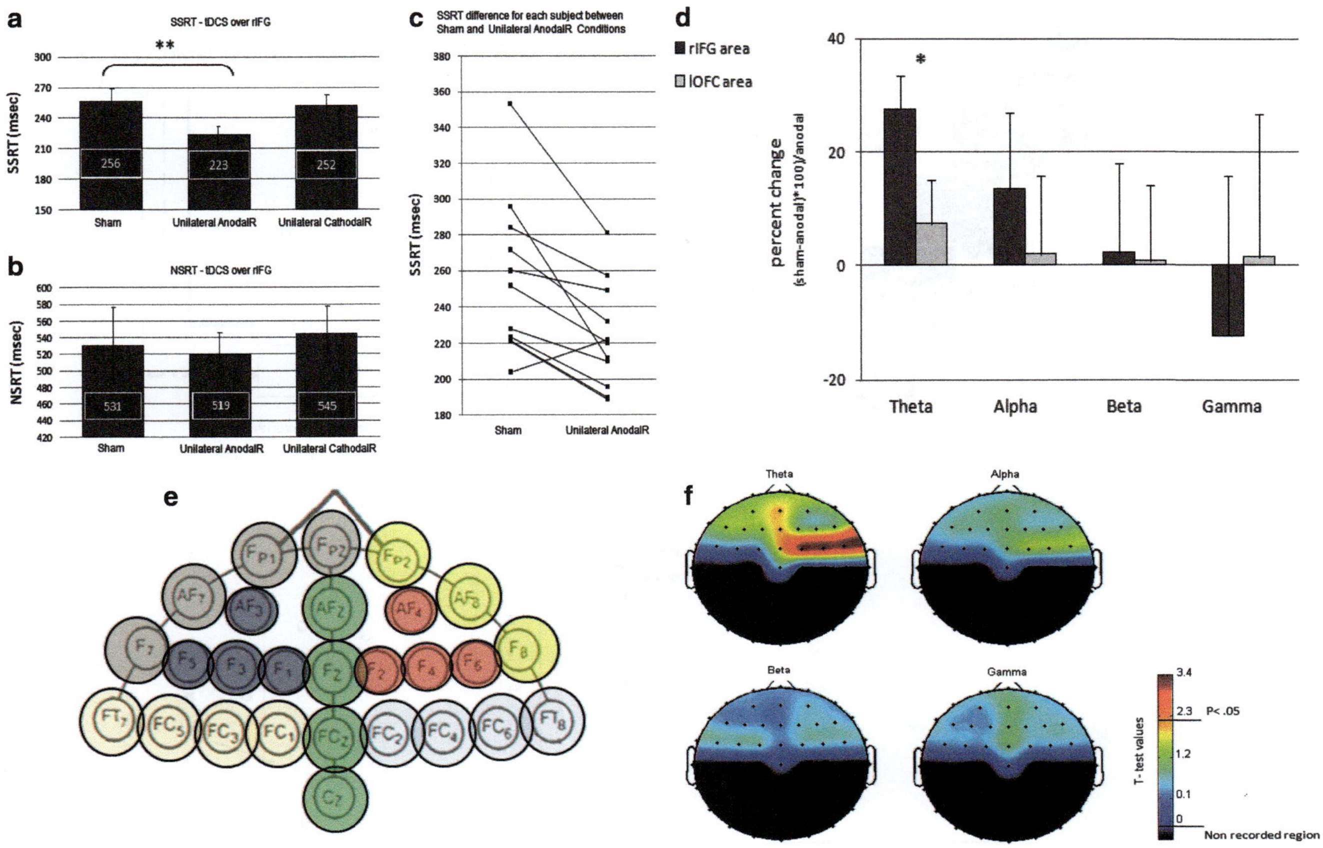

Fig. 18.1 (**a**) Comparison between unilateral simulation conditions of the mean SSRT for 11 subjects. Unilateral AnodalR differed significantly from Sham condition. (**b**) Comparison between unilateral stimulation conditions of the mean NSRT for 11 subjects. This nonsignificant effect of tDCS on general RT indicates Unilateral AnodalR tDCS effect was specific to response inhibition rather than causing a general cognitive improvement. (**c**) The improved inhibition control (SSRT) in the Unilateral AnodalR stimulation compared with Sham in the SST plotted for each subject. Shorter SSRT indicates better ability to inhibit responses, which was found in 10 of the 11 subjects. (**d**) The difference between the power recorded following anodal and sham stimulation conditions presented as percent change [(sham-anodal)*100/anodal; mean ± SEM]; for each band (Theta, Alpha, Beta, and Gamma) and for two clusters represented the rIFG (anode electrode positioning) area (*dark gray*), and the lOFC (cathode electrode positioning) area (*light gray*). * indicates $p < 0.05$. (**e**) Illustration of the 27 recorded channels located over the half front of the head. The different colors refer to the seven different clusters of which the 27 channels were divided to. (**f**) T-maps represented the difference in the power for each of the four analyzed bands (Theta, Alpha, Beta, and Gamma) between anodal and sham stimulation conditions. Data for figures **a–c** taken from [59]; Data figures **d–f** taken from [64]

Sela et al. [69] findings corroborated the hypothesis which was set by Papagno and colleagues [70, 71], showing how the PFC is implicated in selection processes. As Sela et al. [69] proposed, it seemed that the PFC regulates selection processes by using top-down bias based on stimuli characteristics (e.g., idiom predictability), and that individual differences in trait motivations are linked with the magnitude of the effect which is caused by tDCS.

It was also found that tDCS stimulation enhances complex verbal insight problem-solving by anodal tDCS in the left DLPFC. A study by Cerruti and Schlaug [75] tested whether prefrontal stimulation may enhance performance in the remote associates test (RAT). Typically, In RAT problems, subjects are presented with three words, e.g., AGE/MILE/SAND, and must find a common linguistic associate which forms a compound noun or a two-word phrase with each cue word—in this case, STONE (STONE-AGE, MILESTONE, and SANDSTONE). This task requires strong executive function capacities, since lateral associations and internal production of many words is needed until a key decision stage in which the subject must select or generate a single answer.

The Cerruti and Schlaug [75] findings indicated that stimulating the left DLPFC led to increased fluency when it came to the generation of solutions. Their findings prompt interesting questions regarding the influence of tDCS on cognitive control processing and the role the left DLPFC has in supporting the executive control processes that are involved and are necessary in order to solve verbal insight problems. In order to describe the underlying neurocognitive processes that may modulate verbal problem solving, Metuki et al. [76] created a stimulation study with few

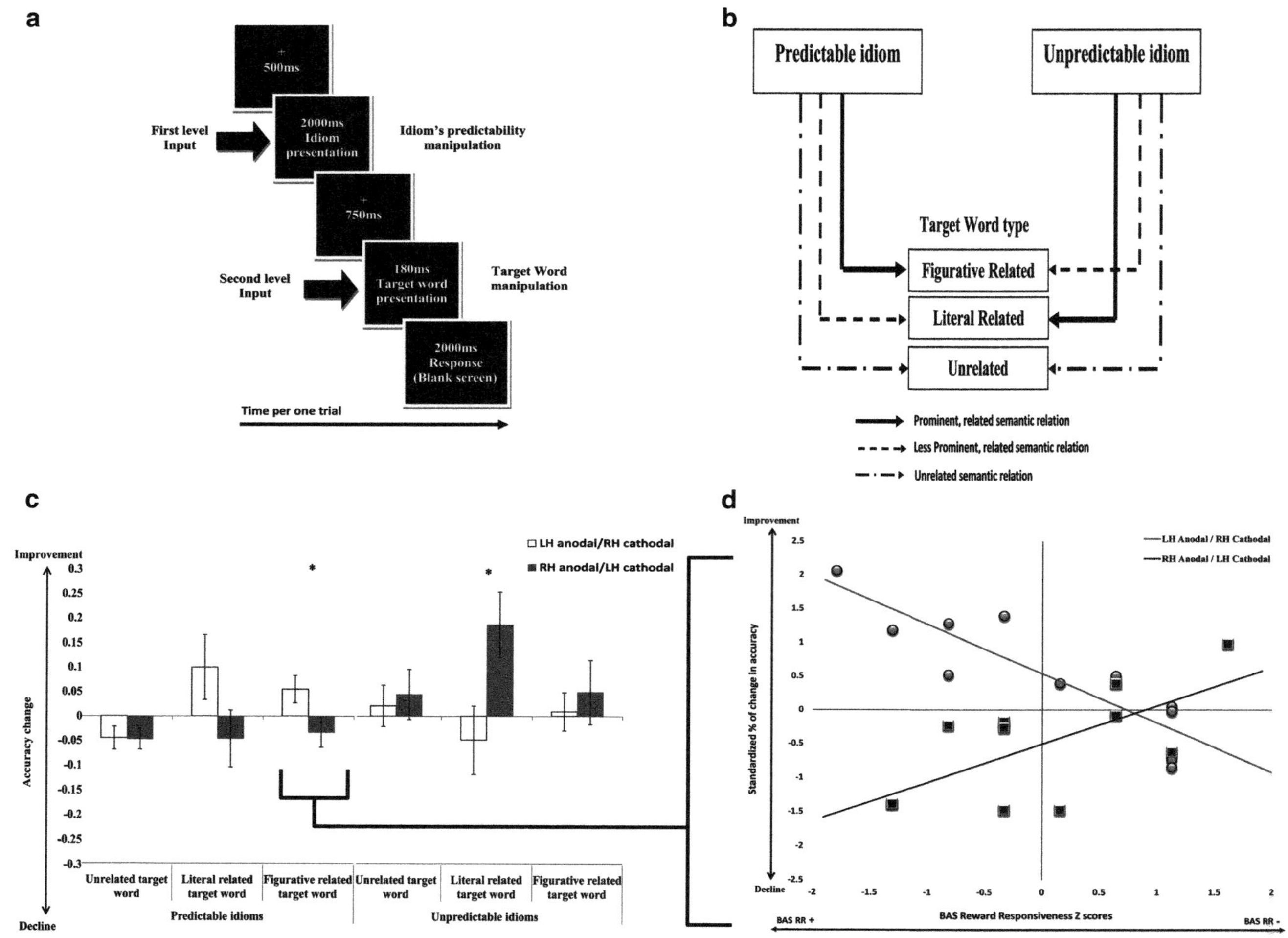

Fig. 18.2 (**a**) Semantic decision task procedure: the trial began with the presentation of a fixation cross for 500 ms. The cross was replaced by an idiom which remained on the screen for 2,000 ms. The participants were instructed to read the idioms silently. The fixation cross reappeared for 750 ms and was followed by the target word for 180 ms. The participants were instructed to indicate whether the idiomatic expression and the target word were related by pressing the right or left mouse keys. They were instructed to respond rapidly while maintaining a high level of accuracy. The next trial began after a 2,000 ms interval. (**b**) Six experimental conditions: two experimental manipulations (2 × 3) have been used—idiom's predictability with two levels (predictable and unpredictable) and target word type with three levels (figurative related, literal related, and unrelated). The conditions were a priori defined as being prominent, related semantic relations (*continuous line*), less prominent, related semantic relations (*dash line*), or unrelated semantic relations (*dash–dot line*). (**c**) Main finding found in [69] is reflected in accuracy change scores (mean ± SE). The 3-way interaction revealed that the tDCS effects were limited to specific idiom–target pairings. *$p < 0.05$. (**d**) DC effects were more pronounced in individuals that were rated as being most sensitive to reward likelihood. Scores on a trait motivation propensity (BAS reward responsiveness; BAS-RR, part of the BIS/BAS scale; [121]) moderated the effects of tDCS for the most canonical form of stimuli (predictable idioms followed by their figurative meaning). Data is taken from [69]

methodological modifications that was compared to the procedure used by Cerruti and Schlaug [75].

The Metuki et al. study employed a sham controlled within design. Twenty-one participants completed two identical experimental sessions that were separated by 1 week. Subjects received 1 mA for 11 min, with anodal electrode over the left DLPFC, and the reference electrode over the right supraorbital region. The results indicated that anodal tDCS over the left DLPFC enhanced solution recognition, but did not enhance solution generation, for difficult problems only (see Fig. 18.3). Metuki et al. suggested that these findings support the idea that prefrontal LH cognitive control mechanisms modulate linguistic processing and specified the conditions by which the facilitation effect were effective and substantial. Both Cerruti and Schlaug [75] and Metuki et al. [76] studies show how the understanding of facilitation effects is constrained by physiological and cognitive hypotheses, in terms of site specification [75] and experimental conditions [76]. This way, the understanding of the improvements that were induced by tDCS stimulation

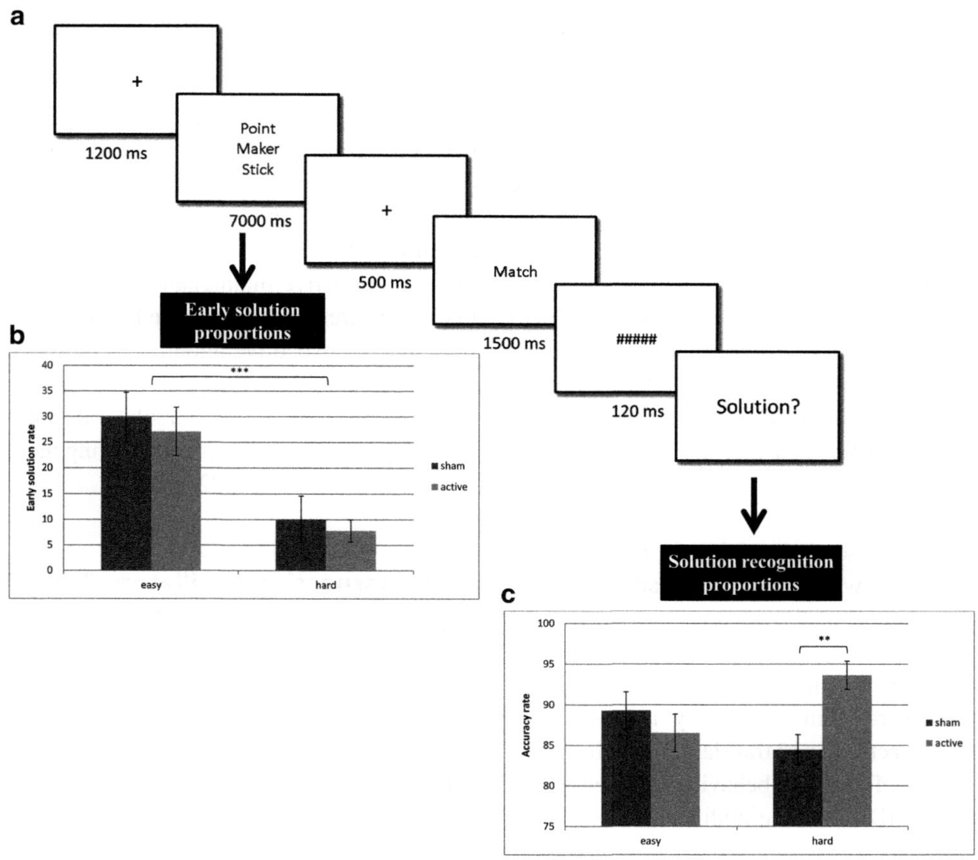

Fig. 18.3 (**a**) Task procedure: Each trial began with a central fixation cross which was presented for 1,200 ms. The three prime words were then presented simultaneously, above, at, and below the center of the screen. The words remained on the screen for 7 s, during which the participants were asked to solve the problem. After a solution was indicated or the time limit was exceeded, a fixation cross reappeared for an additional 500 ms, followed by a presentation of the target word for 1,500 ms. Then, the word "Solution?" appeared on the screen, and the participants were instructed to indicate whether the target word was the correct solution of the problem or not. On half of the trials, the target was the correct solution word, and on the other half—an unrelated distractor. In this example, the correct solution followed the three problem words. (**b**) Solution generation: mean early solution rates and SE, by stimulation condition and item difficulty. $***p < 0.001$. (**c**) Solution generation: mean early solution rates and SE, by stimulation condition and item difficulty. $***p < 0.00$. Data is taken from [76]

is placed within a framework that is built of prediction based on combined cognitive and anatomical hypotheses [77] and enhance the validity of the results.

Enhancing Learning and Memory with tDCS

Floël and colleagues [78] examined tDCS effects on learning and acquisition of novel vocabulary. In their experiment, tDCS stimulation was applied over the posterior part of the left perisylvian area in 19 young right-handed individuals, while the participants had to acquire a miniature lexicon of 30 novel object names. This study employed a double-blind, sham controlled, within design. Each participant was given anodal, cathodal (each 20 min of 1 mA), and sham sessions in a randomized, counterbalanced manner. Results showed that with anodal stimulation, the participants showed better associative learning in the fifth block when compared to sham and cathodal stimulation. Mood ratings, blood pressure, heart rate, discomfort, RTs, and response styles were similar between stimulation conditions. Importantly, transfer of the vocabulary into the participants' native language was also significantly better after learning under anodal tDCS when compared to cathodal tDCS and sham. However, no significant difference between the conditions was found for the lexical knowledge test after 1 week. This study was the first to show that anodal tDCS, when performed on the left hemisphere, significantly improves the acquisition of a novel vocabulary (faster learning and higher overall success) in healthy subjects.

Another study by Liuzzi and others [79] tested the hypothesis that language is embodied in neural circuitry connections between perisylvian language areas and the motor cortex, as based on Hebb's law of association. Liuzzi et al. examined the functional relevance of the left motor cortex for the learning of a novel action word vocabulary by interfering with neural accessibility in the motor cortex by means of tDCS. The study utilized a between design, double-blind, sham-controlled, randomized, matched-samples design in 30 young healthy, right-handed volunteers. In combination with tDCS (anodal, cathodal, or sham), subjects learned a novel vocabulary of 76 concrete, body-related actions by means of an associative learning paradigm. The training of novel action-word learning was spread over four single learning sessions (40 min each), separated by 24 h. Prior to each learning session, subjects received tDCS. Electrode positions over the left motor cortex were determined by TMS, and the anodal or cathodal was placed accordingly. The reference electrode was placed over the right supraorbital region. tDCS was applied at 1 mA for 20 min.

The primary outcome measure was the percentage of novel action words that were correctly translated into German at the end of the training session on day 4. This test was chosen in order to assess whether subjects had established robust semantic associations of the action concepts with the novel words independent of the action photos that were used during training. Compared with sham stimulation, cathodal tDCS reduced success rates in vocabulary acquisition as shown by tests of novel action word translation into the native language. The analysis of learning behavior revealed a specific effect of cathodal tDCS on the ability to associatively couple actions with novel words.

Liuzzi et al. [79] also included different control conditions: the same experiment was conducted with different stimulation conditions (anodal, cathodal, or sham) that were performed on the left DLPFC. Additionally, in another control experiment, subjects learned object-related words instead of action words. No significant effects were found when tDCS was applied to the prefrontal cortex or when subjects learned object-related words.

This study provided direct evidence to the suggestion that the left motor cortex is causally involved in the acquisition of novel action-related words. In addition, this study should be notable for several reasons: first, for its rigorous methodological design. The inclusion of a target stimulation site alongside a control task clearly addressed the main possible alternative explanation and improved the validity of results. Second, although tDCS is not known for being highly precise in terms of localization, Liuzzi et al. [79] demonstrated that with the use of relatively conventional electrodes (25 cm^2), it is possible to distinguish between roughly close areas (motor strip–frontal cortex). This is in line with recent neuroimaging studies that showed that the spread of activation following tDCS stimulation is restricted to the area underneath the electrode [49, 80]. Finally, this study demonstrated that cathodal tDCS reduced success rates in vocabulary acquisition, and could be used to create a TMS like "virtual lesion" [5], thus providing another venue for tDCS usage in future research.

Regarding a different domain, recent studies have demonstrated that tDCS can induce significant effects on working memory function in humans [30]. Working memory (WM) is the ability to temporarily hold and manipulate task-relevant information. WM load is considered to be the amount of temporarily stored WM items prior to WM retrieval and is hypothesized to impose higher demands on executive attention as its value increases. Thus, WM tasks that require active maintenance of temporarily stored high-load items are considered to be highly dependent on DLPFC function and executive attention [81]. Indeed some of these studies revealed that anodal tDCS to the left prefrontal cortex, presumably the dorsolateral prefrontal cortex of healthy participants, improves working memory, specifically its verbal domains [30, 82].

tACS: Harnessing Oscillatory Brain Activity to Explore and Improve Sensory and Cognitive Functions

Another method that allows for investigating and manipulating brain activity is transcranial alternating current stimulation (tACS) tACS provides a powerful approach to establish the functional role of neuronal oscillatory activities in the human brain and to explore the functional role of neural oscillations in cognitive tasks by stimulating the brain with biophysically relevant frequencies during task performance. tACS is supposed to induce regional brain oscillations in a frequency-dependent manner, thereby interacting with specific functions of the stimulated region [39, 83–86]. Oscillatory activity is suggested to play an important role in linking the crosstalk between brain areas [85], and it has been argued that oscillations are particularly instrumental in top-down processing [87] or in a large-scale integration of bottom-up and top-down processes [88].

Although this technique is still largely unexplored and volume conduction effects are not wholly understood [83, 89–91], recent studies have demonstrated tACS efficiency in different domains. For instance, Kanai et al. [83] showed that cortical excitability of the visual cortex as measured by the thresholds for TMS evoked phosphenes exhibits frequency dependency, whereby 20 Hz tACS over the visual cortex enhances the sensitivity of the visual cortex. A recent study demonstrated that stimulation in alpha and gamma bands over the associative sensory cortex induced positive sensory sensations [89]. It has also been demonstrated that tACS at prefrontal sites during sleep-improved procedural memory consolidation [92].

In another study, Sela et al. [73] used tACS to investigate the effects of oscillatory prefrontal theta stimulation on risk-taking [93]. To modulate risk-taking they used a well-established paradigm in the realm of risk-taking known as the Balloon Analog Risk Task (BART; [94]). In this task, participants pump a balloon without knowing when it will explode. The more the pump button is pressed, the more points accumulate while at the same time the risk of losing points with a balloon explosion increases. Subjects are thus pressured to decide whether to adopt a risky behavior and keep pumping, or to use a more conservative strategy and stop. Results showed a remarkable effect of left PFC stimulation, whereas right PFC and sham stimulations failed to produce any substantial effect on task performance. More specifically, the increase of sequential losses during theta stimulation over left PFC suggested that subjects lost the ability to adjust their actions based on negative feedback given to them explicitly during the task (the balloon exploded and they lost all the point they earned in that round). In addition, it was suggested that left PFC stimulation interfered with a hypostasized "left to right theta dependent switch" that may be obligatory in order to switch from an explorative "risk-taking mode" into a "risk-averse" mode.

Most recently, Polanía and others [95] simultaneously applied tACS at 6 Hz over left prefrontal and parietal cortices with a relative 0 ("synchronized") or 180 ("desynchronized") phase difference or a placebo stimulation condition, while healthy subjects performed a delayed letter task. The results showed that induced frontoparietal theta synchronization significantly improved visual memory-matching reaction times as compared to placebo stimulation. In contrast, exogenously induced frontoparietal theta desynchronization deteriorated performance.

Given the enormous potential tACS holds [40], it is expected that in the near future this method would serve to explore basic questions in other domains in cognition by utilizing the huge amount of the electrophysiological data that was gathered so far.

Discussion

The utility of using brain stimulation methods (TMS, tDCS, tACS) to explore novel theoretical hypothesis and to uncover the neural basis of sensory and cognitive functioning is evident. The different studies tackles intriguing questions such as the contribution of prefrontal cortex and motor system to language production, learning, or comprehension (e.g., [44, 75, 79]), questions of connectivity [80], and transcallosal disinhibition [26] using a relatively safe, noninvasive methods. We conclude this chapter a methodological section that specifies the different considerations that one should consider when designing and evaluating brain stimulation experiment (tDCS in particular) in the context of cognitive research. We also emphasize a major future direction in the promising field of rehabilitation, particular in the domain of language recovery.

Enhancing Cognitive Functions: Methodological Considerations

In the following section, we emphasize different methodological consideration and caveats that must be addressed in order to assert that a genuine effect has been found, and as such may be considered as reliable and replicable. We aim to shed more light on what we consider as important steps in order to help direct future experimental work in the research of cognition by using mostly tDCS (see Fig. 18.4 and the following discussion; see also [96, 97] for other types of considerations that need to be addressed in the context of clinical trials).

Different stimulation montages (see Fig. 18.5) have been used in past studies in order to explore cognitive functions. In general, two types of montages have been used: first, the so-called unilateral stimulation method, in which the target location is being excited or inhabited with the "active" electrode while the "reference" electrode is placed in an unrelated area (mostly contralateral frontopolar cortex; cf. [78]). Second, in other studies, a bilateral placement has been used (e.g., [33]). The obvious advantage of the former method is that it guarantees, to some extent, that the stimulation modifies a specific region of interest. The primary caveat of this method is the fact that the usage of the contralateral frontopolar cortex as the default region for "reference" electrode may be reasonable when stimulating the motor cortex [62], but not when the aim is to modify cognitive functions that may be related to the activation of this region or nearby regions. In any case, it is highly suggested to use a large reference electrode (10×10 cm^2) when employing this type of montage, as reported for instance in the Meinzer et al. [80] study, since the increased size of the reference electrode renders stimulation functionally inefficient without compromising tDCS effects under the active electrode [98]. The main advantage of the bilateral placement is based on the idea that if the two electrodes are both placed over cortical areas, tDCS can be used to simultaneously increase excitability in one region and decrease excitability in another region (cf. [73]). This method may be useful if the main hypothesis tackles issues of brain asymmetry and/or the combined involvement of the two cerebral hemispheres (or any other two regions) to a specific function (cf. [33]). This method may suffer from potential confounding effects of two electrodes with opposite polarities over the brain, and may required further stimulation conditions in the form of unilateral stimulation. Alternatively, this shortcoming can be solved with a task design that includes two or more conditions that are expected to produce inverse patterns that may result from the stimulation. Another possible electrode placement that is available, and will probably be in widespread use, is to use multiple

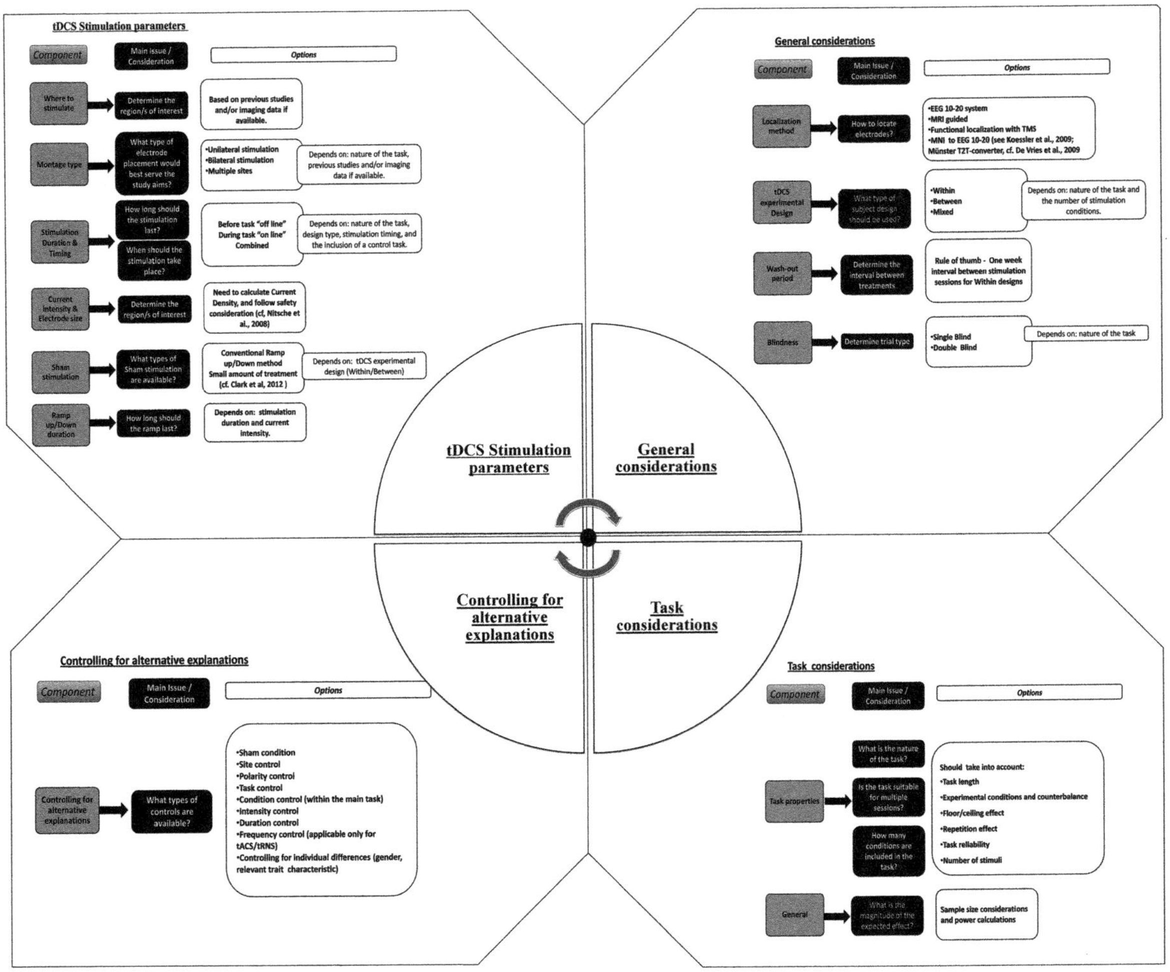

Fig. 18.4 Designing a tDCS experiment: main considerations. Four main themes are presented: tDCS Stimulation parameters, general considerations, task considerations, and controlling for alternative explanations

small electrodes (i.e., around 1.2 cm diameter) in order to achieve effective and targeted stimulation while ensuring safety of stimulation (see [99]). As noted by Holland and Crinion [97], it is not clear what the "best" approach one can use. Deciding which of the above methods of placements to use directly taps on, and is derived from, other important parameters such as stimuli duration, electrode size, and current intensity alongside more general considerations that includes the nature of the function in question, task at hand, and other deign parameters.

Another main consideration should be addressed when it comes to issues of experimental design, which are related to issues such as what would be the best design to use (within/between/mixed), when should we start the stimulation (stimulation timing), how many control conditions should be included, and what is the sample size that should be used. All of these issues inherently interconnect with the nature of the task and the task specifications that are in use. For example, including a control task may be important when the task by itself produces only one primary measure. In this case, it will be most recommended to include a control task in order to verify and specify the effect. Including such a control has implications with respect to stimulation duration, the need to counterbalance tasks presentation and so on. Moreover, task properties should be examined carefully when deciding on the appropriate experimental design. For instance, tasks which are known to produce high inter-subject variability should naturally be tested with a within design. However, what happens if the task involves learning and the subjects' performance is qualitatively changed after one time exposure? There are many ways to cope with these types of questions; naturally, it is impossible to address all possible scenarios here, so the aim is to draw attention to the vast amount of considerations as summed in Fig. 18.5.

Importantly, the issue of controlling alternative explanations should be addressed thoroughly. It is obvious that a single study cannot always cover all the bases, as doing so would result in endless control groups. However,

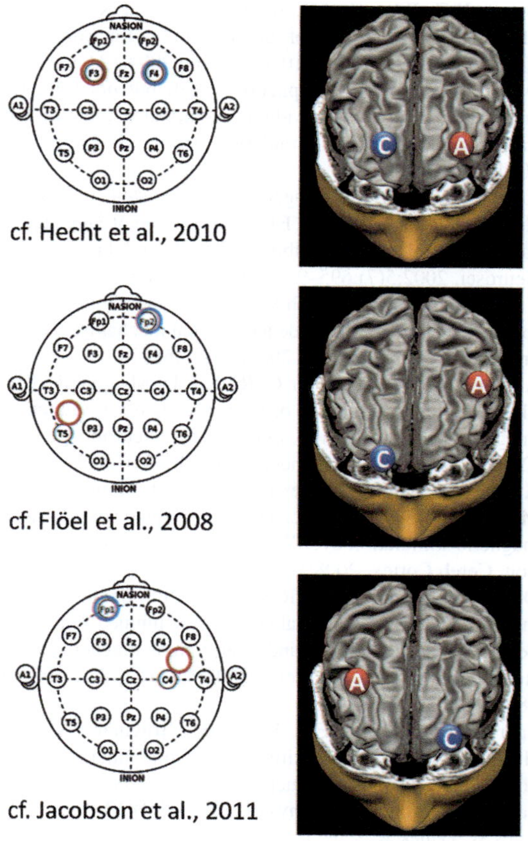

Fig. 18.5 Example of different stimulation montages. The *upper panel* shows a bilateral placement (cf. [33]), which is based on the EEG 10–20 system. The anode electrode was fixed over the F3 (left DLPFC), whereas the cathode electrode was placed over its homologue in the right hemisphere (F4; right DLPFC). The *middle* and *lower panels* shows a bilateral placement (cf. [33]), which is based on the EEG 10–20 system. In the *middle panel* (cf. [78]), the anode electrode was fixed over the CP5 (Wernicke's area), whereas the cathode electrode was placed over the contralateral supraorbital region (FP2). In the *lower panel* (cf. [59]), the anode electrode was fixed over the crossing point between T3-Fz and F7-Cz (right IFG), whereas the cathode electrode was placed over the contralateral supraorbital region (FP1)

it is highly recommended to deal with the alternative explanations that are most critical for the given experiment, and at least use a (1) sham condition, (2) site control, (3) polarity control, and (4) task or condition (within the main task) control. As in other domains of behavioral research, it is clear that any evidence for a "single dissociation" is good, but we should strive to create experimental designs that can produce an evidence for a "double dissociation." Finally, with respect to current intensity and the usage of current density as a possible control (see [96, 100]), it is quite surprising that the Iyer et al. study [44] is almost the only case in which different levels of current intensity were examined (1 and 2 mA), and showed it may affect performance. It is clear that many other tDCS effects may be intensity dependent, so this parameter should be subjected to systematic manipulation in future studies.

Future Direction: tDCS Use in Clinical Contexts and Combining With Training

Cognitive training is being recently the preferred method to affect brain plasticity. In the last 20 years, controlled cognitive training studies have demonstrated that learning of new cognitive skills and improving existing skills is possible across different populations and ages [101]. Successful training was documented in clinical populations (Schizophrenia: [102]; ADHD: [103]). Several brain-imaging studies have recently revealed training-induced plasticity in the healthy human brain (i.e., [104, 105]). Facilitation effects of the integration of the tDCS combined with cognitive training are only beginning to be explored [106, 107]. Most recently, Ditye et al. [108] showed that tDCS-combined cognitive training is an effective tool for improving the ability to inhibit responses. The main aim was to investigate response inhibition in the context of a learning paradigm by giving tDCS over the right IFG repetitively over four consecutive days of training on a behavioral inhibition task (SST). The results showed that the integration of the training and rIFG–tDCS produced a steeper linear learning slope. Additionally, better performance was also found in the active stimulation group in comparison with the control group.

Combining tDCS protocols with language training hold a great promise for future research. It may be used as a tool for enhancing language functions among healthy individuals and among patients. Language training protocols are at vast use among clinicians in verity of fields (e.g., language and speech therapy) and are a standard component of medical care after traumatic brain injury (TBI) or stroke [109].

So far, a small number of controlled studies evaluated the potential of tDCS for language recovery (for a comprehensive review see [96, 97]). For example, Monti and coauthors [110] evaluated the effect of tDCS over the damaged left frontotemporal areas in eight chronic nonfluent post-stroke aphasic patients, and showed that cathodal tDCS significantly improved accuracy of picture naming. In Baker et al. [111] study, ten patients with varying types and severities of chronic aphasia, received 5 days of anodal tDCS over the left frontal cortex, and 5 days of sham stimulation while performing a computerized anomia treatment. Performance in the naming task improved significantly after anodal stimulation, and the effect persisted at least 1 week. Another work by the same group [112] examined the effect of anodal tDCS on reaction time during overt picture naming in eight chronic stroke participants. This time the anode electrode was placed over perilesional brain regions. Anodal tDCS reduced reaction time during naming of trained items immediately after stimulation, and at subsequent testing 3 weeks later. A recent study by Fiori and colleagues [113] showed that 5 days of anodal tDCS over Wernicke's area produced an improvement in naming accuracy that lasted for 3 weeks in three aphasic patients. Kang and colleagues [114] showed that a protocol of cathodal tDCS applied on the right Broca's homologue combined with language therapy improved picture naming in patients with post-stroke aphasia. Flöel and coworkers [115] demonstrated that anodal tDCS applied over the right temporoparietal cortex improved the success of anomia training in a group of 12 post-stroke aphasic left-brain-damaged patients. You and colleagues [116] found that cathodal tDCS over the right superior temporal areas of subacute patients with global aphasia showed significantly greater improvements in auditory verbal comprehension. In sum, tDCS, may be used concomitantly to training protocols to enhance language reacquisition, a potential only touched upon in small patient studies so far [96].

Acknowledgments This chapter presents studies that were supported by the Israel Academy of Sciences grant no. 100/10, the Israeli Center of Research Excellence (I-CORE) in Cognition (I-CORE Program 51/11), the EC ITN-LAN (grant 214570), and an ERC starting grant which was awarded to ML (Inspire 200512).

References

1. Farah MJ, Illes J, Cook-Deegan R, Gardner H, Kandel E, King P, Parens E, et al. Neurocognitive enhancement: what can we do and what should we do? Nat Rev Neurosci. 2004;5(5):421–5. doi:10.1038/nrn1390.
2. Sandberg A, Bostrom N. Converging cognitive enhancements. Ann N Y Acad Sci. 2006;1093:201–27. doi:10.1196/annals.1382.015.
3. Walsh V, Pascual-Leone A. Transcranial magnetic stimulation: a neurochronometrics of mind. Cambridge, MA: Bradford Books; 2003. p. 319.
4. Barker AT, Jalinous R, Freeston IL. Non-invasive magnetic stimulation of human motor cortex. Lancet. 1985;1(8437):1106–7.
5. Walsh V, Cowey A. Transcranial magnetic stimulation and cognitive neuroscience. J Neurosci. 2000;19:5792–801.
6. Paus T. Inferring causality in brain images: a perturbation approach. Philos Trans R Soc Lond B Biol Sci. 2005;360(1457):1109–14. doi:10.1098/rstb.2005.1652.
7. Rounis E, Lee L, Siebner HR, Rowe JB, Friston KJ, Rothwell JC, Frackowiak RSJ. Frequency specific changes in regional cerebral blood flow and motor system connectivity following rTMS to the primary motor cortex. Neuroimage. 2005;26(1):164–76. doi:10.1016/j.neuroimage.2005.01.037.
8. Amassian VE, Cracco RQ, Maccabee PJ, Cracco JB, Rudell A, Eberle L. Suppression of visual perception by magnetic coil stimulation of human occipital cortex. Electroencephalogr Clin Neurophysiol. 1989;74(6):458–62.
9. Töpper R, Mottaghy FM, Brügmann M, Noth J, Huber W. Facilitation of picture naming by focal transcranial magnetic stimulation of Wernicke's area. Exp Brain Res. 1998;121(4):371–8.
10. Pobric G, Mashal N, Faust M, Lavidor M. The role of the right cerebral hemisphere in processing novel metaphoric expressions: a transcranial magnetic stimulation study. J Cogn Neurosci. 2008;20(1):170–81.
11. Huang Y-Z, Edwards MJ, Rounis E, Bhatia KP, Rothwell JC. Theta burst stimulation of the human motor cortex. Neuron. 2005;45(2):201–6. doi:10.1016/j.neuron.2004.12.033.
12. Oliveri M, Romero L, Papagno C. Left but not right temporal involvement in opaque idiom comprehension: a repetitive transcranial magnetic stimulation study. J Cogn Neurosci. 2004;16(5):848–55.
13. Knecht S, Flöel A, Dräger B, Breitenstein C, Sommer J, Henningsen H, Ringelstein EB, et al. Degree of language lateralization determines susceptibility to unilateral brain lesions. Nat Neurosci. 2002;5(7):695–9. doi:10.1038/nn868.
14. Vallesi A, Shallice T, Walsh V. Role of the prefrontal cortex in the foreperiod effect: TMS evidence for dual mechanisms in temporal preparation. Cereb Cortex. 2007;17(2):466–74.
15. Andoh J, Artiges E, Pallier C, Rivière D, Mangin JF, Cachia A, Plaze M, et al. Modulation of language areas with functional MR image-guided magnetic stimulation. Neuroimage. 2006;29(2):619–27. doi:10.1016/j.neuroimage.2005.07.029.
16. Andoh J, Artiges E, Pallier C, Rivière D, Mangin JF, Paillère-Martinot ML, Martinot JL. Priming frequencies of transcranial magnetic stimulation over Wernicke's area modulate word detection. Cereb Cortex. 2008;18(1):210–6.
17. Devlin JT, Matthews PM, Rushworth MFS. Semantic processing in the left inferior prefrontal cortex: a combined functional magnetic resonance imaging and transcranial magnetic stimulation study. J Cogn Neurosci. 2003;15(1):71–84. doi:10.1162/089892903321107837.
18. Sparing R, Mottaghy FM, Hungs M, Brügmann M, Foltys H, Huber W, Töpper R. Repetitive transcranial magnetic stimulation effects on language function depend on the stimulation parameters. J Clin Neurophysiol. 2001;18(4):326–30.
19. Fries W, Danek A, Scheidtmann K, Hamburger C. Motor recovery following capsular stroke. Role of descending pathways from multiple motor areas. Brain. 1993;116(2):369–82.
20. O'Shea J, Johansen-Berg H, Trief D, Göbel S, Rushworth MFS. Functionally specific reorganization in human premotor cortex. Neuron. 2007;54(3):479–90. doi:10.1016/j.neuron.2007.04.021.
21. Kobayashi M, Hutchinson S, Théoret H, Schlaug G, Pascual-Leone A. Repetitive TMS of the motor cortex improves ipsilateral sequential simple finger movements. Neurology. 2004;62(1):91–8.
22. Théoret H, Kobayashi M, Valero-Cabré A, Pascual-Leone A. Exploring paradoxical functional facilitation with TMS. Suppl Clin Neurophysiol. 2003;56:211–9.
23. Hilgetag CC, Théoret H, Pascual-Leone A. Enhanced visual spatial attention ipsilateral to rTMS-induced virtual lesions' of human parietal cortex. Nat Neurosci. 2001;4:953–8.
24. Seyal M, Ro T, Rafal R. Increased sensitivity to ipsilateral cutaneous stimuli following transcranial magnetic stimulation of the parietal lobe. Ann Neurol. 1995;38:264–7.
25. Jung-Beeman M. Bilateral brain processes for comprehending natural language. Trends Cogn Sci. 2005;9(11):512–8.
26. Thiel A, Habedank B, Herholz K, Kessler J, Winhuisen L, Haupt WF, Heiss W-D. From the left to the right: how the brain compensates progressive loss of language function. Brain Lang. 2006;98(1):57–65. doi:10.1016/j.bandl.2006.01.007.
27. Voets NL, Adcock JE, Flitney DE, Behrens TEJ, Hart Y, Stacey R, Matthews PM. Distinct right frontal lobe activation in language processing following left hemisphere injury. Brain. 2006;129(3):754–66.
28. Kapur N. Paradoxical functional facilitation in brain-behaviour research a critical review. Brain. 1996;119(5):1775–90.
29. Weiller C, Chollet F, Friston KJ, Wise RJ, Frackowiak RS. Functional reorganization of the brain in recovery from striatocapsular infarction in man. Ann Neurol. 1992;31(5):463–72. doi:10.1002/ana.410310502.

30. Fregni F, Boggio PS, Nitsche M, Bermpohl F, Antal A, Feredoes E, Marcolin MA, et al. Anodal transcranial direct current stimulation of prefrontal cortex enhances working memory. Exp Brain Res. 2005;166(1):23–30.
31. Boggio PS, Khoury LP, Martins DCS, Martins OEMS, Macedo ECD, Fregni F. Temporal cortex direct current stimulation enhances performance on a visual recognition memory task in Alzheimer disease. J Neurol. 2009;80(4):444–7. doi:10.1136/jnnp.2007.141853.
32. Kincses TZ, Antal A, Nitsche MA, Bartfai O, Paulus W. Facilitation of probabilistic classification learning by transcranial direct current stimulation of the prefrontal cortex in the human. Neuropsychologia. 2004;42(1):113–7.
33. Hecht D, Walsh V, Lavidor M. Transcranial direct current stimulation facilitates decision making in a probabilistic guessing task. J Neurosci. 2010;30(12):4241–5.
34. Jacobson L, Koslowsky M, Lavidor M. tDCS polarity effects in motor and cognitive domains: a meta-analytical review. Exp Brain Res. 2011;216:1–10. doi:10.1007/s00221-011-2891-9.
35. Pope PA, Miall RC. Task-specific facilitation of cognition by cathodal transcranial direct current stimulation of the cerebellum. Brain Stimul. 2012;5(2):84–94. doi:10.1016/j.brs.2012.03.006.
36. Weiss M, Lavidor M. When less is more: evidence for a facilitative cathodal tDCS effect in attentional abilities. J Cogn Neurosci. 2012;24(9):1826–33. doi:10.1162/jocn_a_00248.
37. Antal A, Boros K, Poreisz C, Chaieb L, Terney D, Paulus W. Comparatively weak after-effects of transcranial alternating current stimulation (tACS) on cortical excitability in humans. Brain Stimul. 2008;1(2):97–105. doi:10.1016/j.brs.2007.10.001.
38. Terney D, Chaieb L, Moliadze V, Antal A, Paulus W. Increasing human brain excitability by transcranial high-frequency random noise stimulation. J Neurosci. 2008;28(52):14147–55.
39. Kanai R, Chaieb L, Antal A, Walsh V, Paulus W. Frequency-dependent electrical stimulation of the visual cortex. Curr Biol. 2008;18(23):1839–43.
40. Kuo MF, Nitsche MA. Effects of transcranial electrical stimulation on cognition. Clin EEG Neurosci. 2012;43(3):192–9.
41. Broca P. Sur le siège de la faculté du langage articulé. Bull Soc Anthropol Paris. 1865;6(1):377–93.
42. Wernicke C. Der aphasische Symptomencomplex: eine psychologische Studie auf anatomischer Basis. Breslau: Cohn & Weigert; 1874.
43. Silvanto J, Pascual-Leone A. Why the assessment of causality in brain-behavior relations requires brain stimulation. J Cogn Neurosci. 2012;24(4):775–7. doi:10.1162/jocn_a_00193.
44. Iyer MB, Mattu U, Grafman J, Lomarev M, Sato S, Wassermann EM. Safety and cognitive effect of frontal DC brain polarization in healthy individuals. Neurology. 2005;64(5):872.
45. Sparing R, Dafotakis M, Meister IG, Thirugnanasambandam N, Fink GR. Enhancing language performance with non-invasive brain stimulation—a transcranial direct current stimulation study in healthy humans. Neuropsychologia. 2008;46(1):261–8.
46. Mottaghy FM, Hungs M, Brügmann M, Sparing R, Boroojerdi B, Foltys H, Huber W, et al. Facilitation of picture naming after repetitive transcranial magnetic stimulation. Neurology. 1999;53(8):1806–12.
47. Indefrey P, Levelt WJM. The spatial and temporal signatures of word production components. Cognition. 2004;92(1–2):101–44. doi:10.1016/j.cognition.2002.06.001.
48. Ross LA, McCoy D, Wolk DA, Coslett HB, Olson IR. Improved proper name recall by electrical stimulation of the anterior temporal lobes. Neuropsychologia. 2010;48(12):3671–4. doi:10.1016/j.neuropsychologia.2010.07.024.
49. Holland R, Leff AP, Josephs O, Galea JM, Desikan M, Price CJ, Rothwell JC, Crinion J. Speech facilitation by left inferior frontal cortex stimulation. Curr Biol. 2011;21(16):1403–7.
50. Aron AR, Poldrack RA. The cognitive neuroscience of response inhibition: relevance for genetic research in attention-deficit/hyperactivity disorder. Biol Psychiatry. 2005;57(11):1285–92. doi:10.1016/j.biopsych.2004.10.026.
51. Aron AR, Robbins TW, Poldrack RA. Inhibition and the right inferior frontal cortex. Trends Cogn Sci. 2004;8(4):170–7. doi:10.1016/j.tics.2004.02.010.
52. Logan GD, Cowan WB. On the ability to inhibit thought and action: a theory of an act of control. Psychol Rev. 1984;91(3):295–327. doi:10.1037/0033-295X.91.3.295.
53. Li CR, Huang C, Yan P, Paliwal P, Constable RT, Sinha R. Neural correlates of post-error slowing during a stop signal task: a functional magnetic resonance imaging study. J Cogn Neurosci. 2008;20(6):1021–9. doi:10.1162/jocn.2008.20071.
54. Rubia K, Russell T, Overmeyer S, Brammer MJ, Bullmore ET, Sharma T, Simmons A, et al. Mapping motor inhibition: conjunctive brain activations across different versions of go/no-go and stop tasks. Neuroimage. 2001;13(2):250–61. doi:10.1006/nimg.2000.0685.
55. Chambers CD, Bellgrove MA, Stokes MG, Henderson TR, Garavan H, Robertson IH, Morris AP, et al. Executive “brake failure” following deactivation of human frontal lobe. J Cogn Neurosci. 2006;18(3):444–55. doi:10.1162/089892906775990606.
56. Figner B, Knoch D, Johnson EJ, Krosch AR, Lisanby SH, Fehr E, Weber EU. Lateral prefrontal cortex and self-control in intertemporal choice. Nat Neurosci. 2010;13(5):538–9. doi:10.1038/nn.2516.
57. Bloch Y, Harel EV, Aviram S, Govezensky J, Ratzoni G, Levkovitz Y. Positive effects of repetitive transcranial magnetic stimulation on attention in ADHD subjects: a randomized controlled pilot study. World J Biol Psychiatry. 2010;11(5):755–8.
58. Cho SS, Ko JH, Pellecchia G, Van Eimeren T, Cilia R, Strafella AP. Continuous theta burst stimulation of right dorsolateral prefrontal cortex induces changes in impulsivity level. Brain Stimul. 2010;3(3):170–6. doi:10.1016/j.brs.2009.10.002.
59. Jacobson L, Javitt DC, Lavidor M. Activation of inhibition: diminishing impulsive behavior by direct current stimulation over the inferior frontal gyrus. J Cogn Neurosci. 2011;23(11):3380–7.
60. Li CSR, Huang C, Constable RT, Sinha R. Imaging response inhibition in a stop-signal task: neural correlates independent of signal monitoring and post-response processing. J Neurosci. 2006;26(1):186–92.
61. Hsu T-Y, Tseng L-Y, Yu J-X, Kuo W-J, Hung DL, Tzeng OJL, Walsh V, et al. Modulating inhibitory control with direct current stimulation of the superior medial frontal cortex. Neuroimage. 2011;56(4):2249–57. doi:10.1016/j.neuroimage.2011.03.059.
62. Nitsche MA, Paulus W. Excitability changes induced in the human motor cortex by weak transcranial direct current stimulation. J Physiol. 2000;527(3):633–9.
63. Isoda M, Hikosaka O. Switching from automatic to controlled action by monkey medial frontal cortex. Nat Neurosci. 2007;10(2):240–8. doi:10.1038/nn1830.
64. Jacobson L, Ezra A, Berger U, Lavidor M. Modulating oscillatory brain activity correlates of behavioral inhibition using transcranial direct current stimulation. Clin Neurophysiol. 2012;123(5):979–84. doi:10.1016/j.clinph.2011.09.016.
65. Lansbergen MM, Schutter DJLG, Kenemans JL. Subjective impulsivity and baseline EEG in relation to stopping performance. Brain Res. 2007;1148:161–9. doi:10.1016/j.brainres.2007.02.034.
66. Wienbruch C, Paul I, Bauer S, Kivelitz H. The influence of methylphenidate on the power spectrum of ADHD children—an MEG study. BMC Psychiatry. 2005;5:29. doi:10.1186/1471-244X-5-29.
67. Fecteau S, Knoch D, Fregni F, Sultani N, Boggio P, Pascual-Leone A. Diminishing risk-taking behavior by modulating activity

in the prefrontal cortex: a direct current stimulation study. J Neurosci. 2007;27(46):12500–5.
68. Fecteau S, Pascual-Leone A, Zald DH, Liguori P, Theoret H, Boggio PS, Fregni F. Activation of prefrontal cortex by transcranial direct current stimulation reduces appetite for risk during ambiguous decision making. J Neurosci. 2007;27 (23):6212–8.
69. Sela T, Ivry RB, Lavidor M. Prefrontal control during a semantic decision task that involves idiom comprehension: a transcranial direct current stimulation study. Neuropsychologia. 2012;50 (9):2271–80. doi:10.1016/j.neuropsychologia.2012.05.031.
70. Lauro LJR, Tettamanti M, Cappa SF, Papagno C. Idiom comprehension: a prefrontal task? Cereb Cortex. 2008;18(1):162–70.
71. Papagno C. Idiomatic language comprehension: neuropsychological evidence, Neuropsychology of communication. Milan: Springer; 2010. p. 111–29.
72. Rapp AM, Mutschler DE, Erb M. Where in the brain is nonliteral language? A coordinate-based meta-analysis of functional magnetic resonance imaging studies. Neuroimage. 2012;63 (1):600–10. doi:10.1016/j.neuroimage.2012.06.022.
73. Sela T, Kilim A, Lavidor M. Transcranial alternating current stimulation (tACS) increases risk taking behavior in the balloon analogue risk task. Front Neurosci. 2012;6:22. doi:10.3389/fnins.2012.00022.
74. Romani C, Ward J, Olson A. Developmental surface dysgraphia: what is the underlying cognitive impairment? Q J Exp Psychol. 1999;52(1):97–128.
75. Cerruti C, Schlaug G. Anodal transcranial direct current stimulation of the prefrontal cortex enhances complex verbal associative thought. J Cogn Neurosci. 2009;21(10):1980–7.
76. Metuki N, Sela T, Lavidor M. Enhancing cognitive control components of insight problems solving by anodal tDCS of the left dorsolateral prefrontal cortex. Brain Stimul. 2012;5(2):110–5. doi:10.1016/j.brs.2012.03.002.
77. Fecteau S, Walsh V. Introduction: brain stimulation in cognitive neuroscience. Brain Stimul. 2012;5(2):61–2. doi:10.1016/j.brs.2012.04.001.
78. Flöel A, Rösser N, Michka O, Knecht S, Breitenstein C. Noninvasive brain stimulation improves language learning. J Cogn Neurosci. 2008;20(8):1415–22. doi:10.1162/jocn.2008.20098.
79. Liuzzi G, Freundlieb N, Ridder V, Hoppe J, Heise K, Zimerman M, et al. The involvement of the left motor cortex in learning of a novel action word lexicon. Curr Biol. 2010;20 (19):1745–51.
80. Meinzer M, Antonenko D, Lindenberg R, Hetzer S, Ulm L, Avirame K, Flöel A. Electrical brain stimulation improves cognitive performance by modulating functional connectivity and task-specific activation. J Neurosci. 2012;32(5):1859–66.
81. Kane MJ, Engle RW. The role of prefrontal cortex in working-memory capacity, executive attention, and general fluid intelligence: an individual-differences perspective. Psychon Bull Rev. 2002;9(4):637–71.
82. Zaehle T, Sandmann P, Thorne JD, Jäncke L, Herrmann CS. Transcranial direct current stimulation of the prefrontal cortex modulates working memory performance: combined behavioural and electrophysiological evidence. BMC Neurosci. 2011;12:2. doi:10.1186/1471-2202-12-2.
83. Kanai R, Paulus W, Walsh V. Transcranial alternating current stimulation (tACS) modulates cortical excitability as assessed by TMS-induced phosphene thresholds. Clin Neurophysiol. 2010;121 (9):1551–4.
84. Pogosyan A, Gaynor LD, Eusebio A, Brown P. Boosting cortical activity at beta-band frequencies slows movement in humans. Curr Biol. 2009;19(19):1637–41.
85. Thut G, Miniussi C. New insights into rhythmic brain activity from TMS-EEG studies. Trends Cogn Sci. 2009;13(4):182–9.
86. Zaehle T, Rach S, Herrmann CS. Transcranial alternating current stimulation enhances individual alpha activity in human EEG. PLoS One. 2010;5(11):e13766.
87. Engel AK, Fries P, Singer W. Dynamic predictions: oscillations and synchrony in top-down processing. Nat Rev Neurosci. 2001;2 (10):704–16.
88. Varela F, Lachaux JP, Rodriguez E, Martinerie J. The brainweb: phase synchronization and large-scale integration. Nat Rev Neurosci. 2001;2(4):229–39. doi:10.1038/35067550.
89. Feurra M, Bianco G, Santarnecchi E, Del Testa M, Rossi A, Rossi S. Frequency-dependent tuning of the human motor system induced by transcranial oscillatory potentials. J Neurosci. 2011;31(34):12165–70.
90. Schutter DJLG, Hortensius R. Brain oscillations and frequency-dependent modulation of cortical excitability. Brain Stimul. 2011;4(2):97–103.
91. Zaghi S, Acar M, Hultgren B, Boggio PS, Fregni F. Noninvasive brain stimulation with low-intensity electrical currents: putative mechanisms of action for direct and alternating current stimulation. Neuroscientist. 2010;16(3):285–307.
92. Marshall L, Helgadóttir H, Mölle M, Born J. Boosting slow oscillations during sleep potentiates memory. Nature. 2006;3:6.
93. Christie GJ, Tata MS. Right frontal cortex generates reward-related theta-band oscillatory activity. Neuroimage. 2009;48 (2):415–22. doi:10.1016/j.neuroimage.2009.06.076.
94. Lejuez CW, Read JP, Kahler CW, Richards JB, Ramsey SE, Stuart GL, Strong DR, et al. Evaluation of a behavioral measure of risk taking: the balloon analogue risk task (BART). J Exp Psychol Appl. 2002;8(2):75.
95. Polanía R, Nitsche MA, Korman C, Batsikadze G, Paulus W. The importance of timing in segregated theta phase-coupling for cognitive performance. Curr Biol. 2012;22:1314–8.
96. Flöel A. Non-invasive brain stimulation and language processing in the healthy brain. Aphasiology. 2012;26(9):1082–102. doi:10.1080/02687038.2011.589892.
97. Holland R, Crinion J. Can tDCS enhance treatment of aphasia after stroke? Aphasiology. 2012;26(9):1169–91. doi:10.1080/02687038.2011.616925.
98. Stagg CJ, Nitsche MA. Physiological basis of transcranial direct current stimulation. Neuroscientist. 2011;17(1):37–53.
99. Dmochowski JP, Datta A, Bikson M, Su Y, Parra LC. Optimized multi-electrode stimulation increases focality and intensity at target. J Neural Eng. 2011;8(4):046011. doi:10.1088/1741-2560/8/4/046011. Epub 2011 Jun 10.
100. Nitsche MA, Cohen LG, Wassermann EM, Priori A, Lang N, Antal A, Paulus W, et al. Transcranial direct current stimulation: state of the art 2008. Brain Stimul. 2008;1(3):206–23. doi:10.1016/j.brs.2008.06.004.
101. Green CS, Bavelier D. Exercising your brain: a review of human brain plasticity and training-induced learning. Psychol Aging. 2008;23(4):692–701. doi:10.1037/a0014345.
102. McGurk SR, Twamley EW, Sitzer DI, McHugo GJ, Mueser KT. A meta-analysis of cognitive remediation in schizophrenia. Am J Psychiatry. 2007;164(12):1791–802. doi:10.1176/appi.ajp.2007.07060906.
103. Shalev L, Tsal Y, Mevorach C. Computerized progressive attentional training (CPAT) program: effective direct intervention for children with ADHD. Child Neuropsychol. 2007;13(4):382–8.
104. Erickson KI, Colcombe SJ, Wadhwa R, Bherer L, Peterson MS, Scalf PE, Kim JS, et al. Training-induced plasticity in older adults: effects of training on hemispheric asymmetry. Neurobiol Aging. 2007;28(2):272–83. doi:10.1016/j.neurobiolaging.2005.12.012.
105. McNab F, Varrone A, Farde L, Jucaite A, Bystritsky P, Forssberg H, Klingberg T. Changes in cortical dopamine D1 receptor binding associated with cognitive training. Science. 2009;323 (5915):800.

106. Cohen Kadosh R, Soskic S, Iuculano T, Kanai R, Walsh V. Modulating neuronal activity produces specific and long-lasting changes in numerical competence. Curr Biol. 2010;20(22):2016–20.
107. Reis J, Schambra HM, Cohen LG, Buch ER, Fritsch B, Zarahn E, Celnik PA, et al. Noninvasive cortical stimulation enhances motor skill acquisition over multiple days through an effect on consolidation. Proc Natl Acad Sci U S A. 2009;106(5):1590–5. doi:10.1073/pnas.0805413106.
108. Ditye T, Jacobson L, Walsh V, Lavidor M. Modulating behavioral inhibition by tDCS combined with cognitive training. Exp Brain Res. 2012;219:363–8.
109. Rohling ML, Faust ME, Beverly B, Demakis G. Effectiveness of cognitive rehabilitation following acquired brain injury: a meta-analytic re-examination of Cicerone et al.'s (2000, 2005) systematic reviews. Neuropsychology. 2009;23(1):20–39. doi:10.1037/a0013659.
110. Monti A, Cogiamanian F, Marceglia S, Ferrucci R, Mameli F, Mrakic-Sposta S, Vergari M, et al. Improved naming after transcranial direct current stimulation in aphasia. J Neurol Neurosurg Psychiatry. 2008;79(4):451–3. doi:10.1136/jnnp.2007.135277.
111. Baker JM, Rorden C, Fridriksson J. Using transcranial direct-current stimulation to treat stroke patients with aphasia. Stroke. 2010;41(6):1229–36.
112. Fridriksson J, Richardson JD, Baker JM, Rorden C. Transcranial direct current stimulation improves naming reaction time in fluent aphasia: a double-blind, sham-controlled study. Stroke. 2011;42(3):819–21. doi:10.1161/STROKEAHA.110.600288.
113. Fiori V, Coccia M, Marinelli CV, Vecchi V, Bonifazi S, Ceravolo MG, Provinciali L, et al. Transcranial direct current stimulation improves word retrieval in healthy and nonfluent aphasic subjects. J Cogn Neurosci. 2011;23(9):2309–23. doi:10.1162/jocn.2010.21579.
114. Kang EK, Kim YK, Sohn HM, Cohen LG, Paik N-J. Improved picture naming in aphasia patients treated with cathodal tDCS to inhibit the right Broca's homologue area. Restor Neurol Neurosci. 2011;29(3):141–52. doi:10.3233/RNN-2011-0587.
115. Flöel A, Meinzer M, Kirstein R, Nijhof S, Deppe M, Knecht S, Breitenstein C. Short-term anomia training and electrical brain stimulation. Stroke. 2011;42(7):2065–7. doi:10.1161/STROKEAHA.110.609032.
116. You DS, Kim D-Y, Chun MH, Jung SE, Park SJ. Cathodal transcranial direct current stimulation of the right Wernicke's area improves comprehension in subacute stroke patients. Brain Lang. 2011;119(1):1–5. doi:10.1016/j.bandl.2011.05.002.
117. Nitsche MA, Schauenburg A, Lang N, Liebetanz D, Exner C, Paulus W, Tergau F. Facilitation of implicit motor learning by weak transcranial direct current stimulation of the primary motor cortex in the human. J Cogn Neurosci. 2003;15(4):619–26.
118. Nitsche MA, Paulus W. Sustained excitability elevations induced by transcranial DC motor cortex stimulation in humans. Neurology. 2001;57(10):1899.
119. Liebetanz D. Pharmacological approach to the mechanisms of transcranial DC-stimulation-induced after-effects of human motor cortex excitability. Brain. 2002;125(10):2238–47. doi:10.1093/brain/awf238.
120. Gandiga PC, Hummel FC, Cohen LG. Transcranial DC stimulation (tDCS): a tool for double-blind sham-controlled clinical studies in brain stimulation. Clin Neurophysiol. 2006;117(4):845–50.
121. Carver CS, White TL. Behavioral inhibition, behavioral activation, and affective responses to impending reward and punishment: the BIS/BAS scales. J Pers Soc Psychol. 1994;67(2):319.

19 Conclusive Overview

Dirk Rasche and Helena Knotkova

In this textbook, experts in the field of neuromodulation from all over the world presented an overview of invasive and noninvasive neuromodulatory approaches and its potential for the treatment of various pathological states and conditions.

The book can serve as a structured guide for clinicians, scientific researchers, medical staffs, and students to get an insight, structured overview, as well as specific clinically relevant information about the neuromodulation techniques. Every chapter strived to provide up-to-date information regarding underlying physiological mechanisms, technical aspects, and application protocols in the scope of good clinical practice and safe performance of these methods and procedures. All chapters have an extensive reference list that can serve as an additional source for those interested in more extensive and in-depth information.

The broad overview of invasive and noninvasive neuromodulatory methods presented in this book has indeed demonstrated that neuromodulation is a rapidly growing field of expertise with enormous potential for research and therapy. Although some invasive procedures are performed for more than 30 years, e.g., deep brain stimulation, a revival is witnessed during the past 10 years because of new experimental research, medical experience, controlled trials with new indications, and ongoing technological improvement. Building on the foundations of available up-to-date evidence, each neuromodulatory method can benefit from further technical progress, continuing development, and targeted clinical applications. In specific,

D. Rasche (✉)
Department of Neurosurgery, University Hospital of Schleswig-Holstein, University of Lübeck, Campus Lübeck, Ratzeburger Allee 160, 23538 Lübeck, Germany
e-mail: dirk.rasche@uksh.de

H. Knotkova
MJHS Institute for Innovations in Palliative Care, 39 Broadway, New York, NY, USA
e-mail: hknotkov@mjhs.org

- Existing studies and clinical observations show enormous heterogeneity of protocols, dosages, and devices and therefore results from the studies are difficult to compare and/or reproduce.
- The documentation and reporting of adverse events or negative results in published literature on neuromodulation highly vary, making it difficult to evaluate the methods across the treatment protocols and patient populations.
- Further research is needed to fill gaps in understanding neurophysiological mechanisms underlying the effects of specific neuromodulatory methods. Traditional neurophysiological approaches together with novel disciplines, such as epigenetics, can greatly contribute to this endeavor.
- Large-sample Phase III clinical trials are needed for those neuromodulatory methods that indicated analgesic efficacy in pilot and Phase II clinical studies.
- For methods that have not yet been fully implemented into clinical practice, more evidence is needed not only on efficacy, but also on safety and cost-effectiveness in clinical settings.
- For most of the existing neuromodulatory methods, approaches, and protocols, durability of the effects as well as factors contributing to the treatment responsiveness have yet to be established and need to be evaluated in long-term follow-up.
- Consequently, an effective and patient-friendly use of neuromodulation calls for the dose adjustments for specific populations (for example children), with the ultimate goal of the development of patient-tailored treatment regimens supported by imaging-assisted diagnostic assessment prior to the neuromodulatory procedures.
- Further, technical refinement of neuromodulatory devices and procedures, including miniaturization of electronic devices, further implementation of biotechnologies, robotics, or nanotechnology, can facilitate user-friendly modifications of neuromodulatory devices, general safety, reduction in the complication rate of the invasive neuromodulatory procedures, and availability of novel research and treatment protocols.

H. Knotkova and D. Rasche (eds.), *Textbook of Neuromodulation*,
DOI 10.1007/978-1-4939-1408-1_19, © Springer Science+Business Media, LLC 2015

- Regarding education in the field of neuromodulation, more educational initiatives are needed on all fronts of the field, from educational materials for patients to comprehensive educational and training programs for providers, and topic-relevant education for supporting medical and research personnel. A full integration of neuromodulation into international and national medical education programs needs to be facilitated and supported by all involved disciplines and societies.

Overall, it can be expected that the future initiatives in the field of neuromodulation will encompass developing novel neuromodulatory approaches, methods, devices, and treatment protocols; facilitating basic and clinical research; building evidence base on safety, efficacy, and effectiveness; implementation of neuromodulatory treatment approaches into clinical practice when appropriate; developing and periodically reviewing/updating guidelines for the use of specific neuromodulatory methods; implementing and facilitating educational and/or training programs for both providers and recipients of the neuromodulatory procedures; as well as other activities that will contribute to the overall development of this exciting field of expertise.

Index

H. Knotkova and D. Rasche (eds.), *Textbook of Neuromodulation*,
DOI 10.1007/978-1-4939-1408-1, © Springer Science+Business Media, LLC 2015

V